Medical and Surgical
Management of
MALE INFERTILITY

Editors

Botros RMB Rizk MD MA FRCOG FRCS HCLD FACOG FACS
Professor and Head
Reproductive Endocrinology and Infertility
Department of Obstetrics and Gynecology
University of South Alabama
Mobile, Alabama, USA

Nabil Aziz MD FRCOG
Consultant in Gynecology and Reproductive Medicine
Lead Clinician, Liverpool Women's Hospital and
The University of Liverpool, Liverpool, UK

Ashok Agarwal PhD HCLD
Professor, Lerner College of Medicine
Director, Andrology Laboratory
Center for Reproductive Medicine
Cleveland Clinic, Ohio, USA

Edmund Sabanegh Jr MD
Chairman, Department of Urology
Director, Section of Male Fertility
Glickman Urological and Kidney Institute
Center for Reproductive Medicine
Cleveland Clinic, Cleveland, Ohio, USA

JAYPEE BROTHERS MEDICAL PUBLISHERS (P) LTD

New Delhi • London • Philadelphia • Panama

Jaypee Brothers Medical Publishers (P) Ltd.

Headquarters
Jaypee Brothers Medical Publishers (P) Ltd.
4838/24, Ansari Road, Daryaganj
New Delhi 110 002, India
Phone: +91-11-43574357
Fax: +91-11-43574314
Email: jaypee@jaypeebrothers.com

Overseas Offices

J.P. Medical Ltd.
83, Victoria Street, London
SW1H 0HW (UK)
Phone: +44-2031708910
Fax: +02-03-0086180
Email: info@jpmedpub.com

Jaypee-Highlights Medical Publishers Inc.
City of Knowledge, Bld. 237, Clayton
Panama City, Panama
Phone: +507-301-0496
Fax: +507-301-0499
Email: cservice@jphmedical.com

Jaypee Medical Inc.
The Bourse
111, South Independence Mall East
Suite 835, Philadelphia, PA 19106, USA
Phone: + 267-519-9789
Email: joe.rusko@jaypeebrothers.com

Jaypee Brothers Medical Publishers (P) Ltd.
17/1-B, Babar Road, Block-B
Shaymali, Mohammadpur
Dhaka-1207, Bangladesh
Mobile: +08801912003485
Email: jaypeedhaka@gmail.com

Jaypee Brothers Medical Publishers (P) Ltd.
Shorakhute
Kathmandu, Nepal
Phone: +00977-9841528578
Email: jaypee.nepal@gmail.com

Website: www.jaypeebrothers.com
Website: www.jaypeedigital.com

© 2014, Jaypee Brothers Medical Publishers

Inquiries for bulk sales may be solicited at: jaypee@jaypeebrothers.com

This book has been published in good faith that the contents provided by the contributors contained herein are original, and are intended for educational purposes only. While every effort is made to ensure accuracy of information, the publisher and the editors specifically disclaim any damage, liability, or loss incurred, directly or indirectly, from the use or application of any of the contents of this work. If not specifically stated, all figures and tables are courtesy of the editors. Where appropriate, the readers should consult with a specialist or contact the manufacturer of the drug or device.

Medical and Surgical Management of Male Infertility

First Edition: **2014**
ISBN: 978-93-5025-946-7
Printed at : Ajanta Offset & Packagings Limited, New Delhi

Dedicated to

Our very dear families for their love, support and inspiration

Contributors

Ahmed El-Guindi MD
Assistant Lecturer of Andrology
Faculty of Medicine, Cairo University
Andrology Specialist, The Egyptian IVF Center
Cairo, Egypt

Alan Fryer MD
Consultant Clinical Geneticist
Liverpool Women's Hospital
Liverpool, UK

Ali Ahmady PhD
Department of Reproductive Biology
Case Western Reserve University
MacDonald IVF and Fertility Program
University Hospitals Case Medical Center
Cleveland, OH, USA

Amjad Hossain PhD HCLD
Division of Reproductive Endocrinology and
Infertility
Department of Obstetrics and Gynecology
The University of Texas Medical Branch
Galveston, TX, USA

Antonio Capalbo PhD
Centro GENERA
Clinica Valle Giulia
Rome, Italy

Ashok Agarwal PhD HCLD
Professor, Lerner College of Medicine
Director, Andrology Laboratory
Center for Reproductive Medicine
Cleveland Clinic, OH, USA

Botros RMB Rizk MD MA FRCOG FRCS
HCLD FACOG FACS
Professor and Head
Reproductive Endocrinology and Infertility
Department of Obstetrics and Gynecology
University of South Alabama
Mobile, AL, USA

Brian Le MD
Department of Urology
Northwestern University
Feinberg School of Medicine
Chicago, Illinois, USA

Charles M Lynne MD
Department of Urology
University of Miami Miller School of
Medicine, Miami, FL, USA

Dana A Ohl MD
Department of Urology
University of Michigan
Ann Arbor, MI, USA

David Rizk
Tulane University
New Orleans, LA, USA

Deborah M Spaine MSc PhD
Director of Tissue Bank
Human Reproduction Section
Division of Urology
Department of Surgery
São Paulo Federal University
São Paulo, SP, Brazil

Edmund Sabanegh Jr MD
Chairman, Department of Urology
Director, Section of Male Fertility
Glickman Urological and Kidney Institute
Center for Reproductive Medicine
Cleveland Clinic
Cleveland, OH, USA

Edmund Y Ko MD
Department of Urology
Fellow, Section of Male Fertility
Glickman Urological and Kidney Institute
Cleveland Clinic
Cleveland, OH, USA

Eleonora Bedin Pasqualotto MD PhD
Professor of Gynecology
University of Caxias do Sul, RS, Brazil
Director CONCEPTION
Center for Human Reproduction
Caxias do Sul
RS, Brazil

Fábio Firmbach Pasqualotto MD PhD
Director, Conception
Centro de Reproducao Humana
Caxias do Sul, RS, Brazil

Fnu Deepinder MD
Department of Endocrinology
Cedars Sinai Medical Center and
Greater Los Angeles VA Hospitals
Los Angeles
CA, USA

Giovana Cobalchini
Research Assistant
University of Caxias do Sul
RS, Brazil

Hanhan Li BS
Cleveland Clinic Lerner College of Medicine
of Case Western Reserve University
Cleveland, OH, USA

Hassan N Sallam MD PhD FRCOG
Professor and Head
Department of Obstetrics and Gynecology
University of Alexandria, Alexandria
Clinical Director
Alexandria Fertility and Assisted
Reproduction Center
Alexandria, Egypt

Ibrahim Fahmy MD PhD
Professor of Andrology
Faculty of Medicine, Cairo University
Andrology Consultant
The Egyptian IVF Center
Cairo, Egypt

Iryna Kuznyetsova PhD HCLD
The Toronto Institute for Reproductive
Medicine, ReproMed Toronto
Ontario, Canada

Jason Hedges MD PhD
Department of Urology
Northwestern University
Feinberg School of Medicine
Chicago, Illinois, USA

Jens Sønksen MD PhD
Department of Urology
Herlev Hospital
University of Copenhagen
Denmark

John Phelps MD
Division of Reproductive Endocrinology and
Infertility
Department of Obstetrics and Gynecology
The University of Texas Medical Branch
Galveston, TX, USA

Jorge Haddad Filho MD PhD
Director, Endocrinology Division
Human Reproduction Section
Division of Urology
Department of Surgery
São Paulo Federal University
São Paulo, SP, Brazil

Karen C Baker MD
Department of Urology
Fellow, Section of Male Fertility
Glickman Urological and Kidney Institute
Cleveland Clinic
Cleveland, OH, USA

Karen Schnauffer BSc (Hons) Dip Embryol
Dip RCPath
Consultant Embryologist
Hewitt Center for Reproductive Medicine
Liverpool Women's Hospital
Liverpool, UK

Kashif Siddiqi MD
Fellow, Section of Male Fertility
Glickman Urological and Kidney Institute
Cleveland Clinic Foundation
Cleveland, OH, USA

Keith Jarvi MD
Director of Murray Koffler Urologic
Wellness Center, Head of Urology
Mount Sinai Hospital
Professor of Surgery
Director of Male Infertility Program
University of Toronto
Toronto, ON, Canada

Kirk C Lo MD FRCSC
Assistant Professor
Division of Urology
Department of Surgery
Mount Sinai Hospital
University of Toronto
Toronto, ON, Canada

Laura Rienzi PhD
Direttore del Laboratorio
Centro GENERA, Clinica Valle Giulia
Rome, Italy

Marcia C Inhorn PhD MPH
Yale University Fertility Center
Department of Obstetrics
Gynecology and Reproductive Sciences
New Haven
Connecticut, USA

Martin Olsen MD
Professor and Program Director
Department of Obstetrics and Gynecology
James H Quillen College of Medicine
Johnson City, TN, USA

Marwa Badr MB ChB
Research Assistant
Division of Reproductive Endocrinology and
Infertility
Department of Obstetrics and Gynecology
University of South Alabama
Mobile, AL, USA

Mary K Samplaski MD
Glickman Urological and Kidney Institute
Cleveland Clinic Foundation
Cleveland, OH, USA

Nabil Aziz MD FRCOG
Consultant in Gynecology and Reproductive
Medicine
Lead Clinician, Liverpool Women's Hospital
and The University of Liverpool
Liverpool, UK

Nancy L Brackett PhD HCLD
The Miami Project to Cure Paralysis
University of Miami Miller School of Medicine
Lois Pope Life Center
Miami, FL, USA

Nina Desai PhD
IVF Laboratory Director
Cleveland Clinic Lerner College of Medicine
of Case Western Reserve University
Cleveland Clinic Foundation
Cleveland, OH, USA

Nissankararao Mary Praveena
Center for Cellular and Molecular Biology
Hyderabad, Andhra Pradesh, India

Pasquale Patrizio MD MBE
Professor and Director
Yale University Fertility Center
Department of Obstetrics
Gynecology and Reproductive Sciences
New Haven, Connecticut, USA

Philip Kumanov MD PhD DMSci
Clinical Center of Endocrinology
Medical University of Sofia
Sofia, Bulgaria

Rachel A Jesudasan PhD
Center for Cellular and Molecular Biology
Hyderabad, Andhra Pradesh, India

Rakesh K Sharma PhD
Glickman Urological and Kidney Institute
Cleveland Clinic, Cleveland, OH, USA

Ralf Henkel PhD
Department of Medical Biosciences
University of the Western Cape
Bellville, South Africa

Reecha Sharma
Center for Reproductive Medicine
Glickman Urological and Kidney Institute
Cleveland Clinic, Cleveland, OH, USA

Ricardo Miyaoka MD
Division of Urology
ANDROFERT—Andrology and Human
Reproduction Clinic
Campinas, SP, Brazil

Robert E Brannigan MD
Department of Urology
Northwestern University
Feinberg School of Medicine
Chicago, Illinois, USA

Sajal Gupta MD
Andrology Laboratory
Center for Reproductive Medicine
Glickman Urological and Kidney
Cleveland Clinic, Cleveland, OH, USA

Sandro C Esteves MD PhD
Director, ANDROFERT
Andrology and Human Reproduction Clinic
Campinas, SP, Brazil

Shaikat Hossain MSc
School of Behavioral and Brain Sciences
The University of Texas Dallas
Richardson, TX, USA

Sherman J Silber MD FACS
Medical Director
Infertility Center of St. Louis
St Luke's Hospital
St Louis, MO, USA

Sonja Grunewald MD
Physician, University of Leipzig
Department of Dermatology
Venerology and Allergology
European Training Center of Andrology
Leipzig, Germany

Stefan du Plessis PhD
Division of Medical Physiology
Faculty of Health Sciences
Stellenbosch University
Tygerberg, South Africa

Stephen Troup PhD Dip RCPath
Scientific Director
Hewitt Center for Reproductive Medicine
Liverpool Women's Hospital
Liverpool, UK

Sudha Ranganathan MBBS MD DNB
Research Assistant
Division of Reproductive Endocrinology and
Infertility
Department of Obstetrics and Gynecology
University of South Alabama, Mobile, AL, USA

Tahir Beydola BS
Center for Reproductive Medicine
Glickman Urological and Kidney Institute
Cleveland, OH, USA

Tamer M Said MD PhD
The Toronto Institute for Reproductive
Medicine, ReproMed
Toronto, ON, Canada

Tolou Adetipe MBBS DFRSH MBA
Department of Obstetrics and Gynecology
Liverpool Women's Hospital NHS Trust
Liverpool, UK

Trustin Domes MD
Fellow, Male Reproductive Medicine and
Surgery
Division of Urology, Department of Surgery
Mount Sinai Hospital
University of Toronto
Toronto, ON, Canada

Uwe Paasch MD PhD
Andrologist (EAA)
University of Leipzig
Department of Dermatology
European Training Center of Andrology
Division of Dermatopathology
Division of Aesthetics and Laserdermatology
Leipzig, Germany

Viacheslav Iremashvili MD PhD
Department of Urology
University of Miami Miller
School of Medicine, Miami, FL, USA

Wayne Kuang MD
Assistant Professor
Division of Urology
University of New Mexico
Director, Southwest Fertility Center for Men
Albuquerque, NM, USA

Zsolt Peter Nagy MD PhD
Scientific and Laboratory Director
Reproductive Biology Associates
Atlanta, GA, USA

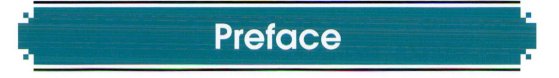

Preface

Scientific advances made in the field of male infertility have surpassed most disciplines of medicine. We would dare to say that the last twenty years have witnessed developments in this field that overshadow all scientific developments in the previous two millennia. The ancient Egyptian physicians were interested in male health including carrying out male circumcision as recorded on the temple walls over 3000 years ago. It is thought that the earliest reference to spermatozoon came from the Egyptian *Ebers Papyrus*, which was written in the XVIIIth dynasty (1500 BC) and recorded that sperm originated from the bones. However, the Greek philosophers had more elaborate thoughts about semen (Greek θεμεν = seed) and spermatozoa (σπερμν = to sow, and ζωον = living thing or animal). Nevertheless, it was Leeuwenhoek, a Dutch tradesman and a maker of microscopes who observed and provided diagrammatic representation of sperm. He wrote a letter to the Medical Society of London in 1696 which he described observing cells with tails when he examined human semen under the microscope. He called sperm 'homunculi', believing they consisted of the same parts of the body of the future male or female individuals, distinguishing two different shapes of sperm corresponding to the two sexes. His attempts to dissect a dried sperm, by brushing, to see the parts of the homunculi were fruitless. He made no mention of pathological forms but noted that sperms were absent in the semen of infertile men. He demonstrated sperm in the genital tracts of domesticated animals after copulation and stated that they lived longer *in vivo* than *in vitro*.

The evaluation of human semen and its relevance to male fertility potential received a significant boost in mid twentieth century through the work of John MacLeod and Ruth Gold that demonstrated clear differences between subfertile and fertile men in sperm count, motility, and morphology. They described seven different forms of sperm head morphology that are used in our present day. From a different perspective, one of the great advances in treating male infertility was the development of intracytoplasmic injection in 1991 at the Vrije Universiteit, Brussels. However, all theses advances in male infertility assessment and treatment were perfected in animals first decades before it was applied in humans.

We ought not forget, however, that male fertility potential is a multifaceted and sperm production represents only one aspect of it. Spermatogenesis is hormonally driven and is dependent on intact genetic complement of the male. It takes place within an environment that is sequestrated from the immune system and is prone to intrinsic and extrinsic environmental factors. The integrity of sperm transport and storage system and an adequate erectile function together with an intact sperm emission mechanism are of paramount importance for natural conception. The loss of integrity of any of these facets will give rise to male infertility.

Male Infertility Practice has been written by leading world authorities in the field who have made the biggest impact in revolutionizing the management of male infertility over the last two decades. Scientific authorities from Europe, South America, USA, South Africa and Egypt have contributed their most valuable practical and research pearls, offering the state of the art knowledge in the field of male factor infertility. The aim behind this volume was to be a one-stop authoritative resource for those who are involved in the management of male infertility irrespective of discipline and clinical specialty. The book is composed of six sections that cover a range of topics incorporating basic and clinic science as applied to the management of male infertility. Besides encompassing the breadth and the depth of the field the volume addresses clinical and ethical challenges faced by today's clinicians and scientists with an eye on potential developments in the future.

Finally, the editors wish to sincerely thank all contributing authors, both clinicians and scientist for their hard work and outstanding contributions, which make this volume a distinguished resource available today in its field.

Botros RMB Rizk
Nabil Aziz
Ashok Agarwal
Edmund Sabanegh Jr

Contents

Section V: Intrauterine Insemination

Section VI: Assisted Reproduction

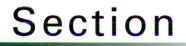

Section I

Physiology

1

The Testis: Development and Structure

Deborah M Spaine, Sandro C Esteves

■ INTRODUCTION

The testis is functionally compartalized into the gamete and endocrine sectors; the process of spermatogenesis occurs in the first where the haploid germ cell is generated, androgen production takes place in the second which is the site of testosterone biosynthesis.[1]

■ TESTIS DEVELOPMENT

Embryonic Development of the Gonadal Sex

The presumptive gonad is only a mass of mesoderm that will eventually differentiate into the somatic elements of the testis. Prior the 7th week of human development, the urogenital tract is identical in both sexes. Genetic males and females have both Wolffian and Mullerian duct systems. At the end of this indifferent phase of phenotypic sexual differentiation, the dual duct system constitutes the primordium of the internal accessory organs of reproduction.[2] Most of the gonad's cell types are derived from the mesoderm of the urogenital ridges. However, the primordial germ cells originate outside the area of the presumptive gonad and are initially identifiable in the endoderm of the yolk sac; they are derived from the primitive ectodermal cells of the inner cell mass.[3] At the 4th week of development, human primordial germ cells are well recognized in the hind-gut epithelium while at the 5th week they are found at the coelomic angle's dorsal mesentery and in the forming germinal ridge after migration. At 6th week of development, most primordial germ cells have already migrated to the gonad and are usually surrounded by and in close association with adjacent somatic cells.[4] The human primordial germ cells are characterized by their large and round nucleus and the presence of considerable number of lipid droplets in the cytoplasm. Histochemically, they have a high content of alkaline phosphatase and glycogen.[5]

The testis arises from the primitive gonad on the medial surface of the embryonic mesonephros. Primitive germ cells, which migrate to this region from the yolk sac, induce coelomic epithelial cells proliferation and formation of the sex cords. Formation of the sex cords gives to this region a raised contour that is called the genital ridge. By the 7th week of fetal development, proliferation of the mesenchyme has split the sex cords

from the underlying coelomic epithelium. During the 16th week, the sex cords become U-shaped and their ends anastomose to form the rete testis.[6,7] The chronology of the male reproductive tract development is depicted in **Figure 1.1**.

Sex Differentiation

Normal male sex differentiation involves a complex mechanism that depends on both genetic and hormonal control. The mechanism by which the germ cells differentiate is not fully understood, but it is known that the process begins early since primordial germ cells can be recognized in the 4 to 5 day-old human blastocyst.[8] At the beginning of the 4th week of development, germ cells begin to migrate by amoeboid movement through the gut endoderm into the mesentery's mesoderm, finally ending up in the coelomic epithelium of the gonadal ridges.[5] The formation of the gonadal blastema is completed during the 5th week of human embryogenesis; at this time the primitive and undifferentiated gonad is composed of three distinct cell types:

1. Germ cells
2. Supporting cells of the gonadal's ridge coelomic epithelium that either give rise to the testicular Sertoli cells or ovarian granulosa cell
3. Stromal (interstitial) cells derived from the mesonchyme of the gonadal ridge.

Sex differentiation is determined by the presence and expression of DNA sequences normally carried on by the Y-chromosome. All placental mammals have an XX female XY male sex determining system although the Y-chromosome differs morphologically and genetically between species.[9] In mammals, both male sex determination and spermatogenesis are controlled by genes located on the Y-chromosome. The testis-determining factor (TDF) is responsible for the transformation of the undifferentiated gonad to a differentiated testis.[10] TDF is produced by the sex-determining gene (SRY) that is located in the short arm of Y-chromosome (Yp). SRY is the first gene known to be involved in the differentiation process and undoubtedly is the main initiator of the gene interactions cascade that determine the development of the testis from the undifferentiated gonad.[11] The biochemical mechanism by which SRY determines testis differentiation appears to involve the binding to A/TAACAAT that is located within a minor DNA groove.[12] It was originally suggested

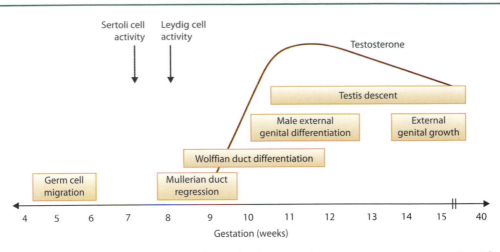

Figure 1.1: Embryologic events in male sex differentiation. The line depicts the increase in serum testosterone concentrations. The word activity refers indirectly to the action of anti-Mullerian hormone in causing Mullerian duct regression and androgens to induce male sex differentiation. (Adapted from Endocrinology 142(8), Hughes, Minireview: sex differentiation, page 3282, copyright 2001, with permission from the publisher, Association for the Study of Internal Secretions)

that SRY directly activates other genes in the testis-determining pathway. SOX9 plays a crucial role in the differentiation because it is up-regulated by SRY and SF1 to initiate differentiation of pre-Sertoli to Sertoli cells.[13] The development of the undifferentiated gonad within the genital ridge is controlled by autossomal genes, such as WT-1, LIM-1, SF-1, DAZ-1, DMTR1/DMTR-2, which act as transcription factors.[14]

Descent of the Testis

In most mammals the testes migrate from their original site. In many, including the humans, they pass through the abdominal wall into an evagination of the peritoneum that forms the scrotum.[15] The descent of the testis occurs in two morphologically and hormonally distinct phases termed transabdominal and inguinoscrotal phases.[16] During the first phase the testis remains anchored to the retroperitoneal inguinal area by the swollen gubernaculum, which prevents its ascent as the fetus enlarges. The gubernaculum is a cylindrical and gelatinous structure attached to the inguinal canal. Prior to the descent of the testis, an increase in the length of the intra-abdominal gubernaculum occurs. The increase of the gubernaculum wet mass plays an important role in the descent of the testis through the inguinal canal while the relative mass of the testis remains constant during this period.[17] The testis receives its neurovascular supply at approximately the T10 medular level. During the 3rd trimester of development, it slips down the posterior wall dragging its neurovascular leash.[18] In the second phase the testis descends from the inguinal area into the scrotum guided by the gubernaculum. The inguinoscrotal phase is androgen-dependent and is possibly mediated indirectly by the release of the neuropeptide calcitonin gene-related peptide (CGRP) from the genitofemoral nerve.[19] The role of the peptide INSL3 (Leydig cell protein product) in the control of testis descent in humans is

not fully understood.[20] At the sixth -month of fetal development, the tip of the gubernaculum protrudes through the external inguinal ring. By the 7th month, it is at the level of the presumptive internal ring of the inguinal canal. Soon thereafter, the lower anterior abdominal wall is evaginated to form the scrotal sac. By birth, or shortly thereafter, the testis has moved into its definitive extra-abdominal location and is covered by the processus vaginalis of the peritoneum.

It appears that the descent of the testis is a time-dependent embryological phenomenon similar to other important events of fetal development. It takes place between the 6th month of intra-uterine life and the first six weeks post-delivery. Thereafter, the forces that drive descent, which have already been diminishing fairly rapidly, fail altogether.[21] Several congenital problems may arise if this development sequence does not proceed normally. For instance, failure in the closure of the superior portion of the processus vaginalis may lead to a congenital inguinal hernia.[18] Cryptorchidism is associated with impaired germ cell development.[15] Androgens are still produced when the testis does not descend properly but the secretion rate is lower than normal particularly if the conditional is unilateral because there is no compensatory stimulation by increased levels of luteinizing hormone (LH).

▉ TESTIS STRUCTURE

Anatomy

The human testis is an ovoid mass that lies within the scrotum. The testes in all mammals are paired encapsulated organs consisting of seminiferous tubules separated by interstitial tissue. The testis weight increases many fold at puberty and it decreases slightly with age.[22] There are very few detailed studies of the spermatogenic function of the testis in aging men. The average testicular volume is 20 cubic centimeters in young men but decreases with age. The right testis is usually 10 percent larger than the left. Normal longitudinal length of the testis is approximately 4.5–5.1 cm. The average weight of human testis is 15 to 19 g with a specific gravity of 1.038 g/mL.[23] Measurement of testicular size is critical in the clinical assessment of the infertile man since seminiferous tubules correspond to approximately 90 percent of the testicular volume. Spermatogenesis probably decreases parallel to the decline in the overall testicular size.[24] Testicular consistency is also of value in determining fertility capacity. A soft testis is likely to reflect degenerating or shrunken spermatogenic components within the seminiferous tubules.

The layers covering the testis and their derivations (**Fig. 1.2**) are as follows:

• Skin
• Dartos fascia which is a continuation of Scarpa's fascia over the scrotum
• External spermatic fascia, derived from the external oblique aponeurosis
• Cremasteric muscle, derived from the internal oblique muscle
• Internal spermatic fascia, derived from fascia transversalis.
• Tunica vaginalis, derived from the processus vaginalis of the abdominal peritoneum.[25] The testis projects into the abdominal peritoneum from the retroperitoneum as it descends into the scrotum. It therefore explains the existence of double tunica vaginalis layers, an outer parietal and an inner visceral, surrounding the testis. Normally, there is a small amount of fluid between the visceral and parietal layers; a hydrocele is an excessive accumulation of fluid between these layers.

The testicular parenchyma is surrounded by a capsule containing blood vessels, smooth muscle fibers and nerve fibers sensitive to pressure. This capsule is often referred to as the tunica albuginea and it consists of fibroblasts and bundles of collagen and smooth-muscle cells.[26] The tunica albuginea is a tough fibrous covering which is composed of three layers:

1. An outer layer of visceral peritoneum—the tunica vaginalis
2. The tunica albuginea itself
3. The tunica vasculosa which is a subtunical extension of the interstitial tissue consisting of blood vessels and some Leydig cells in a loose connective tissue. The functional role of the testicular capsule is unknown but may relate to movement of fluid out through the rete testis or to maintain the interstitial pressure inside the testis.

Structure of the Seminiferous Tubules

In the male, the tunica albuginea and the rete testis combined comprise about 20 percent of the testicular size of young men; this value increases with age.[27] Most of the testis is made up by the seminiferous tubules, where the spermatozoa are formed, and interstitial cells. The seminiferous tubules are long V-shaped tubules; both ends drain toward the central superior and posterior regions of the testis, the rete testis which has a flat cuboidal epithelium. These cells appear to form a valve or plug which may prevent the passage of fluid from the rete into the tubule. The rete lies along the epididymal edge of the testis and coalesces in the superior portion of the testis, just anterior to the testicular vessels, to form 5 to 10 efferent ductules. The ductules leave the testis and travel a short distance to enter the head or caput region of the epididymis providing a connecting conduit to sperm transport to the epididymis. The seminiferous tubules are arranged in about 300 lobules each containing between one and four tubules. The rete testis is located in close proximity to the testicular artery that has part of its course on the surface of the testis. The interstitial tissue fills up the spaces between the seminiferous tubules and contains all the blood and lymphatic vessels and nerves of the testicular parenchyma.

Vasculature

The first description of the human testicular vasculature is dated of 1677. The author demonstrated that the gonadal artery divides into two branches just above the testis. One of them supplies the epididymis and the other branch enters the testis posteriorly, descends to the inferior pole and turns back superiorly along the anterior surface. This classical description remained substantially correct over time.[28] The testes receive their blood supply from the testicular, cremasteric and deferential arteries. The testicular artery is the primary testis blood supply; it arises from the abdominal aorta just inferior to the origin of the renal arteries and courses the retroperitoneum toward the pelvis. By the time the artery reaches the testicular surface, it is comparatively thinwalled to the portion that will course along the surface of the testis. The testicular artery pierces the tunica albuginea at the posterior aspect of the superior pole, courses down to the inferior pole, and then ascends along the anterior surface, just under

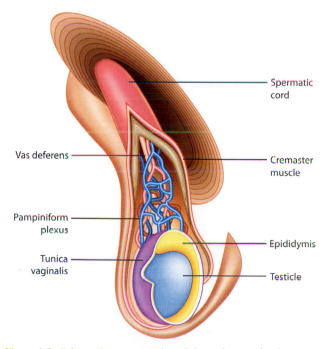

Vas deferens

Pampiniform plexus

Tunica vaginalis

Spermatic cord

Cremaster muscle

Epididymis

Testicle

Figure 1.2: Schematic representation of the male reproductive organs and their related structures

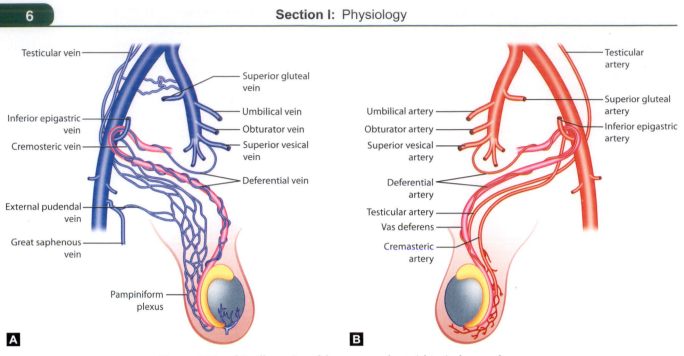

Figures 1.3A and B: Illustration of the venous and arterial testicular vasculature

the tunica albuginea, giving off several branches that course into the testicular parenchyma. The highest density of surface arteries is concentrated in the anterior, medial and lateral surfaces of the inferior pole and the lowest density is found in the medial and lateral aspects of the superior pole. It has been suggested that a myogenic response of subcapsular artery to increases in blood pressure may have an important role in the auto-regulation of the testicular blood supply.[29] The cremasteric arteries, also referred to as the external spermatic arteries, are branches of inferior epigastric artery and originate as branches of the external iliac arteries. The deferential arteries are branches of the internal iliac arteries and traverse much of the length of the vas deferens and supply it with blood (**Figs 1.3A and B**).

The venous anatomy of the testis is a particularly important feature of the male reproductive tract. The veins emerging from the testis form a dense network of intercommunicating branches known as the pampiniform plexus which extends through the scrotum and into the spermatic cord. The arteries supplying the testis pass through this plexus of veins in route to the testis. The venous blood (33°C) cools the arterial blood coming from the abdomen at a temperature of 37°C by the countercurrent heat exchange mechanism. After traversing the inguinal canal, the venous plexus disperses into veins that follow the arterial supply of the testis. The blood drains off the testis via the internal spermatic and the external pudendal veins (**Fig. 1.3**). There are no cross communication between the right and left spermatic venous system in the scrotal, retropubic and pelvic regions.[30] The right testicular vein empties into the inferior vena cava. In contrast, the left testicular vein normally enters the left renal vein (**Fig. 1.4**).

Anatomic dissections in several species have shown that the autonomic nerve supply to the testis is derived from the

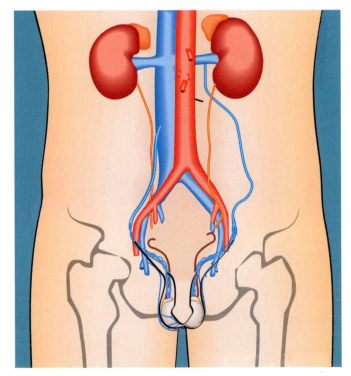

Figure 1.4: Illustration depicting the venous drainage of right and left testes. The right testicular vein empties into the inferior vena cava while the left testicular vein normally enters the left renal vein

spermatic plexus, which is composed of nerve fibers originating at the T10-L11 vertebral levels.

REFERENCES

1. Hales DB. Testicular macrophage modulation of Leydig steroidogenesis. J Reprod Immunol 2002;57(1-2):3-18.

2. Yamamoto M, Turner TT. Epididymis, sperm maturation and capacitation. In: Lipshultz LI and Howards SS, Eds. Infertility in the male. 2nd edn: Mosby Year Book 1991.pp.103-23.

3. Gardner RL, Lyon MF, Evans EP, Burtenshaw MD. Clonal analysis of x-chromosome inactivation and the origin of the germ line in mouse. J. Embryol Exp Morphol 1985;88:349-63.

4. Fujimoto T, Miyayama Y, Fuyuta M. The origin, migration and fine morphology of human primordial germ cells. Anat Rec 1977;188(3):315-30.

5. Mckay DG, Hertig AT, Adams EC, Danziger S. Histochemical observation on the germ cells of the human embryo. Anat Rec 1953;117(2):201-19.

6. George FW, Wilson JD. Sex determination and differentitian. In: Knobill E and Neill JD, (Eds). The physiology of reproduction. Vol. 1 New York: Raven Press 1994.pp.3-25.

7. Mawhinney MG, Tarry WF. Male acessory sex organs and androgen action. Lipshultz LI and Howards SS, (Eds). Infertility in the male. 2nd edn. Mosby Year Book 1991.pp.124-54.

8. Hertig AT, Adams EC, Mckay DG, Rock J, Mulligan WJ, Menkin K. A description of 34 human ova within the first 17 days of development. Am J Anat 1956;98(3):435-93.

9. Waters PD, Wallis MC, Graves JAM. Mammalian sex-origin and evolution of the Y-chromosome and SRY. Semin Cell Dev Biol 2007;18(3):389-400.

10. Welsbons WJ, Russell LB. The Y-chromosome as the bearer of male determining factor in mouse. Proc Natl Acad Sci USA 1959;45(4):560-6.

11. Graves JA. Interactions between SRY and SOX genes in mammalian sex determination. Bioessays 1998;20(3):264-9.

12. Harley VR, Lovell-Badge R, Goodfellow PN. Definition of a consensus DNA binding site for SRY. Nucleic Acids Res 1994;22(8):1500-1.

13. Hughes IA. Minireview: sex differentiation. Endocrinology 2001;142(8):3281-7.

14. Hiort O. Neonatal endocrinology of abnormal male sexual differentiation: molecular aspects. Horm Res 2000;53 (suppl 1): 38-41.

15. Stechell BP, Maddocks S, Brooks IDE. Anatomy, vasculature, innervation and fluids of male reproductive tract. In: Knobill E, Neill JD (Eds). The physiology of reproduction. Vol. 1 New York: Raven Press 1994.pp.1063-175.

16. Virtanen HE, Cortes D, Meytes ER, et al. Development and descent of the testis in relation to cryptorchidism. Acta Paediatr 2007;96(5):622-7.

17. Heyns CF. The gubernaculum during testicular descent in the human fetus. J Anat 1987;153:93-112.

18. Huckins C, Hellerstein DK. Development of the testes and establishment of spermatogenesis. In: Lipshultz LI and Howards SS, (Eds). Infertility in the male. 2nd edn: Mosby Year Book 1991;pp.3-20.

19. Hutson JM, Baker M, Tereda M, Zhou B, Paxton G. Hormonal control of testicular descent and the cause of cryptorchidism. Reprod Fertil Dev 1994;6(2):151-6.

20. Hughes IA, Acerini CL. Factors controlling testis descent. Eur J Endocrinol 2008;159 (suppl 1):S75-S82.

21. Scorer CG. The natural history of testicular descent. Proc R Soc Med 1965;58 (11 part 1):933-4.

22. Johnson L, Petty CS, Neaves WB. Age-related variation in seminiferous tubules in men: a stereologic evaluation. J Androl 1986;7(5):316-22.

23. Handelsman DJ, Staraj S. Testicular size: the effects of aging, malnutrition and illness. J Androl 1985;6(3):144-51.

24. Kothari LK, Gupta AS. Effect of aging on the volume, structure and total Leydig cell content of the human testis. Int J Fertil 1974;19(3):140-6.

25. Roberts KP, Pryor JL. Anatomy and physiology of the male reproductive system. In: Hellstrom WJG, Ed. Male infertility and sexual dysfunction. Springer-Verlag 1997.pp.1-21.

26. Langford GA, Heller CG. Fine structure of muscle cells of the human testicular capsule: basis of testicular contractions 1973;179(73):573-5.

27. Sosnik H. Studies on the participation of tunica albuginea and rete testis (TA and RT) in quantitative structure of human testis. Gegenbaurs Morphol Jahb 1985;131(3):347-56.

28. Jarow JP. Intratesticular arterial anatomy. J Androl 1990; 11(3): 255-9.

29. Davis JR. Myogenic tone of the rat testicular subcapsular artery has a role in autoregulation of testicular blood supply. Biol Reprod 1990;42(4):727-35.

30. Wishasi MM. Anatomy of the spermatic venous plexus (pampiniform plexus) in men with and without varicocele: intraoperative venographic study. J Urol 1992;147(5):1285-9.

2

The Testis: Function and Hormonal Control

Jorge Haddad Filho, Deborah M Spaine, Sandro C Esteves

INTRODUCTION

The hypothalamus, the pituitary and the testes form an integrated system responsible for an adequate secretion of male hormones and for normal spermatogenesis. The endocrine components of the male reproductive system are integrated in a classic endocrine feedback axis loop. The testes require stimulation by the pituitary gonadotropins, luteinizing hormone (LH) and follicle-stimulating hormone (FSH), which are secreted in response to hypothalamic gonadotropin releasing hormone (GnRH). Their action on germ cell development is affected by androgen and FSH receptors on Leydig and Sertoli cells, respectively. While FSH acts directly on the germinative epithelium, LH stimulates secretion of testosterone by the Leydig cells. Testosterone stimulates sperm production and virilization (along with dihydrotestosterone), and also feeds back the hypothalamus and pituitary to regulate GnRH secretion. FSH stimulates Sertoli cells to support spermatogenesis and to secrete inhibin B that negatively feedback FSH secretion.

GENERAL STRUCTURE OF THE TESTIS

Roughly, the testis consists of the seminiferous tubules and, among them, the interstitial space. The seminiferous tubules, containing germ cells, are lined by a layer of Sertoli cells coated by lamina propria. The lamina propria consists of the basal membrane covered by peritubular cells (fibroblasts). The main component of the interstitial space is the Leydig or interstitial cells, but it also contains macrophages, lymphocytes, loose connective tissue and neurovascular bundles.

Testicular Cell Types and Function

Peritubular Cells

The peritubular cells are distributed concentrically in layers around the seminiferous tubules, separated by collagen fibers. They produce extracellular matrix, connective tissue proteins (collagen, laminin, vimentin, fibronectin) and proteins related to cellular contractility such as smooth muscle myosin and actin.[1] They also synthetize adhesion molecules such as nerve growth factor (NGF) and monocyte chemoattractant protein 1 (MCP-1).[2] Secretion of these factors is regulated by tubular necrosis factor-α

(TNF-α), which in turn is produced by mast cells; as such, an interaction between peritubular and mast cells is suggested. It has also been shown that the number of mast cells increases in the testis in some cases of infertility.[3]

Peritubular cells have some contractility properties and are sometimes related as myofibroblasts. Cell contractions aid in the transport of sperm through the seminiferous tubules. Peritubular contractility is regulated by oxytocin, prostaglandins, androgens and endothelin.[4-6] Endothelin is, in turn, modulated by the relaxant peptide adrenomedullin produced by Sertoli cells.[4] Peritubular cells also secrete insulin-like growth factor-1 (IGF-1) and cytoquines that modulates the function of Sertoli cells, particularly the secretion of transferrine, inhibin and androgen-binding protein.[5]

Due to the complex interactions between peritubular cells and other cellular elements, it has been suggested that these cells have a role in male fertility. In fact, loss of contractility markers, tubular fibrosis and sclerosis as well as an increased number of mast cells are seen in some derangements of spermatogenesis leading to subfertility.[3,7,8] Peritubular and interstitial fibrosis, in association to spermatogenic damage, have also been demonstrated in the testis of vasectomized men.[9]

Leydig Cells

Also known as interstitial cells, the Leydig cells produce and secrete the major masculine hormone, testosterone. The differentiation of Leydig cells is determined, at least in part, by peritubular and Sertoli cells, which secrete leukemia inhibitory factor (LIF), platelet-derived growth factor-α (PDGF-α) and other factors that trigger Leydig stem cells to proliferate and migrate into the interstitial compartment of the testis, where they differentiate in the so-called progenitor Leydig cells. After that, growth factors and hormones (LH, IGF-1, PDGF-α, and others) transform them into immature Leydig cells and, finally, into the adult Leydig cell population.[10]

Adult Leydig cells exhibit endoplasmatic reticulum and mitochondria, typical of a steroid producing cell. The major substrate for androgen synthesis is cholesterol; acetate can also be utilized by the Leydig cells to synthetize cholesterol. Mitochondrial enzymes cytochrome P450SCC (side chain cleavage) or CYP11A1 (cytochrome P450, family 11, subfamily A, polypeptide 1) transforms cholesterol into pregnenolone, a process of androgen synthesis limited by the availability of cholesterol substrate. In the so-called delta-4 pathway, pregnenolone is converted to progesterone by 3β-hydroxysteroid dehydrogenase, which in turn is converted to 17α-hydroxyprogesterone and androstenedione by 17α-hydroxylase or CYP17A; androstenedione is finally converted to testosterone by cytochrome P450c17 (**Fig. 2.1**). In the delta-5 pathway, pregnenolone is hydroxylated to 17α-hydroxypregnenolone and dehydroepiandrosterone by 17α-hydroxylase or CYP17A), which in turn are converted to androstenediol by cytochrome P450c17; finally, androstenediol is transformed into testosterone by 3β-hydroxysteroid dehydrogenase (**Fig. 2.1**). Testosterone can be converted to estradiol by aromatase or to dihydrotestosterone by 5α-reductase. LH stimulates the transcription of genes that encode the enzymes involved in the steroidogenic pathways to testosterone.

Sertoli Cells

The Sertoli cells form the structure of the seminiferous tubules; their base rest on the basement membrane and their apex is oriented towards the lumen of the tubule (**Fig. 2.2**). Tight junctions between adjacent cells create a basal compartment that acts as a blood-testis barrier. Spermatogonia and early preleptotene primary spermatocytes are enclosed in the basal compartment while spermatocytes and spermatids are confined to the

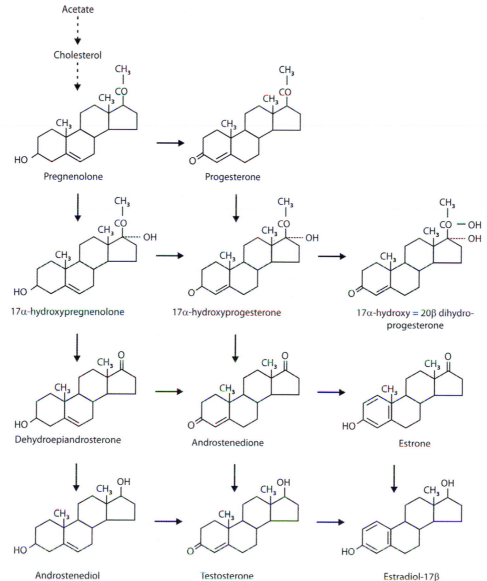

Figure 2.1: Steroidogenic pathways to testosterone

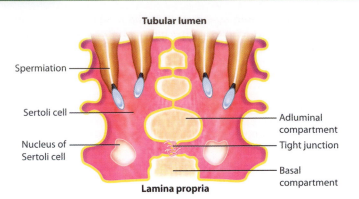

Figure 2.2: Sertoli cells and their relation to the compartments that enclose the germ cells

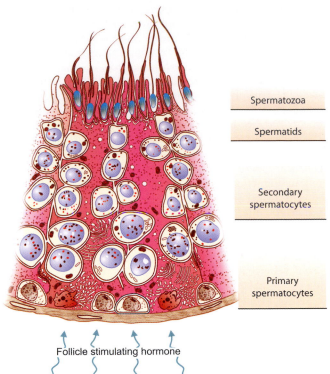

Figure 2.3: Germinative epithelium within the seminiferous tubule. Reprinted from International J Urol. 17(10), Agarwal et al., New generation of diagnostic tests for infertility: review of specialized semen specialized semen tests, page 839, copyright 2010, with permission from the authors and Blackwell Publishing Asia

adluminal compartment.[11] Spermatocytes and spermatids first appear at puberty and, therefore, after the development of the immune system. The blood-testis barrier separates spermatocytes and spermatids from the immune system, thus avoiding the formation of autoantibodies. A continuous remodeling of the tight junctions occurs as the germ cells are transferred from the basal to the adluminal compartment.[12] This process is mediated by proteases and protease inhibitors self-secreted by the Sertoli cells.[13]

Sertoli cells synthetize and secrete a large number of proteins, such as transport proteins (transferrin, ceruloplasmin, androgen binding protein), proteins involved in tight junction remodeling (cadherins, connexins, laminins) and regulatory proteins (antimullerian hormone, seminiferous grown factor), which are crucial for their interaction with germ-cells. Protein secretion is influenced by testosterone and FSH.[14,15] Sertoli cells functions include the regulation of spermatogenesis, by providing support and nutrition to germ cells, and the release of spermatids and spermiation.

Germ Cells

The germinative cells are enclosed within the compartments created by the Sertoli cells and the tubular lumen (**Fig. 2.3**). Three types of spermatogonia are found in the basal compartment:
1. Type A dark (considered as testicular stem cells)
2. Type A pale (replicate by mitosis)
3. Type B (the cell type that will progress into meiosis).[16] Cohorts of type B spermatogonia initiate meiosis by entering the leptotene stage of the first meiotic prophase. Meiosis is initiated after mitotic proliferation of spermatogonia by DNA synthesis that accomplishes precise replication of each chromosome to form two chromatids. Thus, the DNA content doubles but the number of chromosomes remains the same, i.e. diploid. These cells are the primary spermatocytes; they progressively show the nuclear features that identify meiosis I stages of leptotene, zygotene, pachytene and diplotene. During meiosis I, homologous chromosome pair, forming

bivalents, and undergo reciprocal recombination, resulting in new combination of gene alleles. The first meiotic division is reductional, separating the members of each homologous pair and reducing chromosome number from 2N to 1N. The result is two haploid cells, secondary spermatocytes, each with 23 chromosomes, but with each chromosome still comprised of two chromatids. The meiosis II is an equational division that separates the chromatids to separate cells, each containing the haploid number of chromosome and DNA content. The products of these meiotic divisions are four spermatids (**Fig. 2.3**). When meiosis is completed, the haploid round spermatids are conjoined in a syncytium as they initiate the differentiation process of spermiogenesis.

The final stage of spermatogenesis is termed spermiogenesis and involves no cell division. It represents a complex series of cytological changes leading to the transformation of the round spermatids to spermatozoa. This process includes:
• Changes in the position of the nucleus from a central to an eccentric location, together with reduction in the nuclear size and condensation of the nuclear DNA
• Formation of the acrosome from the Golgi complex, which interposes between the nucleus and the cell membrane

- Tail formation from a pair of centrioles lying adjacent to the Golgi complex and the aggregation of mitochondria
- Elimination of most of the cytoplasm which are phagocytosed by Sertoli cells. Once formed, sperm is released into the tubular lumen (spermiation).

Classically, the duration of spermatogenesis from the differentiation of pale spermatogonia to the ejaculation of mature spermatozoa has been estimated to be around 74 days.[17] This concept has been recently challenged by Misell et al. (2006), who showed that the appearance of new sperm in the semen occurred at a mean of 64 days. In their study, men with normal sperm concentrations ingested deuterated (heavy) water (^2H_2O) daily and semen samples were collected every 2 weeks for up to 90 days. ^2H_2O label incorporation into sperm DNA was quantified by gas chromatography/mass spectrometry, allowing calculation of the percent of new cells. The overall mean time to detection of labeled sperm in the ejaculate was 64 ± 8 days (range 42–76 days). They also observed biological variability, thus contradicting the current belief that spermatogenesis duration is fixed among individuals. All subjects achieved greater than 70 percent new sperm in the ejaculate by day 90, but plateau labeling was not attained in most, suggesting rapid washout of old sperm in the epididymal reservoir.[18] Their data also suggested that in normal men, sperm released from the seminiferous epithelium enter in the epididymis in a coordinated manner with little mixing of old and new sperm before subsequent ejaculation.

ENDOCRINE REGULATION

Gonadotropin Releasing Hormone

The hormonal control of testicular activity initiates with secretion of GnRH by the hypothalamus (**Fig. 2.4**). Gonadotropin releasing hormone (GnRH) is a polypeptide secreted by neurons located in the periventricular infundibular region, and its activation is achieved by occupancy of specific receptors (KiSS1-derived peptide receptor, also known as GPR54 or Kisspeptin receptor) by a protein, kisspeptin, also produced in the hypothalamus.[19] Negative feedback of androgens (testosterone and dihydrotestosterone) and estrogens is exerted by activation of their specific receptors located in the kisspeptin secreting neurons of the arcuate nucleus. Other substances also influence GnRH secretion. Noradrenalin and leptin have stimulatory effects, whilst prolactin, dopamine, serotonin, gama-aminobutyric acid (GABA) and interleukin-1 are inhibitory.[19] GnRH has a pulsatile secretion and a half-life of approximately 10 minutes. It is secreted into the hypothalamic-hypophyseal portal blood system to the pituitary gland.[20,21]

Once secreted, GnRH links to specific pituitary cell membrane receptors that results in the production of diacylglycerol and inositol triphosphate, intracellular calcium increase (by mobilization from intracellular stores and extracellular influx) and activation of protein kinase C. As a consequence, gonadotropins (LH and FSH) are released by exocytosis. The complex GnRH-receptor undergoes intracellular degradation; as such,

the cell needs some time to replace the receptors which is in harmony with the 60–90 minutes interval between GnRH secretion pulses. Continuous administration of GnRH leads to desensitization of the cells and decrease of gonadotropin secretion, the so-called "down regulation".[22]

Luteinizing and Follicle-stimulating Hormones

Luteinizing hormone (LH) and follicle-stimulating hormone (FSH) are glycoproteins consisting of alpha and beta polypeptide chains (α and β subunits). They have identical alpha subunits but differ in their beta subunit which determines receptor binding specificity. Thyroid-stimulating hormone (TSH) and human chorionic gonadotropin (hCG) are also glycoproteins that share the same structure. The β-chains of both LH and hCG are very similar, conferring similar properties such as receptor affinity. Once synthesized, LH and FSH are stored in granules at the pituitary. GnRH induces granules exocytosis and hormonal release to circulation. Low GnRH pulse frequency tend to produce preferential release of FSH, whereas higher frequencies are associated with preferential secretion of LH.[23,24] Due to syalization, FSH has longer (2 hours) half-life than LH (20 minutes). FSH and LH target to specific membrane receptors, whose internalization produces cAMP and protein kinase A.

LH exerts its influence on the Leydig cells, stimulating the production of steroids, mainly testosterone (**Fig. 2.4**). The Sertoli cells have receptors for FSH and testosterone. It is therefore believed that both hormones support the initiation of spermatogenesis, and are both needed for the maintenance of quantitatively normal spermatogenesis. Testosterone, or its metabolite dihydrotestosterone, binds to Sertoli cells androgen receptors and then modulate gene transcription. It has been shown that a functional Sertoli cell androgen receptor is a key element for normal spermatogenesis. Intratesticular testosterone levels are ~50 times higher than serum levels; as such, it is suggested that the androgen receptors are fully saturated in the normal testis.[25] FSH, on the other hand, binds to FSH receptors on Sertoli cells and initiates signal transduction events that ultimately lead to the production of inhibin B, which is a marker of Sertoli cell activity.[26] Inhibin B and testosterone, in turn, regulates pituitary FSH secretion (**Fig. 2.4**).[27] FSH receptors are expressed in the seminiferous tubules regions involved in spermatogonia proliferation. The dual hormonal dependence for normal spermatogenesis can be appreciated in hypogonadotropic hypogonadism males. Sperm production is restored to about 50 percent of normal levels with either FSH or hCG (as a surrogate for LH) treatment whereas only the combination of hCG plus FSH lead to quantitative restoration.[28]

It is suggested that testicular function is also regulated by other factors. For instance, Sertoli cells are influenced by factors secreted by the germ cells.[29] Estrogen receptors are found in the efferent ducts, Sertoli cells and most germ cell types. The testes are major sites of estrogen production; however, direct evidence for its role in spermatogenesis is yet to be established. Thyroid hormone receptor is important for Sertoli cell development.[30]

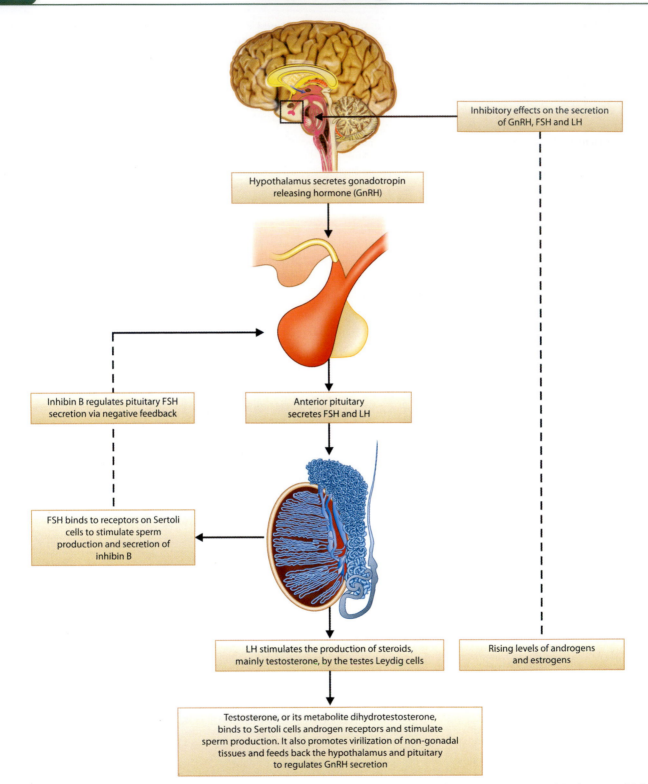

Figure 2.4: Components of the hypothalamic-pituitary-testicular axis and the endocrine regulation of spermatogenesis. Luteinizing hormone (LH) and follicle-stimulating hormone (FSH) are secreted by the pituitary in response to hypothalamic gonadotropin releasing hormone (GnRH). While FSH acts directly on the seminiferous tubules regions involved in spermatogonia proliferation, LH stimulates secretion of testosterone by the Leydig cells. Testosterone stimulates sperm production and also feeds back the hypothalamus and pituitary to regulate GnRH secretion. FSH stimulates Sertoli cells to support spermatogenesis and to secrete inhibin B that negatively feedback FSH secretion

REFERENCES

1. Holstein AF, Maekawa M, Nagano T, Davidoff MS. Myofibroblasts in the lamina propria of human seminiferous tubules are dynamic structures of heterogenous phenotype. Arch Histol Cytol 1996;59(2):109-25.
2. Schell C, Albrecht M, Mayer C, Schwarzer JU, Frungieri MB, Mayerhofer A. Exploring human testicular peritubular cells: identification of secretory products and regulation by tumor necrosis factor-alpha. Endocrinology 2008;149(4): 1678-86.
3. Apa DD, Cayan S, Polat A, Akbay E. Mast cells and fibrosis on testicular biopsies in male infertility. Arch Androl 2002; 48(5):337-44.
4. Romano F, Tripiciano A, Muciaccia B, et al .The contractile phenotype of peritubular smooth muscle cells is locally controlled: possible implications in male fertility. Contraception 2005;72(4):294-7.
5. Verhoeven G, Hoeben E, De Gendt K. Peritubular cell-Sertoli cell interactions: factors involved in PmodS activity. Andrologia 2000;32(1):42-5.
6. Zhang C, Yeh S, Chen Y, et al. Oligozoospermia with normal fertility in male mice lacking the androgen receptor in testis peritubular myoid cells. Proc Natl Acad Sci USA 2006; 103(47):17718-23.
7. Gulkesen KH, Erdogru T, Sargin CF, Karpuzoglu G. Expression of extracellular matrix proteins and vimentin in testes of azoospermic man: an immunohistochemical and morphometric study. Asian J Androl 2002;4(1):55-60.
8. Roaiah MM, Khatab H, Mostafa T. Mast cells in testicular biopsies of azoospermic men. Andrologia 2007;39(5):185-9.
9. Raleigh D, O'Donnell L, Southwick GJ, de Kretser DM, McLachlan RI. Stereological analysis of the human testis after vasectomy indicates impairment of spermatogenic efficiency with increasing obstructive interval. Fertil Steril 2004;81(6):1595-1603.
10. Svechnikov K, Landreh L, Weisser J, et al. Origin, development and regulation of human Leydig Cells. Horm Res Paediatr 2010;73(2):93-101.
11. Waites GMH. Fluid secretion. In: Johnson AD, Gomes WR (Eds). The Testis. Vol. IV New York: Academic Press 1977.pp.91-123.
12. Li MW, Xia W, Mruk DD, et al. Tumor necrosis factor "alpha" reversibly disrupts the blood-testis barrier and impairs Sertoli-germ cell adhesion in the seminiferous epithelium of adult rat testes. J Endocrinol 2006;190(2):313-29.
13. Griswold MD. The central role of Sertoli cells in spermatogenesis. Semin Cell Dev Biol 1998;9(4):411-6.
14. Verhoeven G. A Sertoli cell-specific knock-out of the androgen receptor. Andrologia 2005;37(6):207-8.
15. Gromoll J, Simoni M. Genetic complexity of FSH receptor function. Trends Endocrinol Metab 2005;16(8):368-73.
16. Ehmcke J, Schlatt S. A revised model for spermatogonial expansion in man: lessons from non-human primates. Reproduction 2006;132(5):673-80.
17. Amann RP. The cycle of the seminiferous epithelium: a need to revisit? J Androl 2008;29(5):469-87.
18. Misell LM, Holochwost D, Boban D, et al. A stable isotope-mass spectrometric method for measuring human spermatogenesis kinetics *in vivo*. J Urol 2006;175(1):242-6.
19. Popa SM, Clifton DK, Steiner RA. The role of kisspeptins and GPR54 in the neuroendocrine regulation of reproduction. Annu Rev Physiol 2008;70:213-38.
20. Pinón R, (Ed). Biology of human reproduction. Sausalito: University Science Books 2002.pp.171-2.
21. Filkenstein JS, Whitcomb RW, O'dea LSL, Longscope C, Schoenfeld DA, Crowley WFJ. Sex steroid control of gonadotropin secretion in the human male I. Effects of testosterone administration in normal and gonadotropin-releasing hormone deficient men. J Clin Endocrinol Metab 1991;73(3):609-20.
22. Belchetz PE, Plant TM, Nakai Y, Keogh EJ, Knobil E. Hypophyseal responses to continuous and intermittent delivery of hypothalamic gonadotropin-releasing hormone. Science 1978;202(4368):631-3.
23. Ferris HA, Shupnik MA. Mechanisms for pulsatile regulation of the gonadotropin subunit genes by GNRH1. Biol Reprod 2006;74(6):993-8.
24. Silverman AJ, Livne I, Witkin JW. The gonadotropin-releasing hormone (GnRH) neuronal systems: immunocytochemistry and in situ hybridization. In: Knobil E, Neill JD, (Eds). The physiology of reproduction. 3rd edn. New York: Elsevier Academic Press 2006.pp.1683-1710.
25. Mclachlan RI. How is the production of spermatozoa regulated? Handbook of Andrology, American Society of Andrology, 2nd edn. New Hampshire: Allen Press 2010.pp.1-4.
26. Raivio T, Wikstron AM, Dunkel L. Treatment of gonadotropin deficient boys with recombinant FSH: long term observation and outcome. Eur J Endocrinol 2007;156(1):105-11.
27. Boepple PA, Hayes FJ, Dwyer AA, et al. Relative roles of inhibin B and sex steroids in the negative feedback regulation of follicle-stimulating hormone in men across the full spectrum of seminiferous epithelium function. J Clin Endocrinol Metab 2008;93(5):1809-14.
28. Matsumoto AM, Karpas AE, Bremner WJ. Chronic human chorionic gonadotropin administration in normal men: evidence that follicle-stimulating hormone is necessary for the maintenance of quantitatively normal spermatogenesis in man. J Clin Endocrinol Metab 1986;62(6):1184-92.
29. Griswold MD. Interactions between germ cells and Sertoli cells in the testis. Biol Reprod 1995;52(2):211-6.
30. Maffei L, Murata Y, Rochira V, et al. Dysmetabolic syndrome in a man with a novel mutation of the aromatase gene: effects of testosterone, alendronate and estradiol treatment. J Clin Endocrinol Metab 2004;89(1):61-70.

3

Sperm Transport and Maturation

Deborah M Spaine, Sandro C Esteves

■ INTRODUCTION

Spermatozoa leave the testis neither fully motile nor able to recognize or fertilize the oocytes. To become functional gametes, spermatozoa must migrate through a long duct, the epididymis, and undergo additional maturation processes. The epididymis is a dynamic organ that under the influence of androgens promotes sperm maturation, provides a place for sperm storage, plays a role in the transport of the spermatozoa from the testis to the ejaculatory duct, protects the male gametes from harmful substances and reabsorbs both fluids and products of sperm breakdown. Spermatozoa within the epididymis are held in a quiescent state by luminal fluid factors.[1] Gamete transport is achieved by contractions of the smooth muscle that surrounds the epididymal epithelium and by continuous production and movement of fluid originating from the testis. The manner by which the epididymis protects the spermatozoa from harmful substances is not clear but it seems that the epididymis has evolved elaborate protective mechanisms. The blood-epididymis barrier, for instance, regulates the entry of solutes and ions into the epididymal lumen. The luminal fluid contains antioxidants substances, e.g. glutathione, superoxide dismutase and glutathione-S-transferase that are involved in antioxidant defense and protection against oxygen radicals and xenobiotics. The endpoint resulting from these processes is the sperm ability to fertilize the oocyte and contribute to the formation of a healthy embryo.

■ EPIDIDYMIS

Embryology

The intimately associated urinary and reproductive tracts develop from a common embriologic origin. The primary embryonic kidney generates a single nephric duct (Wolffian) that elongates caudally towards the cloaca. The nephrogenic cords and urogenital ridges appear by 25 days in the human embryo. The nephric duct subsequently forms the second embryonic kidney—the mesonephros. When the nephric duct reaches the metanephric mesenchyme, interactions between both tissues initiate the metanephros development. The newly formed ureter branches and induces mesenchymal-epithelial transitions in the surrounding mesenchyme, initiating the first of numerous cycles of nephron formation.[2] Prior to the 7th week of human development, the urogenital tract is identical in the two sexes. The mesonephric duct is either transformed into the male genital tract (epididymis and vas deferens) or degenerates in female embryos. The mesonephric tubules persist as the ductuli efferentes and unit with the rete testis. The epididymis is derived from the Wolffian duct and at birth consists mainly of mesenchymal tissue. The adult efferent ducts and epididymides share a common origin with the primitive kidney.[3] The epididymis undergoes considerable remodeling including duct elongation and convolution so that by puberty the epididymis has acquired its fully differentiated state consisting of a highly tortuous tubule lined by epithelial cells.[4]

Anatomy

The epididymis is a single highly convoluted duct extending from the anterior to the posterior pole of the testis. It is closely attached to the testis surface by connective tissue and tunica vaginalis which surrounds the testis and the epididymis except for its posterior aspect. The posterior surface is attached to the scrotum and spermatic cord by a fibrofatty connective tissue. Classical gross anatomy uses the terms *globus major* for the proximal epididymis and *globus minor* for the distal epididymis, with the *globus minor* disappearing in the epididymal fat pad.[5]

The epididymis consists of the *ductuli efferentes* and the epididymis duct. Between 10 and 15 *ductuli efferentes* arise from the rete testis. These tubules come together to form the epididymal duct that is extremely long and varies from 3–4 meters in man.[6] This convoluted duct folds repeatedly upon itself and forms the main bulk of the organ. The epididymis is conventionally divided in three anatomic regions or segments: the caput or head, the corpus or body and cauda or tail (**Fig. 3.1**). This nomenclature is commonly used in medicine and reproductive biology. An alternative subdivision has been proposed by Glover and Nicander.[7] This subdivision is based on histologic and functional criteria and it divides the epididymis into three regions: initial, middle and terminal segments. The initial and middle segments are primarily concerned with sperm maturation and the terminal segment coincides with the region where mature sperm are stored before ejaculation.[7,8] The initial segment comprises the region where the *ductuli efferentes* empty while

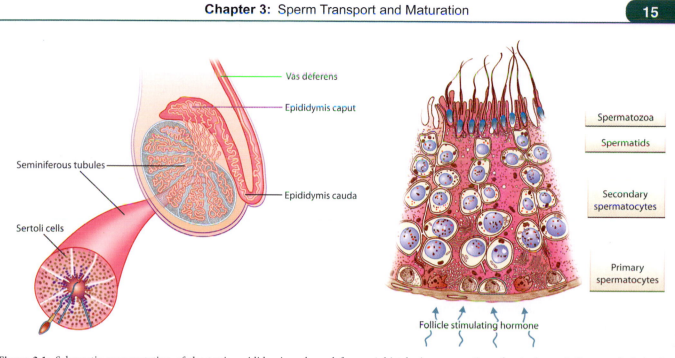

Figure 3.1: Schematic representation of the testis, epididymis and vas deferens. A histologic cross-section of a single seminiferous tubule is also depicted showing the spermatogenesis stages (Reprinted from International J Urol. 17(10), Agarwal et al., New generation of diagnostic tests for infertility: review of specialized semen specialized semen tests, page 839, copyright 2010, with permission from the authors and publisher Blackwell Publishing Asia)

the terminal portion disappears into the epididymal fat making it appear that the epididymis has a minimal cauda region. In fact, the still-coiled human cauda epididymis is 10–12 cm long before becoming the convoluted vas, and the convoluted vas extends for approximately another 7–8 cm.[6]

Histology

The epididymis is remarkably well-developed in the human fetus at 16 week's gestation. The tall pseudostratified epithelium lines a discrete duct with a patent lumen and stereocilia and cilia are seen on the apical surface of principal cells. The duct is surrounded by connective tissue that contains fibroblasts, collagen, elastic fibers, blood vessels, lymphatic vessels, nerve fibers, macrophages, wandering leukocytes and concentric layers of smooth-muscle fibers.[8] The muscle surrounding the epididymal duct gradually increases in thickness from the proximal to the distal regions. At the level of the caput epididymis, longitudinal and obliquely arranged bundles of smooth-muscle cells are added to those that are circularly oriented. A layer of thick smooth muscle is superimposed to the subepithelially located bundles of smooth-muscle cells at the junction of the corpus and cauda.[3]

The epididymal epithelium is composed of several cell types which include the principal, basal, apical, halo, clear and narrow cells (**Fig. 3.2**). The distribution of these cells varies in number and size at different points along the epididymal duct.[5,9] The primary cell type throughout the epididymal tubule is the principal cell which constitutes approximately 80 percent of the epithelium

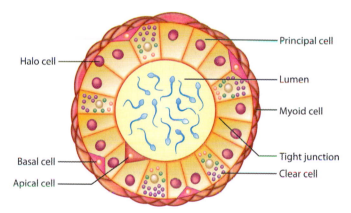

Figure 3.2: A histologic cross-section of the epididymis with the cell elements (Adapted and reprinted from Hum Reprod Update 15(2), Cornwall, New insights into epididymal biology and function, page 216, copyright 2009, with permission from the publisher Oxford University Press)

and is, by far, the most studied since it is responsible for the bulk of proteins secreted into the lumen.[4] The infranuclear compartments of the principal cells are rich in rough endoplasmic reticulum while the supranuclear one have numerous mitochondria and highly developed Golgi complexes. The principal cells are responsible for the secretion of carnitine, glycerylphosphorylcholine and sialic acid, inositol and a variety of glycoproteins.[10] Narrow, apical and clear cells contain vacuolar H^+-ATPase and secrete protons into the lumen, thus participating in its acidification.[11,12] Clear cells are endocytic cells and may be responsible for the clearance of proteins from the epididymal lumen. Basal cells do not access the luminal compartment and are in close association with the overlying principal cells, as indicated by the presence of cytoplasmic extensions with the principal cells, It has been suggested that basal cells regulate the principal cells functions.[13,14] Halo cells appear to be the primary immune cell type in the epididymis, whereas apical cells may also endocytose luminal components. The most detailed study of the epithelia and tubule organization in the human epididymis came from Yeung et al in 1991.[15] The authors described at least seven types of tubules, connected by at least eight types of junctions to form a network, each one characterized by a different epithelium. The differences in the cellular architecture are primarily due to the functional roles of each epithelium within each epididymal region. In the proximal region there is considerable absorption of water, hence the epithelium takes on the classical appearance of a water absorbing surface with long stereocilia and many mitochondria in the basal aspects. The cells at the distal epididymis are much smaller and some are specialized in removing cellular debris.

Physiology

Mammalian spermatogenesis involves proliferation of spermatogonia to give rise to diploid spermatocytes, meiotic division which produces haploid cells, called spermatids, and cytological transformation which leads to mature spermatozoa (**Fig. 3.1**). After being produced in the testis, spermatozoa are transported through the caput and corpus regions of the epididymis, and are then stored in the proximal epididymis cauda. The duration of one human cycle of spermatogenesis and epididymal transit has been estimated to be 64 days and 5.5 days, respectively. These estimates are derived mainly from older kinetic studies performed *in vivo*. Based on sequential biopsy and radiography in men who underwent testicular injections of the radioisotope 3H-thymidine, it was estimated that the production of spermatocytes from spermatogonia takes 16 days, and the duration of all 3 phases of spermatogenesis was estimated to be 64 days, a value exclusive of epididymal transit time.[16] These data form the foundation for our concept that human spermatogenesis requires 2–3 months to complete and they guide the time lines proposed for improvement or recovery in countless infertile couples undergoing male infertility treatment. Misell et al. (2006), however, showed for the first time that the appearance of new sperm in ejaculated semen occurred at a mean of 64 days, and this value included epididymal transit time.[17] In their study, a total of 11 men with normal sperm concentrations ingested ^2H_2O daily for 3 weeks and semen samples were collected every 2 weeks for up to 90 days. ^2H_2O label incorporation into sperm DNA was quantified by gas chromatography/mass spectrometry, allowing calculation of the percent of new cells present. They found that all men had negligible new sperm in the ejaculate (less than 10%) 4 weeks after labeling began. Overall mean time to detection of labeled sperm in the ejaculate was 64 ± 8 days (range 42–76).

They also observed biological variability, since in one subject the time lag was 42 days with greater than 33 percent of new sperm at this time point, although it was at least 60 days in all others. By day 90 all subjects had achieved greater than 70 percent new sperm in the ejaculate, but in most individuals plateau labeling was not attained, suggesting rapid washout of old sperm in the epididymal reservoir (**Fig. 3.3**). Their interesting data has important clinical impact, particularly for assessing the male patient responses to various infertility treatment modalities. Another important observation was the significant biological variability in the time needed to produce and ejaculate sperm in normal men. This contradicts the current belief that spermatogenesis requires approximately 60 days, which is a duration that was believed not to vary among individuals.

Spermatozoa mature during the epididymal transit and acquire functional competence and ability to move. Maturation involves alterations in the plasma membrane, chromatin condensation and stabilization, and possibly some final modifications to the shape of the acrosome.[18] During their development, spermatozoa are continually bathed in fluid secretions provided by the epithelium of seminiferous tubules and epididymal ducts.[9] Although the mechanisms by which the epididymis performs its functions of sperm maturation, transport and storage are not completely understood, the consensus is that these functions are affected by the fluid milieu within the epididymal lumen and the epithelial cells that produce it.[3] Microanalytic studies revealed that several biochemical changes fundamental for sperm maturation and survival occur in the epididymal duct intraluminal

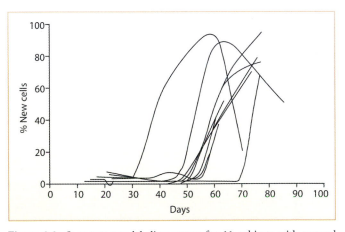

Figure 3.3: Spermatocyte labeling curves for 11 subjects with normal semen analyses. Cases were labeled with 50 ml 70% deuterated (heavy) water (^2H_2O) twice daily for 3 weeks. Semen samples were collected every 2 weeks for 90 days from start on ^2H_2O. Spermatocyte DNA enrichment was measured by gas chromatography/mass spectrometry and compared to that of fully turned over cell (monocyte) to calculate percentage of new cells present. A considerable inter-individual variability between normal subjects were observed (Reprinted from J Urol 175: 242-6, Misell et al, A Stable Isotope-Mass Spectrometric Method for Measuring Human Spermatogenesis Kinetics *in vivo*, pages 242-6, copyright 2006, with permission from Elsevier)

fluid.[19,20] The fluid in the proximal epididymis is quite acidic with pH values in the 6.5 range; it increases to approximately 6.8 in the distal region. A variety of substances are secreted by the epididymis and these substances may influence sperm maturation. The epididymal lumen contains the most complex fluid found in any exocrine gland. It results from the continuous changes in composition as well as the presence of components in unusually high concentration for reasons not yet known.[4] Epididymal tubule segments represent unique physiological compartments, each one possessing distinctive gene expression profiles within the epithelium that dictate segment-specific secretion of proteins into the luminal fluid that affect sperm maturation.

SPERM TRANSPORT

Human spermatozoa released from Sertoli cells into the lumen of seminiferous tubules ride approximately 6 meters in the reproductive tract before leaving the urethral meatus.[3] Sperm movement occurs in part by hydrostatic pressure that originates from fluids secreted into the seminiferous tubules and tubular peristaltic-like contractions. Tunica albuginea contractions play a role in the generation of positive fluid pressure in the head of the epididymis.[5] Transport through the proximal epididymis is facilitated by peristaltic contractions of the smooth muscles surrounding the epididymal duct. Additional mechanisms that aid sperm movement include fluid currents established by the action of cilia along the walls of the efferent ducts and spontaneous rhythmic contractions of the contractile cells surrounding the epididymal duct.[3] Adrenergic and cholinergic mechanisms, and vasopressin, have been proposed as regulating factors for epididymal duct peristaltic activity.[3] Transport rates are estimated to be more rapid in the efferent ducts and proximal epididymis where the fluid is non-viscous and water is rapidly absorbed from the luminal compartment.[5]

Epididymal transit time has been estimated to range from 2 to 6 days. Variation is probably due to the rate of passage through the epididymis cauda which in turn is influenced by ejaculatory frequency.[5,21] It has also been shown that men with high testicular sperm production have shorter epididymal transit time than men with lower testicular sperm output. This difference seems to be explained by a direct association between the production of sperm and fluid; testes that produce more sperm also produce more fluid so the movement of spermatozoa along the epididymal duct is faster.[22] A recent study using direct kinetic measurement of spermatogenesis and time to sperm ejaculation has suggested that in normal men, sperm released from the seminiferous tubules enter the epididymis in a coordinated manner with little mixing of old and new sperm before subsequent ejaculation. This concept is novel because it had been suggested that because of mixing, in any segment of the epididymal duct, the population of sperm would be heterogeneous in age and biological status. Although this may be true with regard to biological status these kinetic data suggest that the epididymal reservoir is purged of old sperm fairly rapidly and completely in normal men.[17]

SPERM MATURATION

Spermatozoa undergo important changes during their passage through the epididymis, many of which are the result of changes in the nature and composition of the plasma membrane. In many species, including humans, a reduction in sperm cholesterol is one of the first steps that triggers signal transduction cascades during capacitation including tyrosine phosphorylation of sperm proteins. Sperm remodeling also involves changes in the dimension and appearance of both acrosome and nucleus, migration of the cytoplasmic droplet along the tail, as well as structural changes in intracellular organelles.[23] Spatially separated lipids and proteins are re-organized during maturation possibly allowing the formation of signaling complexes critical for fertilization. These changes are promoted by the fluid microenvironment within the epididymis and ensure that sperm can traverse the female reproductive tract, and after capacitation, fertilize the oocyte.[24] The epididymal fluid is hyperosmotic and its major constituents are L-carnitine, glutamate, inositol, sialic acid, taurine, glycerophosphorylcholine, and lactate. Concentrations of these substances can range from 20 to 90 mM depending upon the epididymal region. Sodium, potassium, bicarbonate and chloride are also present in the luminal fluid.[24] Organic substances, electrolytes and enzymes are likely to be involved in the acquisition of sperm motility, in epididymal cell metabolism and in the osmoregulation of sperm and epididymal epithelium cells. Several proteins such as albumin, transferrin, immobilin, clusterin (SGP-2), metalloproteins and proenkephalin are also found within the epididymal lumen and are claimed to be associated with sperm maturation.[5]

REFERENCES

1. Hinrichsen MJ, Blaquier JA. Evidence supporting the existence of sperm maturation in the human epididymis. J Reprod Fert 1980;60(2):291-4.
2. Grote D, Souabni A, Busslinger M, Bouchard M. Pax2/8-regulated Gata3 expression is necessary for morphogenesis and guidance of the nephric duct in the developing kidney. Development 2006;133(1):53-61.
3. Yamamoto M, Turner TT. Epididymis, sperm maturation and capacitation. In: Lipshultz LI and Howards SS (Eds). Infertility in the male. 2nd edn. St. Louis: Mosby Year Book 1991.pp.103-23.
4. Cornwall GA. New insights of epididymal biology and function. Hum Reprod Update 2009;15(2):213-27.
5. Turner TT. De Graaf's thread: the human epididymis. J Androl 2008;29(3):237-50.
6. Turner TT. On the epididymis and its role in development of the fertile ejaculate. J Androl 1995;16(4):292-8.
7. Glover TD, Nicander L. Some aspects of structure and function in the mammalian epididymis. J Reprod Fertil Suppl 1971;13(Suppl):39-50.
8. Setchell BP, Maddocks S, Brooks IDE. Anatomy, vasculature, innervations and fluids of the male reproductive tract. In: Knobil E and Neill JD, (Eds). The physiology of reproduction. 2nd edn. Vol.1 New York: Raven Press 1994.pp.1063-175.

9. Hinton BT, Lan ZT, Rudolph DB, Labus JC, Lye RJ. Testicular regulation of epididymal gene expression. J Reprod Fertl Suppl 1998;53 (suppl):47-57.

10. Flickinger CJ. Synthesis and secretion of glycoprotein by the epididymal epithelium. J Androl 1983;4(2):157-61.

11. Pietrement C, Sun-Wada GH, Silva ND, et al. Distinct expression patterns of different subunit isoforms of the V-ATPase in the rat epididymis. Biol Reprod 2006;74(1):185-94.

12. Kujala M, Hihnala S, Tienari J, et al. Expression of ion transport-associated proteins in human efferent and epididymal ducts. Reproduction 2007;133(4):775-84.

13. Veri JP, Hermo L, Robaire B. Immunocytochemical localization of the Yf subunit of glutathione S-transferase P shows regional variation in the staining of epithelial cells of the testis, efferent ducts, and epididymis of the male rat. J Androl 1993;14(1):23-44.

14. Seiler P, Cooper TG, Yeung CH, Nieschlag E. Regional variation in macrophage antigen expression by murine epididymal basal cells and their regulation by testicular factors. J Androl 1999;20(6):738-46.

15. Yeung CH, Cooper TG, Bergmann M, Schulze H. Organization of tubules in the human caput epididymis and the ultrastructure of their epithelia. Am J Anat 1991;191(3): 261-79.

16. Clermont Y. Kinetics of spermatogenesis in mammals: seminiferous epithelium cycle and spermatogonial renewal. Physiol Rev 1972;52(1):198-236.

17. Misell LM, Holochwost D, Boban D, et al. A stable isotope-mass spectrometric method for measuring human spermatogenesis kinetics *in vivo*. J Urol 2006;175(1):242-6.

18. Mortimer ST. Essentials of sperm biology. In: Patton PE and Battaglia DE (Eds). Office Andrology. New Jersey: Humana Press 2005.pp.1-9.

19. Howards SS, Johnson A, Jessee S. Micropuncture and micro-analytic studies of the rat testis and epididymis. Fert Steril 1975;26(1):13-9.

20. Hilton BT. The epididymal microenvironment: a site of attack for a male contraceptive? Invest Urol 1980;18(1):1-10.

21. Amann RP. A critical review of methods for evaluation of spermatogenesis from seminal characteristics. J Androl 1981;2(1):37-58.

22. Johnson L, Varner DD. Effect of daily sperm production but not age on the transit times of spermatozoa through the human epididymis. Biol Reprod 1988;39(4):812-17.

23. Olson GE, Nag Das SK, Winfrey VP. Structural differentiation of spermatozoa during post-testicular maturation. In: Robaire B, Hinton BT (Eds). The Epididymis: From Molecules to Clinical Practice. New York: Kluwer Academic/Plenum Publishers 2002. pp.371-87.

24. Toshimori K. Biology of spermatozoa maturation: an overview with an introduction to this issue. Microsc Res Tech 2003;61(1):1-6.

4

Seminal Plasma: Constitution, Chemistry and Cellular Content

Stefan du Plessis

INTRODUCTION

Seminal plasma is the biggest contributor to the volume of semen. It is a physiological heterogeneous mixture that mediates the chemical function of the ejaculate. Seminal plasma consists of secretions, in varying volume, from the epididymis, seminal vesicles, prostate and bulbourethral glands.[1] The Ampullary, Littre and Tyson's glands also contribute in very small volumes but are barely studied and thus still poorly understood. Products secreted by these various glands are responsible for the nourishment, activation and protection of spermatozoa. Seminal plasma is an alkaline medium that buffer the acidic environment of the vagina, is responsible for coagulation of the ejaculate and provides a medium of transport for the spermatozoa in the female genital tract.[2] In fertile men, about 5 percent of the ejaculate is secreted by the bulbourethral and Littre glands and Littre glands; the prostate contributes between 15–30 percent to the total ejaculate. Some other small contributions come from the ampulla and epididymis. Finally, the seminal vesicles contribute the remainder, and also the majority of the ejaculate.[2]

FLUID CONSTITUTION

The major male accessory glands which are responsible for secreting the bulk of the semen are the seminal vesicles, prostate and Cowper's glands.[2,3] Also contributing very small volumes to semen are the Ampullary, Littre, and Tyson's glands.[4] Products of these glands which are secreted at the beginning of the ejaculatory phase serve to nourish and activate the spermatozoa, clear the urethral tract prior to ejaculation and acts as a vehicle of transport for spermatozoa in the female reproductive tracts.[5]

Bulbourethral Glands

Bulbourethral glands are also known as Cowper glands and exist in pairs. They are found in the majority of male mammals. The two Cowper's glands lie side by side and are located beneath the prostate gland in the urogenital diaphragm, posterior and lateral to the membranous urethra.[3] They secrete clear, alkaline, mucuslike substance. These secretions are commonly known as the pre-ejaculate and enter the urethra during sexual arousal, and may contain small numbers of spermatozoa. The amount of the pre-ejaculate emitted varies widely between individuals, averaging about 0.2 milliliters in most men, but as much as 5 milliliters have been recorded in some men, depending predominantly on the duration of the plateau phase levels of sexual tension.[6] Generally, the bulbourethral secretions contribute less than 1 percent to the total semen composition.[7] Functions of the bulbourethral secretions are lubrication of the urethra to allow for the passage of spermatozoa during ejaculation and the removal of residual urine or other foreign matter.[4]

Prostate Gland

The prostate in a healthy young adult male is a walnut-size gland that weighs up to 20 grams.[8] The gland is located between the urogenital diaphragm and the neck of the bladder and connecting the prostate and bulbourethral glands is the urogenital sinus.[8,9] The prostate completely surrounds both of the ejaculatory ducts as well as the urethra and originates at the neck of the bladder and ends by merging with the ejaculatory ducts.[10,11] It secretes many proteins in a prostatic fluid that combine with the fluid secreted by the seminal vesicles to promote sperm activation and function. Its secretion is a thin, milky, alkaline fluid, which makes up about 18–20 percent of the total ejaculate.[12] The alkaline properties of the prostate secretions provide an important function in neutralizing the acidic vaginal secretions and thus ensure successful fertilization. The prostate is also responsible for the secretion of clotting enzymes.[11] The prostatic component in the seminal plasma can be identified by its major secretary products such as acid phosphatase, citrate and zinc. Secretions from the prostate gland are in the form of both soluble and particulate matter.[13,14] The soluble fraction includes carbohydrates, proteins, electrolytes, polyamines, hormones, lipids and growth factors. The proteins constitute the major biochemical components. Major proteins expressed in both pubertal and adult humans are prostatic acid phosphatase (PAP), prostate specific antigen (PSA), and prostate binding protein (PBP).[14]

Prostate Specific Antigen

Prostate specific antigen (PSA) was first isolated in 1971.[15] PSA has shown to be the most useful tumor marker, not only for the screening and detection of prostate cancer, but also as a follow-up tool after therapy. Prostate specific antigen cleaves the major seminal vesicle protein that is found in the seminal coagulate and is important for the liquefaction of the sample.[15]

Prostatic Acid Phosphatase

Prostatic acid phosphatase (PAP) is a glycoprotein and the most abundant phosphatase in the prostatic seminal fluid.[16] Before the identification of prostate specific antigen (PSA), PAP was used as a marker to identify prostate cancer. Since the development of more sensitive and specific PSA assays, interest in PAP has decreased. Even though the exact biological function of PAP is unknown it is thought to act on phosphorylcholine to produce free cholines.[17]

Citrate

Citrate is one of the most important anions (groups of negatively charged atoms) present in human semen.[18] Secretary epithelial cells of the prostate produce citrate from aspartic acid and glucose. Citrate levels are approximately 100 times higher in the prostate than in any other soft tissues.[17]

Zinc

High levels of Zinc are found in the seminal plasma.[17] Zinc has an important role in testes development and sperm physiological function. Zinc has antioxidant properties and serves an important role in scavenging reactive oxygen species.[19] Zinc has also been implicated to have an antibacterial role in the prostate.[17] Concentrations of Zinc in the prostatic secretion of men with chronic bacterial prostatitis are significantly lower when compared to that of normal men.[20]

Seminal Vesicles

The seminal vesicles are a pair of accessory sexual glands, which provide a variety of secretions vital to the overall composition of semen. Seminal vesicles supply up to 85 percent of the total volume of the seminal plasma and are responsible for the final contribution to the semen.[21] Functions of the seminal vesicle secretions include nourishment and transportation of the ejaculated sperm. As these secretions represent the bulk of the semen, they dilute the spermatozoa and enable them to become motile.[11] Substances secreted by the seminal vesicles include fructose, fibrinogen and prostaglandins.[21]

Fructose

Fructose is the energy source for spermatozoa while they are still in the semen. The lower reference value for the total fructose content is defined by the WHO[22] as 13 μmol or more per ejaculate. Absence of fructose in the semen usually indicates the congenital absence of the seminal vesicles and vas deferens.[22]

Fibrinogen

Another function of the seminal vesicles is to secrete fibrinogen, a precursor of the molecule fibrin. Fibrinogen interacts with enzymes produced by the prostate, ultimately resulting in the clotting of semen. This enables semen to remain in the female reproductive tract during and after the retraction of the penis after coitus.[11]

Prostaglandins

Prostaglandins were first discovered and isolated in 1930 by Ulf von Euler of Sweden. Even though prostaglandins were first identified in semen and believed to originate from the prostate, hence the name, their production and actions are not at all limited to the reproductive system.[11] It is believed that the prostaglandins aid fertilization in the following ways: Reacting with the female cervical mucus to make it more receptive to sperm movement and stimulating smooth muscle contraction in both the male and female reproductive tracts and thus enabling the sperm to be transported from their site of storage in the male reproductive tract to the site of fertilization in the female.[13]

Epididymis

The epididymis is essential for normal reproduction as sperm leaving the testes are incapable of fertilizing an ovum. Epididymal secretions are important for some of the changes maturing spermatozoa undergo. Three low molecular weight secretions are present in the epididymis: glycerophosphocholine (GPC), L-carnitine and myo-inositol.[23] The hydrolytic enzyme, α-glucosidase, is the predominant secretion of the epididymis.[23] Epididymal secretions present in seminal fluid vary greatly between fertile men.[24]

Glycerophosphocholine

Glycerophosphocholine (GPC) is synthesized from circulating or luminal proteins, lipoproteins, and possibly from spermatozoa themselves.[25] Jeyendran et al., reported that glycerophosphocholine provides a low prognostic value for *in vitro* fertilization success rates.[26]

L-carnitine

L-carnitine is not synthesized in the epididymis, but rather taken up by the epithelial cells of the epididymis from the circulating blood plasma.[27] L-carnitine plays an essential role in mitochondrial metabolism by controlling the transport of acetyl and acyl groups across the mitochondrial inner membrane[28] and furthermore acts as an antioxidant, protecting spermatozoa against damaged caused by reactive oxygen species. A study done by De Rosa et al. showed a statistically significant correlation between L-carnitine and the functional sperm parameters and could thus be and appropriate marker for sperm and epididymal function.[27]

Myo-inositol

Myo-inositol is both transported and synthesized in the epididymal epithelium. Myo-inositol can be synthesized from glucose in the testis.[29]

Alpha-glucosidase

Alpha-glucosidase is a hydrolytic enzyme, which in its neutral form is the predominant secretary product of the epididymis. Clinically, the absence of this enzyme from the seminal plasma is a sign of distal ductal occlusion in cases of azoospermia.[23] The exact role or function of α-glucosidase is still unknown, although there are some speculations that neutral α-glucosidase are involved in sperm-zona pellucida interaction,[30] and Viljoen et al., showed a significant positive correlation between α-glucosidase activity and human sperm motility.[31]

■ CELLULAR CONTENT

Cellular components in the normal ejaculate include spermatozoa and other cells that are collectively referred to as "round cells". These include epithelial cells from the genitourinary tract, prostate cells, spermatogenic cells and leukocytes. As defined by the World Health Organization (WHO), round cells in a normal ejaculate should not exceed 5×10^6 /mL.[22]

Round Cells

Leukocytes

Leukocytes, predominantly neutrophils, are present throughout the male reproductive tract and are found in most human semen. Leukocyte content in semen, also known as white blood cells, is a classical measurement of semen quality as defined by the WHO.[22] The reference value for leukocytes in the ejaculate, stipulated by the WHO, should not exceed 1×10^6 /mL.[22] Even though white blood cells are present in almost every semen sample, the clinical significance is still unknown.[32] Leukocytospermia, defined by the WHO, as having more than insert 1×10^6 leukocytes per milliliter in the ejaculate, has a 10–20 percent incidence in the general population and is especially common among infertile men.[33] A study done by Tomlinson et al., reported that leukocytes have a role in removing abnormal spermatozoa from the ejaculate[34] and Kiessling et al., found an improvement in sperm motility in semen samples which had leukocyte concentration larger than 2×10^6 per milliliter.[35] Leukocytes are the primary producers of reactive oxygen species, which negatively impacts spermatozoa.[33]

Immature Germ Cells

Immature germ cells are 'round cells' other than leukocytes. These include round spermatids, spermatocytes, spermatogonia, and exfoliated epithelial cells.[22] A study done by Tomlinson et al., showed that excessive immature germ cells usually results from impaired seminiferous tubule function as observed in hypospermatogenesis, varicocele, and Sertoli cell dysfunction.[36] Thus the presence of large numbers of immature germ cells is associated with reduced fertilization ability and may be an indication of an immature sperm population.[36]

Spermatozoa

A male germ cell undergoes a series of modification processes initiated in primary spermatocytes. These processes include: the formation; development and release of spermatids; maturation of spermatozoa within the epididymis; mixing of spermatozoa with seminal fluid secreted by various accessory sex glands; exposure to the female reproductive tract after ejaculation, and finally the penetration of the oocyte.[37] According to the WHO, males should have a minimum of twenty million sperm per ejaculate to be classified as fertile.[22] A male produces approximately one billion sperm for every ovum ovulated by a female. Spermatozoa are produced in the testes during a process called spermatogenesis. Spermatozoa leaving the testes are incapable of fertilizing an ovum, and hence a series of modification steps need to be achieved before these 'immature spermatozoa' can become 'mature spermatozoa'.[37] Sperm maturation in the epididymis is generally postulated to be a 'series of triggers' each capable of initiating cellular changes either at emission or when the spermatozoa are at or near the oocyte. Each trigger has a safety setting to prevent premature occurrence of the event.[37]

Storage of Spermatozoa

The two testes of the human adult can produce up to 120 million sperm each day. Spermatozoa can be stored and maintain their fertility for at least one month after production. Most of the spermatozoa are stored in the vas deferens, but small quantities are also stored in the epididymis.[22] The storage capacity of the epididymis is small and the transport of sperm through it is rapid.[38] Sperm are not held for long periods in the epididymis, and after about 2 weeks of abstinence, sperm will appear in the urine.[39] During the time spermatozoa are stored in the epididymis, they are most likely protected from lipid peroxidation by secretary products of the epididymis such a superoxide dismutase and glutathione peroxidase[40] and damage from leaking acrosomal enzymes by a secreted acrosin inhibitor.[41]

Maturation of Spermatozoa

Sperm maturation occurs in the proximal (caput and corpus) epididymis and is the process whereby spermatozoa gain the ability to fertilize the ova.[23] This process is associated with many physiological, biochemical and morphological changes in the spermatozoa. For spermatozoa to achieve maturational modifications, certain enzymes and lipid proteins are necessary for sperm survival and not available within the cell.[37] The sperm cell has virtually no biosynthetic capabilities, hence the fluid bathing the cells are responsible for the maturation of the spermatozoa.[37] The epididymal epithelium provides the necessary biocatalyst or ions, since the spermatozoa cannot do it themselves. Thus, for maturation to be achieved, secretions of specialized enzymes and transfer proteins are required together with unique interactions between spermatozoa and their surrounding environments, via luminal fluid.[42] How are these modifications accomplished? This task relies on preprogrammed cleavage of integral molecules coupled with the activation of pre-existing switches present in the luminal fluid.[37]

■ REFERENCES

1. Rossato M, Balercia G, Lucarelli G, Foresta C, Mantero F. Role of seminal osmolarity in the reduction of human sperm motility. Int J Androl 2002;25(4):230-5.

2. Owen DH, Katz DF. A review of the physical and chemical properties of human semen and the formulation of a semen stimulant. J Andrology 2005;26:459-69.

3. Dunker N, Aumuller G. Transforming growth factor-beta 2 heterozygous mutant mice exhibit Cowper's gland hyperplasia and cystic dilations of the gland ducts (Cowper's syringoceles). J Anat 2002;201:173-83.

4. Mortimer S. Practical laboratory Andrology. 1st edn. Oxford University Press, New York, 1993.

5. Chughtai B, Sawas A, O'Malley RL, Naik RR, Ali KS, Pentyala S. A neglected gland. A review of Cowper's gland. Int J Androl 2005;28:74-7.

6. Tikva P. Does preejaculatory penile secretions originating from Cowper's gland contain sperm? Journal of Assisted Reproduction and Genetics 2003;20:157-9.

7. Riva A, Usai E, Cossu M, Lantini MS, Scarpa R, Testa-Riva F. Ultrastructure of human bulbourethral glands and of their main excretory ducts. Arch Androl 1990;24:177-84.

8. Honda GD, Bernstein L, Ross RK, Greenland S, Gerkins V, Henderson BE. Vasectomy, cigarette smoking, and age at first sexual intercourse as risk factors for prostate cancer in middle-aged men. Br J Cancer 1988;57:326-31.

9. Wilson FJ, Kestenbaum MG, Gibney JA, Matta S. Histology Image Review. 1st edn. McGraw Hill-Companies, New York, 1997.

10. Pienta KJ, Esper PS. Risk factors for prostate cancer. Ann Intern Med 1993;118:793-803.

11. Sherwood L. Human Physiology from Cells to Systems. 7th edn. Brooks/Cole, Belmont, 2007.

12. Lalani N, Laniado ME, Abel PD. Molecular and cellular biology of prostate cancer. Cancer Metastasis Rev 1997;16: 29-66.

13. Hafez ESE. Techniques of human Andrology. In: Human Reproductive Medicine. Vol 1. North Holland Biomedical Press, Amsterdam, 1977.

14. Ganong WF. Review of Medical Physiology. 10th edn. Lange Medical Publications, Los Altos, 1981.

15. Hara M, Fukuyama T. Some physical-chemical characterizations of gamma seminoprotein, an antigenic component specific for human seminal plasma. Jap J Legal Med 1971; 25:322-4.

16. Hassan MI, Ahmad F. Structural and functional analysis of human prostatic acid phosphatase. Expert Rev Anticancer Ther 2010;10:1055-68.

17. Fouad RK. Male Reproduction Dysfunction: Pathophysiology and Treatment. Informa Healthcare, 2007.

18. Stenman UH, Leinonen J, Zhang WM, Finne P. Prostate-specific antigen. Semin Cancer 1999;9:83-93.

19. Colagara AH, Marzonya ET, Chaichib MJ. Zinc levels in seminal plasma are associated with sperm quality in fertile and infertile men. Nutrition Research 2009;29:82-8.

20. Fair W, Couch J, Wehner N. Prostatic antibacterial factor identity and significance. Urology 1976;7(2):169-77.

21. Heath JW, Young B. Wheater's Functional Histology. 4th edn. Churchill Livingstone, London, 2000.

22. World Health Organization (WHO). WHO Laboratory Manual for the Examination of Human Semen and Sperm-Cervical Mucus Interaction. Cambridge University Press, Cambridge, 1999.

23. Nieschlag E, Behre H. Andrology. Male reproductive Health and Dysfunction. 2nd edn. Springer, Berlin, 2000.

24. Cooper TG, Jockenhovel F, Nieschlag E. Variations in semen parameters from fathers. Hum Reprod 1991;6(6):856-66.

25. Wang CY, Killian G, Chapman DA. Association of [14C] phosphatidycholine with rat epididymal sperm and its conversion to [14C] glycerylphosphorylcholine by sperm and principal cells. Biol Reprod 1981;25(5):969-76.

26. Jeyendran RS, Van der Ven HH, Rosecrans R, Perez-Pelaez M, al-Hasani S, Zaneveld LJ. Chemical constituents of human seminal plasma: relationship to fertility. Andrologia 1989;21(5):423-8.

27. De Rosa M, Boggia B, Amalti B, Zarrillis S, Vita A, Colao A, Lombardi G. Correlation between seminal carnitine and functional spermatozoa characteristics in men with semen dysfunction of various origins. Drugs R D 2005;6(1):1-9.

28. Jeulin C, Lewin LM. Role of free L-carnitine and acetyl-L-carnitine in post-gonadal maturation of mammalian spermatozoa. Hum Reprod Update 1996;2(2):87-102.

29. Eisenberg F. D-myoinositol 1-phosphate as product of cyclization of glucose 6-phosphate and substrate for specific phosphatase in rat testis. J Biol Chem 1967;242(7):1275-1382.

30. Ben Ali H, Guerin JF, Pinatel MC, Mathieu C, Boulieu D, Tritar B. Relationship between semen characteristics, alpha-glucosidase and the capacity of spermatozoa to bind to the human zona pellucida. Int J Androl 1994;17(3):121-6.

31. Viljoen MH, Bornman MS, van de Merwe MP, du Plessis DJ. Alpha-glucosidase activity and sperm motility. Andrologia 1990;22(3):205-8.

32. Moskovtsev SI, Willis J, White J, Mullen JB. Leukocytospermia: relationship to sperm deoxyribonucleic acid integrity in patients evaluated for male factor infertility. Fertility Sterility 2007;88(3):737-40.

33. Lackner JE, Mahfouz R, Du Plessis SS, Schatzl G. The association between leukocytes and sperm quality is concentration dependent. Reproductive Biology and Endocrinology 2010;8:12.

34. Tomlinson MJ, Barratt CL, Cooke ID. Prospective study of leukocytes and leukocyte subpopulations in semen suggests they are not a cause of male infertility. Fertil Steril 1993;60(6):1069-75.

35. Kiessling AA, Lamparelli N, Yin HZ, Seilbel MM, Eyre RC. Semen leukocytes: friends or foes? Fertl Steril 1995;64(1):196-8.

36. Tomlinson MJ, Barratt CL, Bolton AE, Lenton EA, Roberts HB, Cooke ID. Round cells and sperm fertilizing capacity: the presence of immature germ cells but not seminal leukocytes are associated with reduced success of *in vitro* fertilization. Fertil Steril 1992;58(6):1257-9.

37. Amann RP, Hammerstedt RH, Veeramachaneni DN. The epididymis and sperm maturation: a perspective. Reprod Fertil Dev 1993;5(4):361-81.

38. Bedford JM, Cooper GW, Phillips DM, Dryden GL. Distinctive features of the gametes and reproductive tracts of the Asian musk shrew, Suncus murinus. Biol Reprod 1994;50(4):820-34.

39. Barratt CL, Cooke ID. Sperm loss in the urine of sexually rested men. Int J Androl 1988;11(3):201-7.

40. William K, Frayne J, McLaughlin EA, Hall L. Expression of extracellular superoxide dismutase in the human male reproductive tract, detected using antisera raised against a recombinant protein. Mol Hum Reprod 1998;4(3):235-42.

41. Kirchhoff C. Gene expression in the epididymis. Int Rev Cytol 1999;188:133-202.

42. Turner TT. Spermatozoa are exposed to a complex microenvironment as they traverse the epididymis. Ann N Y Acad Sci 1991;637:364-83.

5

Environment and Male Fertility

David Rizk, Stefan du Plessis, Ashok Agarwal

INTRODUCTION

In recent times male infertility and deteriorating semen quality has been an increasingly prevalent issue; researchers point towards changing environmental and lifestyle conditions as arguably the most significant cause of this phenomenon. Environmental and lifestyle exposure to a wide variety of factors may stress the male reproductive system throughout a man's lifespan, from gestation to advanced adult age (**Fig. 5.1**). Ultimately, male infertility may be the result of exposure to any combination of factors such as chemical toxins, smoking, alcohol, diet, exercise, obesity, different types of stress, and the increasing prevalence of cell phone and ionizing radiation.

While spermatogenesis is a function of only mature testes, the effects of maternal or paternal exposure to adverse environmental factors can be projected to the future offspring, resulting in poor semen quality in the male offspring years later. Parental exposure in conjunction with the exposure of the adult offspring can amplify the affects. While adverse environmental effects during adulthood are believed to be reversible, damage done before and up to puberty is considered by many to be irreversible.[1,2]

Despite the lack of conclusive studies tracking effects of the environment and lifestyle of an individual throughout life, there is reason enough to believe that the environment and lifestyle plays a significant role in the quality of male gamete production and thus male fertility as a whole. This argument is evidenced by the fact that over the last 50 years mean sperm counts in the general population have decreased by 50 percent while dramatic environmental and lifestyle changes have occurred during this same period. The expansion of the chemical industry in every facet of modern life in both developed and developing countries is one such major change.[3-5] While there may be arguments that state otherwise, the implications of these issues are significant and warrant increased awareness and the implementation of precautions that may help reverse diminishing male fertility.

MATERNAL AND INFANT EXPOSURE

Not only male infertility can be caused during adulthood, but also it can be a result of maternal and pre-pubertal toxic exposure (**Fig. 5.1**). Sperm production begins during puberty and continues until death. Due to the complexity of germ cell development, proper sperm manufacturing relies on optimal conditions. During this critical period errors in spermatogenesis are more likely than usual when influenced by environmental factors. Spermatogenesis, only occurring in mature testis, can be disrupted either directly in germ cells throughout adulthood, or indirectly via environmental insults; indirect injuries include maternal exposure during pregnancy that affect events preceding gamete production in the offspring. Early damage may impair testicular development in the male fetus as well as during infancy and these impacts may manifest themselves in adulthood.

In all phases until puberty, any environment that affects Sertoli cell proliferation may lead to impaired spermatogenesis and a diminished final number of cells, thus ultimately impacting sperm counts. Disorders such as cryptochidism, hypospadias, and testicular germ cell cancer have a fetal precursor triggered by testicular malformation, which is a result of insults during developmental stages.[6] While it is difficult to study the final outcomes of maternal exposure in humans because of the time span between the discovery of male infertility and maternal exposure, animal models can be helpful. Results from these animal models supported the theory that environmental injuries that occur during development can determine spermatogenesis and fertility in adulthood.[1] A study conducted by Mocarelli et al. concluded that toxin exposure until puberty affected semen quality while adult exposure revealed no effect, thus making early exposure an especially noteworthy issue.[2]

Since hormones regulate fetal development, outside influences on hormone regulation can have dramatic effects. Maternal lifestyle that involves exposure to environmental chemicals with endocrine-disrupting properties, especially anti-androgenic activity, can influence testicular development and spermatogenesis in the adult offspring. Maternal smoking and obesity are two more factors that reduce sperm counts in developing male offspring. Significant sperm count reductions were reported in male offspring whose mothers smoked substantially during pregnancy.[7,8] It is believed that polycyclic aromatic hydrocarbons (PAHs) and other components of cigarette smoke activate the aryl hydrocarbon receptor and antagonize the androgen receptor mediated action. Thus, smoking during pregnancy reduces Sertoli cell number.[9,10] Meanwhile, maternal obesity during pregnancy can theoretically encroach on testicular development via

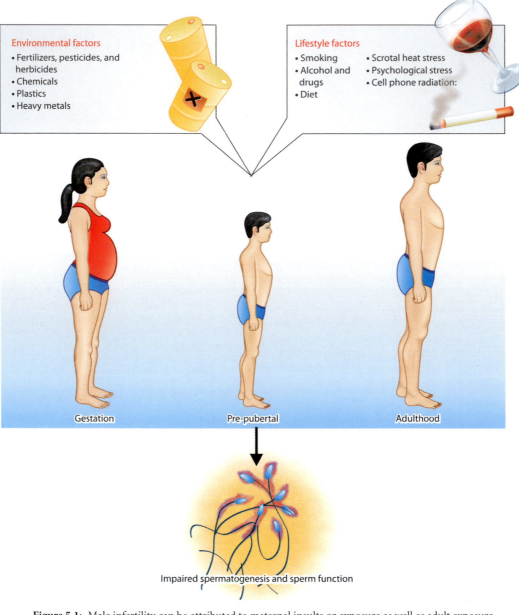

Figure 5.1: Male infertility can be attributed to maternal insults or exposure as well as adult exposure

increased aromatization, thereby disrupting the testosterone/estrogen ratio of the developing fetus. Furthermore, harmful herbicides and pesticides are lipophilic and therefore can accumulate in the fat of obese expecting mothers. During pregnancy and lactation these accumulated compounds can be delivered to the fetus and neonate.[1,11] Maternal diet is yet another area that the environment influences and thus affects the developing fetus. Anabolic steroids can be present in meat consumed by expectant mothers and these steroids have been linked to the reduction of spermatogenesis in the mature testis of the future son.[11]

After gestation damage may still occur. Toxins may still be passed on to an infant via breastfeeding. Also during infancy,

certain types of diapers may cause testicular heat stress. It has been found that disposable plastic lined diapers cause higher scrotal temperatures than reusable cotton diapers. This heat stress may be partially responsible for declining sperm counts.[12,13]

ADULT EXPOSURE

Environmental Effects on Mature Men

The mature human male, unlike females, is capable of reproducing throughout life. In the average fertile male millions of spermatozoa are produced daily until death. Injuries incurred to the reproductive system early on may manifest themselves in the semen produced later. Unfortunately, evaluation of the results of environmental insults on spermatogenesis in human sperm studies is hampered by inconsistencies in biological analytical methods, in controlling factors and study design. Because of the shorter developmental period as well as being less varied in their spermatogenesis profile than humans, animals allow researchers to more clearly observe how external factors influence the reproductive process. It would be exceedingly difficult to isolate one specific environmental factor in the life of an individual who is constantly exposed to a mixture of chemicals and factors, therefore animal testing allows for controlled experiments.

Western lifestyle and worldwide environmental conditions have dramatically changed especially with respect to diet and exercise; dramatic change suggests that these factors may be involved in the etiology of declining male fertility and the impairment of sperm production. It is possible that such change caused this decline in fertility due to its rapid and widespread nature. Several of the following occupational and lifestyle factors to be discussed below are regarded as major areas of concern.

Fertilizers, Pesticides, and Herbicides

With over six and a half billion people populating the world today, food production has been engineered to a large degree. While fertilizers and pesticides have revolutionized food production in recent times, both have also introduced new chemicals and possible toxins to millions. Chemical fertilizers such as nitrogen and ammonia are being extensively used in agriculture today. Nitric oxide has been found to reduce sperm motility, viability, and other semen parameters; it also has been found in some cases to impair the ability of spermatozoa to penetrate the oocyte.[14] Jurewicz suggested that there are consistent indications that pesticides like dichlorodiphenyltrichloroethane, better known as DDT, affect sperm counts in humans.[15] Also, herbicides such as lindane, methoxychlor, and dioxin-TCDD have all been linked with testicular oxidative stress and decreased sperm counts.[16,17] Food preservatives are yet another method for toxins to enter the bloodstream and cause fertility issues. Carbendazim is a systemic broad-spectrum fungicide commonly used on fruit and leather.[18] It has been found to have detrimental effects on male reproduction including decreased mean testicular weight and reduced seminiferous tubule diameters.[19] The vast prevalence of such pesticides, herbicides, and fertilizers utilized by the food industry today is a major fertility concern, one that will be difficult to overcome due to the necessity of large scale production.

Chemicals, Toxins, and Endocrine Active Compounds

Environmental chemicals and toxins have the potential to negatively affect fertility. Some of these chemicals have estrogenic properties and thus are considered toxic because they affect the normal functioning state of the endocrine system. Such compounds can affect LH stimulated Leydig cells which influence androgen secretion and thus interfere with the proper endocrine regulation of spermatogenesis. The ideal ratio of testosterone and estrogen can be shifted as a result of such endocrine disrupters; this can lead to errors in feedback and regulation of the hypothalamus-pituitary-gonadal axis. In addition the pro-oxidant and anti-oxidant system of cells can also be thrown out of harmony. Such a disturbance could lead to the generation of free radicals and Reactive Oxygen Species (ROS). These free radicals could destabilize the electrolytic balance within cells. Spermatozoa are especially susceptible to ROS and lipid peroxidation due to the large amount of polyunsaturated fatty acids found in their membranes. Therefore, chemical toxins that generate ROS in spermatozoa are quite significant.

Chemicals in Plastics

Plastic: The material of modern times. The increasing amount of plastic in contemporary products is a concern because of the toxicity of the chemicals infused to give the products certain desirable qualities. Plasticizers are polyphenolic chemical additives used to enhance the flexibility and toughness of plastic and are found in all clear, heat-resistant and unbreakable plastics. These compounds have been reported to be toxic to the male reproductive system. Another similarly common chemical is Bisphenol A (BPA); it is used to improve polycarbonate plastics and is found in disposable plastic ware, especially in the lids of food containers. BPA from such containers can migrate into food and become circulated in the body.[20,21] It has been estimated that approximately 90 percent of Americans have BPA present in their blood. Since this is such a prevalent chemical that is known to reduce sperm count, motility, and viability, it is a significant environmental threat to male fertility. Chitra reported that BPA generates ROS in various rat tissues including the reproductive organs.[22] BPA was shown to increase hydrogen peroxide levels in testicular tissue. This subsequently leads to the depletion of the antioxidant defense system. Kabuto found that BPA caused an overproduction of hydrogen peroxide in the kidneys, liver, and testes of rats.[23]

Some common plastic products including plastic bags, inflatable recreational toys, blood storage bags, plastic clothing, soaps, and shampoos have phthalate esters in them to improve the flexibility of the plastic. Animal studies concluded that a prevalent phthalate ester commonly used named Di (2-ethyhexyl) phthalate caused testicular atrophy in animals, but the effects on humans is still in question.[24-26]

Yet another commonly found chemical that has been under scrutiny is Nonylphenol. Nonylphenol is a synthetic plastic additive that has estrogenic properties and can accumulate in tissues due to its lipophylic nature. It is often found in detergents, paints, personal care products, food processing, and the packaging industry. Adult exposure to this chemical may reduce sperm counts.

The vast prevalence of such chemicals in numerous facets of daily life is a key concern. Further studies are required to definitively determine the effects of such chemicals, but currently it is believed that these common chemicals and others are harmful to the male reproductive system.

Heavy Metal Toxicity

Several studies reported that heavy metal toxicity in men impaired spermatogenesis and decreased sperm counts.[27-30] Metals such as lead, cadmium, and mercury are three metals of concern while the effects of aluminum and vanadium are being investigated for possible adverse affects on male fertility. Inorganic lead can disturb the pro-oxidant and anti-oxidant balance and cause oxidative stress.[28] Before being banned, lead was found in a variety of common products, the most well known being lead paint; mercury was also found to accumulate in fish, which provides means of over exposure. Like lead, cadmium has been strongly linked to infertility; much higher cadmium levels were found in both the seminal plasma and the blood of infertile men when compared to those of fertile men. A strong negative correlation exists between cadmium and sperm concentrations due to its antisteroidogenic effects that lower testosterone production.[31]

Metal workers and other men who are exposed to such metals through their occupation may be rendered less fertile due to the toxic effects of these metals.

LIFESTYLE EXPOSURE

Exposure to certain lifestyle and occupational factors can influence the adult testis directly and lead to impaired spermatogenesis. A few of the most common issues will be subsequently discussed; often these issues can be avoided by implementing the right precautions.

SMOKING

It is well established that smoking has detrimental effects on spermatogenesis as it has been correlated with significantly lower sperm counts, decreased motility, and impaired morphology.[32-34] Smoking not only interferes with oxygen supply, but also exposes smokers to thousands of potentially harmful substances such as alkaloids, nitrosamines, nicotine, and hydroxycotine to name a few. These substances can lead to the formation of ROS and reactive nitrogen species, which leads to oxidative stress and ultimately infertility.[33-35] Saleh et al. demonstrated that cigarette smoking causes an increase in ROS levels and a decrease in ROS-TAC scores in semen. A 100-fold increase in oxidative stress was observed in the semen of smokers. Cadmium levels were also five times the normal level.[33,35] Furthermore, smokers have decreased levels of seminal plasma antioxidants such as Vitamin C and Vitamin E.[36,37] Besides the numerous other health issues caused by smoking, it has been clearly identified that smoking significantly reduces fertility in men due to the toxins in cigarettes.

ALCOHOL AND DRUGS

There is a growing body of evidence suggesting that alcohol is a lifestyle factor that impacts spermatogenesis. Moderate alcohol consumption has not shown any significant impact on sperm count, however, chronic alcohol consumption appears to harm spermatogenesis and male fertility. Impotence, testicular atrophy, and loss of sexual interest are associated with alcoholism, and reduced FSH, LH, and testosterone levels have been found as a result of excessive drinking.[38] It was also reported that decreased numbers of morphologically normal sperm as well as semen volume were present in alcoholics as apposed to individuals who drank moderately.[39] Alcohol was found to induce oxidative stress; ROS molecules are generated in response to the metabolism of ethanol by the microsomal ethanol-oxidizing system (MEOS).[40,41] Alcohol metabolism results in NADH formation, which enhances activity in the respiratory chain including heightened oxygen use and ROS formation.[42] Tissues are also at increased risk of damage due to the fact that alcohol induces hypoxia.[43]

Like alcohol, certain drugs whether therapeutic, recreational, or performance enhancing can have adverse effects on spermatogenesis. Several prescription drugs used for therapeutic purposes, especially when used chronically, can impact the development of sperm. Antibiotics and chemotherapy can damage germinal epithelium.[44] Many antibacterial drugs (e.g. tetracycline derivatives, sulfa drugs) impair spermatogenesis and chronic use can lead to infertility.[45,46] One especially interesting study showed that men who switched or stopped treatment of the most common medications (allergy relief, antiepileptic, antibiotics) had a 93 percent improvement in semen quality.[46] The class of therapeutic agent used, as well as the dose and duration of the therapy were obviously pertinent factors, but all concluded that these common drugs were contributing in some fashion to infertility whether it was short term reversible infertility or longer lasting.

Concrete evidence for the effect and mechanism of recreational drug abuse such as marijuana and cocaine on sperm production has yet to be found, however, some believe there are links to such drugs and infertility; some studies show endocrine disruption from excessive recreational drug use.[48]

The use of anabolic steroids, predominantly used to enhance body image or improve performance, is on the increase.[47] Steroids often lead to oligozoospermia because they suppress LH secretion and consequently suppress intratesticular testosterone levels. Hypogonadotropic hypogonadism is therefore the most common cause for impairment of sperm production in this group. This damage can be reversed in mature men after a few months of discontinued use.[49] Once again the widespread use of alcohol and such drugs prompt the need for awareness.

DIET AND OBESITY

Diet and obesity are two important lifestyle factors that can influence spermatogenesis. Accompanying modern Westernized lifestyles are changes in diets and eating habits that are a result of a fast paced lifestyle. People are eating more highly refined carbohydrate rich foods and simultaneously consuming less fresh fruits and vegetables. The importance of fresh vegetables in a well balanced diet was noted in a study that decreased subjects' intake of certain nutritional substances, like fruits and vegetables; a correlation between this lack of nutrients and sub fertility was found.[50-53] Besides containing antioxidants and essential nutrients, vitamins and folate are found in fruit and vegetables; these substances are involved in DNA and RNA synthesis and thus play an important role in spermatogenesis by protecting the sperm's DNA from free radical damage.[52]

Nutritionally deficient diets, lacking antioxidant vitamins and synergistic minerals do not enable the quenching of reactive oxygen molecules. For example, vitamin C and vitamin E are essential antioxidants that protect the body's cells from damage due to oxidative stress and free radicals. Vitamin C is the most abundant antioxidant in the semen of fertile men and contributes to the maintenance of healthy sperm by protecting the sperm's DNA from free radical damage.[50-53] Vitamin E is a fat-soluble vitamin that helps protect the sperm's cell membrane from damage. Studies show that vitamin E improves sperm motility and morphology while vitamin C regenerates vitamin E; thereby these vitamins work together to improve sperm function.[50-53] Selenium is a mineral that also functions as an antioxidant; Selenium supplements have also been shown to increase motility. Combinations of these three nutrients have been shown to improve sperm parameters in infertile men.[54]

Obese and overweight individuals with high body mass index (BMI) are at risk of infertility.[55-57] Men with a BMI higher than 25 are considered three times more at risk of infertility due to the reduction in sperm count and increase of DNA fragmentation.

There are many links between obesity and infertility: firstly, excess adipose tissue leads to the conversion of more testosterone to estrogen. This subsequently results in the development of secondary hypogonadism through hypothalamic-pituitary-gonadal axis inhibition, thereby decreasing the levels of circulating testosterone and increasing the levels of estradiol.[58] This decrease in testosterone is most likely responsible for impaired spermatogenesis. Secondly, accumulation of suprapubic and inner thigh fat in severely obese men can lead to infertility due to the insulating effects of fat deposits near the scrotum, which causes testicular heat stress. Fat deposits around scrotal blood vessels can impair blood cooling and elevate temperatures. Obese men also tend to be more sedentary which would exacerbate any temperature increases. Finally, obesity and several of its accompanying complications, namely insulin resistance and dyslipidemia, are associated with systemic proinflammatory states and increased oxidative stress.[59,60] Oxidative stress causes sperm membrane lipid peroxidation, which results in the impairment of sperm motility, DNA damage, and impaired sperm-oocyte interaction.[61,62] Conversely, adipose tissue releases pro-inflammatory adipokines that increase leukocyte production of ROS, which negatively impacts sperm function.[63]

Poor endocrine and exocrine functions of the testis are believed to be directly proportional to increased BMI and obesity in men around the world. Lowering BMI in obese men can be a solution to some infertility issues.

SCROTAL HEAT STRESS

The exteriorization of the male gonads in the scrotum is a uniquely mammalian feature. The most plausible evolutionary explanation is that optimal spermatogenesis requires a temperature approximately 2°C cooler than core body temperature (37°C). It is widely accepted that increased scrotal temperatures impair spermatogenesis. In rats, testicular temperatures elevated via exposure to warm bath water showed deterioration in spermatogenesis.[64]

During puberty the testes descend into the very bottom of the scrotum—as far as possible from the higher temperature of the body's core. Also, counter-current blood exchange evolved to reduce the temperature of blood coming towards the testes and heating the cooled blood returning to the core of the body. Finally, the corrugated scrotal surface is a third mechanism through which heat is dissipated to cool the testes.

The lower temperature leads to reduced rates of oxidative DNA damage and consequently fewer mutations in resulting sperm cells.[65] Sperm are stored in the epididymis for many days or even weeks. Storage occurs specifically in the cauda epididymis, which by no coincidence is the coolest area of the scrotum, thereby reducing metabolic rates and oxidative damage of these spermatozoa.[66]

Scrotal pathologies such as varicocele and cryptorchidism can increase testicular temperature excessively, however, lifestyle and occupation can also lead to chronically elevated scrotal temperatures that can contribute to the global trend in declining male reproductive parameters.[67]

Occupational exposure in certain professions, for example bakers, welders, furnace operators, and professional drivers, has been shown to directly relate to levels of infertility because of the increase in scrotal temperatures, often for extended periods of time. Such workers have been found to have poor semen quality compared to men with similar lifestyles, but who are not exposed to such temperatures during work.[68] Some studies show short lasting infertility or no infertility caused by this type of heat stress, but if there is the possibility it is worth implementing precautions such as cooling breaks for these workers.

Another area of study is the boxers versus briefs dilemma. The tightness of underpants has been determined to cause scrotal heating. Constantly wearing tighter underpants that leads to elevated scrotal temperatures in conjunction with the effects of obesity, sedentary lifestyle, and certain occupations mentioned above compound and exacerbate potential heat stress and infertility. Loose fitting underpants and clothing have been found to keep scrotal temperatures at an optimal compared to the elevating effects of restrictive clothing.[69]

Other lifestyle factors like hot baths, sauna use, and excessive exercise can cause testicular heat stress especially in combination with previously mentioned conditions. Moderate exercise has been found to allow air circulation and thus cooling of the scrotum, but on the other hand extreme exercise may raise temperatures, for example, moderate biking and walking was found to be beneficial, whereas very competitive levels of biking were found to generate heat stress.[70]

Testicular heat stress can be an easily avoidable phenomenon with the implementation of a few simple lifestyle changes. Daily modifications may reduce previous heat stress and allow the return of any lost fertility.

PSYCHOLOGICAL STRESS

One issue that is unfortunately all too prevalent in societies across the globe is mental stress. Not only can it reduce your quality of life, but also impair the quality of your semen. Mental stress is associated with lower levels of antioxidants such as glutathione (GSH) and SOD, as well as higher levels of pro-oxidants, which can create oxidative stress.[71] Various studies have shown correlations between poor semen quality and stress: one study showed that students have lower sperm counts and quality during highly stressful periods of exams.[72] Eskiocak was able to link intervals of psychological stress with a reduction in sperm quality mediated by an increase in seminal plasma ROS generated and a reduction in antioxidant protection. It has also been said that stress can lead to increased levels of glucocorticoids and decreased levels of testosterone.[73]

Numerous individuals struggle with psychological stress each day as a result of work, home life, and a variety of issues. This psychological phenomenon can be an acute stress on reproductive functions and has adverse affects on general health.

CELL PHONE RADIATION

Another health concern is the use of cell phones and the effects of ionizing radiation on male fertility. Since cell phones are constantly being used across the globe and are often placed in the pockets of pants, mere centimeters from the testes, these phones are a very noteworthy topic.

Stopczyk demonstrated that radiofrequency electromagnetic waves (RF-EMW) produced by cell phones significantly deplete SOD-1 activity, thereby increasing the concentration of malonyldialdehyde (MDA) after 1, 5, and 7 minutes of exposure in a suspension of human blood platelets.[74] This team concluded that oxidative stress after exposure to microwaves may be the reason for many adverse changes in cells and could cause a number of systemic disturbances in the human body.

Various epidemiological studies proposed that cell phone usage might cause decreases in sperm count and other sperm parameters.[75,76] A study by Friedman et al. revealed that cell phone radiation could lead to generation of ROS.[77] Results showed a significant increase in ROS production and a decrease in sperm motility, viability, and ROS-TAC score in exposed semen samples. A possible explanation for the production of ROS is the stimulation of the plasma membrane redox system of spermatozoa due to this radiation. Furthermore, the electromagnetic wave-dependent decrease in melatonin can predispose sperm to oxidative stress, which as mentioned results in poor semen quality.[78]

Considerable research is still required to conclude the exact effects of cell phones on male fertility. The close proximity of cell phones to the testes in men is a factor that may increase the risks of radiation. Since cell phones are constantly sending and receiving data regardless of whether they are actually being operated at the time by the owner, men may be constantly exposed to potentially harmful waves that could have negative effects on their reproductive success.

CONCLUSION

The increase in defective spermatogenesis, testicular cancer, cryptorchidism, and numerous other male fertility issues over the course of the past few decades is a great cause of concern and has prompted the investigation of environmental and lifestyle factors that may be responsible. As societies increasingly introduce new chemical and potentially toxic substances into daily life, adverse effects may be amplified from one generation to the next. This is an issue that both developed and developing countries face.

These environmental factors can disrupt endocrine functions eventually leading to fertility problems. Exposure to certain toxins can lead to DNA damage, oxidative stress, and a host of other issues. Whether it occurred during gestation, the pre-pubertal age, or during adulthood, such exposure can affect fertility. The effects of exposure during each period are not fully understood, but information from animal models reveals that exposure itself and exposure at certain times is a topic worth investigating.

While assisted reproductive techniques have advanced in recent years and allows couples to bypass semen quality issues by directly injecting sperm into an egg, this only treats the symptom and not the issue itself. By eliminating or reducing certain environmental or lifestyle factors male fertility as a whole may increase.

REFERENCES

1. Sharpe RM. Environmental/lifestyle effects on spermatogenesis. Philosophical transactions of the Royal Society of London. May 27;365(1546):1697-712.
2. Mocarelli P, Gerthoux PM, Patterson DG, Jr, Milani S, Limonta G, Bertona M, et al. Dioxin exposure, from infancy through puberty, produces endocrine disruption and affects human semen quality. Environmental Health Perspectives 2008;116(1):70-7.
3. Irvine DS. Declining sperm quality: a review of facts and hypotheses. Bailliere's Clinical Obstetrics and Gynecology 1997;11(4):655-71.
4. Andersen HR, Schmidt IM, Grandjean P, Jensen TK, Budtz-Jorgensen E, Kjaerstad MB, et al. Impaired reproductive development in sons of women occupationally exposed to pesticides during pregnancy. Environmental Health Perspectives 2008;116(4):566-72.
5. Swan SH, Liu F, Overstreet JW, Brazil C, Skakkebaek NE. Semen quality of fertile US males in relation to their mothers' beef consumption during pregnancy. Human Reproduction (Oxford, England) 2007;22(6):1497-502.
6. Skakkebaek NE, Rajpert-De Meyts E, Main KM. Testicular dysgenesis syndrome: an increasingly common developmental disorder with environmental aspects. Human Reproduction (Oxford, England) 2001;16(5):972-8.
7. Storgaard L, Bonde JP, Ernst E, Spano M, Andersen CY, Frydenberg M, et al. Does smoking during pregnancy affect sons' sperm counts? Epidemiology (Cambridge, Mass) 2003;14(3):278-86.
8. Jensen MS, Mabeck LM, Toft G, Thulstrup AM, Bonde JP. Lower sperm counts following prenatal tobacco exposure. Human Reproduction (Oxford, England) 2005;20(9):2559-66.
9. Kizu R, Okamura K, Toriba A, Kakishima H, Mizokami A, Burnstein KL, et al. A role of aryl hydrocarbon receptor in the

antiandrogenic effects of polycyclic aromatic hydrocarbons in LNCaP human prostate carcinoma cells. Archives of Toxicology 2003;77(6):335-43.

10. Barnes-Ellerbe S, Knudsen KE, Puga A. 2,3,7,8-Tetrachlorodibenzo-p-dioxin blocks androgen-dependent cell proliferation of LNCaP cells through modulation of pRB phosphorylation. Molecular Pharmacology 2004;66(3):502-11.

11. Ramlau-Hansen CH, Nohr EA, Thulstrup AM, Bonde JP, Storgaard L, Olsen J. Is maternal obesity related to semen quality in the male offspring? A pilot study. Human Reproduction (Oxford, England) 2007;22(10):2758-62.

12. Toppari J, Larsen JC, Christiansen P, Giwercman A, Grandjean P, Guillette LJ, Jr., et al. Male reproductive health and environmental xenoestrogens. Environmental Health Perspectives 1996;104(Suppl)4:741-803.

13. Hughes PI. How vulnerable is the developing testis to the external environment? Archives of Disease in Childhood 2000;83(4):281-2.

14. Wu TP, Huang BM, Tsai HC, Lui MC, Liu MY. Effects of nitric oxide on human spermatozoa activity, fertilization and mouse embryonic development. Archives of Andrology 2004;50(3):173-9.

15. Jurewicz J, Hanke W, Radwan M, Bonde JP. Environmental factors and semen quality. International Journal of Occupational Medicine and Environmental Health 2009;22(4):305-29.

16. Chitra KC, Sujatha R, Latchoumycandane C, Mathur PP. Effect of lindane on antioxidant enzymes in epididymis and epididymal sperm of adult rats. Asian Journal of Andrology 2001;3(3):205-8.

17. Latchoumycandane C, Mathur PP. Induction of oxidative stress in the rat testis after short-term exposure to the organochlorine pesticide methoxychlor. Archives of Toxicology 2002;76(12):692-8.

18. Selmanoglu G, Barlas N, Songur S, Kockaya EA. Carbendazim-induced haematological, biochemical and histopathological changes to the liver and kidney of male rats. Human and experiMental Toxicology 2001;20(12):625-30.

19. Carter SD, Hess RA, Laskey JW. The fungicide methyl 2-benzimidazole carbamate causes infertility in male Sprague-Dawley rats. Biology of Reproduction 1987;37(3):709-17.

20. Korasli D, Ziraman F, Ozyurt P, Cehreli SB. Microleakage of self-etch primer/adhesives in endodontically treated teeth. Journal of the American Dental Association (1939). 2007;138(5):634-40.

21. Le HH, Carlson EM, Chua JP, Belcher SM. Bisphenol A is released from polycarbonate drinking bottles and mimics the neurotoxic actions of estrogen in developing cerebellar neurons. Toxicology Letters 2008;176(2):149-56.

22. Chitra KC, Latchoumycandane C, Mathur PP. Induction of oxidative stress by bisphenol A in the epididymal sperm of rats. Toxicology 2003;185(1-2):119-27.

23. Kabuto H, Amakawa M, Shishibori T. Exposure to bisphenol A during embryonic/fetal life and infancy increases oxidative injury and causes underdevelopment of the brain and testis in mice. Life Sciences 2004;74(24):2931-40.

24. Gesler RM. Toxicology of di-2-ethylhexyl phthalate and other phthalic acid ester plasticizers. Environmental Health Perspectives 1973;3:73-9.

25. Ishihara M, Itoh M, Miyamoto K, Suna S, Takeuchi Y, Takenaka I, et al. Spermatogenic disturbance induced by di-(2-ethylhexyl) phthalate is significantly prevented by treatment with antioxidant vitamins in the rat. International Journal of Andrology 2000;23(2):85-94.

26. Peakall DB. Phthalate esters: Occurrence and biological effects. Residue Reviews 1975;54:1-41.

27. Acharya UR, Acharya S, Mishra M. Lead acetate induced cytotoxicity in male germinal cells of Swiss mice. Industrial health 2003;41(3):291-4.

28. Hsu PC, Guo YL. Antioxidant nutrients and lead toxicity. Toxicology 2002;180(1):33-44.

29. Naha N, Chowdhury AR. Inorganic lead exposure in battery and paint factory: effect on human sperm structure and functional activity. Journal of UOEH 2006;28(2):157-71.

30. Xu DX, Shen HM, Zhu QX, Chua L, Wang QN, Chia SE, et al. The associations among semen quality, oxidative DNA damage in human spermatozoa and concentrations of cadmium, lead and selenium in seminal plasma. Mutation Research 2003;534(1-2):155-63.

31. Benoff S, Auborn K, Marmar JL, Hurley IR. Link between low-dose environmentally relevant cadmium exposures and asthenozoospermia in a rat model. Fertility and Sterility 2008;89(2 Suppl):e73-9.

32. Kunzle R, Mueller MD, Hanggi W, Birkhauser MH, Drescher H, Bersinger NA. Semen quality of male smokers and nonsmokers in infertile couples. Fertility and Sterility 2003;79(2):287-91.

33. Saleh RA, Agarwal A, Sharma RK, Nelson DR, Thomas AJ Jr. Effect of cigarette smoking on levels of seminal oxidative stress in infertile men: a prospective study. Fertility and Sterility 2002;78(3):491-9.

34. Vine MF, Tse CK, Hu P, Truong KY. Cigarette smoking and semen quality. Fertility and Sterility 1996;65(4):835-42.

35. Saleh RA, Agarwal A. Oxidative stress and male infertility: from research bench to clinical practice. Journal of Andrology 2002;23(6):737-52.

36. Mostafa T, Anis TH, El-Nashar A, Imam H, Othman IA. Varicocelectomy reduces reactive oxygen species levels and increases antioxidant activity of seminal plasma from infertile men with varicocele. International Journal of Andrology 2001;24(5):261-5.

37. Fraga CG, Motchnik PA, Wyrobek AJ, Rempel DM, Ames BN. Smoking and low antioxidant levels increase oxidative damage to sperm DNA. Mutation Research 1996;351(2):199-203.

38. Boyden TW, Pamenter RW. Effects of ethanol on the male hypothalamic-pituitary-gonadal axis. Endocrine Reviews 1983;4(4):389-95.

39. Goverde HJ, Dekker HS, Janssen HJ, Bastiaans BA, Rolland R, Zielhuis GA. Semen quality and frequency of smoking and alcohol consumption—an explorative study. International Journal of Fertility and Menopausal Studies 1995;40(3):135-8.

40. Dahchour A, Lallemand F, Ward RJ, De Witte P. Production of reactive oxygen species following acute ethanol or acetaldehyde and its reduction by acamprosate in chronically alcoholized rats. European Journal of Pharmacology 2005;520(1-3):51-8.

41. Lieber CS. The discovery of the microsomal ethanol oxidizing system and its physiologic and pathologic role. Drug Metabolism Reviews 2004;36(3-4):511-29.

42. Agarwal A, Prabakaran SA. Mechanism, measurement, and prevention of oxidative stress in male reproductive physiology. Indian Journal of Experimental Biology 2005;43(11):963-74.

43. Wiseman H, Halliwell B. Damage to DNA by reactive oxygen and nitrogen species: role in inflammatory disease and progression to cancer. The Biochemical Journal 1996;313 (Pt 1):17-29.

44. Shalet SM. Effects of cancer chemotherapy on gonadal function of patients. Cancer Treatment Reviews 1980;7(3):141-52.

45. Schlegel PN, Chang TS, Marshall FF. Antibiotics: potential hazards to male fertility. Fertility and Sterility 1991;55(2):235-42.

46. O'Morain C, Smethurst P, Dore CJ, Levi AJ. Reversible male infertility due to sulphasalazine: studies in man and rat. Gut 1984;25(10):1078-84.

47. Sikka SC, Wang R. Endocrine disruptors and estrogenic effects on male reproductive axis. Asian Journal of Andrology 2008;10(1):134-45.

48. Fronczak CM, Kim ED, Barqawi AB. The Insults of Recreational Drug Abuse on Male Fertility. Journal of Andrology, 2011.

49. Knuth UA, Maniera H, Nieschlag E. Anabolic steroids and semen parameters in bodybuilders. Fertility and Sterility 1989;52(6):1041-7.

50. Eskenazi B, Kidd SA, Marks AR, Sloter E, Block G, Wyrobek AJ. Antioxidant intake is associated with semen quality in healthy men. Human reproduction (Oxford, England) 2005;20(4):1006-12.

51. Fraga CG, Motchnik PA, Shigenaga MK, Helbock HJ, Jacob RA, Ames BN. Ascorbic acid protects against endogenous oxidative DNA damage in human sperm. Proceedings of the National Academy of Sciences of the United States of America 1991;88(24):11003-6.

52. Song GJ, Norkus EP, Lewis V. Relationship between seminal ascorbic acid and sperm DNA integrity in infertile men. International Journal of Andrology 2006;29(6):569-75.

53. Therond P, Auger J, Legrand A, Jouannet P. alpha-Tocopherol in human spermatozoa and seminal plasma: relationships with motility, antioxidant enzymes and leukocytes. Molecular Human Reproduction 1996;2(10):739-44.

54. Hawkes WC, Turek PJ. Effects of dietary selenium on sperm motility in healthy men. Journal of Andrology 2001;22(5):764-72.

55. Koloszar S, Fejes I, Zavaczki Z, Daru J, Szollosi J, Pal A. Effect of body weight on sperm concentration in normozoospermic males. Archives of Andrology 2005;51(4):299-304.

56. Kort HI, Massey JB, Elsner CW, Mitchell-Leef D, Shapiro DB, Witt MA, et al. Impact of body mass index values on sperm quantity and quality. Journal of Andrology 2006;27(3):450-2.

57. Nguyen RH, Wilcox AJ, Skjaerven R, Baird DD. Men's body mass index and infertility. Human Reproduction (Oxford, England) 2007;22(9):2488-93.

58. Fejes I, Koloszar S, Zavaczki Z, Daru J, Szollosi J, Pal A. Effect of body weight on testosterone/estradiol ratio in oligozoospermic patients. Archives of Andrology 2006;52(2):97-102.

59. Dandona P, Aljada A, Chaudhuri A, Mohanty P, Garg R. Metabolic syndrome: a comprehensive perspective based on interactions between obesity, diabetes, and inflammation. Circulation 2005;111(11):1448-54.

60. Davi G, Falco A. Oxidant stress, inflammation and atherogenesis. Lupus 2005;14(9):760-4.

61. Kodama H, Yamaguchi R, Fukuda J, Kasai H, Tanaka T. Increased oxidative deoxyribonucleic acid damage in the spermatozoa of infertile male patients. Fertility and Sterility 1997;68(3):519-24.

62. Twigg J, Fulton N, Gomez E, Irvine DS, Aitken RJ. Analysis of the impact of intracellular reactive oxygen species generation on the structural and functional integrity of human spermatozoa: lipid peroxidation, DNA fragmentation and effectiveness of antioxidants. Human reproduction (Oxford, England) 1998;13(6):1429-36.

63. Singer G, Granger DN. Inflammatory responses underlying the microvascular dysfunction associated with obesity and insulin resistance. Microcirculation 2007;14(4-5):375-87.

64. Jung A, Schuppe HC. Influence of genital heat stress on semen quality in humans. Andrologia 2007;39(6):203-15.

65. Werdelin L, Nilsonne A. The evolution of the scrotum and testicular descent in mammals: a phylogenetic view. Journal of Theoretical Biology 1999;196(1):61-72.

66. Bedford JM. Anatomical evidence for the epididymis as the prime mover in the evolution of the scrotum. The American Journal of Anatomy 1978;152(4):483-507.

67. Ivell R. Lifestyle impact and the biology of the human scrotum. Reprod Biol Endocrinol 2007;5:15.

68. Thonneau P, Bujan L, Multigner L, Mieusset R. Occupational heat exposure and male fertility: a review. Human Reproduction (Oxford, England) 1998;13(8):2122-5.

69. Jung A, Leonhardt F, Schill WB, Schuppe HC. Influence of the type of undertrousers and physical activity on scrotal temperature. Human Reproduction (Oxford, England) 2005;20(4):1022-7.

70. Jung A, Schuppe HC. Influence of genital heat stress on semen quality in humans. Andrologia 2007;39(6):203-15.

71. Eskiocak S, Gozen AS, Kilic AS, Molla S. Association between mental stress and some antioxidant enzymes of seminal plasma. The Indian Journal of Medical Research 2005;122(6):491-6.

72. Eskiocak S, Gozen AS, Yapar SB, Tavas F, Kilic AS, Eskiocak M. Glutathione and free sulphydryl content of seminal plasma in healthy medical students during and after exam stress. Human Reproduction (Oxford, England) 2005;20(9):2595-600.

73. Eskiocak S, Gozen AS, Taskiran A, Kilic AS, Eskiocak M, Gulen S. Effect of psychological stress on the L-arginine-nitric oxide pathway and semen quality. Brazilian journal of medical and biological research = Revista brasileira de pesquisas medicas e biologicas/Sociedade Brasileira de Biofisica et al 2006;39(5):581-8.

74. Stopczyk D, Gnitecki W, Buczynski A, Kowalski W, Buczynska M, Kroc A. Effect of electromagnetic field produced by mobile phones on the activity of superoxide dismutase (SOD-1)- in vitro researches. Annales Academiae Medicae Stetinensis 2005;51(Suppl)1:125-8.

75. Agarwal A, Desai NR, Makker K, Varghese A, Mouradi R, Sabanegh E, et al. Effects of radiofrequency electromagnetic waves (RF-EMW) from cellular phones on human ejaculated semen: an in vitro pilot study. Fertility and Sterility, 2008.

76. Deepinder F, Makker K, Agarwal A. Cell phones and male infertility: dissecting the relationship. Reproductive Biomedicine Online 2007;15(3):266-70.

77. Friedman J, Kraus S, Hauptman Y, Schiff Y, Seger R. Mechanism of short-term ERK activation by electromagnetic fields at mobile phone frequencies. The Biochemical Journal 2007;405(3):559-68.

78. Burch JB, Reif JS, Yost MG, Keefe TJ, Pitrat CA. Nocturnal excretion of a urinary melatonin metabolite among electric utility workers. Scandinavian journal of work, environment and health 1998;24(3):183-9.

Section II

Diagnostic Evaluation

6

Male Infertility: When and How to Start the Evaluation?

Sandro C Esteves, Ricardo Miyaoka

INTRODUCTION

In the last decades extraordinary advances have been achieved in the field of assisted reproduction technology (ART). Specifically in the male infertility field, significant progress has been made regarding both diagnostic and treatment techniques. Novel genetic tests made it possible to correctly classify cases of nonobstructive azoospermia previously believed to be idiopathic. Microsurgery has allowed for increasing success rates in reproductive tract reconstruction and sperm retrieval either from the testicle or the epididymis. With the advent of gamete micromanipulation previously infertile men with severe oligozoospermia or azoospermia were given the chance to father children of their own.

Infertility is a common scenario at the urologist's office and the procurement for specialized centers is increasingly rising in the latest years. Currently, approximately 8 percent of men within reproductive age seek medical attention for infertility issues. Of these, 1–10 percent presents a treatable cause affecting their fertility potential. Varicocele represents 35 percent of these cases.[1] Therefore, the evaluation of the male partner must be incorporated systematically in every infertile couple assessment.

Around 80 percent of couples are able to achieve pregnancy within the first year of attempt. A couple should only be diagnosed as infertile after one year of regular sexual activity without using any contraceptive method. Traditionally, investigation starts at this point. However, longer infertility duration periods are related to smaller chances of success, regardless of the treatment strategy adopted. As such, it is recommended that investigation is initiated earlier whenever risk factors are present including advanced maternal (>35 years) or paternal age (>45 years), history of urogenital surgery, cancer, cryptorchidism, varicocele, orchitis, use of gonadotoxins, genital infections, among others.

From a couple's perspective, infertility is classified as primary when no pregnancy has ever been achieved up to the moment of the medical evaluation; and secondary when a pregnancy has been achieved at least once.

The role of the urologist in the management of the subfertile male cannot be underestimated. He/she is responsible for diagnosing, counseling and treating whenever possible the existing cause. When no specific treatment is available the urologist is still responsible to refer the patient to a specialized ART center or for extracting the male gamete from the testicle or epididymis as a member of the ART center's multi-professional team.

EPIDEMIOLOGY

For healthy young couples, the probability of achieving pregnancy per reproductive cycle is about 20–25 percent. The cumulative probabilities of conception are 60 percent within the first 6 months, 84 percent within the first year and 92 percent within the second year of fertility-focused sexual activity.[2]

Infertility is a common clinical problem and affects 13–15 percent of couples worldwide.[3] The prevalence varies throughout developed and underdeveloped countries being higher in the latter where limited resources for diagnosis and treatment exist.[4] In the United Kingdom, infertility is believed to reach one in six couples.[5] According to Kamel, it should be regarded as a public problem, as it affects not only the health care system but also the social environment. The infertile couple faces feelings such as depression, grief, guilt, shame and inadequacy with social isolation.[2]

PHYSIOPATHOLOGY

The reproductive male system is composed of the testicles and seminiferous tubules, efferent ducts and rete testis, epididymis, deferent ducts, ejaculatory ducts, seminal vesicles, prostate and accessory glands, penis and urethra (**Fig. 6.1**). The testicles are responsible for producing the gametes (spermatozoa) within the seminiferous tubules and sexual hormones (testosterone and androstenedione) in the interstitial cells. Recent data suggests that the duration of spermatogenesis is less than 60 days, instead of 70 ± 4 days as previously thought for over 40 years.[6] As such, seminal parameters of an individual actually represent the result of influencing biological, physical and occupational factors which acted within the past 2 months from the semen collection. Daily sperm production is about 40 million and declines progressively with aging. Spermatogenesis hormonal control involves the hypothalamus gonadotropin releasing hormone (GnRH), anterior pituitary gland (gonadotropins—FSH and LH), and testicles (testosterone and inhibin). Storage and maturation of spermatozoa occur in the epididymis. This process is, however,

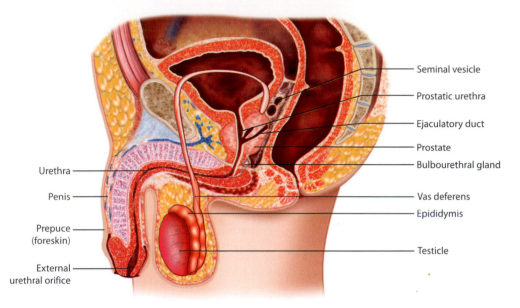

Figure 6.1: Male reproductive tract structures

only fully completed within the female reproductive tract. Spermatozoa transit throughout the epididymis is about 12 days long. The epididymides are in continuity with the vasa deferentia which in turn join the emerging ducts from the seminal vesicles to form the ejaculatory ducts. They enter the prostate, a gland responsible for producing a fluid enriched with zinc, citric acid, acid phosphatase and proteases that assure liquefaction and that accounts for approximately 0.5 mL of the ejaculate. The seminal vesicles produce an line fluid with prostaglandins and fructose that composes 1.5–2.0 mL of the seminal fluid. Both the seminal vesicles and vas deferens have a common embryologic origin. As such, when congenital bilateral absence of vas deferens (CBAVD) is diagnosed it is associated with seminal vesicles hypoplasia/ agenesia. This is an important aspect of the differential diagnosis of azoospermia. In CBAVD, no fructose can be found in the seminal fluid and the ejaculate volume is low. Under normal conditions, spermatozoa are not stored in the seminal vesicles but in the epididymides. At the time of ejaculation, ductal and epididymal muscle contractions under sympathetic stimulation conduct the spermatozoa towards the prostatic urethra where they join fluids excreted by both the prostate and seminal vesicles to form the semen. Periurethral muscle contraction is responsible to expel semen out. Interference in any of these steps may lead to male infertility. Herein, the physiopathological mechanism involved is dependent on which organ or regulatory system is afflicted.

ETIOLOGY

Any process negatively impacting sperm production and sperm quality is potentially harmful to male fertility. We can didactically outline the major causes for male infertility according to their prevalence: varicocele, obstruction, testicular failure, cryptorchidism, idiopathic, gonadotoxin exposure, genetic, infectious, hormonal dysfunction, immunological, ejaculatory/ sexual dysfunction, cancer and systemic diseases. In a group of 2,383 male infertility patients attending our tertiary center for male reproduction, potentially surgically or medically correctable conditions were identified in 48.4 percent of the individuals. The other half comprised candidates for assisted reproduction, particularly assisted reproductive technologies (ART) involving *in vitro* fertilization (IVF) coupled to intracytoplasmic sperm injection (ICSI) (**Table 6.1**).

CLINICAL PRESENTATION

The typical clinical presentation is an infertile couple within reproductive age that is sexually active and does not use any contraceptive methods but is unable to achieve pregnancy whatsoever. In general, the female partner is evaluated by a gynecologist who orders a semen analysis for the male. If the semen analysis results are abnormal then male infertility is suspected.

DIFFERENTIAL DIAGNOSIS

In approximately 1 percent of cases, male infertility may be the clinical presentation of a more serious and potentially fatal disease such as testicular cancer, brain cancer, medullary spinal cancer, endocrinopathies, genitourinary malformation, systemic disease and genetic syndromes.[7,8] Testicular cancer is about 50 times more prevalent in infertile men than in those not affected by this condition.[9] It is important for the urologist to keep in mind that infertility may be solely the initial manifestation of a more severe medical condition.

Table 6.1: Distribution of diagnostic categories in a group of infertile men attending a male infertility clinic

Category	N	Percentage (%)
Varicocele	629	26.4
Infectious	72	3.0
Hormonal	54	2.3
Ejaculatory dysfunction	28	1.2
Systemic diseases	11	0.4
Idiopathic	289	12.1
Immunologic	54	2.3
Obstruction	359	15.1
Cancer	11	0.5
Cryptorchidism	342	14.3
Genetic	189	7.9
Testicular failure	345	14.5
TOTAL	2,383	100.0

Source: Androfert, Center for Male Reproduction, Campinas, Brazil

■ CLINICAL ASSESSMENT

Initial Workup

Medical History

A thorough medical history must be inquired on any factor that may impact the fertility potential. Information should be collected regarding: prior fertility, previous diseases during childhood and puberty such as viral orchitis and cryptorchidism; surgeries performed, especially those involving the pelvic and inguinal regions and genitalia; genital traumas; infections such as epididymitis and urethritis; physical and sexual development; social and sexual habits; exposure to gonadotoxic agents such as radiotherapy or chemotherapy, recent fevers or heat exposures, and current or recent medications; family history of birth defects, mental retardation, reproductive failure or cystic fibrosis. In **Table 6.2** we present a summary of what should be considered when assessing the infertile male.

Physical Examination

Physical examination should evaluate appropriate sexual development, body habitus, pattern of hair distribution, gynecomastia.

Table 6.2: Clinical male infertility history

Infertility history	Age of partners, time attempting to conceive Contraceptive methods/duration Previous pregnancy (actual partner/other partner) Previous treatments Current treatments/evaluation of female partner
Sexual history	Potency, libido, lubricant use Ejaculation, timed intercourse, frequency of masturbation
Childhood and development	Cryptorchidism, hernia, testicular trauma Testicular torsion, infection (e.g. mumps orchitis) Sexual development, puberty onset
Personal history	Systemic diseases (diabetes, cirrhosis, hypertension) Sexually transmitted diseases, tuberculosis, viral infections
Previous surgeries	Orchidopexy, herniorraphy, orchiectomy (testicular cancer, torsion) Retroperitoneal and pelvic surgery Other inguinal, scrotal and perineal surgery Bariatric surgery, bladder neck surgery, transurethral resection of the prostate
Gonadotoxin exposure	Pesticides, alcohol, cocaine, marijuana abuse Medication (chemotherapy agents, cimetidine, sulfasalazine, nitrofurantoin, allopurinol, colchicine, thiazide, β-and α-blockers, calcium-channel blockers, finasteride) Organic solvents, heavy metals Anabolic steroids, tobacco use High temperatures, electromagnetic energy Radiation (therapeutic, nuclear power plant workers),etc.
Family history	Cystic fibrosis, endocrine diseases Infertility in the family
Current health status	Respiratory infection, anosmia Galactorrhea, visual disturbances Obesity

In the presence of diminished corporal hair distribution, gynecomastia or eunuchoid proportions inadequate virilization must be suspected as a consequence of androgen deficiency. In this case, delayed maturation and endocrine abnormalities are to be ruled out.

Genital examination can reveal the presence of a hypospadic urethral meatus, pathologic curvature of the phallus or even an active sexually transmitted disease. These factors may ultimately result in misplacement of spermatozoa inside the vaginal vault following ejaculation.

Testicular volume can be estimated with the aid of an orchidometer or be measured using a pachymeter (**Fig. 6.2A**). A normal sized adult testicle should have a 4 cm length and a 2.5 cm width resulting in a volume around 20 mL. They should present firm consistency. Eighty-five percent of the testicular parenchyma is involved with spermatogenesis. There is no lower limit for testicular volume to exclude the presence of spermatozoa. As such, testicle size cannot be relied on as a clinical marker to preclude a trial of sperm retrieval.[10]

Bilateral testicular atrophy may be caused by primary or secondary testicular failure. When serum testosterone is low seminal fluid is often of small volume as well. Endocrine workup helps to distinguish both conditions. High FSH levels accompanied by normal or low testosterone levels imply primary testicular failure. These patients should be offered genetic evaluation for chromosomal abnormalities and Y-chromosome microdeletions. Low serum FSH levels and testosterone levels combined suggest hypogonadotropic hypogonadism especially if bilateral atrophic testicles are present. In this scenario, serum LH is also often low. These men should undergo cranial imaging and serum prolactin measurement to exclude pituitary gland disease as in Kallmann syndrome.[11]

The epididymides have to be evaluated according to their size and consistency as well. The obstructed epididymis is enlarged and soft. A healthy epididymis free of trauma, infection or obstruction should be firm. Partial depletion of an epididymis may represent a scenario of CBAVD. The vasa are easily palpable inside the posterior aspect of the spermatic cord as a distinct, firm, round, 'spaghetti-like' structure. Unilateral or bilateral congenital absence of the vas result in oligozoospermia or azoospermia, respectively. Narrow areas of the vasa deferentia may represent an infection sequelae or a traumatic one.

Absence of the vasa deferentia or vasal agenesis is a clinical diagnosis and does not depend on any complementary imaging study. However, 25 percent of men with unilateral vasal agenesis and about 10 percent of those with CBAVD also have unilateral renal agenesis and should undergo an abdominal ultrasonography to identify this condition.[12]

Each spermatic cord has to be inspected to assess volume and consistency and to detect existing lipomas or varicocele.

Physical examination is the method of choice for the diagnosis of varicocele and should be performed with the patient

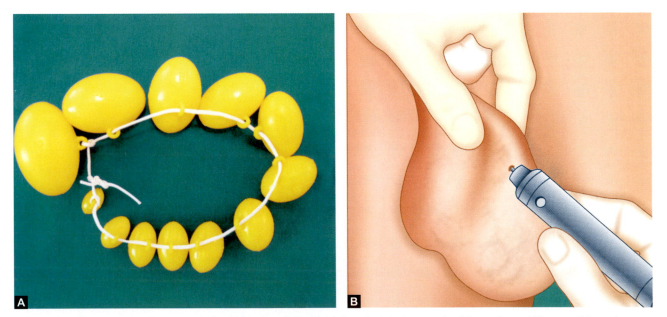

Figures 6.2A and B: Useful tools for the physical examination of the subfertile male: (A) Photograph of the prader orchidometer. It is used to measure the volume of the testicles and consists of a chain of 12 numbered beads of increasing size from 1 to 25 mL. The beads are compared with the testicles of the patient and the volume is read off the bead which matches most closely in size. Pre-pubertal sizes are 1 to 3 mL, pubertal sizes are 4 to 12 mL and adult sizes are 15 to 25 mL; (B) Schematic illustration depicting the use of the 9 Mhz pencil-probe Doppler stethoscope for varicocele examination. The patient is examined in the upright position and the conducting gel is applied at the upper aspect of scrotum. A venous 'rush' may be listened during Valsalva maneuver indicating blood reflux. Reproduced with permission from Clinics (Sao Paulo). 2011 April; 66(4): 691-700. Copyright © 2011 Hospital das Clínicas da FMUSP. Esteves SC, Miyaoka R, Agarwal A: An update on the clinical assessment of the infertile male.

standing in a warm room.[13] It provides a sensitivity and specificity of approximately 70 percent.[14] Varicoceles diagnosed by this method are termed "clinical" and may be graded according to their size. Valsalva maneuver may reveal differences in blood volume in each cord. Spermatic internal veins and cremasteric veins are filled up whenever the patient stands. In varicocele patients a venous dilation exists and may be enhanced during Valsalva maneuver. Large varicoceles (grade III) are varicose veins seen through the scrotal skin (**Fig. 6.3**). Moderate (grade II) and small-sized varicoceles (grade I) are dilated veins palpable without and with the aid of the Valsalva maneuver, respectively.[15] No standardized diagnostic method has been defined for the identification of varicocele.[16]

Inguinal and genital regions must be carefully examined in order to identify scars from previous surgical interventions such as hydrocele correction and inguinal hernia repairs. They may account for damage to the testicular blood supply and to the vas deferens.

Digital rectal exam should account for any palpable masses including prostatic cysts.

Semen Analysis

The semen analysis is the cornerstone of the laboratorial evaluation, although it is not a sperm function test.[17] It provides

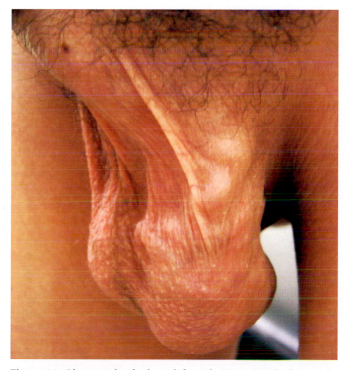

Figure 6.3: Photograph of a large left grade III varicocele that can be seen through the scrotal skin. Reproduced with permission from Clinics (Sao Paulo). 2011 April; 66(4): 691-700. Copyright © 2011 Hospital das Clínicas da FMUSP. Esteves SC, Miyaoka R, Agarwal A: An update on the clinical assessment of the infertile male.

information on the functional status of the seminiferous tubules, epididymides and accessory sexual glands. Semen analysis is of great value on the male initial investigation and its results are often taken as surrogate measures of male fecundity and pregnancy risk. Reference intervals for semen parameter values from a fertile population may provide data from which prognosis of fertility or diagnosis of infertility can be extrapolated. Therefore, it is recommended that evaluation should be undertaken in a specialized andrology laboratory and analyzed by well trained technicians under rigorous quality control standards.[18] Nonetheless, the prognostic value of semen components such as sperm number, motility and morphology, as surrogate markers of male fertility, is confounded in several ways; the fertility potential of a man is influenced by sexual activity, the function of accessory sex glands and other, defined as well as yet unrecognized, conditions. Routine semen analysis itself has its own limitations, and does not account for putative sperm dysfunctions such as immature chromatin or a fragmented DNA. Results from at least two, preferably three, separate semen analyses must be obtained before a definitive conclusion can be drawn as wide biological variability may exist within the same individual. The interval between the analyses is arbitrary and is generally recommended to be 1–2 weeks. Ejaculatory abstinence should be a minimum of 2 days to a maximum of 5 days, ideally 2–3 days.[19] Longer abstinence periods lead to higher ejaculatory volumes and increased spermatozoa quantity but motility is usually decreased. The specimen is generally collected by masturbation inside a sterile cuntainer with a wide opening in order to avoid spillage outside the container which can be misinterpreted as hypospermia. Collection should be preferentially done in a proper collection room and no lubricant should be used. If collected at home, the specimen should be brought to the lab within 30 minutes and kept close to the body in an effort to maintain physiological temperature during transportation. The specimen must be identified and allowed to liquefy for 30–60 minutes before analysis is undertaken. Routine seminal analysis should include:

- Physical characteristics of semen, including liquefaction, viscosity, pH, color and odor
- Specimen volume
- Sperm count
- Sperm motility and progression
- Sperm morphology
- Leukocyte quantification
- Fructose detection in cases where no spermatozoa is found especially if total volume is less than 1 mL.

The criteria used for normality according to the World Health Organization (WHO) have recently been updated,[19] as shown in **Table 6.3**. Approximately 2,000 men from eight countries whose partners had a time-to-pregnancy of ≤ 12 months were chosen as individuals to provide reference distributions for semen parameters. One-sided lower reference limits (the fifth centile) were generated and have been proposed to be considered the lower cutoff limits for normality (**Table 6.3**). Apart from total sperm number per ejaculate, the lower limits of these distributions are lower than the previously presented 'normal' or 'reference' values[20-22] but are in agreement with recent observations.[23-25]

Table 6.3: Cut-off values for semen parameters as published in consecutive WHO manuals

Semen parameters	WHO, 1992	WHO, 1999	WHO, 2010*
Volume	$\geq$ 2 mL	$\geq$ 2 mL	1.5 mL
Sperm concentration/mL	$\geq 20 \times 10^6$/mL	$\geq 20 \times 10^6$/mL	15×10^6/mL
Total sperm concentration	$\geq 40 \times 10^6$	$\geq 40 \times 10^6$	39×10^6
Total motility (% motile)	$\geq$ 50%	$\geq$ 50%	40%
Progressive Motility**	$\geq$ 25% (grade a)	$\geq$ 25% (grade a)	32% (a + b)
Vitality (% alive)	$\geq$ 75%	$\geq$ 75%	58%
Morphology	$\geq$ 30%#	(14%)##	4%$
Leukocyte count	$< 1.0 \times 10^6$/mL	$< 1.0 \times 10^6$/mL	$< 1.0 \times 10^6$/mL

*Lower reference limit obtained from the lower fifth centile value.
**Grade a = rapid progressive motility (> 25 μm/s); grade b = slow/sluggish progressive motility (5-25 μm/s); Normal = 50% motility (grades a + b) or 25% progressive motility (grade a) within 60 min of ejaculation.
#Arbitrary value.
##No actual value given, but multicenter studies refer to > 14% (strict criteria) for *in vitro* fertilization (IVF).
$Normal shaped spermatozoa according to Tygerberg (Kruger) strict criteria.

The morphometric description of spermatozoa according to the strict criteria, described by Kruger et al.,[26] was definitely incorporated to the new WHO guidelines. The low proportions of normal-shaped spermatozoa, as defined by those retrieved from the endocervical mucus, inevitably produce the reference limits for a fertile population. With this method, similar values of 3–5 percent normal forms have been found by others to be the optimal cut-off point with predictive value for pregnancy in *in vitro* fertilization,[27] intrauterine insemination[28] and in spontaneous pregnancies.[29] Interpretation of the reference ranges requires an understanding that they provide a description of the semen characteristics of recent fathers. The reference limits should not be over-interpreted to distinguish fertile from infertile men accurately, but they do represent semen characteristics associated with a couple's chance of achieving pregnancy within 12 months of unprotected sexual intercourse; as such, the limits provide only a standardized guide regarding a given man's fertility. None of these values were able to solely distinguish fertile and infertile men, although morphology was suggested to be the most important. The coexistence of more than one altered seminal parameter significantly increases the risk for infertility.[23] A man's semen characteristics need to be interpreted in conjunction with his clinical information. The reference limits provided by the WHO manual are from semen samples initiating natural conceptions. Values below cutoff may indicate the need for infertility treatment but such values should not be used to determine the nature of that treatment.

Leukocyte count has also been added to routine semen analysis as leukocytospermia represents a frequent cause of male infertility. Leukocytospermia (> 1 million leukocytes/mL of semen) prevalence in infertile men vary between 3 and 23 percent and has been correlated with clinical and subclinical genital infections, elevated levels of oxygen reactive species, antisperm antibodies and deficient spermatic function.[30] Neutrophils predominate among inflammatory cells and may be both identified and quantified through different methods and staining techniques. The Endtz test is one of the most used as it is a simple low cost option to detect the presence of peroxidase within neutrophils.[31] In azoospermic patients, diagnosis must be confirmed by the lack of any spermatozoa on the examination of the centrifuged seminal fluid on two separate occasions. The WHO recommends centrifugation for 15 minutes at 3000 *g* or greater.[11] Azoospermia with low ejaculate volume (<1.0 mL) not related to hypogonadism or CBAVD can be caused by ejaculatory dysfunction, although the most common cause is ejaculatory duct obstruction (EDO). When suspected, EDO can be confirmed by assessing seminal pH and fructose as seminal vesicle secretions are alkaline and contain fructose.

Complementary Workup

Endocrine Evaluation

Should be performed in the following scenarios:
- Sperm concentration < 10 million/mL
- Erectile dysfunction
- Hypospermia (volume <1 mL)
- Signs and symptoms of endocrinopathies or hypogonadism.

Minimal evaluation includes serum follicle-stimulating hormone (FSH) and total testosterone. They reflect germinative and Leydig cells status, respectively. If testosterone level is low repeated analysis is recommended along with free testosterone, LH and prolactin measurements. Isolated FSH elevation is usually indicative of severe spermatogenesis damage. Highly elevated FSH and LH levels when associated with low normal or below normal testosterone levels implicate diffuse testicular failure which may have a congenital (e.g. Klinefelter syndrome) or acquired cause. Concomitant low levels of FSH and LH indicate hygonadotropic hypogonadism. This may also be congenital, or secondary to a prolactin-producing pituitary tumor. In these cases, a complete workup of pituitary function is recommended including serum measurement of adrenocorticotropic hormone, thyroid-stimulating hormone, growth hormone and brain magnetic resonance imaging.[32] Gonadotropin values within normal range suggest extraductal obstruction in azoospermic subjects. However, patients with maturation arrest and 10 percent of those diagnosed with Sertoli cell-only syndrome may show non-elevated hormonal measurements. Serum estradiol determination should be done in obese patients and in those presenting the gynecomastia. Infertile patients in whom testosterone to estradiol ratio is less than 10 can harbor significant but reversible seminal alterations.[33] Vaucher and Cols[34] suggested that hyperestrogenism secondary to a higher conversion of testosterone to estradiol in Klinefelter syndrome (KS) patients inhibits testosterone production via a negative feedback pathway and may indicate overexpression of aromatase CYP19 in the testis at a molecular level. As such, there would be scientific rationale for using aromatase inhibitors in such patients.[33]

In azoospermic men with normal ejaculate volume, FSH level greater than two times the upper limit of normality is a reliable marker of dysfunctional spermatogenesis. In such cases, diagnostic testicular biopsy is usually unnecessary although no consensus exists in this matter.[11] If FSH level is normal, unilateral biopsy on the larger testis is recommended as there is no guarantee of normal spermatogenesis.

Hyperprolactinemia is a rare cause of infertility in healthy men and is more commonly related to erectile dysfunction and hypospermia. These men may present with micro- or macropituitary prolactin-secreting adenomas. Prolactin levels should be determined in infertile men with a complaint of concomitant sexual dysfunction and in those with clinical and/or laboratorial evidence of pituitary disease. Although hormonal alterations may be present in approximately 10 percent of men who undergo investigation, clinically significant changes affect less than 2 percent of the subjects (**Table 6.1**).[35]

Genetic Evaluation

Genetic factors commonly associated with male infertility include chromosomal aberrations, genetic alterations and Y-chromosome microdeletions. Chromosomal aberrations are assessed through peripheral blood lymphocyte culture and Giemsa band staining (G-band karyotype). Genetic mutations and Y-chromosome microdeletions assessments are also performed by analyzing lymphocytes obtained from peripheral blood sampling. DNA is amplified using polymerase chain reaction (PCR) biomolecular technique. **Table 6.4** summarizes the indications and recommended tests for genetic evaluation.

Chromosomal abnormalities can be found in about 6 percent of infertile men and its prevalence inversely correlates with sperm count. Azoospermic men can present chromosomal alterations in as much as 16 percent of cases.[36] Sex chromosomal aneuploidy (Klinefelter syndrome; 47,XXY) is the most frequent chromosomal disorder present in infertile men and is generally associated with hypotrophic or atrophic testicles, elevated serum FSH levels and azoospermia, although spermatogenesis can be differently affected in patients with a mosaic karyotype (46,XY/47,XXY). Among genetic disorders, the mutation of the cystic fibrosis gene (cystic fibrosis transmembrane conductance regulator - CFTR) located in the long arm

Table 6.4: Indications for genetic testing in the infertile male

Indications	Recommended tests
Men with infertility of unknown etiology and sperm concentration < 10 million/mL who are candidates for assisted reproductive technology (ART)	Y-chromosome microdeletion and G-band karyotype
Nonobstructive azoospermia in a male considering testicular sperm retrieval and ART	Y-chromosome microdeletion and G-band karyotype
Azoospermic or oligozoospermic men with absence of at least one vas deferens at physical examination	CFTR gene mutation
Azoospermic men with signs of normal spermatogenesis (e.g. obstructive azoospermia of unknown origin)	CFTR gene mutation
History of recurrent miscarriage or personal/familiar history of genetic syndromes	G-band karyotype

of chromosome 7 is the most commonly found. According to the extension of the mutation, cystic fibrosis can be manifested in its full clinical presentation (an autosomic recessive potentially fatal disease) or in a mild form, where congenital bilateral absence of the vasa deferentia (CBAVD) is found. CBAVD affects approximately 1.3 percent of infertile men. CFTR gene mutations compromise the development of Wolffian ducts-derived structures (efferent ducts, epididymis and vasa deferentia) and may even be implicated in seminal vesicles hypoplasia or agenesis and unilateral renal agenesis. Approximately 80 percent of men presenting with CBVAD have a CFTR mutation. As the diagnostic methods routinely used are not 100 percent sensitive, a man with CBAVD should be assumed to harbor a CFTR mutation. Testing should be offered to his female partner to exclude the possibility that she may also be a carrier (approximately 4% risk) before using his sperm for assisted conception. Genetic counseling should be offered after genetic testing.[11] Recent data suggest that azoospermic men with idiopathic obstruction and those presenting the triad composed by chronic sinusitis, bronchiectasis and obstructive azoospermia (Young syndrome) have an elevated risk for CFTR mutations.[36] The long and short arms of Y-chromosome are respectively related to spermatogenesis and testicle development. The Y-chromosome region related to infertility is named azoospermia factor *locus* (AZF – *azoospermia factor*). The *locus* may harbor complete or partial microscopic deletions, isolated or in combination, and in non-overlapping subregions called AZFa, AZFb, AZFc and AZFd (**Fig. 6.4**). These subregions contain multiple genes controlling different steps of spermatogenesis.

The most common Y-chromosome deletion in infertile men is the one affecting the DAZ gene (*deleted in azoospermia*) located

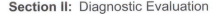

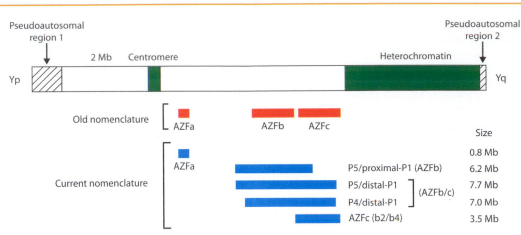

Figure 6.4: Illustration of the Y-chromosome in humans and the regions involved in fertility and infertility (Adapted from Am J Hum Genet. 71(4), Repping S et al., Recombination between Palindromes P5 and P1 on the Human Y-chromosome Causes Massive Deletions and Spermatogenic Failure, pages: 906–22, Copyright 2002, with permission from Elsevier). Interstitial or terminal deletions that include AZFa usually produce the severe phenotype of Sertoli-cell-only syndrome. Interstitial or terminal deletions that include AZFb and/or AZFb+c) are mediated by recombination between palindromic repeats, either P5/proxP1, P5/distP1, or P4/distP1. These deletions are associated to the maturation arrest phenotype and azoospermia. Interstitial or terminal deletions that include AZFc only are mediated by recombination between the b2/b4 palindromic repeats and result in a variable phenotype, ranging from azoospermia and SCOS to severe or mild oligozoospermia

in AZFc region. Severe oligozoospermia or azoospermia is often seen in such cases. Y-chromosome microdeletions can be found in 6 percent of men presenting with severe oligozoospermia (<1 million/mL) and in 15 percent of those with azoospermia.[36] For sperm counts between 1 and 5 million/mL the detection rate drops to 1.7 percent.[37] Detection of Y-chromosomal microdeletions provides predictive information on the success of obtaining spermatozoa from the testicle for intracytoplasmic sperm injection (ICSI). AZFa and/or AZFb microdeletions almost invariably present clinically as azoospermia and are usually associated with germ cell aplasia and maturation arrest, respectively. In such cases, sperm retrieval attempt is not indicated because there is no chance of finding testicular sperm.[38,39] In azoospermic men with AZFc microdeletion sperm can be retrieved in approximately 71 percent of patients.[37] In these cases, the clinical pregnancy rates after ICSI are virtually the same compared to idiopathic azoospermic patients who had their sperm retrieved.

Testing results also provides information for genetic counseling as sons of men with Y-chromosomal microdeletion will inherit the abnormality and may also be infertile.[40,41]

The prevalence of structural abnormalities in the autosomes, such as inversions and translocations, is also higher in infertile men than in the general population. Gross karyotypic abnormalities are related to an elevated risk for miscarriages and for having children with both chromosomal and congenital defects. As such, men with nonobstructive azoospermia or severe oligozoospermia should be karyotyped before their sperm are used for ICSI.[11]

Transrectal, Scrotal and Renal Ultrasonography

Indications for transrectal ultrasonography (TRUS) include:
- Low semen volumes (<1.5 mL)
- Abnormal digital rectal examination (DRE)

- Ejaculatory disorders (anejaculation, hematospermia, painful ejaculation).

Trus allows for the evaluation of the distal extraductal system (seminal vesicles and ejaculatory ducts). EDO can be identified with TRUS by the presence of seminal vesicles enlargement and by visualization of cysts at the level of ejaculatory ducts.[42] When CBAVD is diagnosed, TRUS can reveal abnormalities at the level of seminal vesicles such as hypoplasia or agenesis. A recent study has suggested that combination of scrotal and TRUS may not only distinguish obstructive from nonobstructive azoospermia (NOA) but also determine the etiologic classification of obstructive azoospermia (OA). Ultrasonographic abnormalities are more commonly seen in OA than in NOA patients (92.2% versus 2.8%, p < 0.001). Sensitivity, specificity and accuracy of combined assessments for discriminating between OA and NOA were 95.3, 97.2 and 96.0 percent, respectively.[43] Seminal vesicle aspiration and seminal vesiculography may be performed under TRUS guidance and may help to establish the diagnosis of EDO.[44] In azoospermic patients, large amounts of sperm in the seminal vesicles strongly suggest EDO. Concomitant seminal vesiculography can determine the site of obstruction.

The indication for scrotal ultrasonography is to evaluate palpable nodules or testicular masses. Its use for subclinical varicocele diagnosis is controversial, as several studies demonstrated no clinical benefit for surgical treatment in this situation.[45] When there is a doubtfuly physical examination, such as in obese patients and in difficult cases to assess the contralateral side of a clinically detectable varicocele, scrotal ultrasonography is useful. The commonly accepted color-Doppler ultrasonography criterion for varicocele (maximum vein diameter of 3 mm or greater) has a sensitivity of about 50 percent and specificity of 90 percent compared to physical examination.[46] A pencil-probe Doppler (9 Mhz) stethoscope is an inexpensive tool that may aid in the diagnosis of the varicocele. The patient is examined in the upright position, and a venous "rush" representing blood reflux is heard with or without the Valsalva maneuver (**Fig. 6.2B**). Although simple and easily performed in the office, Hirsh et al. demonstrated that more than 50 percent of men without clinical varicoceles exhibited a Valsalva-maneuver Doppler-positive reflux.[47] None of these adjunctive diagnostic methods can differentiate between clinical and subclinical varicoceles. The significance of a positive test result using any of these adjuvant techniques in infertile men remains uncertain.

Urinary tract ultrasonography is indicated to evaluate the renal status in patients diagnosed with CBAVD. Renal agenesis may be present in 10 percent of patients with CBAVD and 25 percent of those with unilateral absence of vas deferens.[48]

Magnetic resonance imaging: Use of MRI in infertility investigation has gained importance in recent years. Varicocele, EDO, seminal vesicle agenesis and undescended testis are examples of conditions that can be studied by MRI.[49]

Pelvic MRI helps to clarify in detail pictorial changes initially seen at TRUS (**Fig. 6.5**). Moreover, MRI has traditionally been used to exclude cranial pathologies manifested by hormonal alterations (low serum LH and FSH; hyperprolactinemia).

There is evidence of the optimized usefulness of pituitary MRI in men with hypogonadism when prolactin levels are greater than twice the normal range or with symptoms suggesting a worrisome intracranial abnormality (headache, visual disturbances, diffuse metabolic derangements and other).[50] In general, pituitary abnormalities can be identified in 25 percent of hypogonadal men. Of these, however, empty sella and pituitary nonfunctional microadenomas require no specific treatment and make one wonder about the cost-effectiveness of their diagnosis.

Nuclear magnetic resonance spectroscopy has been recently proposed as a possible tool to identify metabolic signatures associated with various histological states in infertile men. Based on ex-vivo analysis of testicular biopsy specimens, concentrations of 19 tissue metabolites were acquired and then reassessed in men with a diagnosis of NOA. A singular pattern could be determined for two testis histological states: normal and Sertoli cell-only (SCO) syndrome. Proliferating germ cells are related to high phospholipid synthesis and with elevated phosphocoline. Normal spermatogenesis spectroscopic pattern presents high peaks of phosphocoline as opposed to SCO. Further research in this area may aid in the identification of a distinct metabolic signature for sperm presence, regardless of testis histopathology.[51]

Sperm Function Laboratory Tests

In 10–20 percent of infertile couples who undergo basic investigation, all diagnostic workup will yield normal results and couples will be classified as having unexplained infertility. Additional tests have been developed to identify functional disorders and other spermatic abnormalities which are not addressed by conventional semen analysis. While some of them are mainly used as research tools (computer-assisted semen analysis, acrosome reaction, oxidative stress evaluation using chemiluminescence, hamster egg sperm penetration test, hemizona assay),[52] others, such as sperm DNA fragmentation and anti-sperm antibodies testing, have already been implemented in clinical practice.

Sperm DNA fragmentation seems to be one of the most important causes of reduced fertility potential.[9] Advanced paternal age, inadequate diet intake, drug abuse, pesticide environmental exposure, tobacco use, varicocele, medical disease, hyperthermia, air pollution, genital inflammation and infectious diseases can be cited as possible causes, some of which are reversible. Fragmentation can be secondary to internal factors such as apoptosis and oxidative stress (a physiological mechanism secondary to a high concentration of free radicals), or external factors such as the presence of leukocytes. Assessment of sperm DNA integrity is indicated in the following situations:

- To investigate infertility in men presenting with normal semen analysis as determined by conventional methods
- Cases of recurrent spontaneous abortion
- To aid determining the most appropriate reproductive assisted technology when necessary.

  Elevated proportions of sperm with fragmented DNA can be found in 5 percent of infertile men with normal semen analyses and in 25 percent of infertile men with abnormal semen analyses, but is rarely seen in fertile men.[9] Among the available methods the most to detect sperm DNA fragmentation common are TUNEL, Comet, sperm chromatin dispersion, acridine orange test and SCSA (sperm chromatin structure assay). The TUNEL technique (transferase-mediated dTUP nick-end labeling) offers the possibility to precisely identify all existing endogenous breaks in sperm DNA. It combines both enzymatic and immunohisto chemical techniques for direct observation of DNA fragmentation using a fluorescence microscope or flow cytometry. Elevated sperm DNA

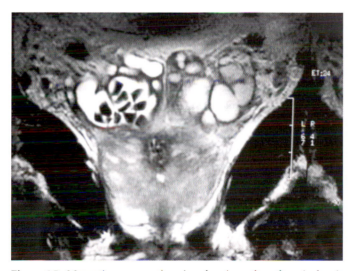

Figure 6.5: Magnetic resonance imaging showing enlarged seminal vesicles with calculosis. Reproduced with permission from Clinics (Sao Paulo). 2011 April; 66(4): 691-700. Copyright © 2011 Hospital das Clínicas da FMUSP. Esteves SC, Miyaoka R, Agarwal A: An update on the clinical assessment of the infertile male.

Family History

A family history of infertility problems, including recurrent miscarriages, may give a clue to a genetic etiology of a man's infertility. Known genetic disorders associated with infertility, such as cystic fibrosis or karyotypic anomalies, should also be sought.

Evaluation of the Female Partner

It is important to inquire about the female partner's fertility potential and what investigations and assessments she has undergone. Specific questions regarding previous pregnancies and their outcome (with current or previous partner), age at menarche, menstrual cycle history and gynecologic/general medical health are important to ask.

Physical Examination (see Flow chart 7.3)

The physical examination should focus on general appearance and the genital exam. Additional elements should be examined based on history, for example an assessment of visual fields if the patient has onset of blurred vision or suspicion of a pituitary tumor. The degree of virilization should be assessed, based on facial and body hair distribution and body habitus. Patients with inadequate virilization or bilateral testicular atrophy should have a hormonal profile to assess for hypogonadism. A eunuchoid body stature (tall stature with arm span exceeding body length) is associated with classic Klinefelter syndrome and is due to delayed epiphyseal closure. Conversely, Prader-Willi syndrome is associated with short stature, severe obesity, hypopigmentation and muscular hypotonia. Patients with Kallman syndrome will have craniofacial asymmetry, cleft palate and micropenis. An assessment for gynecomastia should be made and a formal breast exam for masses is required if there is a history of galactorrhea or Klinefelter syndrome, due to the significant increased risk of breast cancer in this population.[48]

The genital exam is critical. The penis should be examined for abnormalities, including micropenis (stretched penile length less than 2.5 standard deviation below the mean), chordee, penile plaques and hypospadias.[49] Physical examination of the scrotal contents is the most effective means of diagnosing clinically significant pathology. The testes should be carefully palpated for size, consistency and masses. Patients that have a challenging or indeterminate physical examination, either due to body habitus or a significantly contracted scrotum, should undergo a scrotal ultrasound. As well, any palpable abnormality of the testis needs to be assessed with a scrotal ultrasound and should be considered testicular cancer until proven otherwise. Testis size can be estimated with a Prader orchidometer, with the average testis size being approximately 18–20 cc.[50] Testicular failure is indicated by smaller than normal testes. Small and firm testes are seen in Klinefelter syndrome, while small and soft testes are seen in hypogonadotropic hyogonadism, anabolic androgen abuse and testicular failure secondary to chemotherapy. The testicular adnexa, including the vas deferens, epididymis and pampiniform venous plexus should be assessed. Palpation for the vas deferens

is critical, as CBAVD is the cause of infertility in approximately 1.4 percent of infertile males and indicates a CFTR gene mutation in approximately 80 percent of those affected.[51] The epididymis should be palpated for size, tenderness and masses. Epididymal width should be less than 1 cm and if enlarged may indicate epididymal or vasal obstruction.[52] Clinical varicoceles should be assessed in the standing position with and without Valsalva. The vast majority of varicoceles are left-sided.[53] Patients with isolated right-sided varicoceles require abdominal imaging to rule out retroperitoneal pathology. Grade I varicoceles are palpable only with Valsalva, grade II are palpable without Valsalva and grade III are visibly obvious with the typical "bag of worms" appearance. A digital rectal exam may be indicated in patients with lower urinary tract symptoms to assess the prostate or in patients with a low volume ejaculate to assess for palpable seminal vesicles and midline cystic structures. A transrectal ultrasound (TRUS) should confirm these findings and if ejaculatory duct obstruction or cysts are identified, the patient requires CFTR testing.

Semen Analysis (see Flow chart 7.4)

The semen analysis is the most important laboratory test to measure in men undergoing an infertility evaluation, as it assists the clinician in formulating a differential diagnosis and guides what further tests need to be performed. The World Health Organization (WHO) has published standardized procedures for semen analysis.[54] A minimum of two properly collected samples, separated by more than seven days but not more than three weeks, should be obtained from all patients. Specific patient instructions regarding collection and transportation to the laboratory are important. Patients should have a 2–5 days abstinence period prior to collection. Samples may be collected by masturbation or by special condoms used during intercourse, but not by coitus interruptus. Samples collected at home should be kept at body temperature and brought to the laboratory ideally within 1 hour to be analyzed.

There is considerable individual variability in semen analysis results, due to biological and technical factors. Since the total duration of spermatogenesis is 74 days, a recovery from a temporary insult on spermatogenesis may take around 3 months to be reflected on the semen analysis. In addition, semen parameters, especially concentration, can vary considerably in an individual over time.[55] Lastly, inter and intra-observer variability is seen when analyzing semen parameters.[56] A trend of semen analysis results is much more useful than a single result.

The basic semen analysis assesses the physical characteristics of the semen (volume, liquefaction, appearance, consistency, pH and agglutination), sperm concentration (in million of sperm/cc), motility, morphology, vitality and the presence of pyospermia (greater than 1 million white blood cells (WBCs)/cc). Abnormalities in semen volume, sperm concentration, sperm motility and the presence of pyospermia require additional investigations.

Semen volume is characterized as either low (<1.5 cc) or normal volume. A patient with a low volume ejaculate requires a transrectal ultrasound (TRUS) and post-ejaculatory urinalysis.[57]

TRUS can detect abnormalities of the seminal vesicles and prostate, presence of utriclar and müllerian duct cysts and other etiologies of ejaculatory duct obstruction. Obstructive azoospermia is associated with CFTR mutations in 47 percent of men, therefore men with obstructive lesions in the epididymis or ejaculatory ducts (including ejaculatory duct cysts) require CFTR testing.[58] A post-ejaculatory urinalysis is important to detect retrograde ejaculation, an important and easily treated cause of low semen volume.

Patients with severe oligospermia and azoospermia require a hormonal evaluation. The yield of finding an endocrinopathy is exceedingly low if the sperm concentration is more than 10 million/cc, with only 1 in 1034 infertile men with counts greater than this having an endocrinopathy identified in one study.[59] Initial evaluation of FSH and testosterone is the most efficient, cost-effective and revealing hormonal survey for male infertility and hypogonadism.[59] If the FSH or testosterone levels are abnormal, then LH should additionally be evaluated. If LH and testosterone are found to be low, prolactin should be evaluated as hyperprolactinemia causes LH suppression and resulting low testosterone.

Men with non-obstructive azoospermia and severe oligospermia (<5 million sperm/cc) should undergo both karyotypic and Y-chromosomal microdeletion analyses because approximately 15 percent of these patients will have a genetic mutation or abnormality.[60,61] While the technique to definitively diagnosis non-obstructive azoospermia is not included in this chapter, we will in general perform genetic testing for all non-obstructive azoospermic men (those with elevated FSH and/or small, softer testis). Identifying the genetic abnormality is important to not only explain why the patient is infertile but also to identify which genetic abnormalities may be passed onto future offspring. Referral for genetic counselling in these cases is critical.

Adequate sperm motility is essential for conception via sexual intercourse and intrauterine insemination. Asthenospermia has multiple etiologies, including varicocele, antisperm antibodies (ASA), genitourinary infections and ultrastructural anomalies of the sperm tail.[62] ASAs may develop with ductal obstruction, testicular infections, trauma, torsion and previous vasovasotomy/vasoepididymostomy. An assessment for ASA should be made if there is isolated asthenospermia with normal sperm concentration or the presence of sperm agglutination. There are multiple assays available to detect ASA, including direct methods that detect ASA directly on sperm and indirect methods that detect ASA in the serum, seminal plasma or cervical fluid. The direct mixed agglutination and immunobead assays are most commonly performed.[63] The effect of ASA on pregnancy rates is controversial,[64] although the presence of ASA has been associated with decreased pregnancy rates in some series.[65] Sperm with absent or near absent motility and high viability may have ultrastructural anomalies of the sperm tail, which can be confirmed with electron microscopy.[66]

Pyospermia may or may not be associated with bacteriospermia, however, all men with pyospermia should have a semen culture performed. Pyospermia can impaired semen parameters,[67] however, this has not uniformly been seen.[68]

A recent international study by Cooper et al[69] on semen parameters in fertile men has set new benchmarks for the fifth edition of the WHO Laboratory Manual for the Examination of Human Semen. The 5th percentile from this study is now used as the new lower reference limits for fertile men set by the WHO. A comparison between the 5th and 50th percentile in Cooper's study and previous 1999 WHO reference values demonstrates the discrepancy in semen parameters between the "barely fertile" and the "average" (**Table 7.2**).

■ CONCLUSION

Male factor infertility is an important aspect of the couple's infertility that requires specific evaluation. A step-wise approach is critical, by starting with a basic evaluation of all patients inclusive of history, physical examination and semen analyses and conducting additional investigations when indicated. By following this logical schema, the male patient can be adequately and efficiently evaluated without undergoing unnecessary, costly and stressful investigations.

Table 7.2: Semen parameter comparisons between 1999 WHO lowest reference values[54] and the 5th and 50th percentile from Cooper et al. study, World Health Organization reference values for human semen characteristics[69]

Semen parameter	1999 WHO lowest reference values	5th percentile from cooper et al. study	50th percentile from cooper et al. study
Volume (cc)	2	1.5	3.7
Concentration (10^6/cc)	20	15	73
Total number (10^6/ejaculate)	40	39	255
Progressive motility (%)*	50	32	55
Normal forms (%)**	14	4	15
Vitality (%)	75	58	79

* Progressive motility as outlined in WHO 1999 (54), Grades a + b
** Normal forms determined by the strict Tygerberg method

■ REFERENCES

1. Gunnell DJ EP. Infertility prevalence, needs assessment and purchasing. J Public Health Med 1994;16:29-35.
2. Page H. Estimation of the prevalence and incidence of infertility in a population: a pilot. Fertil Steril 1989;51:571-7.
3. Jensen TCE, Jorgensen N, Berthelsen J, Keiding N, Christensen K, Petersen J, Knudsen L, Skakkebaek N. Poor semen quality may contribute to recent decline in fertility rates. Human Reproduction 2002;17(6):1437-40.
4. Jensen TST, Hansen M, Pedersen A, Lutz W, Skakkebaek N. Declining trends in conception rates in recent birth cohotrs of native Danish women: a possible role of deteriorating male reproductive health. Int J of Andrology 2008;31:81-92.
5. Report on optimal evaluation of the infertile male. Fertil Steril 2006;86(5 Suppl 1):S202-9.
6. Shindel AW, Nelson CJ, Naughton CK, Ohebshalom M, Mulhall JP. Sexual function and quality of life in the male partner of infertile couples: prevalence and correlates of dysfunction. J Urol 2008;179(3):1056-9.
7. Van Balen F, Trimbos-Kemper TC. Factors influencing the well-being of long-term infertile couples. J Psychosom Obstet Gynaecol 1994;15(3):157-64.
8. Jarvi K, Lo K, Fischer A, Grantmyre J, Zini A, Chow V, et al. CUA Guideline: The workup of azoospermic males. Can Urol Assoc J 2010;4(3):163-7.
9. Molitch ME. Drugs and prolactin. Pituitary 2008;11(2): 209-18.
10. Nielsen J, Wohlert M. Chromosome abnormalities found among 34,910 newborn children: results from a 13-year incidence study in Arhus, Denmark. Hum Genet 1991;87(1):81-3.
11. Brugh V, Matschke H, Lipshultz L. Male factor infertility. Endocrinol Metab Clin North Am 2003;32:689-707.
12. Mak V, Jarvi K. The genetics of male infertility. J Urol 1996;156:1245-46.
13. Brugh VM ND, Lipshultz LI. What the urologist should know about the female infertility evaluation. Urol Clin North Am 2002;29(4):983-92.
14. Levitas E, Lunenfeld E, Weisz N, Friger M, Potashnik G. Relationship between age and semen parameters in men with normal sperm concentration: analysis of 6022 semen samples. Andrologia 2007;39(2):45-50.
15. Valentin J. Exclusions and attributions of paternity: practical experiences of forensic genetics and statistics. Am J Hum Genet 1980;32:209-17.
16. Wilcox A, CR W, DD B. Timing of sexual intercourse in relation to ovulation. Effects on the probability of conception, survival of the pregnancy, and sex of the baby. N Engl J Med 1995;333(23):1517-21.
17. Agarwal A, Deepinder F, Cocuzza M, Short R, Evenson D. Effect of vaginal lubricants on sperm motility and chromatin integrity: a prospective compartive study. Fertil Steril 2008;89(2):375-9.
18. Ostrer H. Sexual differentiation. Semin Reprod Med 2000;18(1):41-9.
19. Woodhouse CR, Snyder HM, 3rd. Testicular and sexual function in adults with prune belly syndrome. J Urol 1985;133(4):607-9.
20. Stein R, Fisch M, Stockle M, Hohenfellner R. Treatment of patients with bladder exstrophy or incontinent epispadias. A long-term follow-up. Eur Urol 1997;31(1):58-64.
21. Berkowitz GS, Lapinski RH, Dolgin SE, Gazella JG, Bodian CA, Holzman IR. Prevalence and natural history of cryptorchidism. Pediatrics 1993;92(1):44-9.
22. Lee P. Fertility after cryptorchidism: epidemiology and other outcome studies. Urology 2005;66:427-31.
23. Cendron M, Keating MA, Huff DS, Koop CE, Snyder HM, 3rd, Duckett JW. Cryptorchidism, orchiopexy and infertility: a critical long-term retrospective analysis. J Urol 1989;142(2 Pt 2):559-62; discussion 72.
24. Albanese A, Stanhope R. Investigation of delayed puberty. Clinical Endocrinology 1995;43:105-10.
25. Bar-Chama N, Fisch H. Infection and pyospermia in male infertility. World J Urol 1993;11(2):76-81.
26. Pellati D, Mylonakis I, Bertoloni G, Fiore C, Andrisani A, Ambrosini G, et al. Genital tract infections and infertility. Eur J Obstet Gynecol Reprod Biol 2008;140(1):3-11.
27. Everaert K, Mahmoud A, Depuydt C, Maeyaert M, Comhaire F. Chronic prostatitis and male accessory gland infection—is there an impact on male infertility (diagnosis and therapy)? Andrologia 2003;35(5):325-30.
28. Wise GJ, Shteynshlyuger A. An update on lower urinary tract tuberculosis. Curr Urol Rep. 2008;9(4):305-13.
29. Gallegos G, Ramos B, Santiso R, Goyanes V, Gosalvez J, Fernandez JL. Sperm DNA fragmentation in infertile men with genitourinary infection by *Chlamydia trachomatis* and *Mycoplasma*. Fertil Steril 2008;90(2):328-34.
30. Heyns CF, Fisher M. The urological management of the patient with acquired immunodeficiency syndrome. BJU Int 2005;95(5):709-16.
31. Umapathy E, Simbini T, Chipata T, Mbizvo M. Sperm characteristics and accessory sex gland functions in HIV-infected men. Arch Androl 2001;46(2):153-8.
32. Scott LS. Mumps and male fertility. Br J Urol 1960;32:183-7.
33. Ver Voort SM. Infertility in spinal-cord injured male. Urology 1987;29(2):157-65.
34. Bycroft JA, Hamid R, Shah J, Craggs M. Management of the neuropathic bladder. Hosp Med 2003;64(8):468-72.
35. Jarow JP. Endocrine causes of male infertility. Urol Clin North Am 2003;30(1):83-90.
36. Amaral S, Oliveira PJ, Ramalho-Santos J. Diabetes and the impairment of reproductive function: possible role of mitochondria and reactive oxygen species. Curr Diabetes Rev 2008;4(1):46-54.
37. Agbaje IM, Rogers DA, McVicar CM, McClure N, Atkinson AB, Mallidis C, et al. Insulin dependant diabetes mellitus: implications for male reproductive function. Hum Reprod 2007;22(7):1871-7.
38. Xu LG, Xu HM, Zhu XF, Jin LM, Xu B, Wu Y, et al. Examination of the semen quality of patients with uraemia and renal transplant recipients in comparison with a control group. Andrologia 2009;41(4):235-40.
39. Howell S, Shalet S. Testicular function following chemotherapy. Hum Reprod Update 2001;7(4):363-9.
40. Handelsman DJ, Conway AJ, Boylan LM, Turtle JR. Young's syndrome. Obstructive azoospermia and chronic sinopulmonary infections. N Engl J Med 1984;310(1):3-9.
41. Amory JK. Drug effects on spermatogenesis. Drugs Today (Barc) 2007;43(10):717-24.
42. Kom C, Mulholland SG, Edson M. Etiology of infertility after retroperitoneal lymphadenectomy. J Urol 1971;105(4):528-30.

43. Ramlau-Hansen CH, Thulstrup AM, Aggerholm AS, Jensen MS, Toft G, Bonde JP. Is smoking a risk factor for decreased semen quality? A cross-sectional analysis. Hum Reprod 2007;22(1):188-96.

44. Muthusami KR, Chinnaswamy P. Effect of chronic alcoholism on male fertility hormones and semen quality. Fertil Steril 2005;84(4):919-24.

45. Weinberg CR. Infertility and the use of illicit drugs. Epidemiology 1990;1(3):189-92.

46. Brinkworth M, Handelsman D. Environmental Influences on Male Reproductive Health. In: Nieschlag E, (Ed). Andrology. Verlag, Berlin, Heidelberg: Springer 2010.pp.365-83.

47. Knuth UA, Maniera H, Nieschlag E. Anabolic steroids and semen parameters in bodybuilders. Fertil Steril 1989;52(6):1041-7.

48. Giordano SH, Buzdar AU, Hortobagyi GN. Breast cancer in men. Ann Intern Med 2002;137(8):678-87.

49. Taran I, Hartke DM, Palmer JS. Congenital genitourinary anomalies and sexual function. Int J Impot Res 2007;19(2):115-8.

50. Behre HM, Yeung CH, Holstein AE, Weinbauer GF, Gassner P, Nieschlag E. Diagnosis of Male Infertility and Hypogonadism In: Nieschlag E (Ed). Andrology: Male Reproductive Health and Dysfunction. 2nd edn. Berlin: Springer-Verlag, 2001.

51. Anguiano A, Oates R, Amos J, et al. Congenital bilateral absence of the vas deferens. A primarily genital form of cystic fibrosis. JAMA 1992;267(13):1794-7.

52. Paduch D, Fuchs F. Office evaluation of male infertility. In: Patton P, Battaglia D, (Eds). Office Andrology. Totowa, New Jersey: Humana Press Inc.; 2005.

53. Report on varicocele and infertility. Fertil Steril 2008;90 (5 Suppl):S247-9.

54. WHO Laboratory Manual for the Examination of Human Semen and Sperm-Cervical Mucus Interaction, 4th edn, Cambridge University Press, 1999.

55. Alvarez C, Castilla JA, Martinez L, Ramirez JP, Vergara F, Gaforio JJ. Biological variation of seminal parameters in healthy subjects. Hum Reprod 2003;18(10):2082-8.

56. Carrell DT, Cartmill D, Jones KP, Hatasaka HH, Peterson CM. Prospective, randomized, blinded evaluation of donor semen quality provided by seven commercial sperm banks. Fertil Steril 2002;78(1):16-21.

57. Roberts M, Jarvi K. Steps in the investigation and management of low semen volume in the infertile man. Can Urol Assoc J 2009;3(6):479-85.

58. Jarvi K, Zielenski J, Wilschanski M, Durie P, Buckspan M, Tullis E, et al. Cystic fibrosis transmembrane conductance regulator and obstructive azoospermia. Lancet 1995;345(8964):1578.

59. Sigman M, Jarow JP. Endocrine evaluation of infertile men. Urology 1997;50(5):659-64.

60. Reijo R, Alagappan RK, Patrizio P, Page DC. Severe oligozoospermia resulting from deletions of azoospermia factor gene on Y-chromosome. Lancet 1996;347(9011):1290-3.

61. Gekas J, Thepot F, Turleau C, Siffroi JP, Dadoune JP, Briault S, et al. Chromosomal factors of infertility in candidate couples for ICSI: an equal risk of constitutional aberrations in women and men. Hum Reprod 2001;16(1):82-90.

62. Sigman M, Jarow J. Male Infertility. In: Wein A (Ed). Campbell-Walsh Urology. 9th en. Philadelphia: Saunders Elsevier, 2007.

63. Andreou E, Mahmoud A, Vermeulen L, Schoonjans F, Comhaire F. Comparison of different methods for the investigation of anti-sperm antibodies on spermatozoa, in seminal plasma and in serum. Hum Reprod 1995;10(1): 125-31.

64. Vujisic S, Lepej SZ, Jerkovic L, Emedi I, Sokolic B. Antisperm antibodies in semen, sera and follicular fluids of infertile patients: relation to reproductive outcome after in vitro fertilization. Am J Reprod Immunol 2005;54(1):13-20.

65. Ayvaliotis B, Bronson R, Rosenfeld D, Cooper G. Conception rates in couples where autoimmunity to sperm is detected. Fertil Steril 1985;43(5):739-42.

66. Williamson RA, Koehler JK, Smith WD, Stenchever MA. Ultrastructural sperm tail defects associated with sperm immotility. Fertil Steril 1984;41(1):103-7.

67. Jarvi K, Noss MB. Pyospermia and male infertility. Can J Urol 1994;1(2):25-30.

68. Rodin DM, Larone D, Goldstein M. Relationship between semen cultures, leukospermia, and semen analysis in men undergoing fertility evaluation. Fertil Steril 2003;79 Suppl 3:1555-8.

69. Cooper TG, Noonan E, von Eckardstein S, Auger J, Baker HW, Behre HM, et al. World Health Organization reference values for human semen characteristics. Hum Reprod Update 2010;16(3):231-45.

Testing Beyond the Semen Analysis: The Evolving Role of New Tests

Mary K Samplaski, Rakesh Sharma, Ashok Agarwal, Edmund Sabanegh Jr

INTRODUCTION

While the semen analysis (SA) is the cornerstone of the assessment of male factor infertility, it remains imperfect in predicting fecundity.[1,2] There are a subset of patients in which there is a deficiency in one of the tasks necessary for spermatozoa to reach and fertilize an ovum, which is not detected by the standard SA, estimated at 40–50 percent of men presenting for subfertility.[3] To try and determine the precise functional impairment, specialized semen tests evaluate specific aspects of spermatozoa function. This chapter reviews selected specialized semen tests, outlining the principals of each, as well as clinical data to support or refute their clinical utility. For the purposes of this chapter, more commonly utilized assays will be listed first, closing with emerging tests.

SEMEN ANALYSIS

The traditional belief that there are a discrete number of spermatozoa with certain characteristics that are necessary to achieve fertilization has been debunked in the last decade with the realization that a normal spermiogram does not necessarily correlate with fertility potential because it does not assess sperm function. Some factors, including sperm count and morphology, have been clearly found to relate to conception,[1-3] however, there are still a significant proportion of patients with normal SAs exhibiting unexplained infertility.[2] As one classic example, Guzick et al. reviewed the semen parameters of 765 subfertile men, and found there was significant overlap between fertile and infertile men with respect to sperm concentration, motility and morphology,[2] a finding which has been corroborated by others.[1-4] These studies illustrate that the SA cannot independently predict male fertility, as it does not evaluate spermatozoa functional competence. For this reason, specialized semen tests have been developed in an attempt to evaluate individual aspects of spermatozoal function.

Computer-assisted Sperm Assessment

Computer-assisted sperm assessment (CASA), the use of computer analysis of videomicrography to assess sperm kinetic parameters, was developed in an attempt to more precisely analyze sperm head and flagellar kinematics. The microscopic field is digitized and kinematic values are determined for each spermatozoon, which are then computer analyzed.[5] Classic SA parameters are generated, as well as sperm trajectory characteristics and straight-line velocity, which cannot be determined by standard microscopic evaluation. While these characteristics have been positively correlated with IVF fertilization rates, CASA cannot reliably predict spontaneous fertilization outcomes.[6]

Viability Assays

When a semen sample has a motility of < 30 percent, viability testing is indicated to distinguish between necrospermia and an ultrastructural defect. Low motility and high viability suggests living sperm with an ultrastructural defect, such as primary ciliary dyskinesia or Kartagener's syndrome, which may be further evaluated with electron microscopy. Immotile sperm may also be seen after testicular extraction, when they have not acquired motility in the epididymis. In this situation, viability testing may be useful in selecting viable sperm, to be used for assisted reproductive techniques (ART).[7]

Living sperm have an intact cytoplasmic membrane, which is the basis for viability assays such as evaluation of hypo-osmotic swelling or dye exclusion. Hypo-osmotic testing (**Fig. 8.1A**) evaluates spermatozoa response to hypo-osmotic fluid, which enters the cytoplasm of living cells to reach osmolar equilibrium, causing viable sperm to visibly swell, best visualized in the tail. Dye exclusion (**Fig. 8.1B**) tests sperms' ability to resist the absorption of certain dyes, including Eosin, Nigrosin, or Trypan blue. These tests are considered normal if ≥ 60 percent of sperm are viable.[8] During dye exclusion sperm are air dried (killed), and thus cannot be used for ART. In contrast, the hypo-osmotic swelling assay does not lyse cells, allowing for the selection of sperm for ART.[9]

Leukocytospermia Testing

Seminal leukocytes are a frequent finding in patients both with and without subfertility. Quantification in the standard SA may be inaccurate since under light microscopy it is difficult to differentiate leukocytes from immature germ cells. The Endtz test stains for peroxidase within polymorphonuclear leukocytes, allowing for this distinction.

Seminal leukocytes are powerful generators of reactive oxygen species (ROS), and their full role in fecundity is still being

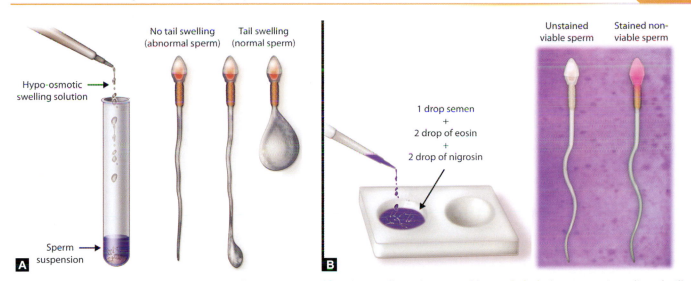

Figures 8.1A and B: (A) Hypo-osmotic sperm swelling test: Sperm with an intact cell membrane are able to exclude the hypo-osmotic media and will not swell; (B) Microscopic image of dye exclusion: spermatozoa with dark pink heads are considered dead (membrane-damaged), whereas spermatozoa with white or light pink heads are considered alive (membrane-intact)

elucidated. Leukocytospermia, defined as $>1 \times 10^6$ WBC/mL, is negatively associated with multiple parameters of spermatozoa function.[10] However, levels as low as 20.2×10^6 WBC/mL have been associated with elevated ROS, suggesting that lower levels of leukocytes are pathologic.[10] Leukocytospermia has been correlated with sperm tail defects, acrosomal damage, teratospermia, and impaired motility.[10,11] Functionally, men with leukocytospermia have a lower chance of spontaneous pregnancy as compared with fertile counterparts,[10] and antibiotic treatment for men with leukocytospermia and genital infections has been shown to reduce seminal leukocyte and ROS levels, leading to an improvement in sperm motility and natural conception rates.[11]

Antisperm Antibodies

Sperm autoantibodies are present in 10 percent of infertile men, compared with 2 percent of fertile men.[12] Sperm agglutination, impaired motility, an atypical postcoital test, or abnormalities of cervical mucus interaction, may prompt ASA testing. Routine semen parameters are often normal, leading some authors to recommend ASA testing in all men undergoing infertility work-up.[3]

Only antibodies that bind to sperm membrane antigens are of functional significance, and thus only tests which examine sperm antibody presence are clinically useful. The immunobead test consists of incubating spermatozoa with microbeads coated with IgG class-specific secondary antibodies, and the observing microscopically for agglutination (**Fig. 8.2**). Antibodies are considered significant when > 50 percent of spermatozoa are coated, when sperm are unable to penetrate the preovulatory human cervical mucus, or demonstrate impaired fertilizing capacity.[8] ASA agglutinate, immobilize, and opsonize sperm, which may interfere with sperm differentiation, migration,

capacitation, zona penetration, or sperm-oocyte membrane interactions.[13] Because of this, the presence of ASA may lead to impaired spontaneous and IVF pregnancy rates and higher miscarriage rates.[13,14] Steroids may be given to lower ASA titers prior to IUI, but are unnecessary if ICSI is used.[13] Isotype specificity and spermatozoa localization of ASA is possible, however, there are currently no tests to determine the quantity of antibody molecules bound. Research is ongoing to determine the stimuli for and effects of specific ASA on individual sperm proteins, which may lead to targeted therapies.[13]

Seminal Fluid Testing

The prostate, seminal vesicles, and epididymis each produce unique seminal components, which may then serve as surrogates for the glands that produce them:
- *Prostate*: Citric acid, zinc, calcium, magnesium, gamma glutamyl-transferase, PSA, acid phosphatase[15]
- *Seminal vesicles*: Fructose, semenogelin, prostaglandin, seminal plasma motility inhibitor[15]
- *Epididymis*: Free L-carnitine, glycerophosphocoline, α-glucosidase[15]

Of these, zinc and citric acid are commonly assayed for the prostate, fructose and semenogelin for the seminal vesicles, and α-glucosidase for the epididymis. Levels of these compounds may highlight the pathogenesis of some semen samples. For example, α-glucosidase and L-carnitine can be used to distinguish ductal obstruction from primary testicular failure,[16,17] and they may also serve as indicators of IVF success.[17] In reality, biomarkers are best interpreted with respect to each other. One example of this involves semenogelin, a coagulum released by the seminal vesicles, and PSA, from the prostate. PSA rapidly cleaves semenogelin, leading to semen liquefaction and sperm motility. An abnormality in either of these components would lead to hyperviscous semen, preventing sperm motility and fertilization.[18]

Acrosomal Integrity and Function

Spermatozoa lacking an acrosome, either never having one or due to spontaneous release, will not bind to or penetrate the zona pellucida. Acrosomal integrity can be assessed by staining with fluorescent lectins that selectively bind to either the outer membrane or acrosomal contents (**Figs 8.2A to C**).[4] If the acrosome is intact, the timing of enzymatic release can also be assessed. A proportion of sperm from any sample will exhibit 'acrosomal prematurity', or spontaneous enzymatic release. Normally, this comprises < 4 percent of the sample,[4] however, men with repeated IVF failure have been shown to have > 20 percent of spermatozoa with acrosomal prematurity.[19] Because acrosomal release can be due to sperm death, these tests are often used in conjunction with viability testing.

To test the acrosomal release of its contents, enzymatic release is induced, either by ionophore A23187, progesterone, or human zona pellucida, and the proportion of reacting spermatozoa is measured. This value, the stimulated acrosomal reaction (SAR) score, ranges from 20–98 percent in fertile men and lower values have been correlated with impaired IVF rates, although predictive values vary.[20] As such, acrosomal testing is primarily used after repeated IVF failure, and has limited utility in the initial assessment of subfertility.

Post-Coital Test

Also known as the cervical mucus reaction, the post-coital test evaluates sperm motility within the cervical environment and its ability to access the uterus. It is indicated in the settings of hyperviscous semen or unexplained infertility. Anatomic abnormalities, including hypospadias, or inappropriate sexual technique may result in the absence of sperm in the cervical mucus.[9] The test is conducted when the cervical mucus is thinnest, just prior to ovulation; the number and motility of sperm in the cervical mucus is assessed 2–8 hours after intercourse. Greater than 10–20 motile sperm per high-powered field is considered normal[9] and has then been positively correlated with spontaneous and *in vitro* pregnancy rates.[21] However, while interesting in theory, a thorough history and SA can predict the results of the post-coital test in half of infertile couples,[22] and thus its true clinical utility is limited.

▌HEMIZONA ASSAY

Binding of spermatozoa to the species-specific zona pellucida triggers the acrosome reaction, wherein the enzymatic contents of the acrosome are released.[9] This reaction is evaluated using the hemizona assay and sperm-zona binding ratio. The former (**Fig. 8.3**) utilizes human oocytes from which the zona pellucida is isolated and split. One half is incubated with fertile donor sperm and the other with patient sperm. The ratio of fertile to donor binding is measured, with < 30 percent considered abnormal.[9] For the sperm-zona binding ratio, different fluorochromes are used to label fertile donor sperm and patient sperm. Sperm are then incubated with zona-intact oocytes, and the ratio of bound to unbound spermatozoa are quantified.[9]

Defects in sperm-zona binding and penetration are among the most common causes of IVF failure,[23] IUI failure,[24] and impaired spontaneous pregnancy in infertile men.[24] These tests are primarily used to elucidate the origin of IVF failure, rather than as part of the initial infertility evaluation, and men found to have abnormal binding should be counseled to consider ICSI.[24]

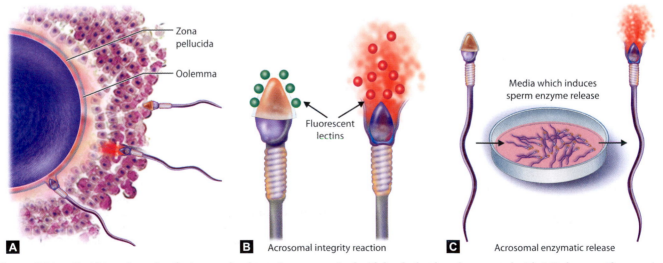

Figures 8.2A to C: ASA testing using the immunobead test: Sperm are mixed with beads that have been coated with IgG class-specific secondary antibodies: (A) Normal physiology: Proteolytic enzymes in the acrosome digest through the zona pellucida, allowing for sperm-oolemma fusion; (B) Assessing acrosomal integrity: Different fluorescent lectins are applied to label either the outer membrane or acrosomal contents; (C) Assessing acrosomal enzymatic release: Enzymatic release is induced and the proportion of reacted spermatozoa are assessed

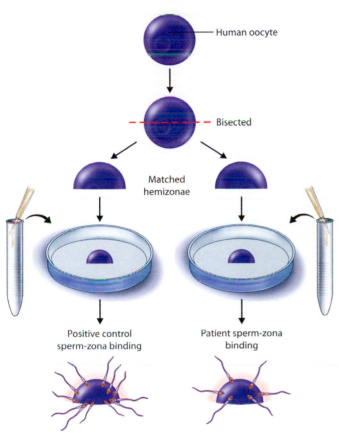

Human oocyte

Bisected

Matched
hemizonae

Positive control
sperm-zona binding

Patient sperm-zona
binding

Figure 8.3: Hemizona assay: The zona pellucida is isolated and divided in half. One-half is incubated with fertile donor sperm (positive control) and the other half is incubated with patient sperm. The ratio of fertile to donor binding is measured

Sperm Penetration Assay

The sperm penetration assay (SPA) tests a sperms ability to undergo capacitation, acrosomal release, fusion and penetration with the oocyte vitelline membrane, and decondensation within the oocyte. The zona pellucida is stripped from a hamster oocyte, which is then incubated with human spermatozoa. The percentage of ova penetrated or average number of sperm penetrations per ovum is used to score the assay, which in limited studies has been shown to correlate with spontaneous pregnancy outcomes[25] and IVF fertilization rates.[26] However, the SPA is hampered by a wide range of sensitivities and specificities,[26] and therefore is not commonly used.

Tests of Spermatozoal Reactive Oxygen Species (ROS)

Human spermatozoa are exquisitely sensitive to damage by ROS.[27] While small amounts of ROS are necessary for the acrosome reaction and capacitation, high levels can overwhelm the limited spermatozoal antioxidant defenses Elevated levels of ROS are detected in the semen of 25–40 percent of infertile men.[27] This excess has been associated with seminal leukocytes,

smoking, varicocele, alcohol, infection, and radiation exposure.[9,28] Functionally, elevated levels of ROS have been correlated with decreased motility, impaired DNA integrity, impaired spontaneous pregnancy rates, and impaired IVF potential.[29]

The chemiluminescent assay is used to directly measure ROS levels within spermatozoa. Luminol or lucigenin probes bind to ROS, including that in leukocytes, seminal fluid, and spermatozoa, are then assessed using a luminometer.[10] The intensity of the signal produced is negatively associated with sperm function,[10,30] and reflects the fertilizing potential of human spermatozoa *in vivo* and *in vitro*.[30] Seminal leukocyte levels are also assessed to determine their contribution to the total ROS.

The ROS levels have been negatively associated with impaired spontaneous,[31] and IVF pregnancy rates.[28] Men with elevated levels of ROS should be considered for antioxidant therapy with vitamins A, C, or E as these agents have been shown to improve semen quality, pregnancy and implantation rates after ICSI.[32] As the full ramifications of oxidative stress on male fertility are still being elucidated, these tests will likely play an expanding role.

Tests of DNA Damage

Excessive ROS levels induce germ cell DNA damage, manifested as DNA fragmentation.[27] While early embryos can repair some spermatozoal DNA damage, there appears to be an upper limit beyond which pregnancy loss occurs.[33] The spermatozoa of infertile men has been shown to possess more DNA damage than fertile counterparts,[33] leading to the suspicion that ROS induced DNA damage may play a role in infertile males. Over 30 assays to assess oxidative stress have been described, which can be largely grouped into direct, indirect, and implied.[27]

Direct assays measure the net sum of ROS production and degradation. Two of the most commonly tests are the lipid peroxidation and 8-oxo-7,8-dihydro-2'-deoxyguanoside (8-OHdG) assays. The former uses sperm cell membrane lipid peroxidation as a surrogate for cell membrane oxidation,[34] and the latter measures levels of 8-OHdG, a byproduct of oxidant induced DNA damage. Also used is the comet assay, in which electrophoresis is applied to fluorochrome-stained spermatozoal DNA,[35] causing the DNA fragments to form a characteristic comet shaped streak, the pattern of which is indicative of DNA fragmentation levels. Another assay is, the sperm chromatin structural assay, which measures sperm DNA susceptibility to acid induced conformational structural changes, as measured using flow cytometry.[36] Finally, the terminal deoxynucleotidyl transferase dUTP nick end labeling (TUNEL) assay (**Figs 8.4A and B**) uses flow cytometry or immunohistochemistry to detect the fragmentation of nuclear chromatin, one of the hallmarks of late stage apoptosis. DNA breaks are tagged with fluorescent-tagged deoxyuridine triphosphate nucleotides (F-dUTP), which binds to exposed 3'-hydroxyl ends, and is then quantified. This can be refined further by also staining for nuclear propidium iodide, which can distinguish sperm from other contaminating cells.[37]

Oxidative damage can also be measured indirectly using the nitroblue tetrazolium assay, in which superoxide radicals within sperm react and become visible under light microscopy. A cutoff value of 30 percent for DNA fragmentation index (DFI) has been

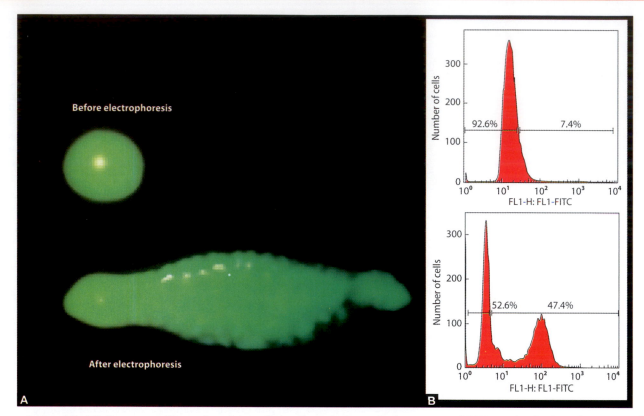

Figures 8.4A and B: (A) Comet assay: Electrophoresis is applied to fluorochrome-stained spermatozoal DNA, causing the DNA fragments to form a characteristic comet shaped streak, the pattern of which is indicative of DNA fragmentation levels, (B) TUNEL assay: DNA breaks are tagged with F-dUTP, which binds to exposed 3'-hydroxyl ends, and is then quantified using flow cytometry. The first frame shows 7.4% damage (negative) and the second shows 47.4% damage (positive)

suggested to correlated with spontaneous, IUI, and IVF pregnancy outcomes.[38]

Approximately 8 percent of subfertile men with normal semen parameters will have high levels of abnormal DNA.[31] Corroborating this, subfertile men have been shown to have abnormal DNA denaturation and fragmentation rates of 25 and 28 percent, respectively, as compared with 10 and 13 percent in fertile men.[33] Oxidative damage in the male germ line has been associated with leukocytospermia, oligoasthenozoospermia,[39] and negatively correlated with sperm concentration, motility, and morphology.[29] With respect to pregnancy, ROS have been linked to impaired preimplantation development, spontaneous abortion, and an increased incidence of disease in the offspring.[27,40] Men with a high percentage of spermatozoa with DNA damage have a reduced potential for natural fertility,[41] and poorer outcomes after IUI, IVF, and ICSI.[42]

At this time, DNA testing is most helpful in cases of unexplained infertility, recurrent pregnancy loss, prognostication of ART outcome, and assessment of genetic integrity in post-chemotherapy patients or those of advanced age. Extensive DNA fragmentation may also suggest the need for testicular sperm extraction, as testicular sperm often have lower levels of DNA fragmentation than ejaculated sperm.[32] Assays of

DNA damage may also be useful in identifying sperm with an optimal quality to be used for ICSI.[27] As DNA testing becomes more standardized, less expensive, more accessible, and more reliable, its role in clinical practice will likely continue to expand.

Microarray Technology

Spermatozoa RNA provides a historical record of spermatogenesis, based on constructs obtained using transcriptional profiling, and these are being investigated as markers of fertility.[43] This technology may be used to investigate the response of cells to conditions that alter mRNA expression,[43] allowing insight into the mechanisms and effects of specific diseases. Microarrays from fertile and infertile men may also allow for the identification of genes which are important for successful fertilization and pregnancy, or biomarkers for infertility. Similarly, comparing transcriptomes at different stages of spermatogenesis, may allow for the identification of genetic aberrations which may provide some insight for couples with recurrent spontaneous abortions.[44] Finally, this technology may have implications for ART, as spermatozoa used for ICSI bypass the bodies natural selection process, and may therefore transmit flawed genes.[44]

Proteomics

Gel electrophoresis is being investigated to identify individual proteins allows from semen samples from fertile men to be compared with infertile men. Currently, seminal fluid has been found to contain 923 proteins, at least 101 of which have an altered expression pattern in infertile men.[45] Examples include protamine 2 precursors, which have been shown to accumulate in some infertile patients,[46] as well as the structural protein, actin, which is altered in asthenozoospermic men.[47] These proteins may prove to be diagnostic markers in understanding some of the pathogenic mechanisms involved in male infertility.

Metabolomics

Metabolites are breakdown products from intracellular metabolic processes which may provide insight into their biochemical precursors.[48] In the evaluation of male infertility, this area may serve as an indirect measure any number of physiologic processes, including oxidative stress by comparing either ROS byproducts or antioxidant levels in fertile and infertile men.[48] The noninvasive nature of this test makes it attractive, and other markers will emerge in the coming years.

High Magnification Microscopy

High magnification microscopy allows for the analysis of sperm morphology at great magnification, up to X8000.[49] As mentioned earlier, the relationship between sperm morphology and pregnancy is not universally predictive. Ultrafine microscopy may be able to detect subtle ultrastructural malformations which are not currently identifiable, which may impact fertilization.[49] Currently this technology is being used to select sperm with the highest morphologic integrity for intracytoplasmic morphologically selected sperm injection (IMSI).[50] In general, the morphologic features most important include the degree of chromatin condensation, which precludes a liability to DNA fragmentation, and nuclear vacuole presence.[49] Studies in which spermatozoa were selected based on high resolution microscopy have demonstrated higher pregnancy rates as compared with conventional ICSI,[50] and the use of this technology in andrology will likely continue to expand.

◼ CONCLUSION

A carefully performed SA remains the cornerstone of the evaluation of male factor infertility. However, there remains a subset of men in which the standard SA is unable to detect an innate functional defect. In these men specialized semen testing may provide insight into the impairment which is preventing fertilization. This may in turn lead to targeted management of a specific defect. Emerging technologies will likely to incorporate an increasing amount of genetic testing, as well as non-invasive testing using biomarkers. These tests will likely hold promise in the continued advancement toward the diagnosis and management of the multitude of causes for male infertility. Finally, with the increasing use of ICSI, which bypasses many of the sperm requirements for egg fertilization, more commonly used tests will be those that select for the optimal spermatozoa lead to a successful pregnancy with IVF or ICSI.

◼ REFERENCES

1. Bonde JP, Ernst E, Jensen TK, Hjollund NH, Kolstad H, Henriksen TB, et al. Relation between semen quality and fertility: a population-based study of 430 first-pregnancy planners. Lancet 1998;352(9135):1172-7.
2. Guzick DS, Overstreet JW, Factor-Litvak P, Brazil CK, Nakajima ST, Coutifaris C, et al. Sperm morphology, motility, and concentration in fertile and infertile men. N Engl J Med 2001;345(19):1388-93.
3. McLachlan RI, Baker HW, Clarke GN, Harrison KL, Matson PL, Holden CA, et al. Semen analysis: its place in modern reproductive medical practice. Pathology 2003;35(1):25-33.
4. Aitken RJ. Sperm function tests and fertility. Int J Androl 2006;29(1):69-75; discussion 105-8.
5. Mortimer ST. CASA--practical aspects. J Androl 2000;21(4):515-24.
6. Macleod IC, Irvine DS. The predictive value of computer-assisted semen analysis in the context of a donor insemination programme. Hum Reprod 1995;10(3):580-6.
7. Wilcox AJ, Weinberg CR, Baird DD. Timing of sexual intercourse in relation to ovulation. Effects on the probability of conception, survival of the pregnancy, and sex of the baby. N Engl J Med 1995;333(23):1517-21.
8. WHO laboratory manual for the examination and processing of human semen. 5 edn. Geneva, Switzerland: World Health Organization, 2009.
9. Sigman M, Baazeem A, Zini A. Semen analysis and sperm function assays: what do they mean? Semin Reprod Med 2009;27(2):115-23.
10. Athayde KS, Cocuzza M, Agarwal A, Krajcir N, Lucon AM, Srougi M, et al. Development of normal reference values for seminal reactive oxygen species and their correlation with leukocytes and semen parameters in a fertile population. J Androl 2007;28(4):613-20.
11. Keck C, Gerber-Schafer C, Clad A, Wilhelm C, Breckwoldt M. Seminal tract infections: impact on male fertility and treatment options. Hum Reprod Update 1998;4(6):891-903.
12. Munuce MJ, Berta CL, Pauluzzi F, Caille AM. Relationship between antisperm antibodies, sperm movement, and semen quality. Urol Int 2000;65(4):200-3.
13. Bohring C, Krause W. Immune infertility: towards a better understanding of sperm (auto)-immunity. The value of proteomic analysis. Hum Reprod 2003;18(5):915-24.
14. Chiu WW, Chamley LW. Clinical associations and mechanisms of action of antisperm antibodies. Fertil Steril 2004;82(3):529-35.
15. Andrade-Rocha FT. Semen analysis in laboratory practice: an overview of routine tests. J Clin Lab Anal 2003;17(6):247-58.
16. Comhaire F, Mahmoud A, Schoonjans F, Kint J. Why do we continue to determine alpha-glucosidase in human semen? Andrologia 2002;34(1):8-10.
17. Sigman M, Glass S, Campagnone J, Pryor JL. Carnitine for the treatment of idiopathic asthenospermia: a randomized, double-blind, placebo-controlled trial. Fertil Steril 2006;85(5):1409-14.

specific sperm function test or test series that may be essential for a subject. A large number of SFT have been developed and reported in literature. A select few of such tests of high clinical relevance are illustrated bellow.[2,6,10,15,44,48,56,60,62,68,72,75,76]

Stress Tolerance

Idea of a sperm stress test was first proposed by Alvarez et al in 1996.[4] Concept behind this is that spermatozoa may face some physiological stress such as temperature, pH, or osmolarity fluctuations during the course of meeting their counterpart, oocyte. Sperm that handle such stress well can be considered better prepared to make fertilization happen either *in vivo* or *in vitro*. Spermatozoa derived from different individuals may exhibit different levels of stress tolerance. Stress tolerance values of sperm samples of previously proven fertile males can be used as a control in assessing the stress handling capabilities of sperm under investigation.

Alvarez et al and several others documented the poor stress tolerance of a sperm population having dual negative impacts. First, sperm failing in stress tolerance may also fail to penetrate the external barrier (zona pellucida) of egg due to their poor vigor. Secondly, sperm with inferior stress handling ability may lose motility and die. If such sperm accumulate in large quantities surrounding an oocyte, they may contribute to creating an unhealthy micro environment for the oocyte. In Alvarez's proposed stress test, sperm are exposed briefly to elevated temperature and purportedly shows different subsets of sperm exhibiting motility of different grades. They proposed that relative abundance of sperm of different degrees of stress tolerance (as reflected in motility) in a sperm sample may have clinical significance.[2,4,31,56,71]

Sperm Longevity

Fertile life of a spermatozoon can be measured by the duration of it's motility. If spermatozoa prematurely lose motility, they also lose their natural fertilization potential since they cannot travel to meet oocyte. Therefore, how long sperm can sustain its motility is important to investigate. Some investigators think that longevity assessment may provide a valuable insight into the potential etiology of male infertility. Sperm longevity can be assessed using washed sperm maintained in culture. Some investigators have predicted higher fertilization potential of sperm exhibiting longer motility duration in culture. Unfortunately, no defined sperm longevity assessment assay has yet been established that could be amenable to routine use in a diagnostic andrology laboratory.[31,39,53,54,56]

Membrane Integrity

Integrity of sperm membrane assures the longevity of spermatozoa. Sperm possessing a weaker membrane may fail the task of fertilization by failing to reach oocyte due to motility loss owing to premature membrane integrity failure. Sperm membrane quality determines the osmoregulatory ability of spermatozoa. A simple test called hypo-osmotic swelling test (HOS-test), introduced by Jeyendran et al in 1984,[45] to assess membrane

integrity, got wide acceptance in human andrology laboratories. HOS-test in fact measures the sperm osmotic fragility. Live spermatozoa with a normal healthy membrane are able to withstand moderate hypo-osmotic stress and swell upon exposure to hypo-osmotic solution. Dead sperm, on other hand, whose plasma membranes are no longer intact, do not swell. Instead, they let solution pass through. In addition, dead sperm that still retain intact membranes as well as senescent spermatozoa with poor osmoregulatory capacity show uncontrolled swelling that rapidly results in rupture of over distended plasma membrane.[6,45,56]

World health organization (WHO) included HOS-test as a sperm function test in its laboratory manual for examination of human semen. This is most likely due to its procedural simplicity. A hypo-osmotic swelling solution is prepared for HOS-test by dissolving 0.735 g sodium citrate and fructose in 1 liter of distilled water. According to WHO (4th edition), HOS test is considered to be normal for a semen sample if more than 60 percent of spermatozoa undergo tail swelling indicating an intact membrane. If less than 50 percent of spermatozoa show tail swelling, the semen specimen is considered abnormal.[6,45,56,72,73]

Acrosome Reaction

For successful invasion of zona pellucida of oocyte, acrosome of sperm head must be functional. Functional site of physiological acrosome reaction is the zona pellucida. It is understood that after binding with zona, sperm releases acrosomal enzyme which helps penetration through zona. Acrosomal morphology is considered to be related to successful or unsuccessful invasion of sperm through the zona pellucida. In the assessment of acrosome reaction, acrosome dysfunction is identified. In this assessment, presence of outer acrosomal membrane, acrosomal contents, and inner acrosomal membrane are evaluated by employing various staining methods using a light or fluorescence microscope. Flow cytometry is also used to examine acrosome. In flow cytometry, fluorescent-labelled lectins and antibodies are applied to visualize different components of the acrosome. Calcium ionophores or progesterone are used for evaluating the competence of spermatozoa to initiate acrosome reactions. Acrosome assessment is specially recommended in cases of abnormal head morphology.[2,10,45,47,48,56,60,65,73,74]

Sperm-Cervical Mucus Interaction

Interactions between sperm and cervical mucus have been studied and reported under different title headings. Postcoital test, sperm-mucus interaction, mucus penetration test and *in vitro* sperm-mucus interaction are some notable examples. Sperm-cervical mucus interaction tests have also been designated by individual researcher's name such as Kremer test, Kurzrok-Miller test. Cervical mucus is considered as the doorway which the sperm have to pass through to get access into internal reproductive tract. Cervical mucus is a hydrogel, that by controlling its viscosity, can regulate the entrance of sperm into reproductive tract. In other words, cervical mucus can be hostile to sperm at times while favorable to them at others. Similarly, some sperm population may be better fit to pass through mucus compared to others. Therefore, in sperm-cervical mucus interaction studies, ability of sperm to penetrate cervical mucus is assessed in order to predict whether the sperm population under investigation has potential power to pass through the reproductive gate (cervix). Cervical mucus works as a biological gate of reproductive tract by providing favorable receptivity to sperm penetration at or near ovulation while interfering with entry at other times in each menstrual period.[2,56,60,73]

Cervical mucus is a heterogenous secretion which contains more than 90 percent water, a large portion of which is bound with the matrix of mucin. Two ovarian hormones regulate secretion and constituents of cervical mucus. Estradiol (estrogens) stimulates mucus production while progesterone (progestrogens) inhibits. Therefore, in a menstrual cycle, the amount and consistency of cervical mucus varies with the different phases (follicular, ovulatory, luteal) of the cycle.[23,48,65,70]

In sperm-mucus interaction studies, the relative ability of different sperm samples passing the cervical mucus are assessed as possible cause(s) of infertility. The purpose of post coital test (PCT) is to determine the number of spermatozoa in cervical mucus, as well as their survival and behavior during the hours after coitus. In a test like PCT, cervical mucus is examined 2–8 hours after intercourse. American Society of Reproductive Medicine (ASRM) specifically recommends PCT for males having hyperviscous semen, low volume semen, and unexplained infertility.[2,10,56,60,70,73]

In *in vitro* cervical mucus penetration assay, a detail assessment of sperm-cervical mucus interaction may be undertaken. When performing such tests, use of fresh semen no older than one hour post ejaculation is recommended. Mortimer[56] suggested that semen samples are liquefied 30 minutes post-ejaculation, which is an ideal standard starting time. According to WIIO,[72,73] when there are difficulties in obtaining human cervical mucus, bovine estrus mucus provides a suitable alternative. One of the advantages of the *in vitro* interaction assay is that it allows detection of possible presence of antisperm antibody in either semen or cervical mucus. It should be pointed out that since antisperm antibodies in cervical mucus are locally secreted they may not be easily detected by analyzing female serum. When a positive antisperm antibody test is obtained using husband's semen and wife's mucus, a crossover test using donor semen and donor mucus is required to confirm whether the antibodies are in semen or in cervical mucus.[30,58,72]

Cervical mucus is collected from exocervical and endocervical canal. It can be aspirated with a tuberculin syringe (of course without needle), pipette, polyethylene tube, catheter or specially designed forceps. It is preferable to conduct the test with fresh mucus. Mucus can be preserved in a refrigerator for a period of up to five days but the issue of dehydration should be taken into consideration. Use of frozen-thawed mucus is highly discouraged.

In evaluating cervical environment, mucus is assessed for its volume, consistency, ferning, spinnbarkeit, cellularity and pH. A grading system of mucus quality was first proposed by Insler et al in 1972[72,73] considering five parameters. Later on mucus cellularity was added to grading system.

Sperm-Zona Pellucida Binding and Penetration

Once spermatozoa manage to reach the vicinity of oocyte, they need to have ability to successfully interact with zona pelucida of oocyte so that they can penetrate into ooplasm for forming pronucleus. This particular aspect of the spermatozoa's potential is evaluated by studying sperm-zona pellucida binding and penetration. Binding of sperm to zona pellucida leads to initiation of acrosome reaction, release of lytic acrosomal components and penetration through the zona matrix. Sperm fuses with outer sheath of zona and releases acrosomal enzyme which makes it's penetration easier through zona pellucida. There are several ways, reported in literature, to assess the ability of sperm penetrating zona. Considering the significance of species specificity issue, direct assessment of interactions between human spermatozoa and human zona pellucida is essential. For sperm-zona binding tests (ZBT), human oocytes from pathological specimen, discarded ovaries or spare oocytes from IVF cycles can be used. However, proper consent and institutional approval must be obtained. Complete failure of binding sperm to the zona of a particular oocyte may indicate abnormality either of sperm or of oocyte.

Incorporation of an adequate control is essential for a valid ZBT. In some ZBT like hemizona assay (HZA), zona is divided into equal halves and exposure of each half is made to equal concentration of test (patient) and control (fertile) sperm. Alternatively, patient and control sperm populations can be labeled with dye (fluorochromes) and then mixed for testing in binding to the same intact zona. In this case, a few or no sperm of patient bound to zona compared to binding of control sperm usually indicates a sperm defect in the patient.

There will always be practical problem of getting fresh human zona pellucida. To circumvent this difficulty, some have come forward with idea of cryopreserving or storing zona in salt solution. Literatures show that zona stored in such ways preserve the functional capacity in binding spermatozoa.[56] Some laboratories may have access to spare uninseminated oocytes (with proper concept and institutional approval) but others may not have such opportunity. To overcome this obstacle, obtaining zona from ovarian tissue either during gynecological surgery or postmortem can be an option but still requires proper approval.[48,55,56,65]

Sperm Maturity

The concepts of sperm maturity in fertilization and subsequent developmental consequences have been emphasized by many investigators. Developmentally immature sperm are incompetent in taking part in fertilization though they are able to meet oocyte. Even fertilization by immature sperm occurs; it may result in poor embryonic development, decreased implantation, lower pregnancy rates, and recurrent pregnancy losses. According to a Yale group of investigators, mature and immature sperm are different with respect to morphological and morphometric attributes, creatine kinase, HspA2 level, chromosomal aneuploides, DNA degradation, zona pellucida binding properties and more. Studies show that during spermiogenesis, sperm plasma membrane undergoes a maturation-related transformation

2. Agarwal A, Bragais F, Sabanegh E. Assessing sperm function. Urol Clin N Am 2008;35:157-71.

3. Agarwal A, Said T. Role of sperm chromatin abnormalities and DNA damage in male infertility. Hum Reprod Update 2003;9(4):331-45.

4. Alvarez J, Minaretzis D, Barrett C, Mortola J, Thompson I. The sperm stress test: a novel test that predicts pregnancy in assisted reproductive technologies. Fertil Steril 1996;65:400-5.

5. American Association of Bioanalyst (AAB): www.aab-pts.org/statistical-summaries.

6. Anzer M, Kroefsch T, Buhr M. Comparison of different methods for assessments of sperm concentration and membrane integrity with bull semen. J Androl 2009;30:661-8.

7. Balhorn R, Reed S, Tanphaichitr N. Aberrant protamine 1/protamine 2 ratios in sperm of infertile human males. Experientia 1988;44:52-5.

8. Bavister B, Andrews J. A rapid sperm motility bioassay procedure for quality-control testing of water and culture media. J In Vitro Fert and Embryo Trans 1988;2:67-72.

9. Bavister B. The effect of variations in culture conditions on the motility of hamster spermatozoa. J Reprod and Fert 1974;38:431-40.

10. Bjorndhal L, Giwercman A, Touurnaye H, Weidner W. Clinical Andrology: EAU/ESAU Course Guidelines. 444 pages, 1st edn., Informa Healthcare, 2010.

11. Brackett N, Ibrahim E, Grotas J, Lynne C. Higher sperm DNA damage in semen from man with spinal cord injuries compared with controls. J Androl 2008;29:93-9.

12. Bungum M, et al. Sperm DNA integrity assessment in prediction of assisted reproduction technology outcome. Hum Reprod 2007;22(1):174-9.

13. Carrell D. The clinical implementation of sperm chromosome aneuploidy testing: Pitfalls and Promises. J Androl 2008;29:124-33.

14. Carrell D, Liu L, Peterson C, Jones K, Hatasaka H, Erickson L. Sperm DNA fragmentation is increased in couples with unexplained recurrent pregnancy loss. Arch Androl 2003;49:49-55.

15. Check J, Check M, Katsoff D. Prognosis for sperm fertilizability: analysis of different variables in men. Arch Androl 2002;48(1):73-83.

16. Chohan K, Griffin J, Lafromboise M, DeJonge C, Carrell D. Comparison of cromatin assays for DNA fragmentation evaluation in human sperm. J Androl 2006;27:53-59.

17. Claassens O, Wehr J, Harrison K. Optimizing sensitivity of the human sperm motility assay for embryo toxicity testing. Hum Reprod 2000;15(7):1586-91.

18. Corson S, et al. The human sperm–hamster egg penetration assay: prognostic value. Fertil Steril 1988;49(2):328-34.

19. Critchlow J, Matson P, Newman M. et al. Quality control in an in vitro fertilization laboratory: use of human sperm survival studies. Hum Reprod 1989;4(5):545-9.

20. Davidson A, Vermesh M, Lobo R, Paulson R. Mouse embryo culture as quality control for human in vitro fertilization: the one-cell versus the two-cell model. Fertil Steril 1989;49(3):516-21.

21. DeJonge C, Centola G, Reed M, et al. Human sperm survival assay as a bioassay for the assisted reproductive technologies laboratory, J Androl 2003;24:16-8.

22. Edwards R, Steptoe P. A matter of life: A medical break through. Hutchinson, London 1980.pp.1-234.

23. Edwards R, Stepto P, Purdy J. Establishing full-term human pregnancies using cleaving embryos grown in vitro. Br J Obstet and Gynaecol 1980;87(9):737-56.

24. Ergur A, Dokras A, Giraldo J, et al. Sperm maturity and treatment choice of IVF or ICSI: Diminished sperm HspA2 chaperone levels predict IVF failure. Fertil Steril 2002;77:910-8.

25. Evenson D, Wixon R. Meta-analysis of sperm DNA fragmentation using the sperm chromatin structure assay. Reprod Biomed Online 2006;12(4):466-72.

26. Evenson D, Larson K, Jost L. Sperm chromatin structure assay: its clinical use for detecting sperm DNA fragmentation in male infertility and comparisons with other techniques. J Androl 2002;23(1):25-43.

27. Evenson D, Wixon R. Clinical aspects of sperm DNA fragmentation detection and male infertility. Theriogenology 2006;65:979-91.

28. Evenson D, Darzynkiewicz Z, Melamed M. Relation of mammalian sperm chromatin heterogeneity to fertility. Science 1980;210:1131-3.

29. Fleetham J, Pattinson H, Mortimer D. The mouse embryo culture system: improving the sensitivity for use as a quality control assay for human in vitro fertilization. Fertil Steril 1993;59:192-6.

30. Francavilla F, et al. Naturally occurring antisperm antibodies in men: interference with fertility and clinical implications. An update. Front Biosci 2007;12:2890-2911.

31. Franco J, Mauri A, Petersen C, Baruffi R, Oliveria J. Efficacy of the sperm survival test for the prediction of oocyte fertilization in culture. Hum Reprod 1994;8:916-8.

32. Gardner D, Reed L, Linck D, Sheehan C, Lane M. Quality control in human in vitro fertilization. Seminar in Reprod Med 2005;23:319-24.

33. Gil-Villa A, Cardona W, Agarwal A, Sharma R, Cadavid A. Assessment of sperm factors possibly involved in early recurrent pregnancy loss. Fertil Steril 2010;94:1465-72.

34. Handelsman D, Swerdloff R. Male gonadal dysfunction. Clinics in Endocrinology and Metabolism 1985;14:89-124.

35. Hinsch E, Ponce A, Hedrich A, Hinsch K. A new combined in vitro test model for the identification of substances affecting essential sperm functions, Hum Reprod 1991;12:1673-81.

36. Hong C, Chaput D, Turner P. A simple method to measure drug effects on human spermatozoa motility. Br Clin Pharm 1981;11:385-7.

37. Hossain A, Helvacioglu A, Huff C, Yeoman R, Aksel S. Pattern of changes in motility, vitality and morphology of human sperm in different in vitro segments of the ejaculate. Mol Androl 1995;7(1):13-20.

38. Hossain A, Huff C, Helvacioglo A, Thorneycroft I. Human sperm bioassay has potential in evaluating the quality of cumulus oocyte complexes. Arch Androl 1996;37:7-10.

39. Hossain A, Osuampke C, Nagamani M. Extended culture of human spermatozoa in the laboratory may have practical value in the assisted reproductive procedures. Fertil Steril 2008;89(1):237-9.

40. Hossain A, Osuampke C, Phelps J. Spontaneously developed tail swelling (SDTS) influences the accuracy of the hypo-osmotic swelling test (HOS-test) in determining membrane integrity and viability of human spermatozoa. JARG 2010;27(2):83-5.

41. Hossain A, Subhash A, Osuampke C, Phelps J. Human sperm bioassay for reprotoxicity testing in embryo culture media: some

practical considerations in reducing the assay time. Advances in Urology, 2010.

42. Huszar G, Ozenci C, Cayli S, Hansch E, Vigue L. Hyaluronic acid binding by human sperm indicates cellular maturity, viability, and unreacted acrosomal status. Fertil Steril 2003;79:1616-24.

43. Huszar G, Ozkavukcu S, Jakab A, Sati L, Cayli S. Hyaluronic acid binding ability of human sperm reflects cellular maturity and fertilizing potential: selection of sperm for intracytoplasmic sperm injection. Current Opinion in Obstetrics and Gynecology 2006;18:260-7.

44. Jequier AM. Male infertility: A guide for the clinician. Blackwell Science Ltd, London pages 2000.pp.67-76.

45. Jeyendran R, Van der Ven H, Perez M, Crabo B, Zaneveld L. Development of an assay to assess the functional integrity of the human sperm membrane and its relationship to the other semen characteristics. J Reprod Fertil 1984;70:219-28.

46. Jouannet P, et al. Male factors and the likelihood of pregnancy in infertile couples I. Study of sperm characteristics. Int J Androl 1988;11(5):379-94.

47. Langlois M, et al. Discrepancy between sperm acrosin activity and sperm morphology: significance for fertilization *in vitro*. Clin Chim Acta 2005;351:121-9.

48. Lars B, Mortimer D, Barrat C, Castilla J, Menkveld R, Kvist U, Alveraz J, Haugen T. A practical guide to basic laboratory andrology. Cambridge University Press, New York, 1st edn., 2010.

49. Li Z, et al. Correlation of sperm DNA damage with IVF and ICSI outcomes: a systematic review and meta-analysis. J Assist Reprod Genet 2006;23(9-10):367-76.

50. Liu Y, Baker H. Assessment of human sperm function and clinical management of male infertility. Zhonghua Nan Ke Xue 2007;13(2):99-109.

51. Meeker J, Singh N, Hauser R. Serum concentrations of E2 and free T4 are inversely correlated with sperm DNA damage in man from an infertility clinic. J Androl 2008;29:379-88.

52. Miller J, Morgan K, McAlister A, Freeman M. A comparison between the human sperm bioassay and the mouse embryo bioassay. Fertil and Steril 2001;76:104-5.

53. Monsour R, Aboulghar M, Serouri G, et al. The life span of sperm motility and pattern in cumulus coculture. Fertil Steril 1995;63: 660-2.

54. Morimoto Y, Hayashi E, Ohno T, Kanzaki H. Quality control of human IVF/ ICSI program using endotoxin measurements and sperm survival test. Human Cell 1997;10:271-6.

55. Mortimer D, Mortimer S. Quality and risk management in the IVF laboratory. Cambridge University Press, Cambridge, 1 edn. 240 pages, 2005.

56. Mortimer D. Practical laboratory andrology. 1st edn, 393 pages, Oxford University Press, Oxford, 1994.

57. Mortimer D. The essential partnership between diagnostic andrology and modern assisted reproductive technologies. Hum Reprod 1994;9(7):1209-13.

58. Munuce M, et al. Relationship between antisperm antibodies, sperm movement, and semen quality. Urol Int 2000;65(4):200-3.

59. Nallella K, et al. Significance of sperm characteristics in the evaluation of male infertility. Fertil Steril 2006;85:629-34.

60. Nieschlag E, Behre H, Nieschlag S. Andrology: male reproductive health and dysfunction. 3rd edn, 629 pages, Springer, New York, 2009.

61. Nijs M, Franssen K, Cox A, Wissmann D, Ruis H, Ombelet W. Reprotoxicity of intrauterine insemination and *in vitro* fertilization-embryo transfer disposables and products: a 4-year survey, Fertil Steril 2009;92(2):527-35.

62. Oehninger S, et al. Sperm function assays and their predictive value for fertilization outcome in IVF therapy: a meta-analysis. Hum Reprod Update 2000;6(2):160-8.

63. Quinn P, Keel B, Serafy N, et al. Results of the American Association of Bioanalysts (AAB) embryology proficiency testing (PT) program, Fertil Steril 1998;70:S100(O-267).

64. Rinehart J, Bavister B, Gerrity M. Quality control in the *in vitro* fertilization laboratory: comparison of bioassay systems for water quality, J *In Vitro* Fert and Embr Trans 1988;5:335-42.

65. Rogers B. The sperm penetration assay: its usefulness reevaluated. Fertil Steril 1985;43:821-40.

66. Seli E, Sakkas D. Spermatozoal nuclear determinants of reproductive outcome: implications for ART. Hum Reprod Update 2005;11:337-49.

67. Sharma R, Said T, Agarwal A. Sperm DNA damage and its clinical relevance in assessing reproductive outcome. Asian J Androl 2004;6(2):139-48.

68. The American Society of Andrology. Handbook of Andrology. Second edn, 2010.

69. Van den A, Vitrier S, Lebrun F, Van Steirteghem A. Optimized bioassays for the detection of embryology contaminants. Hum Reprod 1999;14:205-6.

70. Van der Steeg J, et al. Should the postcoital test (PCT) be part of the routine fertility work-up? Hum Reprod 2004;19:1373-9.

71. Veeck L. Enhancing sperm fertilizing capacity *in vitro*: indications and limitations. ACTA Europaea Fertilitatis 1993;24:267-75.

72. World Health Organization (WHO). Laboratory manual for the examination and processing of human semen. Fifth edn. 271 pages, Switzerland, 2010.

73. World Health Organization (WHO). WHO laboratory manual for the examination of human semen and sperm-cervical mucus interaction. Fourth edn, Cambridge University Press 1999 pp.128.

74. Xu S, Zhan B. Analysis of relationship between semen quality and sperm acrosin activity. Zhonghua Nan Ke Xue 2006;12(5): 438-40.

75. Zini A, Sigman M. Are tests of sperm DNA damage clinically useful? Pros and Cons. J Androl 2009;30:219-29.

76. Zini A, Libman J. Sperm DNA damage: importance in the era of assisted reproduction. Curr Opin Urol 2006;16(6):428-34.

recently available data suggest that men with incidental findings of testicular microlithiasis but who have otherwise normal testes have no increased risk of developing testicular cancer and for them no form of regular surveillance is required.[15] There is a developing consensus that regular self-examination is recommended in men at high-risk of developing testicular cancer, including infertile men with bilateral microlithiasis and men with history of cryptorchidism or history of contralateral testicular tumor.[12,15,16]

Hydrocele: A hydrocele is the accumulation of an abnormally large amount of serous fluid between the two layers of the tunica vaginalis (**Fig. 11.9**). The accumulation of a limited amount of fluid is found in as many as 65 percent of men and is bilateral in 10 percent cases. Hydroceles may be primary (idiopathic) or secondary to other scrotal disease process. A hydrocele may be communicating with peritoneal cavity in which case it becomes be smaller in size on pressing on the testis or larger on standing up. Non-communicating hydrocele remains of the same size in any position.

Cryptorchidism (Undescended testicles): In cryptorchidism one or both testes are not found in the scrotum but are located somewhere along the course of testicular descent which stretches

between the lower pole of the kidney and the external inguinal ring. By far the inguinal canal is the most common place where undescended testes are found (75–80% of cases). Ultrasound scanning is utilized to locate the testicle in the inguinal canal and to evaluate its size and the appearance of its parenchyma. There is up to a 50 times higher frequency of carcinoma in undescended testes compared to orthotopic testes.[11] Generally, the malignancy rate correlates with increasing distance of the testis from the scrotum; thus, malignant change is six times more common in the abdominal testis than in the inguinal testis.[17] It is reported that 10 percent of all testicular neoplasms occur in undescended testes or in testes treated for cryptorchidism.

Abnormalities of the Epididymis

Epididymal cysts: Epididymal cysts can be single or multiple simple cysts, very tiny in size (1–2 mm) but occasionally larger. These cysts are more commonly found in the head compared to the body and tail and do not contain sperm (**Fig. 11.4**) They may cause anxiety because of abnormal palpation although they are painless. They are reported in as many as 70 percent of men who undergo scrotal US.

Spermatoceles: Spermatocele are benign cysts arising from the epididymis and may vary in size between a few millimeters to several centimetres (**Fig. 11.10**). Unlike the simple epididymal cysts, spermatoceles contain nonviable sperm. A spermatocele is most often incidentally noted by a patient or detected during a physical examination. Most spermatoceles are located within the epididymal head and palpated above the testicle. They are usually asymptomatic. They may originate as diverticuli from the epididymis or rete testis and may also be caused by epididymal scarring and obstruction caused by infection or physical trauma to the testis.[18] Ultrasonically, these cysts have internal echoes because of the presence on nonviable sperm. For the same reason the "falling snow" sign was recently described when color Doppler sonography is used to evaluate spermatocele.[19]

Obstructive azoospermia: Ultrasonographic abnormalities of the epididymis are significantly higher in obstructive azoospermia compared to nonobstructive azoospermia[20] and may include

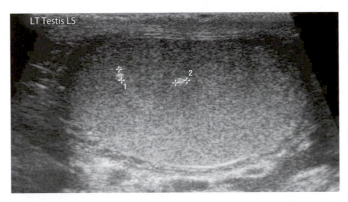

Figure 11.8: Testicular microlithiasis appears as 1–2 mm diameter hyperechoic foci that are randomly distributed

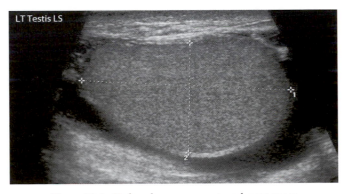

Figure 11.9: Hydrocele appears as a translucent space surrounding the testis

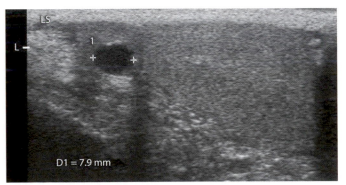

Figure 11.10: Spermatocele is seen in the region of the epididymal head

partial or complete absence of the epididymis. Obstruction in the rete testis secondary to trauma or inflammation may lead to a tapering appearance of the whole of the epididymis. A tapering epididymal body with absent epididymal tail may also indicate proximal obstruction in the epididymis. Equally, absent or atrophic distal portion of the epididymis may noted in azoospermic men diagnosed with combined bilateral absence of the vas deferens.[21] However, acquired obstruction of the vas deferens may be associated with epididymal dilatation (**Fig. 11.11**). The presence of a mass-like enlargement of any of the three epididymal regions caused by inflammation may by itself explain the cause of obstructive azoospermia. In cases of inflammatory-associated obstruction, cystic changes in the rete testis may be seen on ultrasound scanning, usually in association with epididymal obstruction.[22]

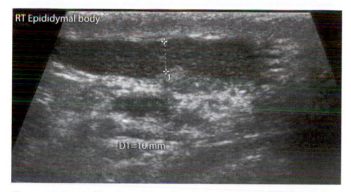

Figure 11.11: A dilated epididymal body is suggestive of acquired distal (Vas deferens) obstruction

Varicocele

It is estimated that 15 percent of men have idiopathic varicocele and this incidence increase to 37 percent in patients with subfertility. Thus, the majority of men with varicoceles are still fertile. Varicoceles are commonly found on the left side and are bilateral in up to 30 percent of patients. The varicocele is idiopathic when it is not related to the presence of a mechanical venous obstruction such as renal masses or other retroperitoneal tumors.

Clinical varicoceles are diagnosed by physical examination and classified into three grades.[23] Grade 1 varicoceles are small and palpable only with the Valsalva maneuver due to the engorgement and the expansion of the pampiniform plexus. Grade 2 varicoceles are moderate in size and are palpable without the Valsalva maneuver. Grade 3 varicoceles are large and visible through the scrotal skin, and are often described as a "bag of worms". Subclinical varicocele is not recognized on palpation and may only be detectable by ultrasonography. It has been demonstrated that spermatic veins become clinically palpable when their diameter in grayscale ultrasonography (**Figs 11.12A and B**) exceeded 2 mm.[24] However, other studies have challenged the relationship between the diagnosis of subclinical varicocele and semen quality by demonstrating that the upper limit of spermatic veins diameters in healthy normozoospermic men with normal scrotal palpation reach 3.8 mn.[25]

The size of the spermatic veins aside, the presence of reversed venous flow (reflux) with Valsalva on color Doppler ultrasound is deemed essential to the diagnosis of a varicocele (**Figs 11.13A and B**). Once again there are studies that have demonstrated reversal of flow in varicoceles diagnosed in healthy men with normal sperm parameters.[26] Nevertheless, there is a consensus

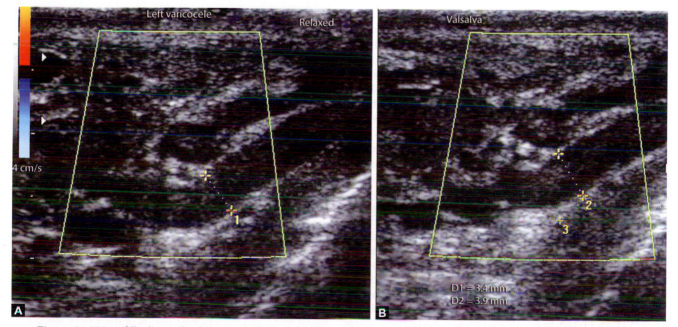

Figures 11.12A and B: Grayscale ultrasonography is used in the assessment of varicocele to demonstrate an increase in veins diameter during Valsalva maneuver

■ VASOGRAPHY

Indications

Vasography remains the definitive test for assessing the patency of the male ductal system. While procedures such as TRUS and seminal vesiculography described above offer minimally invasive imaging, vasography provides unequalled anatomic detail of the vas deferens, seminal vesicles, and ejaculatory ducts. It is indicated for precise anatomic localization of ductal obstruction in the azoospermic patient with confirmed normal spermatogenesis on testicular biopsy. In one of the largest series on vasography in the evaluation for male infertility, Payne et al noted that 92 percent of subfertile men had normal vasograms, including 90 percent of men with azoospermia.[41] It is also occasionally utilized for the severely oligospermic patient in whom there is high suspicion for a unilateral vasal obstruction from iatrogenic injury such as prior inguinal hernia repair.[42] Vasography is also indicated for patients with ejaculatory pain to rule out occult ejaculatory duct obstruction.

Technique

Vasography should be performed at the time of anticipated surgical reconstruction due to the potential for focal vasal scarring postprocedure although this has not been observed in a large series.[42] While vasography can be performed in either a retrograde or antegrade fashion, most reproductive surgeons prefer the antegrade approach to avoid the potential risk of epididymal injury from retrograde flow. For antegrade vasography, a straight portion of the vas deferens is isolated immediately adjacent to the convoluted area, taking great care to avoid interruption of the vassal blood supply. Vasography may be performed either via a puncture or vasotomy technique (**Fig. 11.16**). The puncture method offers advantages since it avoids a full thickness vasal incision and the subsequent need for microsurgical repair. Utilizing a 30-gauge lymphangiogram need, the vasal lumen is entered by direct puncture. Alternatively, the vasotomy utilizes a microsurgical scalpel under loupe or operating microscope magnification to perform a hemi-vasotomy incision through the anterior vasal wall to expose the lumen. A 25-gauge or small angiocatheter is used to cannulate the lumen and perform the vasogram. Once the vasal lumen has been intubated, 5–10 cc or radiographic contrast is injected with subsequent static X-ray images or fluoroscopy. In suspected EDO, methylene blue or indigo carmine may be mixed with the radiographic contrast to allow cystoscopic confirmation of patency during a transurethral resection of the ejaculatory duct. If a hemi-vasotomy incision is utilized, vasal reconstruction should be performed with standard microsurgical technique.

Findings

A normal vasogram will allow visualization of the scrotal and inguinal sections of the vas deferens with subsequent filling of the ipsilateral seminal vesicle and the bladder (**Fig. 11.17**). Lack of contrast in the bladder may be due to insufficient injection of contrast or in fact, evidence of obstruction. With patients who have a history of an inguinal hernia repair, obstruction when present is usually at the level of the internal inguinal ring, showing a sharp cutoff of contrast in the region of the prior repair

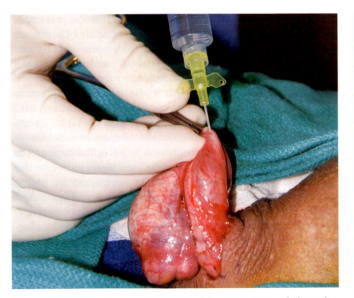

Figure 11.16: Vasogram technique: Vasal lumen is exposed through a hemi-vasotomy incision through the anterior vasal wall. A 25-gauge angiocatheter is used to cannulate the lumen and perform the vasogram. 5–10 cc or radiographic contrast is injected with subsequent static X-ray images or fluoroscopy

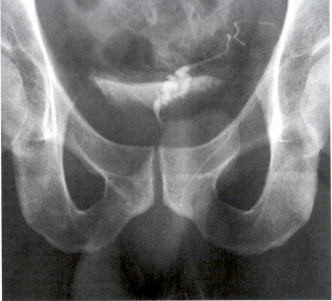

Figure 11.17: Normal vasogram: Vasogram demonstrating complete visualization of scrotal, inguinal, and retroperitoneal vas deferens, seminal vesicle with contrast spill into bladder

(**Fig. 11.18**). With complete EDO, vasography demonstrates a dilated seminal vesicle and/or ejaculatory duct (**Fig. 11.19**) with lack of contrast in the bladder. If some contrast enters the bladder but injection pressure into the vas is higher than normal, one should be suspicious for partial EDO as described previously. Filling of a congenital midline cyst may be quite large and can be misinterpreted as contrast flow into the bladder.

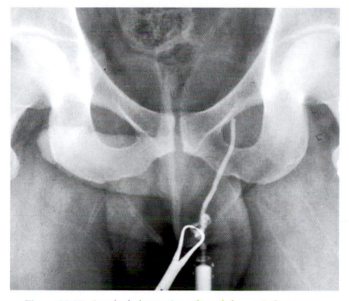

Figure 11.18: Inguinal obstruction of vas deferens: Left vasogram demonstrating complete obstruction in the inguinal vas deferens

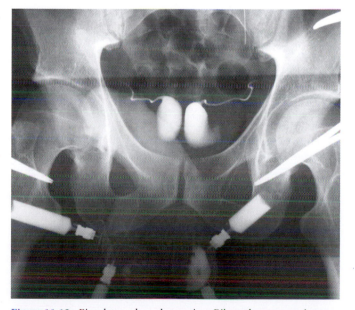

Figure 11.19: Ejaculatory duct obstruction: Bilateral vasograms in azoospermic man with large bilateral ejaculatory duct cysts and no contrast visualization in bladder

VENOGRAPHY

Venograms of the internal spermatic veins have been described for the diagnosis and embolization treatment of scrotal varicoceles. From a diagnostic aspect, venography is arguably the most sensitive imaging modality but test specificity remains problematic. While nearly all clinical varicocele patients will have demonstrated venous reflux on venographic examination, left internal spermatic vein reflux occurs in up to 70 percent of patients without palpable varicoceles.[43] False positive studies have been attributed to a number of exam technique factors to include high pressure contrast instillation and placement of the catheter tip through the valve in the proximal portion of the internal spermatic vein. Because of the high false-positive rate and the invasive nature of this test, venography is not indicated for routine screening in the infertile male. It does have a role in the postvaricocele recurrence situation in which the procedure confirms the diagnosis and allows concurrent embolization of persistent vessels.

CONCLUSION

Available imaging studies offer exquisite delineation of the male reproductive tract, often allowing precise localization of pathology for potential surgical reconstructions. Additionally, scrotal and transrectal ultrasonography allow the identification of potentially significant medical pathology in the patient himself.

REFERENCES

1. Nashan D, Behre HM, Grunert JH, Nieschlag E. Andrologia. Diagnostic value of scrotal sonography in infertile men:report on 658 cases 1990;22:387-95.
2. Behre HM, Kliesch S, Schädel F, Nieschlag E. Clinical relevance of scrotal and transrectal ultrasonography in andrological patients. Int J Androl 1995;(18 Suppl)2:27-31.
3. Pierik FH, Dohle GR, van Muiswinkel JM, Vreeburg JT, Weber RF. Is routine scrotal ultrasound advantageous in infertile men? J Urol 1999;162:1618-20.
4. Sakamoto H, Saito K, Shichizyo T, Ishikawa K, Igarashi A, Yoshida H. Color Doppler ultrasonography as a routine clinical examination in male infertility. Int J Urol 2006;13:1073-8.
5. Qublan HS, Al-Okoor K, Al-Ghoweri AS, Abu-Qamar A. Sonographic spectrum of scrotal abnormalities in infertile men. J Clin Ultrasound 2007;35(8):437-41.
6. Hricak H, Filly RA. Sonography of the scrotum. Invest Radiol 1983;18:112-21.
7. Sakamoto H, Saito K, Ogawa Y, Yoshida H. Testicular volume measurements using Prader orchidometer versus ultrasonography in patients with infertility. Urology 2007;69:158-62.
8. Sakamoto H, Yajima T, Nagata M, Okumura T, Suzuki K, Ogawa Y. Relationship between testicular size by ultrasonography and testicular function: measurement of testicular length, width, and depth in patients with infertility. Int J Urol 2008;15:529-33.
9. Tammela TL, Karttunen TJ, Mattila SI, Makarainen HP, Hellstrom PA, Kontturi MJ. Cysts of the tunica albuginea - more common testicular masses than previously thought? Br J Urol 1991;68:280-4.

10. Rouvière O, Bouvier R, Pangaud C, Jeune C, Dawahra M, Lyonnet. Tubular ectasia of the rete testis: a potential pitfall in scrotal imaging. Eur Radiol 1999;9:1862-8.

11. Oyen RH. Scrotal ultrasound scan. Eur Radiol 2002; 12:196-34.

12. Janzen DL, Mathieson JR, Marsh JI, Cooperberg PL, del Rio P, Golding RH, Rifkin MD. Testicular microlithiasis: sonographic and clinical features. AJR Am J Roentgenol 1992;158:1057-60.

13. Costabile RA. How worrisome is testicular microlithiasis Curr Opin Urol 2007;17:419-23.

14. Backus ML, Mack LA, Middleton WD, King BF, Winter TC 3rd, True LD. Testicular microlithiasis: imaging appearances and pathologic correlation. Radiology 1994;192:781-5.

15. Laviopierre AM. Ultrasound of the prostate and testicles. Word J. Surg 2000;24:198-207.

16. Jaganathan K, Ahmed S, Henderson A, Rané A. Current management strategies for testicular microlithiasis. Nat Clin Pract Urol 2007;4:492-7.

17. Korde LA, Premkumar A, Mueller C, Rosenberg P, Soho C, Bratslavsky G, Greene MH. Increased prevalence of testicular microlithiasis in men with familial testicular cancer and their relatives. Br J Cancer 2008;99:1748-53.

18. Nguyen HT, Coakley F, Hricak H. Cryptorchidism: strategies in detection. Eur Radiol 1999;9:336-43

19. Davis RS. Intratesticular spermatocele. Urology 1998; 51(suppl): 167-9.

20. Sista AK, Filly RA. Color Doppler sonography in evaluation of spermatoceles: the "falling snow" sign. J Ultrasound Med 2008;27:141-3.

21. Moon MH, Kim SH, Cho JY, Seo JT, Chun YK. Scrotal US for evaluation of infertile men with azoospermia. Radiology; 2006;239:168-73.

22. Jequier AM, Ansell ID, Bullimore NJ. Congenital absence of the vasa deferentia presenting with infertility. J Androl 1985;6:15-9.

23. Brown DL, Benson CB, Doherty FJ, Doubilet PM, DiSalvo DN, Van Alstyne GA, Vickers MA, Loughlin KR. Cystic testicular mass caused by dilated rete testis: sonographic findings in 31 cases. AJR Am J Roentgenol 1992;158(6): 1257-9.

24. Dubin L, Amelar RD. Varicocele size and results of varicocelectomy in selected subfertile men with varicocele. Fertil Steril 1970;21:606-9.

25. Chiou RK, Anderson JC, Wobig RK, Rosinsky DE, Matamoros A Jr, Chen WS, Taylor RJ. Color Doppler ultrasound criteria to diagnose varicoceles: correlation of a new scoring system with physical examination. Urology 1997;50:953-6.

26. Cina A, Minnetti M, Pirronti T, Vittoria Spampinato M, Canadè A, Oliva G, Ribatti D, Bonomo L. Sonographic quantitative evaluation of scrotal veins in healthy subjects: normative values and implications for the diagnosis of varicocele. Eur Urol 2006;50:345-50.

27. Cvitanic OA, Cronan JJ, Sigman M, Landau ST. Varicoceles: postoperative prevalence—a prospective study with color Doppler US. Radiology 1993;187(3):711-4.

28. Trum JW, Gubler FM, Laan R, van der Veen F. The value of palpation, varicoscreen contact thermography and colour Doppler ultrasound in the diagnosis of varicocele. Hum Reprod 1996;11:1232-5.

29. Petros JA, Andriole GL, Middleton WD, Picus DA. Correlation of testicular color Doppler ultrasonography, physical examination and venography in the detection of left varicoceles in men with infertility. J Urol 1991;145(4):785-8.

30. Lee J, Binsaleh S, Lo K, Jarvi K. Varicoceles: The Diagnostic Dilemma. J Andrology 2006;29:143-6.

31. Cornud F, Belin X, Amar E, Delafontaine D, Helenon O, Moreau JF. Varicocele: strategies in diagnosis and treatment. Eur Radiol 1999;9:536-45.

32. Meacham RB, Townsend RR, Rademacher D, Drose JA. The incidence of varicoceles in the general population when evaluated by physical examination, gray scale sonography, and color Doppler sonography. J Urol 1994;151:1535-8.

33. Kocakoc E, Kiris A, Orhan I, Bozgeyik Z, Kanbay M, Ogur E. Incidence and importance of reflux in testicular veins of healthy men evaluated with color duplex sonography. J Clin Ultrasound 2002;30:282-7.

34. Belenky A, Avrech OM, Bachar GN, Zuckerman Z, Ben Rafael Z, Fisch B, Cohen M. Ultrasound-guided testicular sperm aspiration in azoospermic patients: a new sperm retrieval method for intracytoplasmic sperm injection. J Clin Ultrasound 2001;29: 339-43.

35. Vazquez-Levin MH, Dressler KP, Nagler HM. Urine contamination of seminal fluid after transurethral resection of the ejaculatory ducts. J Urol 1994;152:2049-52.

36. Carter SSC, Shinohara K, Lipshultz LI. Transrectal ultrasonography in disorders of the seminal vesicles and ejaculatory ducts. Urol Clin North Am 1989;16:773-90.

37. Smith JF, Walsh TJ, Turek PJ. Ejaculatory duct obstruction. Urol Clin North Am 2008;35(2):221-7.

38. Jarow JP. Seminal vesicle aspiration in the management of patients with ejaculatory duct obstruction. J Urol 1994; 152(3): 899-901.

39. Jarow JP. Seminal vesicle aspiration of fertile men. J Urol 1996;156(3):1005-7.

40. Purohit RS, Wu DS, Shinohara K, et al. A prospective comparison of 3 diagnostic methods to evaluate ejaculatory duct obstruction. J Urol 2004;171(1):232-6.

41. Eisenberg ML, Walsh TJ, Garcia MM, Shinohara K, Turek, PJ. Ejaculatory duct manometry in normal men and in patients with ejaculatory duct obstruction. J Urol 2008;180:255.

42. Payne SR, Pryor JP, Parks CM. Vasography, its indications and complications. Br J Urol 1985;57:215.

43. Matsuda, T. Diagnosis and treatment of post-herniorrhaphy vas deferens obstruction. Int J Urol 2000;7 Suppl:S35.

12

The Assessment of Azoospermia

Jason Hedges, Brian Le, Robert E Brannigan

INTRODUCTION

Nearly 15 percent of couples are unable to achieve pregnancy after one year of unprotected intercourse. A male factor is solely responsible in about 20 percent of infertile couples and contributory in another 40 percent.[1] The prevalence of azoospermia is approximately 1 percent among all men and ranges between 10–15 percent in infertile men.[2] Azoospermia is defined as the complete absence of sperm in the ejaculate; aspermia is distinct from azoospermia and is defined as the complete absence of an antegrade ejaculate. In this chapter, we will highlight the important distinction between obstructive azoospermia and nonobstructive azoospermia. While sharing the common finding of no sperm in the ejaculate, these are otherwise two very dissimilar clinical conditions, with very different approaches to evaluation and treatment.

THE PRELIMINARY DIAGNOSIS OF AZOOSPERMIA

A routine semen analysis lacking sperm is not sufficient to confirm the diagnosis of azoospermia. In addition to this first test, a second semen analysis should be obtained to verify the initial findings. As part of the routine testing, each sample should be centrifuged at $3,000 \times g$ for 15 minutes with subsequent inspection of the resultant pellet.[3] Clinicians should be aware that many labs do not routinely perform this second step, but it is an essential aspect of the semen analysis in this setting. Careful evaluation of the centrifuged pellet helps to distinguish true azoospermia from samples with cryptozoospermia (sperm found only after centrifugation and inspection of the pellet). In 1998, Jaffe et al. reported that 16 (23%) of 70 men originally considered to have a clinical diagnosis of nonobstructive azoospermia were subsequently found to have cryptozoospermia after semen centrifugation.[4] In another study, Ron-El et al. similarly found sperm in the pellet after semen centrifugation in 35 percent of men diagnosed initially with nonobstructive azoospermia.[5] To be clear, the initial diagnosis of azoospermia is only confirmed when no spermatozoa are detected on high-powered microscopic examination of the original semen sample and the post-centrifugation semen pellet on at least two separate specimens.

AZOOSPERMIA PARADIGMS

The evaluation of a patient with azoospermia is aimed at defining and determining the underlying cause of his condition. A concept that must be stressed at this time is the importance of clarifying if the patient has an obstructive or a nonobstructive cause of his azoospermia. However, in addition to providing this information, the patient's evaluation also allows for the assessment of medical conditions that might be the underlying cause of azoospermia. Two separate studies have shown that male infertility is sometimes the only sign of more serious yet undiagnosed medical issues (i.e. testicular tumors, pituitary tumors, genetic anomalies, etc.) in some men.[6,7] In certain instances, these associated medical conditions can be life-threatening.

In addition to the classifications of obstructive and nonobstructive azoospermia, a paradigm that categorizes azoospermia into pretesticular, testicular, and post-testicular causes is also quite helpful.[8] Pretesticular causes of azoospermia are relatively rare and include endocrine abnormalities which adversely affect spermatogenesis. This is also known as secondary testicular failure, and such conditions can either be congenital or acquired. These endocrinopathies commonly involve the hypothalamus and/or the pituitary gland. Testicular causes of azoospermia, also known as primary testicular failure, include disorders of spermatogenesis that are intrinsic to the testes. One such example is a patient with a history of chemotherapy for lymphoma who now has no sperm production due to the gonadotoxic exposure. Post-testicular etiologies of azoospermia include obstruction of the sperm delivery pathway and ejaculatory dysfunction. Pretesticular and post-testicular causes of azoospermia are frequently correctable; in contrast, testicular causes of azoospermia are typically more challenging and are rarely correctable. With the use of assisted reproductive techniques, though, many of these conditions that are not *correctable* are nonetheless *treatable*.

EVALUATION OF THE AZOOSPERMIC MALE

History of the Azoospermic Patient

To help determine the etiology of azoospermia and clarify appropriate therapeutic options, the urologist performs a full medical evaluation. This workup includes detailed medical and reproductive histories, as well as a physical examination. This approach is essential in the setting of azoospermia, just as it is a necessary component in the work-up of any other medical condition. Areas of emphasis in the history should include symptoms of androgen deficiency (erectile dysfunction, low libido, decreased energy, or depression), the timing of pubertal development, exposures to potential gonadotoxins (including radiation or chemotherapy), history of previous trauma, or any scrotal or inguinal surgery. Conditions such as cryptorchidism, postpubertal mumps orchitis, infections (epididymoorchitis, urethritis), recent fevers, and environmental heat exposures (> 101°) should all be noted. A family history assessing for reproductive failure, congenital anomalies, mental retardation, and cystic fibrosis should be included. The initial evaluation should also incorporate the patient's prior fertility history, his partner's age, and her reproductive history.

Physical Examination of the Azoospermic Patient

As with any medical condition, a complete physical examination should be performed on the patient with azoospermia. The examination should be conducted in a warm room with the patient in both the supine and standing positions. Physical examination often provides essential clues to differentiate between obstructive and nonobstructive causes of azoospermia, as will be further discussed below. The physical exam should have a particular emphasis on overall androgenization (hair distribution, penile development, scrotal rugation) and assess for the presence of gynecomastia. A thorough scrotal examination should evaluate for the presence and characteristics of the vas deferens and epididymides. Evaluation of the testes should include an assessment of volume and consistency, and care should be taken to detect abnormal testicular masses that might represent neoplasm. The presence and grade of varicoceles should be documented, as these can certainly hamper sperm production. This portion of the exam is best conducted with the patient in a standing position, with the Valsalva maneuver being performed in the course of the assessment. Finally, prostate or seminal vesicle abnormalities detected on rectal examination should also be noted. These might suggest prostate cysts or prostatic neoplasms, and seminal vesicle absence may be a sign of unilateral or bilateral vasal agenesis.

Laboratory Evaluation of the Azoospermic Patient

At least two semen analyses with 2–3 days of abstinence prior to semen collection are needed. For semen analyses with low volume (< 1 mL), retrograde ejaculation should be excluded with a post-ejaculate urinalysis. The presence of sperm in the centrifuged urine sample confirms retrograde ejaculation. A transrectal ultrasound should follow if no sperm are present in the postejaculate urine specimen to help rule out ejaculatory duct obstruction as the etiology. Semen pH and semen fructose are also useful parameters in specific azoospermic settings, and these will both be discussed later in this chapter.

The laboratory evaluation of the patient with azoospermia is also critical to detect potential endocrinopathy. The initial laboratory evaluation, at a minimum, should include a serum FSH level and a morning serum testosterone level.[3] Other lab tests that may be helpful in determining the endocrine status, especially if testosterone is low, include serum LH, prolactin and estradiol. Bioavailable testosterone is preferred by some clinicians and may be calculated from total testosterone, sex hormone binding globulin, and albumin levels, and online calculators are readily available for clinician use.[9,10] Recent studies demonstrate a higher than previously recognized prevalence of hypogonadism in the azoospermic population (particularly men with nonobstructive azoospermia), which may provide an opportunity for medical therapy before surgical sperm retrieval.[11]

As genetic conditions may also be the root cause of nonobstructive azoospermia, laboratory testing for genetic anomalies with a karyotype analysis and a Y-chromosome microdeletion assay should be offered to men with suspected nonobstructive azoospermia who are contemplating IVF/ICSI, in accordance with recommendations from the American Urological Association and the American Society for Reproductive Medicine.[3,8] For men with suspected congenital absence of the vas deferens, cystic fibrosis transmembrane regulator (CFTR) gene testing should be offered. These issues are examined in more depth later in this chapter.

In the past, when a patient presented with presumptive nonobstructive azoospermia, urologists typically performed a testicular biopsy to confirm the diagnosis. The extracted tissue was sent to the pathology laboratory for histological examination; this biopsy was essentially another "laboratory test" to help determine the patient's underlying diagnosis. A recent, important manuscript by Schoor et al reported that FSH levels and testicular longitudinal axis considered together provide an accurate means to distinguish between nonobstructive and obstructive azoospermia without the need for a diagnostic testicular biopsy.[12] The authors reported that a patient with a serum FSH ≥ 7.6 mIU/mL and a testicular longitudinal axis ≤ 4.6 cm has an 89 percent chance of having spermatogenic dysfunction as the cause of azoospermia (i.e. nonobstructive azoospermia). In contrast, a patient with a serum FSH < 7.6 mIU/mL and a testicular longitudinal axis > 4.6 cm has a 96 percent likelihood of having intact spermatogenesis but excurrent ductal blockage as the cause of his azoospermia (i.e. obstructive azoospermia). Thus, diagnostic biopsy before surgical sperm retrieval, purely to discriminate between obstructive azoospermia and nonobstructive azoospermia, is no longer recommended. In other words, testicular biopsy should generally coincide with sperm retrieval, with extracted sperm being used for concurrent IVF/ICSI or cryopreserved for future clinical use.

▌OBSTRUCTIVE AZOOSPERMIA

Obstructive azoospermia accounts for approximately 40 percent of cases of azoospermia.[13] Causes can be quite varied, including congenital and acquired etiologies. Congenital causes include congenital absence of the vas deferens, adult polycystic kidney disease, and Young's syndrome, while acquired causes include trauma, infection, inflammation, and iatrogenic etiologies.

Congenital Bilateral Absence of the Vas Deferens

Congenital bilateral absence of the vas deferens (CBAVD) is most often due to a mutation of the cystic fibrosis transmembrane conductance regulator (CFTR) gene.[14,15] Almost all males with clinical cystic fibrosis have CBAVD, while conversely approximately 70 percent of men with CBAVD have no clinical evidence of cystic fibrosis but do have an identifiable abnormality of the CFTR gene.

The vas deferens are usually palpable within the scrotum, and the diagnosis of vasal agenesis, either unilateral or bilateral, is made by physical examination. Imaging studies are generally not necessary to confirm the diagnosis, but these may be useful for diagnosing abnormalities associated with vasal agenesis.[8] There is an embryological association between the vas deferens and seminal vesicles, and thus most patients with vasal agenesis also have ipsilateral seminal vesicle hypoplasia or absence. The majority of semen volume is derived from the seminal vesicles. This explains the finding that almost all patients with CBAVD also have low semen volume. The seminal vesicle secretions are alkaline, while the prostate secretions are acidic in pH. This accounts for the fact that patients with CBAVD tend to have acidic pH semen, as the acidic prostatic secretions are the predominant seminal component in the absence of the alkaline seminal vesicle secretions.

In the azoospermic patient who has clinical evidence of unilateral vasal agenesis, transrectal ultrasonography may be useful to evaluate the ampullary portion of the contralateral vas deferens and the contralateral seminal vesicle. In some cases of unilateral vasal agenesis, contralateral segmental atresia of the vas deferens and seminal vesicle hypoplasia may also be present, resulting in bilateral excurrent ductal obstruction and azoospermia.[15,16]

When unilateral or bilateral absence of the vas deferens is suspected, both the patient and his partner should undergo genetic counseling and testing of the CFTR gene to rule out abnormalities. Many CFTR mutations may not be detected by routine testing methods, and it should be assumed that men with congenital bilateral absence of the vas deferens harbor a CFTR genetic abnormality. Whether the result of the male testing is positive or negative, it is important to test the female partner for CFTR gene abnormalities. This should be done prior to offering a treatment that utilizes his sperm because of the risk that she may be a carrier. Genetic counseling should be offered in conjunction with genetic testing for both partners.[8]

Finally, clinicians should be aware of the strong association between unilateral vasal agenesis and ipsilateral renal anomalies. This association is due to the vas deferens and kidneys sharing a common mesonephric duct embryological origin. Imaging of the kidneys with ultrasound to assess for ipsilateral renal agenesis is thus helpful in men with unilateral or bilateral vasal agenesis who do not have mutations in the CFTR gene.[8]

Epididymal and Vasal Obstruction

The epididymis and vas deferens facilitate sperm transport and are thus essential components of the male reproductive tract. A number of conditions can lead to their blockage, including inflammation, infection, trauma, and iatrogenic factors, such as prior scrotal or inguinal surgery. Physical examination findings that suggest a possible blockage include fullness or enlargement of the epididymis, palpable gaps or missing segments of the vas deferens, and sperm granulomas. The most common iatrogenic cause of obstructive azoospermia is vasectomy. Interestingly, approximately 5 percent of men undergoing this procedure subsequently wish to pursue efforts at paternity, thus presenting to urologists for treatment of their iatrogenic obstructive azoospermia.[17]

As was detailed above, testicular volume and serum FSH levels are key parameters in delineating obstructive from nonobstructive azoospermia.[12] Additionally, semen volume, semen pH, and semen fructose are also potentially helpful in specifying the root cause of azoospermia. With this in mind, it is important to note that men with epididymal obstruction (unilateral or bilateral) typically harbor no changes in any of these latter three parameters. Along these same lines, men with isolated vasal obstruction (unilateral or bilateral) typically exhibit no changes in semen volume, semen pH, or semen fructose.

Ejaculatory Duct Obstruction

The ejaculatory ducts are paired structures that commence at the ampullary portion of the vas deferens, where the vas deferens and ipsilateral seminal vesicle merge at the level of the prostate gland. The ejaculatory duct travels anterosuperiorly and terminates in the prostatic urethra, where it deposits the collective vasal and seminal vesicular fluid.

Ejaculatory duct obstruction can arise from intrinsic ductal calculi, prostate cysts compressing the ejaculatory duct, and primary intrinsic stenosis. Patients with ejaculatory duct obstruction share many of the seminal parameter findings seen in men with CBAVD: low ejaculate volume, abnormally low (acidic) semen pH, and absent seminal fructose. All of these findings are due to absence of characteristically alkaline seminal vesicle fluid in the ejaculate.

Clinicians should be mindful of the fact that azoospermic patients with low ejaculate volume, normal FSH, and normal sized testes may have ejaculatory duct obstruction, ejaculatory dysfunction, or simply might have had incomplete collection of the ejaculated semen sample. In this setting, seminal pH, seminal fructose, and a postejaculate urinalysis can each be quite helpful at specifying the azoospermia etiology.

Transrectal ultrasonography (TRUS) is minimally invasive and indicated to help rule out the diagnosis of ejaculatory duct obstruction in men with low ejaculate volume and palpable vas deferens. While vasography is an alternative diagnostic test that could be used in these patients, it is more invasive and risks resultant iatrogenic vasal stenosis or atresia.[18] The findings of dilated ejaculatory ducts, midline cysts, and/or dilated seminal vesicles (>1.5 cm in anteroposterior diameter) on TRUS are suggestive of ejaculatory duct obstruction. Of note, the finding of normal seminal vesicle size does not completely rule out the possibility of obstruction. Therefore, seminal vesicle aspiration and seminal vesiculography may be performed under TRUS guidance to confirm a suspected diagnosis of ejaculatory duct obstruction.[19] The presence of large numbers of sperm in the seminal vesicle aspirate from an azoospermic patient is highly suggestive of ejaculatory duct obstruction.[19] Seminal vesiculography performed after seminal vesicle aspiration can further help determine the anatomical site of the obstruction.

Additional Causes

Other conditions can also lead to obstructive azoospermia. Young's syndrome is characterized by the triad of sinusitis, bronchiectasis, and obstructive azoospermia. Men with this condition suffer from obstruction of their reproductive tract duct with thick, inspissated secretions. While the specific cause of Young's syndrome has not yet been determined, the etiology is suspected to be genetic. The condition is usually diagnosed in middle-aged men who undergo evaluation for infertility. At this time, there is no known effective treatment for Young syndrome. Although there is no "cure" for the characteristic azoospermia associated with Young's syndrome, sperm from these men can be extracted and used in the setting of IVF/ICSI.

Adult-Onset Polycystic Kidney Disease (APKD) is typically due to a point mutation in the genes PKD1, PKD2, or PKD3. This condition affects up to 1 in 1000 people, and it is characterized by the presence of bilaterally enlarged kidneys, each with numerous, large renal cysts. Some patients with this condition have been observed to have concurrent seminal vesicle cysts. A study by Pryor et al., however, suggests that the seminal vesicle "cysts" noted in these patients may actually represent large, distended, hypodynamic seminal vesicles which contribute to or are associated with overall excurrent ductal obstruction.[20] In either case, sperm production in these patients is typically intact. Again, while there is no underlying "cure" for the excurrent ductal obstruction in APKD, successful treatment with sperm extraction for use in IVF/ICSI can rendered.

◼ NONOBSTRUCTIVE AZOOSPERMIA

Etiologies of nonobstructive azoospermia include endocrinopathy, testicular failure, genetic anomaly, and idiopathic factors. Endocrinopathies such as Kallmann syndrome and non-anosmic, idiopathic, hypogonadotropic hypogonadism are fairly rare but are important to correctly diagnose as they may be medically treated. Testicular causes of nonobstructive azoospermia include cryptorchidism, gonadotoxin exposure (including chemotherapy and radiation therapy), varicocele, and infections such as mumps orchitis. Finally, genetic causes of nonobstructive azoospermia include Klinefelter's syndrome, Y-chromosome microdeletions, various chromosomal structural abnormalities, and other specific gene mutations.

Endocrinopathy

Disorders of the male endocrine system are potentially reversible causes of nonobstructive azoospermia. The classic endocrine disorders affecting sperm production include congenital idiopathic hypogonadotropic hypogonadism either with anosmia (Kallmann syndrome) or without anosmia. Other disorders include panhypopituitarism, hyperprolactinemia, and exogenous anabolic steroid use.

The key to diagnosing endocrinopathies lies in the serum hormone values. As mentioned above, at a minimum testing should include serum FSH and testosterone levels. If either of these values is abnormally low, additional testing with serum LH and prolactin should be pursued. Finally, although it is highly unlikely to cause azoospermia in isolation, consideration should be given to serum estradiol testing. Schlegel and colleagues reported that abnormally low testosterone: estradiol ratio (<10:1) suggests that medical therapy, in the form of an aromatase inhibitor, may provide benefit in optimizing the testosterone: estradiol ratio and thus sperm concentration.[21] They also noted in a subsequent publication the potential benefits of hCG, FSH, and clomiphene citrate therapy in the more specific setting of Klinefelter's syndrome.[22]

Varicocele

Varicoceles are present in 35–40 percent of infertile men[23,24] and in 4.3–13.3 percent of these men the varicocele is associated with azoospermia or severe oligozoospermia.[24] The diagnosis is made on physical examination, with grade I/III varicoceles being detectable by palpation with Valsalva maneuver, grade II/III varicoceles being detectable by palpation alone (without Valsalva maneuver), and Grade III/III varicoceles being detectable visually. Varicoceles lead to impairment of the countercurrent heat exchange mechanism in the scrotum, which in turn can cause a number of changes including testicular hyperthermia, germ cell sloughing, and testicular atrophy. Clinicians need not order "screening" scrotal ultrasounds in search of subclinical varicoceles in patients, as several studies have clearly shown that correction of subclinical varicoceles is of "questionable benefit" in this setting. In Jarow's study, an equal number of patients had improvement and decline in semen parameters postoperatively, and the mean sperm count remain unchanged.[25]

A dilemma facing the urologist treating patients with varicocele and nonobstructive azoospermia is whether to repair the varicocele or not. An early study by Matthews et al showed that varicocele correction in patients with nonobstructive azoospermia led to return of sperm in the ejaculate in 4 (17%) out of 22 men.[26] Subsequent studies at other centers revealed the return of sperm in the ejaculate in 12 (43%) out of 28 men and 3 (31%) out of 31 men.[27,28] A cost analysis by Schlegel et al found that microsurgical TESE is more cost effective than varicocelectomy for treatment of varicocele-associated nonobstructive azoospermia.[29] As noted by Schlegel even more recently, most studies assessing the efficacy of varicocele correction in men with nonobstructive azoospermia are observational in design without control arms. He calls for controlled trials at centers adept at processing and evaluating cryptozospermic samples to better address this controversy. Although there is little dispute over the potential benefits of varicocele correction in infertile men overall, at this time controversy does exist as to the role of varicocele correction in the specific setting of nonobstructive azoospermia.[30]

Cryptorchidism

Cryptorchidism is a condition diagnosed on physical exam, although sometimes imaging studies such as ultrasound, CT scan, or MRI can help delineate whether a testis is truly undescended or altogether absent. Fortunately, the vast majority of males born with cryptorchidism undergo orchidopexy at a young age, with only rare patients having ongoing cryptorchidism when they present for a fertility evaluation.

Men with a history of an undescended testis (unilateral or bilateral) are at risk for azoospermia, with cryptorchidism accounting for 27 percent of all cases of azoospermia.[31] Some authors suggest that the increased heat exposure in the undescended position leads to permanent impairment of sperm production, while others assert that an underlying primary disorder of spermatogenesis is present in these testes.

Sperm retrieval rates for azoospermic men with a history of cryptorchidism range from 52–74 percent with live birth rates via IVF/ICSI of 22.6–43 percent.[32] Raman and Schlegel reported improved success in sperm retrieval if cryptorchidism was unilateral (100%) rather than bilateral (68%). Mean patient age at orchidopexy was significantly different between the successful (mean age 10.5 +/– 7.6 years) and unsuccessful (21.8 +/– 10.8 years) retrieval groups.[33]

Ejaculatory Dysfunction

Ejaculation is a highly integrated reflex that can be triggered by a variety of stimulatory input, including visual, tactile, and auditory stimuli. Ejaculation can be disrupted by a number of factors, including neuropathy due to medical conditions or prior surgery, and medications. Disrupted ejaculation can be further subcategorized as an ejaculation or retrograde ejaculation. In the setting of azoospermia, the patient typically suffers from retrograde ejaculation, with a small portion of the semen (often the "pre-ejaculate from the Cowper's glands") emanating from the urethra with the bulk of seminal fluid transiting into the bladder during climax. While ejaculatory dysfunction more commonly leads to aspermia or low ejaculate volume with oligospermia, on occasion low ejaculate volume azoospermia may be found.

Overview of Genetic Etiologies of Nonobstructive Azoospermia

Genetic factors causing nonobstructive azoospermia include chromosomal abnormalities, Y-chromosome microdeletions, and individual gene mutations. The workup for these genetic causes of infertility includes karyotype testing, Y-chromosome microdeletion analysis, various chromosomal structural abnormalities, and specific gene mutation studies. However, clinicians and patients alike must be aware that there may be additional unidentified or unknown genetic factors contributing to nonobstructive azoospermia that will not be detected with currently available genetic tests.

Investigators estimate the prevalence of chromosomal disorders in men with nonobstructive azoospermia to be 10–15 percent, and the most common chromosomal disorder is Klinefelter's syndrome, which accounts for 2/3 of karyotypic chromosome abnormalities in infertile men.[3]

Y-chromosome microdeletions are also commonly diagnosed genetic disorders causing male infertility, with a prevalence of 10–15 percent in men with severe oligospermia or azoospermia.[34] Numerous other structural (deletions, duplications, inversions and translocations) and numerical chromosomal anomalies may also cause nonobstructive azoospermia.

Y-Chromosome Microdeletions

The Y-chromosome is the smallest human chromosome with 60 million bases, and it consists of a short arm and a long arm. The short arm carries the SRY gene which is responsible for male differentiation. The long arm houses many genes that code for spermatogenesis. The missing areas on the long arm of the Y-chromosome in azoospermic men were discovered by Tiepolo and Zuffardi in 1976, and they were named "microdeletions" because the areas were too small to be seen on a routine karyotype.[35] Further investigation led to the description of the 3 different areas called *AZFa*, *AZFb* and *AZFc*. *AZFa* is a distinct region as later analysis revealed that *AZFb* and *AZFc* overlap. Microdeletions in these segments lead to varying degrees of decreased spermatogenic activity.[36,37] More specifically, men with complete *AZFa*, *AZFb*, *AZFb/c* and *AZFabc* deletions typically have either Sertoli cell only or maturation arrest histological patterns and a poor prognosis for sperm retrieval.[37] The *AZFc* microdeletion can be seen in 6 percent of men with severe oligozoospermia as well as up to 13 percent of those with nonobstructive azoospermia, with successful sperm retrieval rates typically > 50 percent.[37]

Y-chromosome microdeletion analysis should be offered to all men with severe oligospermia (< 5–10 million sperm/mL) or suspected nonobstructive azoospermia.[3] This testing provides diagnostic information which may provide insight as to the root cause of the patient's infertility. Additionally, the specific type of microdeletion detected may serve as a prognostic factor in gauging the likelihood of successful sperm retrieval during sperm extraction procedures. Finally, genetic information may be useful to some patients as they consider transmission of this anomaly with its associated male infertility along to male offspring.

Klinefelter's Syndrome

Klinefelter's syndrome is a chromosomal genetic disorder characterized by an extra X-chromosome (47, XXY), although this condition is occasionally is found in its mosaic form (46, XY/47, XXY). The syndrome has a reported incidence of 1 in 660 men but may represent up to 3.1 percent of the infertile male population and 10 percent of men with nonobstructive azoospermia.[22,38] While most men with Klinefelter's syndrome display characteristic small, firm testes, the classically described phenotype of a tall male with a pear shaped body habitus and gynecomastia may not be present. Semen analysis typically reveals azoospermia or severe oligospermia. Laboratory testing usually detects hypergonadotropic hypogonadism with elevated FSH and LH levels, and low to normal testosterone. Many patients with Klinefelter's syndrome also exhibit an abnormally low testosterone-to-estradiol ratio.[21] Because of the endocrinopathy typically associated with this genetic disorder, it is important to consider medical therapy for men with Klinefelter's syndrome in advance of sperm retrieval procedures. Ramasamy et al. reported that increasing serum testosterone to $\geq$ 250 ng/dL before microsurgical testicular sperm extraction yielded a 77 percent retrieval rate for men with Klinefelter's syndrome compared to 55 percent for those men with testosterone levels < 250 ng/dL.[22] In this study, men with Klinefelter's syndrome on exogenous testosterone replacement therapy had only a 25 percent sperm retrieval rate during sperm extraction procedures. The authors stopped any exogenous testosterone, and they placed men with Klinefelter's syndrome and abnormally low baseline testosterone levels on an oral aromatase inhibitor (either 1 mg anastrazole daily or 50–100 gm testolactone twice daily) and added hCG (1500 IU twice weekly, titrated to a maximum dose of 2500 IU 3 times weekly) if the aromatase inhibitor failed to normalize the testosterone. Additionally, if men presented on alternative medication (either clomiphene citrate or hCG alone) with satisfactory testosterone levels, the therapy was continued. After a median duration of medical therapy of 163 days before micro-TESE, the overall sperm retrieval rate was 66 percent, clinical pregnancy rate 57 percent and live birth rate 45 percent with IVF. This study highlights the benefit of medical optimization of this subpopulation of men with nonobstructive azoospermia.

Individual Gene Mutations

While many gene mutations may lead to medical conditions that are indirectly associated with nonobstructive azoospermia, one gene defect is directly associated with spermatogenic failure: point mutations in the androgen receptor gene. The androgen receptor gene is located on the long arm of the X-chromosome.[39] Androgens play key roles in sexual differentiation and spermatogenesis, and mutations affecting the androgen receptor can lead to markedly impaired sperm production. Androgen receptor mutations are relatively rare, occurring in an estimated 2 percent of infertile men.[39] Two polymorphisms, CAG and GGC, are associated with male factor infertility. Longer lengths of the CAG polymorphism are generally associated with decreased transcriptional activity of the androgen receptor gene in infertile men, leading to reduced sperm concentration, decreased motility, and in some cases azoospermia. However, these findings do not hold across all populations of men, with racial and ethnic differences noted in some studies.[40]

Genetic Counseling

Genetic counseling in the setting of azoospermia has several roles. First, it provides information about genetic risks as couples consider pursuit of assisted reproductive technologies. The psychosocial impact of potentially passing genetic anomalies along to offspring is an important consideration for many couples. Genetic counseling also provides valuable information as some couples may consider options of prenatal diagnosis, genetic testing of family members, and preimplantation genetic diagnosis.

■ REFERENCES

1. Thonneau P, Marchand S, Tallec A, et al. Incidence and main causes of infertility in a resident population (1,850,000) of three French regions (1988-1989). Hum Reprod 1991;6:811-6.
2. Stephen EH, Chandra A. Declining estimates of infertility in the United States: 1982-2002. Fertil Steril 2006;86:516-23.
3. Male Infertility Best Practice Policy Committee of the American Urological Association and Practice Committee of the American Society for Reproductive Medicine: Report on optimal evaluation of the infertile male. Fertil Steril, suppl 2006;86:S202-9.
4. Jaffe TM, Kim ED, Hoekstra TH, et al. Sperm pellet analysis: a technique to detect the presence of sperm in men considered to have azoospermia by routine semen analysis. J Urol 1998;159:1548-50.
5. Ron-El R, Strassburger D, Friedler S, et al. Extended sperm preparation: an alternative to testicular sperm extraction in nonobstructive azoospermia. Hum Reprod 1997;12:1222-6.
6. Honig SC, Lipshultz LI, Jarow J. Significant medical pathology uncovered by a comprehensive male infertility evaluation. Fertil Steril 1994;62:1028-34.
7. Kolettis PN, Sabanegh ES. Significant medical pathology discovered during a male infertility evaluation. J Urol 2001;166:178-80.
8. Male Infertility Best Practice Policy Committee of the American Urological Association and Practice Committee of the American Society for Reproductive Medicine: Report on evaluation of the azoospermic male. Fertil Steril, suppl 2006;86:S210-5.
9. Plymate SR, Tenover JS, Bremner WJ. Circadian variation in testosterone, sex hormone binding globulin, and calculated non-sex hormone binding globulin bound testosterone in healthy young and elderly men. J Androl 1989;10:366-71.
10. www.issam.ch/freetesto.htm (web site accessed 4/23/2011).
11. Sussman EM, Chudnovsky A, Niederberger CS. Hormonal evaluation of the infertile male: has it evolved? Urol Clin North Am 2008;35:147-55.
12. Schoor RA, Elhanbly S, Niederberger CS, Ross LS. The role of testicular biopsy in the modern management of male infertility. J Urol 2002;167:197-200.
13. Jarow JP, Espeland MA, Lipshultz LI. Evaluation of the azoospermic patient. J Urol 1989;142:62-5.
14. Anguiano A, Oates RD, Amos JA, et al. Congenital bilateral absence of the vas deferens. A primarily genital form of cystic fibrosis. JAMA 1992;267:1794-7.
15. Chillon M, Casals T, Mercier B, et al. Mutations in the cystic fibrosis gene in patients with congenital absence of the vas deferens. N Engl J Med 1995;332:1475-80.

16. Hall S, Oates RD. Unilateral absence of the scrotal vas deferens associated with contralateral mesonephric duct anomalies resulting in infertility: laboratory, physical and radiographic findings, and therapeutic alternatives. J Urol 1993;150:1161-4.

17. Sabanegh ES Jr, Thomas AJ Jr. Microurgical treatment of male infertility. In: Lipshultz LI, Howards S, Niederberger CS (Eds). Infertility in the Male, 4th edn. New York, NY: Cambridge University Press, 2009.

18. Belker AM, Steinbock GS. Transrectal prostate ultrasonography as a diagnostic and therapeutic aid for ejaculatory duct obstruction. J Urol 1990;144:284-6.

19. Jarow JP. Role of ultrasonography in the evaluation of the infertile male. Semin Urol 1994;12:274-82.

20. Hendry WF, Rickards D, Pryor JP, et al. Seminal megavesicles with adult polycystic kidney disease. Hum Reprod 1998;13:1567-9.

21. Raman JD, Schlegel PN. Aromatase inhibitors for male infertility. J Urol 2002;167:624-9.

22. Ramasamy R, Ricci JA, Palermo GD, Gosden LV, Rosenwaks Z, Schlegel PN. Successful fertility treatment for Klinefelter's syndrome. J Urol 2009;182:1108-13.

23. Khera M, Lipshultz LI. Evolving approach to the varicocele. Urol Clin North Am 2008;35:183.

24. Esteves SC, Glina S. Recovery of spermatogenesis after microsurgical subinguinal varicocele repair in azoospermic men based on testicular histology. Int Braz J Urol 2005;31:541-8.

25. Jarow JP, Ogle SR, Eskew LA. Seminal improvement following repair of ultrasound detected subclinical varicoceles. J Urol 1996;155:1287-90.

26. Matthews GJ, Matthews ED, Goldstein M. Induction of spermatogenesis and achievement of pregnancy after microsurgical varicocelectomy in men with azoospermia and severe oligoasthenospermia. Fertil Steril 1998;70:71-5.

27. Kim ED, Leibman BB, Grinblat DM, Lipshultz LI. Varicocele repair improves semen parameters in azoospermic men with spermatogenic failure. J Urol 1999;162:737-40.

28. Schlegel PN, Kaufmann J. Role of varicocelectomy in men with nonobstructive azoospermia. Fertil Steril 2004;81:1585-8.

29. Lee R, Li PS, Goldstein M, et al. A decision analysis of treatments for nonobstructive azoospermia associated with varicocele. Fertil Steril 2009;92:188-96.

30. Schlegel PN. The role of varicocele repair in nonobstructive azoospermia must be evaluated with controlled trials rather than observational studies. Fertil Steril 2011;95:486.

31. Fedder J, Cruger D, Oestergaard B, et al. Etiology of azoospermia in 100 consecutive nonvasectomized men. Fertil Steril 2004;82: 1463-5.

32. Karpman E, Williams IV DH. Techniques of sperm retrieval. In: Lipshultz LI, Howards S, Niederberger CS (Eds). Infertility in the Male, 4th edn. New York, NY: Cambridge University Press, 2009.

33. Raman JD, Schlegel PN. Testicular sperm extraction with intracytoplasmic sperm injection is successful for the treatment of nonobstructive azoospermia associated with cryptorchidism. J Urol 2003;170: 287-90.

34. Pryor JL, Kent-First M, Muallem A, Van Bergen AH, Nolten WE, Meisner L, et al. Microdeletions in the Y-chromosome of infertile men. N Engl J Med 1997;336:534-9.

35. Tiepolo L, Zuffardi O. Localization of factors controlling spermatogenesis in the nonfluorescent portion of the human Y-chromosome long arm. Hum Genet 1976;34:119-24.

36. Reijo R, Alagappan RK, Patrizio P, et al. Severe oligozoospermia resulting from deletions of azoospermia factor gene on Y-chromosome. Lancet 1996;347:1290-3.

37. Hopps CV, Mielnik A, Goldstein M, Palermo GD, Rosenwaks Z, Schlegel PN. Detection of sperm in men with Y-chromosome microdeletions of the AZFa, AZFb and AZFc regions. Hum Reprod 2003;18:1660-5.

38. Bojesen A, Gravholt C. Klinefelter syndrome in clinical practice. Nat Clinic Pract Urol 2007;4:192-204.

39. Ferlin A, Vinanzi C, Garolla A, Selice R, Zuccarello D, Cazzadore C, et al. Male infertility and androgen receptor gene mutations: clinical features and identification of seven novel mutations. Clin Endocrinol 2006;65:606-10.

40. Gottlieb B, Lombroso R, Beitel LK, et al. Molecular pathology of the androgen receptor in male (in) fertility. Reprod Biomed Online 2005;10:42-8.

13

New Insights into the Genetics of Male Infertility

Alan Fryer

INTRODUCTION

Genetic material consists of DNA that is packaged in the human into 46 chromosomes (22 pairs of autosomes and 2 sex chromosomes). This packaging is achieved by complexing the DNA with DNA-binding proteins called histones. This complex of DNA and histones is termed chromatin. For each autosome there is disomy (two copies present) in each DNA-containing cell apart from the gametes, which should contain one copy of each autosome and one sex chromosome. There are about 21,000 protein-coding genes located on these 46 chromosomes and 1 in 25 of all mammalian genes are specifically expressed in the male germline.[1] Spermatogenesis is thus governed by the actions of many genes and, in theory, alterations in any of these genes (or their expression) or the chromosomes that carry them may affect fertility. Such alterations may be classified as follows:

- *Chromosome disorders*: These may be numerical (e.g. 47 chromosomes instead of 46) or structural (deletions, translocations, inversions, etc.)
- *Single gene disorders*: Of either nuclear genes or mitochondrial genes
- *Multi-genic disorders*: The clinical effect is caused by a combination of genetic alterations with or without environmental interactions—each individual alteration being insufficient to cause the disorder on its own but they "predispose" the individual to the condition in question.
- *Epigenetic factors*: These are non-inherited changes in the DNA (e.g. methylation of the DNA bases) or in the folding or position of the chromatin within the nucleus that do not affect the structure of a gene but influence its expression (i.e. whether it is switched on or off).

KNOWN GENETIC CAUSES OF MALE INFERTILITY

Some of the chromosome and single gene disorders associated with male infertility can have manifestations outside of the reproductive system, e.g. cystic fibrosis, myotonic dystrophy. Such conditions may be termed "syndromic" forms of male infertility. In assessing the infertile patient it is important to take a full personal and family history and perform a full general clinical examination in order to try and identify such causes.

Chromosome Disorders

In pooled data from 11 publications, of 9766 sub-fertile men, 5.7 percent had a microscopically-visible chromosome abnormality of which 4.2 percent had a sex chromosome abnormality and 1.5 percent had an autosomal abnormality. The frequency with which chromosome abnormalities are detected varies with the severity of impaired sperm production. Of the subgroup of azoospermic men, 13.7 percent have chromosome abnormalities—mainly sex chromosome abnormalities, most notably 47XXY (Klinefelter syndrome) which is found in 10 percent of azoospermic men. In 47XXY the testes are devoid of germ cells. Other sex chromosome abnormalities are also over-represented in this group of patients, e.g. 47XYY, 46 XX males, 45X/46XY, etc. In addition to sex chromosome anomalies, complex rearrangements and ring chromosomes typically represent an insurmountable obstacle to cell division in the spermatocyte, resulting in azoospermia.[2]

Low level sex chromosome mosaicism could also be a factor in a significant proportion of subfertile men. Such mosaicism may not be detected unless significant numbers of cells are counted. In a recent study of 101 infertile men, low-level sex chromosome mosaicism was found in 34 percent of those presenting for evaluation.[3] The men in this study with low-level mosaicism were significantly older and it is possible that low-level mosaicism may emerge with advancing age and may help to explain the decline in fertility potential seen in older men.

In older studies of severely oligozoospermic men, 4.6 percent have had chromosome abnormalities—mainly chromosomal translocations. Reciprocal translocations are 5 times more common in this group of men than in newborns and those involving an acrocentric chromosome are especially associated.[2] Similarly, Robertsonian translocations are found in 1.6 percent of the oligozoospermic group compared to 0.08 percent of the population. Other rearrangements such as pericentric inversions and extra structurally abnormal (marker) chromosomes also occur at increased frequency. It should however be remembered that most men who carry reciprocal translocations and inversions have normal fertility and that these rearrangements are infrequently associated with severe hypospermatogenesis and moderate to severe oligozoospermia.

Why might these translocations cause spermatogenic arrest in some men? In many animal male meiosis the presence of unaligned chromosomes will trigger apoptotic arrest (programmed cell death) at or before metaphase in cell division. There is a much more extensive system of error detection in male meiosis than female meiosis. Male meiosis contains checkpoints that detect mis-aligned or unpaired chromosomes before the first meiotic division and then direct the cell towards apoptosis.

Could meiotic errors be important causes of male infertility even in men with a normal karyotype? One way of investigating this problem is to look for increased sperm aneuploidy. Early studies using the human sperm + hamster ovum pseudofertilization test suggested a 10 percent background rate of chromosomally abnormal human sperm (aneuploidy in 1–3% and structural anomalies in 5–10%). Studies using fluorescent *in situ* hybridization (FISH) probes showed that considerable variation existed between individuals but there was an average disomy rate for each autosome of 0.1–0.2 percent though higher for chromosomes 21 and 22 and for X and Y disomy. There was no consistent correlation with paternal age, except possibly with XY disomy.[2]

Three strands of evidence suggest that meiotic errors may be important in some men:

1. Studies of sperm from fathers of aneuploid children showed that most had levels of disomic sperm that were little different from controls but there were a few men with a significantly higher level. It is possible therefore that a sub-group of men may be predisposed to meiotic errors.

2. Among infertile men with low sperm count and a normal karyotype, there is an increase in the sperm aneuploidy/diploidy rate.[2] This is particularly notable in men with severe oligospermia and those over 40 years of age. Both sperm count and sperm motility correlated with the level of sperm disomy. Testicular and epididymal biopsy studies from azoospermic men also show increased disomy rates. Furthermore, one small study of testicular biopsies showed that 42 percent (5/12) of men with impaired spermatogenesis displayed reduced genome-wide recombination when compared to the fertile men[4]—reduced recombination being a feature of abnormal meiosis.

3. A few studies in men with abnormal sperm morphology—double headed, large heads, multiple tails etc.—have shown high incidences of sperm aneuploidy.[3] In addition, some single gene disorders affecting meiotic processes have resulted in abnormal sperm morphology.[5]

Currently sperm karyotyping is a discretionary investigation if it is available.[2] In our lab referrals have related to patients with abnormal sperm morphology. A high correlation has been reported between sperm aneuploidy rates and sperm head anomalies. Our lab have used FISH probes for X, Y, 13, 18, 21 and report abnormal if >10 percent cells have the same disomy or if >30 percent of cells have any of the above disomies.

Y-chromosome Infertility

A very important group of patients are those with structural abnormalities of the Y-chromosome. The Y-chromosome alterations may be cytogenetically visible rearrangements (e.g. terminal deletions of Yq, isodicentric Yp, ring Y) or sub-microscopic deletions of the "male-specific region" (MSY).

The Y-chromosome has two "pseudoautosomal" regions that pair with the X-chromosome. It also has a "male-specific region" (MSY) that constitutes 95 percent of the Y-chromosome and consists of 23 million base pairs of DNA and 83 genes. Major components of the MSY are the so-called "ampliconic sequences" consisting of repetitive DNA (sequences with pronounced similarity to other sequences in the MSY). The ampliconic sequences contain 64 of the 83 MSY genes.[6] The amplicons are arranged in direct and inverted repeats, including 8 major palindromes. Palindromes are segments of DNA in which the nucleotide sequence in one strand read from one end is the same as the sequence in the complementary strand read from the opposite end. For example, the sequence GGTACC is a palindrome when the complementary strand sequence is CCATGG. Eight palindromes, designated P1–P8, are present in the MSY and together they comprise one-quarter of the euchromatic (transcriptionally active) DNA of the MSY.[7] These palindromes exhibit 99.97 percent intra-palindromic (arm-to-arm) sequence identity. They are large, with arm lengths that range from 9 kilobases (P7) to 1.45 megabases (P1). The paired arms of each palindrome are separated by a non-duplicated spacer that measures 2–170 kb in length. The palindromes harbour mirror-image gene pairs in the palindrome arms (none in the spacers) and all are expressed predominantly or exclusively in testes. Similar to the palindrome arms in which they reside, these gene families are characterized by extremely low sequence divergence between the copies found in a single Y-chromosome. The amplicons maintain this sequence identity through Y-Y-chromosome gene conversion (non-reciprocal transfer from one copy of the amplicon to another).

However, the presence of such repetitive DNA in the MSY predisposes to the occurrence of deletions. Throughout the genome, large deletions often seem to result from homologous recombination between direct repeat sequences (unequal exchange between repeats on homologous chromosomes or sister chromatids). In the case of the Y-chromosome, the deletions are intrachromosomal rather than interchromosomal and result from mis-alignment of sister chromatids[8] (**Fig. 13.1**).

Males with Y-chromosome infertility usually have no obvious symptoms, although physical examination may reveal small testes and/or cryptorchidism. Short stature may occur in individuals with Yq deletions that extend close to the centromere in a region containing a putative growth-controlling gene GCY.[9] A single study suggested that one of the deletions of the Y-chromosome (designated gr/gr) also causes an increase in susceptibility to testicular germ cell tumors.[10]

In Y-chromosome infertility, testicular biopsy may reveal either one of the following:

- Sertoli-cell-only syndrome (SCOS), in which azoospermia is associated with the absence of germ cells
- Hypospermatogenesis associated with reduced number of germ cells or arrest of germ cells at different developmental stages (spermatogenic arrest, SGA).

The search for "azoospermia factors" (AZF) focussed on the regions of the MSY found to be deleted in infertile males. In particular, three regions were identified known as AZFa, AZFb

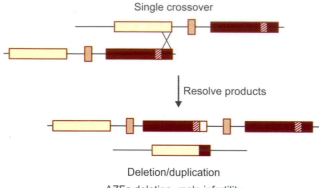

Figure 13.1: Mechanism of intrachromosomal recombination resulting in an AZFa deletion. In the case of AZFa, a deletion results from a single homologous recombination between two well-separated viral HERV15 sequences. The white box represents the proximal HERV and the black box the distal HERV. As these sequences are 94% identical, they may misalign and a single crossover between them can result in a deletion or duplication as shown. If a deletion occurs, there will be loss of the intervening testis-specific genes USP9Y and DDX3Y, shown as the shaded box. (Reproduced from Ref. 8 with permission)

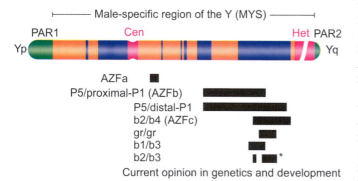

Figure 13.2: Structure of Y-chromosome showing sites and sizes of some recurrent deletions Legend: the centromere (Cen) separates the short arm (Yp) from the long arm (Yq). The male specific region (MSY) is flanked by the two pseudoautosomal regions (PAR1 and PAR2) that pair with the X-chromosome. The area marked "Het" is a long block of heterochromatin that varies in size between men. The euchromatic ampliconic sequences are indicated in blue. The position and size of the recurrent Y deletions are shown as black bars. The asterix indicates that the b2/b3 deletion can only occur on those chromosomes where there is an inverted variant of the AZFc region. (From Ref. 6, figure reproduced with permission)

and AZFc, which map on Yq in order from the centromere to the telomere. Subsequent studies showed that AZFb and AZFc overlap. As the deletions occur between repeat sequences, a more appropriate nomenclature for the types of recurrent deletions has developed using the names of the flanking repeats (**Fig. 13.2**). Currently 7 recurrent submicroscopic deletions have been described—AZFa, P5/proximal P1, P5/distal P1, AZFc (also known as b2/b4) and 3 partial AZFc deletions known as b1/b3, b2/b3 and gr/gr.[6]

Deletions of the AZF region of Y-chromosome have been found in 10–15 percent of men with non-obstructive azoospermia and 5–10 percent of men with severe oligozoospermia.[11] The prevalence of such microdeletions is even greater when patients are selected on testicular structure, reaching 30 percent in patients with Sertoli cell-only syndrome or severe hypospermatogenesis (i.e. complete loss or severe absence of germ cells in both testes).[12] The deletions are usually *de novo* and therefore not present in the father of the proband. Rarely within a family, the same deletion can cause infertility in some individuals but not others; hence, some fertile males with deletion of the AZF regions have fathered sons who are infertile. Theoretically, a father could be mosaic for a deletion of the AZF regions.

The most commonly seen deletion is AZFc (at Yq11.23) accounting for more than 80 percent of all reported Y microdeletions. AZFa deletions are relatively uncommon (1–5%) and generally associated with SCOS type 1 (no spermatogonia develop). AZFb deletions tend to cause spermatogenic arrest usually at the spermatocyte stage and deletions in AZFc are associated with a more variable phenotype ranging from type II SCOS (absence of germ cells in most tubules) to hypospermatogenesis.[13] These observations have to be used with caution as the phenotype may change with time—some patients who initially have oligozoospermia may later become azoospermic. Nevertheless, as a rule AZFa and AZFb deletions are more severe in their effects than AZFc and the finding of AZFa, AZFb or AZFb/c microdeletions predicts little chance of successful sperm retrieval by testicular sperm extraction.[14]

The incidence of these deletions is roughly correlated with the size of the targets for homologous recombination—AZFc deletions have large recombination targets of approximately 229 kb compared to P5/P1 (recombination targets approx. 100 kb) and AZFa (approximately 10kb). The length of identity rather than the degree of homology is the more important determinant of homologous recombination.[6] A summary of the deletions is given in **Table 13.1**.

- AZFa results from a single homologous recombination between two well-separated (800 kb apart) viral HERV15 sequences that are 94 percent identical 8. The deleted region contains 2 testis-specific genes USP9Y and DDX3Y—a case has been reported with a point mutation in USP9Y. All other cases have been deletions.

- P5/P1—account for 2 percent azoospermia cases (1 percent each of P5/proximal P1 and P5/distal P1). They do not always lead to SCOS but can cause maturation arrest. The prime candidate gene in the region is RBMY but the deletion affects other genes as well.

- AZFc consists entirely of amplicons. In AZFc, homologous recombination between two members of the blue amplicon family b2 and b4 (which are direct 229 kb repeats and show 99.9 percent nucleotide identity) causes the common deletion (**Fig. 13.3**). The prevalence of this deletion is estimated at 1 in 4000 males in the general population. Its frequency varies between studies but it probably accounts for 6–12 percent

Table 13.1: Summary of recurrent deletions in the MSY (Reproduced from Ref. 6 with permission)

Deletion	Size (Mb)	Number of genes affected	Phenotypic effect	Frequency	
				Azoo-spermia	Oligozoo-spermia
AZFa	0.8	2	Azoospermia (SCO syndrome)	<1%	0%
P5/proximal-P1 (AZFb)	6.2	23	Azoospermia (SCO syndrome / maturation arrest)	1%	0%
P5/distal-P1	7.6	31	Azoospermia (SCO syndrome / maturation arrest)	1%	0%
AZFc (b2/b4)	3.5	13	Azoospermia / severe oligozoospermia	6%	5%
gr/gr	1.6	6	Variable (risk factor for spermatogenic failure)	3%	3%
b1/b3	1.6	7	Unknown	-	-
b2/b3	1.7	7	Unknown	-	-

Abbreviations: SCO syndrome, Sertoli-cell-only (i.e. complete absence of germ cells in the testis).

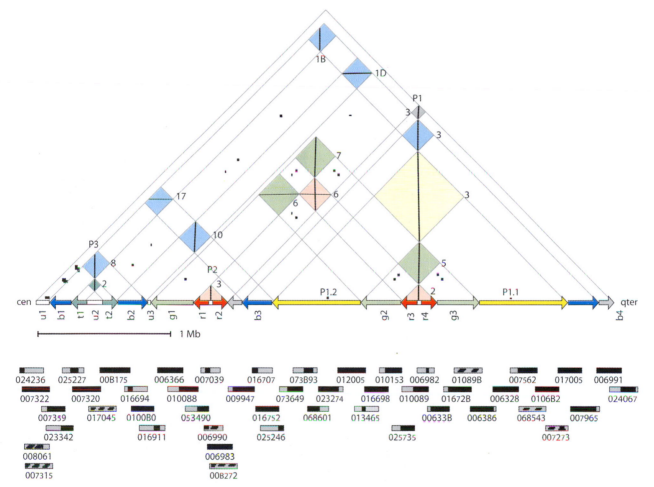

Figure 13.3: Structure of AZFc region with palindromes — The AZFc region consists of the palindromes P1, P2 and P3. Two smaller palindromes P1.1 and P1.2 lie within P1. Selected amplicons are identified (b1, t1, t2, b2, g1, r1, r2, b3, g2, r3, r4, g3 and b4) along with their orientation with respect to the centromere (cen) and long arm telomere (qter). The common deletion involves b2 and b4 which are direct repeats with 99.9% nucleotide identity. Other deletions involve recombination between the direct repeats b1 and b3 and between g1/r1/r2 and gr/r3/r4 (gr/gr deletion). Repeats b2 and b3 are not "direct repeats" as they are in opposite orientation and so deletions involving these amplicons only occur on chromosomes with an inverted repeat polymorphism (Reproduced from Ref. 15 with permission)

of non-obstructive azoospermia and 5–6 percent severe oligozoospermia cases.[6,15] The phenotype varies from SCOS to severe oligozoospermia. Variation probably results from other genetic and environmental factors.

There are also partial AZFc deletions—b1/b3, gr/gr and b2/b3.

- The prevalence of b1/b3 is low.
- The gr/gr deletion seems to be common in certain Y-chromosomes—indeed one branch of the Y-chromosome genealogical tree occurring primarily in Japan contains only gr/gr deleted chromosomes—this deletion removes 1.6 Mb but not the entire AZFc gene family—it reduces the copy number of 5 such families. Phenotype is very variable and can be associated with normal sperm counts and so should be considered a risk factor for spermatogenic failure.[16] Variation probably results from other genetic and environmental factors.
- b2/b3 occurs on inverted variants of the AZFc region in one branch of the Y-chromosome tree.

These deletions all remove multiple genes and it is largely unknown which genes or combinations of genes in these areas are important in causing the associated spermatogenic failure. The role of these genes in male fertility can be judged indirectly by studies of gene expression in animal models. For example, the DAZ gene family in AZFc (these genes reside exclusively in the arms of palindromes P1 and P2) has been shown to be transcribed predominantly in testes and transcripts of the mouse homologue Dazh were not detected in testes of mice that lacked germ cells. In the normal mouse, Dazh transcription was detectable 1 day after birth (when the only germ cells are prospermatogonia). Transcription increased steadily as spermatogonial stem cells appeared, plateaued as the first wave of spermatogenic cells entered meiosis (10 days after birth) and remained at this level thereafter. This unique pattern of expression suggests that Dazh participates in differentiation, proliferation, or maintenance of germ cell founder populations before, during, and after the pubertal onset of spermatogenesis. Such functions could readily account for the diverse spermatogenic defects observed in human males with AZFc deletions.

It is essential that the Y-chromosome has a system for repairing these spermatogenesis genes for the preservation of reproductive function. Indeed, the Y-chromosome in the testis is at high-risk of spontaneous mutation given the large numbers of cell divisions undertaken during gametogenesis and the highly oxidative environment of the testis. The palindromic structure of much of the MSY is particularly beneficial in this respect. A palindrome structure allows the Y-chromosome to repair itself by bending over at the middle (**Fig. 13.4A**). It is then capable of donating an intact gene to fix a defective copy on the neighboring section (**Fig. 13.4B**)—a process called gene conversion. Comparisons of sequence divergence in both human and chimpanzee palindromes suggests a steady-state balance between new mutations that create differences between arms and gene-conversion events that erase these differences.[15]

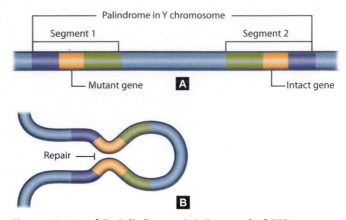

Figures 13.4A and B: Palindromes: (A) Composed of DNA segments that are mirror images—facilitate self-repair of the Y-chromosome. The Y can correct a mutation in one of the segments; (B) By bending and coying the intact version from the other segment. (Reproduced with permission. *Source*: universe-review.ca/R11-14-Ychromosome.htm)

Gene conversion is a frequent process that maintains the >99.9 percent arm-to-arm sequence identity. Such gene conversion results from double-strand breaks followed by noncross over resolution of the breaks either between sister chromatids or within one chromatid (**Fig. 13.5**). The downside of this system is that if the double strand breaks resolve with crossing over a structurally abnormal Y-chromosome can result. Lange et al. found evidence of an idic Yp or isoYp in 8 of 293 men (2.7%) with nonobstructive azoospermia but 0 of 288 men with severe or moderate oligozoospermia. In the large majority of cases therefore idicYp or isoYp formation precludes sperm production. They showed evidence that such isochromosomes arose from crossover between sister chromatids in inverted repeats (**Fig. 13.5**). The creation of such unstable dicentric chromosomes can result in infertility (due to deletion of spermatogenesis genes in distal Yq), Turner syndrome (due to mitotic instability and loss of isoYp leading to 45X) or sex reversal (mitotic instability resulting in 45X/46XisoY mosaicism).[17]

In clinical practice, many units will screen for these Y submicroscopic deletions by deletion/duplication analysis of DNA (usually extracted from leukocytes) in men with non-obstructive azoospermia or severe oligozoospermia (<5 million/mL) where other causes such as Klinefelter syndrome have been excluded. It is unlikely that a Y microdeletion will be found in men with lesser degrees of oligozoospermia (>5–10 million per mL). Finding a deletion provides information about risk of transmission to offspring if a pregnancy is achieved by ICSI (if this is a concern) and may, as indicated above, predict the likelihood of successful sperm retrieval. In addition, studies of men with AZFc deletions have shown some to have 45X/46XY mosaicism—thus, if loss of the Y-chromosome can occur, this may result in sex chromosome mosaicism or Turner syndrome (45X) in a pregnancy conceived by ICSI.[18]

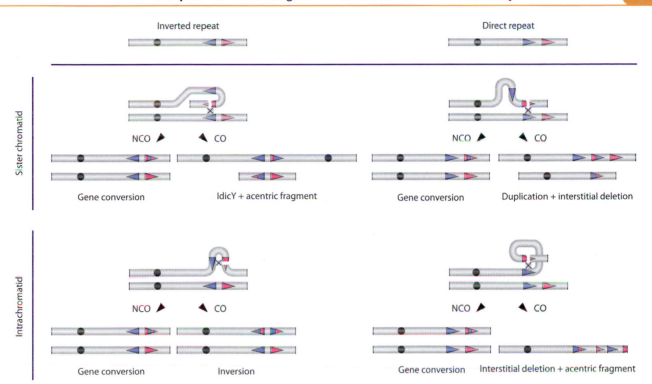

Figure 13.5: Model of double-strand break (DSB) resolution in inverted repeats of sister chromatids. If a double strand break occurs and resolves with no cross over (NCO), gene conversion occurs and this maintains sequence identity. However if the DCB resolves with a cross over event (CO), the result is an idicY and a acentric fragment. (Reproduced from Ref. 17 with permission)

Single Gene Disorders

These may be sub-classified:

- Genetic disorders of sexual differentiation and development—these may include those disorders associated with abnormal testis development, ambiguous genitalia at birth or with cryptorchidism or absence of the vas deferens (e.g. cystic fibrosis).
- Disorders associated with sperm production and function—e.g. myotonic dystrophy, Noonan syndrome, primary ciliary dyskinesia, hemoglobinopathies, CATSPER-related male infertility (deafness-infertility syndrome).
- Genetic endocrinopathies, e.g. hypogonadotrophic hypogonadism (e.g. KAL, FGRF1), pituitary disorders (e.g. HESX1), steroid biosynthetic defects, disorders of steroid metabolism and disorders of steroid action (e.g. of androgen receptor).

One of the reasons for researching rare "syndromic" forms of male infertility is that genes may be uncovered that may, in some circumstances lead to or predispose to "non-syndromic" male infertility. For example, in the autosomal recessive deafness-infertility syndrome, males inheriting two CATSPER1 mutations will be infertile whereas males inheriting two contiguous deletions involving CATSPER and the neighboring gene STRC will be both infertile and deaf. Similarly, investigators have considered whether normal variants (polymorphisms) in candidate genes

such as the androgen receptor may predispose to infertility if present in combination with other variants (i.e. multi-genic model).

Of the recognised single gene disorders, cystic fibrosis (CF) is the most important given its association with CBAVD. CBAVD accounts for 1–2 percent male infertility and cystic fibrosis gene (CFTR) mutations are the most important cause. CF is an autosomal recessive disease and affected patients have mutations in both of their copies of the CF gene. Pooled data from several studies identified at least one CF mutation in nearly 80 percent of cases of CBAVD. Where only one mutation is identified, there clearly is a strong possibility that the expression of the other allele is also sub-optimal, even though the cause of this reduced expression avoids detection. As seen in **Table 13.2**,[19] in many cases the alteration identified in the CF gene is the "5T allele". This describes a poly T tract, a string of thymidine bases, located in intron 8 of the *CFTR* gene. This poly T tract can be associated with *CFTR*-related disorders depending on its size. The three common variants of the poly T tract are 5T, 7T, and 9T. Both 7T and 9T are considered polymorphic variants but 5T is considered a mutation of reduced penetrance (i.e. it does not produce a full CF phenotype unless in conjunction with another mutation in the same allele). The 5T variant is thought to decrease the efficiency of intron 8 splicing. In addition, there is a TG tract lying just 5' of the poly T tract. It consists of a short string of TG repeats

Table 13.2: Frequency of CFTR mutations in CBAVD
(Reproduced from Ref. 19 with permission)

Mutant CFTR Alleles		Percentage in CBAVD Cases
Other than 5T	5T	%
2	0	26
0	2	2
1	1	26
1	0	17
0	1	8
0	0	22

Source: Reproduced from CFTR-Related Disorders [Includes: Cystic Fibrosis (CF, Mucoviscidosis) and Congenital Absence of the Vas Deferens (CAVD)] PMID: 20301428 by Samuel M Moskowitz, MD, James F Chmiel, MD, Darci L Sternen, MS, Edith Cheng, MS, MD, Garry R Cutting, MD. Initial Posting: March 26, 2001. Last Update: February 19, 2008 with kind permission of www.genetests.org copyright University of Washington, Seattle

that commonly number 11, 12, or 13. A longer TG tract (12 or 13) in conjunction with a shorter poly T tract (5T) has the strongest adverse effect on proper intron 8 splicing.[19]

Epigenetic Causes

Concern has been raised that assisted reproductive technologies (ART) may increase the incidence of children being born with the epigenetic disorders Beckwith-Wiedemann syndrome (BWS) and Angelman syndrome (AS). Differential methylation of cytosine in specific regions of DNA known as CpG islands is a mechanism of gene regulation. This process underlies "genomic imprinting" whereby only one of the two parental alleles of some genes is expressed. This imprinting is erased in embryonic germ cells and reset later according to the sex of the embryo. It is thought that ART may cause imprinting disorders BWS and AS through loss of maternal methylation in the oocyte or during embryo culture.

One study examined methylation patterns at two imprinted genes (one maternally and one paternally imprinted) in sperm from 27 normozoospermic and 96 oligozoospermic men under investigation for infertility.[20] In 23 of the oligozoospermic men, incomplete methylation profiles were identified at the paternally imprinted locus whereas the maternal imprint was correctly erased in all cases. This observation suggests an association between abnormal genomic imprinting and hypospermatogenesis but what is cause and effect is not known. One possibility is that altered DNA methyltransferase activity (whether caused by genetic or environmental factors) could be a cause of hypospermatogenesis.

DISSECTING THE GENETIC CAUSES OF IDIOPATHIC MALE INFERTILITY

What about the large number of men with "idiopathic" infertility? Whilst most studies have focussed on the Y-chromosome, the prevalence of families with more than one infertile member suggests that genetic factors are common and important.[21] These genetic causes are likely to be a combination of a number of rare single gene disorders and the added effects of common alterations in several genes (multi-genic model). Which genes may be involved? A variety of approaches have been adopted to try and identify these genes:

Genome-wide Linkage Studies

In rare familial cases, mapping the gene to a chromosome can be attempted—especially in rare consanguineous families. Once a gene is mapped, candidate genes in the region can be identified for mutation searching. Such an approach identified mutations in the AURKC gene in rare families of North African descent.[5]

Candidate Gene Analysis

Pathogenic mutations in genes that may be considered as likely candidates may be sought in cohorts of affected males. This was discussed above in consideration of genes associated with syndromic forms of infertility (e.g. CATSPER) and there are other examples such as mutations in dynein genes (selected as they are important in primary ciliary dyskinesia, a disorder associated with reduced sperm motility in most cases).[22] The most recent example is NR5A1 gene—a gene that has been implicated in disorders of male sexual development. Seven out of 315 men with idiopathic spermatogenic failure were found to carry missense mutations in this gene.[23]

Alternatively case-control studies may be undertaken to identify predisposing genes by looking for variation (polymorphisms) in these genes that are more common in cases than controls. The methodology applied to these case-control studies needs to be very careful as indicated by Visser and Repping.[24] These authors point out that:

- Many studies have been undertaken based on reported fertility rather than semen quality. Such studies may therefore have been confounded by containing subfertile, normozoospermic cases and oligozoospermic but fertile controls.
- Where sperm counts have been part of the inclusion criteria, classification has sometimes been based on only one sample and hence participants may have been erroneously placed into the normozoospermic or oligozoospermic groups.
- Studies that dichotomise men as normozoospermic or oligozoospermic do not consider the quantitative nature of spermatogenesis that may be affected by a genetic risk factor. Visser and Repping argue for a "cohort approach" i.e. assembling a large cohort of men with varying sperm counts and comparing the sperm counts of men with and without the genetic variant.[24]
- Some studies have not adequately matched the cases and controls for factors such as ethnic groups as some studies have shown ethnic differences in spermatogenesis.

How are candidate genes selected? In general, three approaches have been taken;

- Select genes based on their known association or possible association with fertility

- Select genes that are associated with infertility in animal models (notably the mouse)
- Select genes based on their expression or reduced expression in the testes of the mouse or infertile males.

In terms of the first of these groups, several avenues have been explored:

- Genes associated with endocrine function such as the androgen receptor gene and the FSH and LH genes or the genes encoding their receptors, etc. Recently for example 3 mutations were identified in two cohorts (one Japanese and one Irish) of 90 azoospermic patients in the FKBPL gene which encodes a steroid receptor chaperone.[25]
- Genes may also be sought in chromosomal regions identified as possibly carrying spermatogenesis genes. An example is chromosome 1q44 where a deletion patient had SCOS.[26]
- Some genes may be considered because of homology to genes in the MSY region, e.g. the DAZ gene has an autosomal homologue, DAZL (DAZ-Like), on chromosome 3 (3p24) and one Taiwan study found a polymorphism in this gene in severely infertile patients[27] though this was not found in a subsequent study of Italian men.
- Genes associated with "syndromic" forms of infertility.
- Genes known to be testis-specific.
- Other genes postulated reflect the consideration of possible gene-environment interactions. The presence of reactive oxygen species or free radicals in the testes will be expected to cause oxidative damage or mutation to the mitochondrial genome (mtDNA). The key nuclear enzyme involved in the elongation and repair of mtDNA strands is DNA polymerase gamma, mapped to the long arm of chromosome 15 (15q25), and includes a CAG repeat region. Researchers have considered whether variants within this gene might influence fertility.[28] Similarly, researchers have found associations between the glutathione-S-transferase deletion mutation and infertility in various studies as this enzyme has antioxidant activity.

Animal models have been used in many complex disorders to identify candidate genes and rodent models have been heavily investigated in fertility. Visser and Repping[24] advise some caution. Whilst spermatogenesis is similar in mice and men, there are also many different processes that are likely to be governed by different sets of genes. Nevertheless, studying mouse models has identified a large number of candidate genes and aided our understanding of the mechanisms of infertility. A full review of these studies is given by Marzuk and Lamb[29] who categorise the genes involved in male fertility based on the cells where they function and the roles they play:

- Testicular cells (Sertoli, peritubular, Leydig and/or interstitial cells)—genes that encode growth factors and receptors, gonadotrophin receptors, cell-cell adhesion molecules, steroids and receptors, signal transduction molecules, junctional complexes.
- Spermatogonial proliferation—the rate of this process is carefully regulated. Genes involved in growth (e.g. *Kit, Csf, Bmp8b*) and genes involved in apoptosis are all important in the mouse. Defects in the balance of cell

proliferation and cell death could contribute to the pathology of hypospermatogenesis.

- Spermatocyte production (meiosis)—genes affecting meiotic processes such as chromosome pairing, synapsis, recombination, DNA replication and repair, etc.
- Spermatid formation (the process of differentiation)—genes involved in cell remodelling, cytoplasmic extrusion, chromatin packaging, nuclear condensation and spermiation.
- Spermatozoa maturation, motility and egg penetration. Numerous genes affect these various processes.

In addition to these categories, Marzuk and Lamb list a series of genes that cause "other fertility defects".

Mutations in some of the genes identified in mouse models have been found in male infertility patients. One example is SYCP3. Mice deficient in SYCP3 have azoospermia with meiotic arrest. In a study of 19 azoospermic patients, a 1 bp deletion was identified in 2 patients and none in 75 fertile controls.[30] However, as Visser and Repping point out, two subsequent studies reported that mutations in this gene appear to be rare causes of azoospermia.[24] It may be of course that patients with mutations in this gene have a specific phenotype and that most studies involve patients with phenotypes (azoospermia and oligozoospermia) that are too heterogeneous. Other examples of mutations identified in mouse models that have been found in some patients include SPATA16 in some men with globozoospermia,[31] as well as some genes in fibrous sheath of flagellum associated with sperm motility such as AKAP4 and AKAP3[32] and genes involved in flagellar assembly (e.g. TEKT1).[33] The role of CATSPER genes has already been alluded to regulating calcium and potassium currents in sperm. A positive association has been found between a polymorphism in the testis-specific serine/threonine kinase gene and infertility—this gene leads to infertility in the knockout mouse.[34]

The few examples listed above have made a very limited impact on our understanding of human male infertility given the hundreds of potential candidate genes. As Visser and Repping point out, nearly all studies have looked at the effect of a single gene on spermatogenesis but now with the advent of high-throughput screening methods the possibility of studying thousands of genes at the same time is open—either by sequencing many candidate genes (or even whole exonomes or genomes) using new generation sequencing technology or high throughput analysis of genomic variation as employed in genome-wide association studies.[24]

Expression studies aim to detect differences in the expression (or non-expression) of genes in the testes of infertile males (mouse and human) using microarray technology. For example, Okada et al. performed genome-wide gene expression analyzes on human testis specimens from 47 nonobstructive azoospermia (NOA) and 11 obstructive azoospermia (OA) patients and the genes that showed the most significantly differential expression were then subject to case-control association studies. For one gene in this study, ART3, a significant association was found for non-obstructive azoospermia.[35] Visser and Repping caution that interpretation of differential expression data is difficult because the expression can simply mirror the presence or absence of

14

Preimplantation Genetic Screening: Unraveling the Controversy

Antonio Capalbo, Laura Rienzi, Zsolt Peter Nagy

■ DEFINITION AND BACKGROUND

It has been a goal of reproductive medicine and science to diagnose diseases as early as possible in the reproductive process. Since Gregor Johann Mendel elucidated genetic inheritance theories in the 1860s,[1] there has been an understanding that the random assortment of genes leads to a certain percentage of the offspring expressing a given trait. These notions were important to define the reproductive risk for a specific disease or syndrome. Preimplantation testing of embryo is the newest of a series of reproductive technologies that allows for diagnosis or screening at the earliest possible juncture, even before an embryo is placed within the womb and in complete absence of phenotype. This technique has altered our conception of disease prediction, diagnosis, and prevention. Especially in genetics we have entered a new era, the one of predictive medicine. As noted by Jean Dausset, the Nobel laureate who discovered HLA antigens, ". . . medicine was, in its history, first of all curative, then preventive and finally predictive, whereas today the order is reversed: initially predictive, then preventive and finally, only in desperation, curative".[2] Preimplantation genetic diagnosis (PGD), is a well established and efficient clinical diagnostic procedure originally developed as an alternative to prenatal diagnosis (PND) to reduce the transmission of severe genetic disease for fertile couples with a well-known reproductive risk.[3] Virtually any genetically inherited disease with known mutation in human can be identified efficiently in a single cell of preimplantation embryo. As such, the applications of PGD are myriad and well established. In contrast to this specific and restricted application, a related technology has recently been used more frequently to improve *in vitro* fertilization (IVF) success for infertile couples by screening embryos for common or age-related aneuploidies. The latter procedure has been designated as PGD-AS (aneuploidy screening) by the European Society on Human Reproduction and Embryology (ESHRE) consortium[4] or preimplantation genetic screening (PGS) by the Human Fertilization and Embryology Authority (HFEA), but it has been included in the definition of PGD in the United States.[5] Preimplantation genetic diagnosis-aneuploidy screening (PGD-AS) is mainly applied when a low IVF success rate might be attributable to chromosomal aneuploidies in the embryos. Aneuploidy is extremely common in human embryos and leads to developmental arrest, implantation failure and spontaneous abortion. The inadvertent transfer of chromosomally abnormal embryos is believed to explain a significant proportion of failed IVF cycles. In addition, aneuploidy is the leading cause of inborn mental and developmental disabilities, so women over 36 years of age, who are at increased risk of producing a child with Down syndrome, or with other age-related chromosomal abnormalities, and who have already opted for IVF/ICSI because of their infertility, might wish to have their embryos screened for these more common viable abnormalities rather than go through prenatal diagnosis (PND) and possible abortion.

Two main differences help to distinguish between PGD and PDG-AS: the first is the degree of reproductive risk that the couple has. The PGD group consists of patients at high risk of having a child with a genetic disease, e.g. carriers of a monogenic disease or of chromosomal structural aberrations with viable unbalanced genotype—who already have an affected child or repeatedly opted to terminate their pregnancies on the basis of results of prenatal tests. In practice PGD is just another arm of a genetic service which utilizes the skills of the Assisted Conception Unit to obtain the diagnostic material (and most of these couples are not infertile; thus IVF treatment is only performed for the reason to be able to test embryos prior to implantation). PGD-AS patients, on the other hand, who have a low genetic risk are already being treated with *in vitro* fertilization (IVF) and the genetic screening could be seen as a complementary embryo selection process. The second difference is that PGD tests for the diagnosis of single gene disorders or structural chromosome anomalies, are generally patient specific, while in the case of PGD-AS, an identical protocol is employed for all patients and there is no need for a preliminary molecular work-up.

Preimplantation chromosomal testing of embryos is not new in reproductive technology.[6] In 1968, Gardner and Edwards were able to sex rabbit embryos using a sex-specific chromatin pattern in blastocyst biopsies, before their transfer to the uterus. Preimplantation testing of embryos is also used routinely in animal husbandry to produce animals of the preferred sex. In the early 90s, a method that allowed single-cell analysis at the chromosomal level was described; fluorescence *in situ* hybridization (FISH) that has replaced PCR as a reliable method for the sexing of embryos, and has been widely used for PGD-AS and for detection of imbalanced forms of chromosomal structural abnormalities.[7] This technology has had an impressive growth in its clinical application so that at the moment it is becoming apparent that the main demand for embryo biopsy will come from infertile patients seeking to improve their chances of successful IVF treatment. PGD-AS has become so popular that of all the preimplantation genetic testing related procedures, ~75 percent (in USA) and 65 percent (in Europe) of all indications for embryo screening are to identify embryos with aneuploidy.[8,9] PGD-AS is however, a continuing evolving technology with uncertain clinical benefit at the moment but that represents one of the most attracting and promising application in human reproductive medicine with the potential of significantly improve clinical outcomes compared to other embryo selection methods. Moreover it is of critical importance in basic research providing main insight on human meiotic recombination, pathogenesis mechanisms of aneuploidy and their role in human infertility.

INDICATIONS

"Hypotheses nonfingo" I. Newton *Principia* (1713)

The most relevant and recent evidences suggest that failed implantation due to embryo aneuploidy rather than failed conception is the primary cause of low human fertility.[10] Some of the earlier studies underestimate chromosome abnormalities in spontaneous miscarriage because conventional karyotyping requires tissue culture, which is prone to maternal contamination. More recent studies employing molecular cytogenetic techniques suggest the true incidence of aneuploidy may be exceed 65 percent.[11] Chromosome studies in spontaneous abortions of ART patients also indicate a higher rate of chromosome abnormalities,[12] with 65–71 percent of spontaneous abortions being chromosomally abnormal, and increasing with maternal age.[13] Considering these data, researchers soon realized that embryo selection based on chromosome complement would possibly increase IVF efficacy. Preliminary observations showed that many aneuploidies are able to develop during the entire preimplantation period *in vitro*, providing support for the introduction of PGD-AS.

Therefore the assumption behind PGD-AS is to screen embryos in couples with a significantly increased reproductive risk, taken as the increased likelihood of producing embryos that will fail to implant or will establish a pregnancy in which a fetus miscarries or could produce a child with chromosomal syndrome. Several categories of patients presenting such an increased risk in IVF population can be identified.

Advanced-female Reproductive Age

The most significant variable related to the production of aneuploid embryos is the age of the female partner. It is well known that the female age is associated with an increase in aneuploidy rate, correlated with a reduced implantation and a higher abortion rates. Direct cytogenetic analysis of human oocytes demonstrates that oocyte aneuploidy rates could reach even 50 percent some women over 40 years of age and that almost all chromosomes are involved in meiotic errors albeit with different frequencies.[14-16] In addition, with older women it has been proposed that at the embryo stage defective postzygotic mitosis

can give rise to even increased chromosomal abnormalities.[17] Oocyte derived factors play a critical role in maintaining chromosome stability and euploidy in early-cleavage embryogenesis. An age-related defective cytoplasmic maturation during the antral follicle growth in older women could probably induce an alteration in spindle assembly, chromosome alignment and spindle assembly checkpoint (SAC) in a transcriptionally quiescence state of embryonic genome and in the absence of strong cell cycle control mechanisms.[18] Since standard FISH probes combination can detect 72–83 percent of the chromosomally abnormal fetuses routinely detected by karyotyping in women of advanced maternal age it was proposed that PGD-AS should eliminate close to 80 percent of all chromosomally abnormal embryos at risk of causing a miscarriage.[19] These data are supported by oocyte donation programs showing that older women failing to conceive with their own oocytes may conceive by using donor oocytes from younger women.[20] Therefore, advanced-female reproductive age (ARA) (cut off varies between 35 and 40 years of age, depending on the center) was the primary indication proposed for PGD-AS in order to improve IVF outcomes and reduce chromosomal syndromes as an alternative to PND.

Recurrent Pregnancy Loss

Recurrent pregnancy loss (RPL), is defined when three or more consecutive spontaneous abortions of less than 20–28 weeks' gestation occur, which affects 1 percent of couples trying to conceive.[21] There is little evidence of endometrial rejection or a defective endometrium and 50 percent of cases remain classified as having unknown etiology even after an appropriate infertility work-up.[22] The number of miscarriages stands out as a predictor of the chromosome abnormality rate, which is directly proportional to the number of miscarriages. However, when the number of miscarriages is much higher fetal aneuploidy incidence is reduced and the etiology is probably of a different nature. Up to 75 percent of recurrent miscarriages are associated with fetal chromosomal aberrations.[10] Studies employing molecular cytogenetic techniques report even higher rates.[23] The most common cause of spontaneous abortions in karyotipically normal patients is *de novo* numerical abnormalities, in particular autosomal trisomies for chromosomes 13, 14, 15, 16, 21 and 22, followed by monosomy X. Autosomal monosomies are rarely found in spontaneous abortions and are thought to be responsible for preclinical abortions or failed implantation.[24]

Multiple investigators have reported high rates of aneuploidy also in embryos of couples with RPL with rates approaching 80 percent.[25,26] Anomalies for chromosomes 16 and 22 were significantly higher in RPL cases.[27] Moreover in 22 percent of these couples, the incidence of chromosomal aberrations affects all the embryos, and the percentage of abnormal embryos is similar in subsequent attempts.[27] This result suggested that aneuploidy is a common cause of RPL with idiopathic etiology, and led to the idea that PGD-AS may be beneficial in these patients. The success of oocyte donation program in women with RPL supports the idea that the oocyte may be the origin of infertility in most of these couples.[28] However, a paternal contribution cannot be ruled out, since same common gonosomal aneuploidies in abortive samples are paternally biased and an increased incidence of sex chromosome disomy and diploidy has been reported in sperm samples from couples with unexplained recurrent miscarriage.[26,29,30]

Recurrent pregnancy loss (RPL) could also arise from a carrier of a balanced structural chromosomal abnormalities, in particular translocations. Reciprocal translocations are a type of chromosome rearrangement involving the exchange of chromosome segments between nonhomologous chromosomes with an incidence of about 1 in 500 in newborns. This rearrangement are unique and give rise a different rate of unbalanced gamete in carriers. Robertsonian translocations instead, originate from the centromeric fusion of acrocentric chromosome and are recognized to be the most common structural chromosomal rearrangements in the general population and in infertile men, with an incidence of 0.1 percent and 0.7–3 percent, respectively.[31]

Among couples with recurrent miscarriage, about 4.5 percent are carriers of translocations.[32] Individuals with translocations are generally asymptomatic and known to have high rates of unbalanced gametes, impaired or reduced gametogenesis and are therefore at risk for infertility and pregnancy loss.[33] When conceiving naturally, these individuals experience loss in most pregnancies. The prevailing attitude among various medical specialties is that, because most of the unbalanced pregnancies will miscarry and seldom reach term, further interventions other than idiopathic recurrent pregnancy loss (RPL) treatments are unnecessary. However, this attitude does not take into account the pain and suffering caused by RPL. Although the ultimate goal of translocation carriers is to achieve a viable pregnancy free of chromosome abnormalities, reducing the risk of miscarriage is a parallel goal. Additionally, PGD-AS can reduce time to success in these patients.

Moreover, it has been suggested that such rearrangements can also influence the segregation of uninvolved chromosomes. As a result, an increased aneuploidy in the sperm or oocyte may be observed for chromosomes not involved in the rearrangement, a phenomenon known as an interchromosomal effect (ICE), and chromosome translocations have been shown to affect meiotic segregation of uninvolved chromosomes in mice[34] and in Drosophila.[35] An ICE was first described in humans by Lejeune (1963),[36] but the existence of an ICE has remained a source of controversy and the origin hypothesized mechanisms are largely speculative.

Homologous Robertsonian translocations are a very rare form of rearrangement and according to meiotic segregation, gamete cells are either nullisomic or disomic for the translocated chromosome,[37] without chance of having a karyotypically normal embryo unless there is uniparental disomy (UPD) of the translocated chromosomes. Typical genetic counseling for carriers would not suggest assisted reproduction treatments but rather adoption or donation. A recent report using sperm FISH analysis revealed 13 percent normal sperm cells for chromosome 14 in the homologous 14;14 Robertsonian translocation carrier and in subsequent PGD-AS cycle one euploid blastocyst was transferred.[38] In this patient the occurrence of a germline mosaicism or chimerism could explain the presence of normal sperm. This has significant implications genetic counseling of homologous translocation male carriers in which a meiotic segregation analyses could be recommended before suggesting adoption or donation.

Recurrent Implantation Failure

Repeated implantation failure (RIF), defined as the failure of a couple to conceive after the transfer of 10 or more good-quality embryos or after three IVF cycles, is another potential indication proposed for PGD-AS in young patients.[39] Repeated implantation failure (RIF) can be the result of several uterine pathologic conditions, such as intrauterine adhesions, and submucous myomas, disturbed uterine receptivity, autoimmune conditions, thrombophilia, or inadequate ET methods. But even in successful units with high pregnancy and delivery rates, some couples experience repeated IVF failure. Although multiple etiologies have been proposed, increased incidence of numerical chromosomal abnormalities is obviously the most common cause. Indeed, an increased incidence of aneuploidy has been observed in the embryos generated from couples with repeated implantation failure. Using comparative genomic hybridization (CGH), chromosome abnormalities have been detected in about 60 percent of single blastomeres biopsied from embryos before implantation in 20 women with RIF.[40] Significantly higher incidence of complex chromosome abnormalities was also found in RIF patients.[41] The disruption of normal replication sequence and chromosomal segregation in early human embryos, probably caused by maternal cytoplasmic factors or defective cell cycle control mechanisms, might be a common cause for RIF.

Severe Male Factor

In recent years intracytoplasmic sperm injection (ICSI) has been used to achieve pregnancy in couples with severe male factor (SMF) infertility. Two main findings have focused the attention on whether the paternal contribution to aneuploidy could be especially relevant in cases of severe male factor, suggesting it as indication for PGD-AS: first, the increased incidence of *de-novo* chromosomal abnormalities in the children born after ICSI with a notable rise in sex chromosome aneuploidy[42] (1.6% versus 0.45%) according to Liebaers et al.[43] and second, a higher aneuploidy rate in spermatozoa from patients with severe oligoasthenoteratospemia (OAT) or azoospermia compared to normozoospermic men.[44,45] Moreover, prenatal testing in ICSI pregnancies has shown 2.1 percent of *de novo* chromosome abnormalities in men with oligozoospermia, with an incidence of 0.6 percent for gonosomes.[46] These elevated rates have been associated rather with the sperm quality than with the ICSI procedure itself. FISH analysis of sperm from normal karyotype infertile men has shown increased levels of aneuploid and diploid spermatozoa in which the sex chromosomes are mainly affected. This increase is higher in severe OAT men with less than 5×10^6 sperm/mL and in azoospermic men, particularly in non-obstructive ones, (NOA) with many authors reporting a 10–30-fold increase in the most extreme cases.[47]

Defective sex chromosome recombination during meiosis were observed in the sperm of chromosomally normal OAT and NOA population which could be pathogenetic mechanism of the higher rate of gonosomal aneuploidy in these men. Defects in synapsis or recombination may be caught by meiotic checkpoints, leading to a loss of germ cells and subsequent infertility. However, some cells may be able to progress through meiosis, resulting in an increased proportion of sperm with chromosomal abnormalities.

Other than gonosomes, there is little information on the chromosome-specific patterns of recombination in infertile men. However, the reduced levels of both genome-wide and chromosome-specific recombination that have been observed in infertile men may increase their risk of producing autosomal aneuploid sperm and chromosomally abnormal offspring.

Moreover, sperm centrosomal dysfunction has been reported from ultrastructural studies in pathological spermatozoa and could cause aberrant embryonic development.[48] Accordingly, the occurrence of mosaicism in preimplantation embryos is one of the major consequences.[49,50] Generally the observed absolute increase in sperm aneuploidy is modest, with mean value less than 1–2 percent disomy rate per chromosome in male infertility samples. However, we have to consider disomy data only (not nullisomy) are reported as, ordinarily, it is difficult to distinguish nullisomy from failure of hybridization in any given sperm head. In theory, the total aneuploidy rate for any given chromosome can be calculated as twice the disomy rate and we should not forget only a selected panel of chromosomes were evaluated in previous reports. Total aneuploidy rates in OAT and NOA patients considering the 24 chromosomes has been estimated to be higher on a per chromosome disomy frequencies for autosomes and gonosomes.[51] In addition, similar incidences of aneuploid and diploid sperms were described in swim-up motile sperm fractions compared with the pellet fractions in infertile males. So it has been assumed that sperm selection techniques are not able to improve capability of injecting euploid ones. In clinical setting the presence of chromosomally abnormal sperm has been related to recurrent miscarriage.[26] Therefore, the implementation of PGD-AS in these patients could constitute an effective tool to reduce the increased frequency of *de-novo* numerical and structural chromosomal disorders in children born after ICSI and improve IVF outcomes.

Other Potential Indications

Preimplantation genetic diagnosis-aneuploidy screening (PGD-AS) for constitutional mosaic karyotype has been suggested because of recurrence of numerical chromosomal abnormalities.[52] The relationship between low-grade mosaicism and infertility or implantation failure is still controversial because the real incidence of mosaicism in the general population is still unknown. It was claimed that mosaicism has been underestimated as a cause of repeated failure in assisted reproduction. Scholtes et al, report a high incidence of minor mosaicism among infertile patients and a low implantation rate in IVF cycles.[53] No required minimum percentage of abnormal cells has been established to define true versus "low-grade" mosaicism. Thus, the

importance of low-grade mosaicism and its impact on fertility is still to be determined and deserve attention.

Other reasonable indications in female patients could be identified in ovarian pathological conditions that can cause a premature ovarian aging or a deficient oocyte maturation, such as polycystic ovary syndrome PCOS and premature ovarian insufficiency POI. PCOS is associated with higher oocyte yield, poorer oocyte quality, low fertilization rate, and an increased risk of spontaneous pregnancy loss in comparison to women with normal ovarian function.[54] A widely held perception, therefore, suggests that oocytes, and embryos, from patients with PCOS are of poorer overall quality. There is, however, little information on whether PCOS results in increased aneuploidy rates. A small number of studies analyzing oocyte or embryo aneuploidy rate in these patients didn't find evidence of increased susceptibility to numerical chromosomal abnormalities compared to controls.[55]

In POI patients an increased risk of Down syndrome and aged ovarian phenotype has been reported, resembling that of ARA group.[56] Moreover infertility is one of the first clinical phenotype observed in these patients. Accordingly, aneuploidy screening in patients with a family history of POI with an incompletely manifested clinical phenotype could be beneficial.

Being used as an embryo selection method, PGD-AS could be also regarded as an IVF technique for single-embryo transfer with the aim of reduce multiple implantations. Considering that numerical chromosomal abnormalities are abundant even in ovum-donation programs and in the absence of ovarian stimulation,[57,58] PGD-AS could be beneficial for all patients undergoing IVF cycles.

It is important to notice that since patients considering IVF with PGD-AS have no specific identifiable genetic abnormality and PGD-AS is intended to detect aneuploidies which, in most cases, will result in preclinical loss, genetic counseling is challenging but nonetheless extremely important. Counseling before PGD-AS must include the following key points, in addition to the information of IVF: the possibility of a false positive result that may lead to the discard of a normal embryo; the possibility of a false negative result that may lead to the transfer of an abnormal embryo; the possibility that testing may yield inconclusive results and the fate of undiagnosed embryos; the estimated likelihood (on a per couple basis) that no embryos may be transferred and the expected frequencies of embryo aneuploidies; the nature and quality of the available evidence with regard to live-birth rates after IVF with PGD-AS. Probably the importance of counseling is underestimated in IVF-PGD-AS clinics. From a recent report evaluating the accuracy and completeness of the portrayal of PGD on websites clinics advertise PGD online, but the scope and quality of information about it varies widely, emphasizing benefits while minimizing risks.[59] So, a correct information is an essential step to employ when a couple is seeking for aneuploidy screening.

Mechanisms of Aneuploidy Induction in Human Gametogenesis and Early Embryogenesis

Genesis of chromosomal abnormalities in human preimplantation embryos are of meiotic or mitotic origin or both. While chromosomal abnormalities and genetic lesions that arise in the gametes are inherited by all daughter cells and will almost result in an implantation failure or abortion, those acquired in one or a few blastomeres during cleavage are inherited in a mosaic pattern with a portion of cells being of normal ploidy whereas others may be chromosomally abnormal. It is predicted that the earlier in cleavage a genetic lesion occurs, greater will be the number of daughter cells that inherit the genetic defect. Therefore, maintenance of genomic integrity during gametogenesis, fertilization and cleavage is essential for normal human embryogenesis and fetal disorders.

Aneuploidy of meiotic origin is the most common evident chromosomal abnormality in humans, occurring in 5 percent of all pregnancies and 0.3 percent of live births.[60] For reasons that are as yet unclear chromosome segregation in meiosis is surprisingly error prone in our species while in other mammals such as the mouse the overall incidence of aneuploidy among fertilized eggs does not exceed 1–2 percent. Despite this high frequency and clinical importance, we know surprisingly little about factors that modulate the risk of meiotic nondisjunction.

About 50 years ago, Robin Holliday has described the molecular basis of homologous recombination that triggers the origin of genetic diversity among life species.[61] Holliday junctions are not only being identified as an intermediate in genetic recombination but are also discovered and studied in recent years for their importance in maintaining genomic integrity from the dictyotene stage until bivalent separation. The successful segregation of homologues at the first division requires unique chromosome behaviors that include the maintenance of physical connections between homologues until anaphase I, and some form of physical constraint on the centromeres of sister chromatids so that they form attachments to the same, rather than opposing, spindle poles. Chiasmata, the physical manifestations of genetic recombination, have a crucial role in tethering homologous chromosomes during the first meiotic division and their orientation in the metaphase plate. So, it is not surprising that, in all model organisms studied so far, induced disturbances in the recombination pathway are associated with abnormalities in chromosome segregation at MI. In addition to an effect of the number of recombination events, the location of the exchanges also seems to be important, indicating that absent or reduced and suboptimally positioned recombination events increase the likelihood of nondisjunction. By using genetic mapping techniques to study the inheritance of DNA polymorphisms in trisomic conceptuses, it was possible to observe a significant reduction in recombination as a feature of all MI-derived trisomies.[62] The relatively recent introduction of immunofluorescence methodology provides a simple, straightforward approach to the analysis of human meiosis, making it possible to monitor the formation of meiosis-specific structures (e.g. the synaptonemal complex, SC) and to visualize interactions between bivalents as they pair, synapse and recombine during meiotic prophase. Although there are important differences in the recombination rate between male and female gametogenesis, direct evidence of the relationship between reduced recombination and nondisjunction has been obtained in the analysis of human spermatozoa

and more recently in the direct analysis of human MI oocytes. By studying recombination in the pseudoautosomal region in X- and Y-chromosomes, the lack of recombination in this region was established, in association with XY nondisjunction and production of aneuploid spermatozoa.[63] Other than gonosomes, there is little information on the chromosome-specific patterns of recombination in infertile men. However, the reduced levels of both genome-wide and chromosome-specific recombination that have been observed in infertile men may increase their risk of producing autosomal aneuploid sperm and chromosomally abnormal offspring. Indeed, a greater proportion of chromosome 21 bivalents that completely lack a crossover in the NOA and OAT groups has been observed.

The direct analyses of crossover events in human fetal oocytes revealed vulnerable configurations that should exhibit chromosome specificity consistent with data from trisomic conceptions (e.g. for chromosome 16 distally located exchanges and for chromosome 21, proximal and distal exchanges, as well as achiasmate chromosomes). Recently the direct analysis of human MI oocytes from young women have shown that a proportion of bivalents are either achiasmate or tethered by suboptimally located crossovers.[64] With increasing maternal age, these configurations become more likely to nondisjoin. It is interesting to note that most of the achiasmate configurations observed correspond to chromosome 16 which is the trisomie for excellence of female meiosis 1 derivation.[65] The mechanisms by which these susceptibilities are translated into nondisjunction events years later are not clear, nor is the way in which maternal age acts on the different aberrant exchange configurations. Oogenesis is more error-prone as a result of the prolonged arrest at the dictyotene stage in a process that begins during fetal life and becomes complete only after ovulation. In fact beside recombination events and cohesions between bivalents, to date, the only factor that has been unequivocally associated with the genesis of aneuploidies is maternal age with an extraordinary magnitude of the effect and with unclear influence of race, geography, or socioeconomic status. It has been proposed that the checkpoint regulating the transition from metaphase I to anaphase I is more permissive in oogenesis than in spermatogenesis. As a consequence spermatogenesis is usually blocked when an error occurs in bivalent alignment, while oogenesis continues yielding aneuploid gametes.[66] This is the second mechanism believed to be responsible of aneuploidy genesis.

One of the questions that has received considerable attention relates to the way in which meiotic chromosomes 'misbehave' in humans female meiosis; that is, via classical nondisjunction, where both homologues are segregated to the same pole or because of premature separation of sister chromatids (PSSC), where the connection between sister chromatids is abnormally lost at meiosis I and missing or extra chromatids are found in the oocyte. The most recent evidences suggest that both mechanisms are involved in the origin of aneuploidies during the first meiosis, however the occurrence of PSSC is higher than nondisjunction phenomenon [64,67] as previously suggested in mouse model.[68]

First meiotic aneuploidies can derived also from aneuploid oogonia. It has been reported that about 15 percent of the oocytes from young donors had noncomplementary aneuploidy when 1 polar body and oocyte are concurrently analyzed by CGH. Most probably it was during the proliferative stage of oogenesis, when multiple, consecutive mitotic divisions occur and, as a consequence of an abnormal mitotic segregation, the corresponding aneuploid oogonium was produced[69] (**Fig. 14.1**).

The second meiotic division, although similar to a mitosis, follows the first one without S-phase in between the two. So, to orchestrate the orderly separation of sister chromatids at MII, cohesion must be released along the chromosome arms at anaphase I (to allow the separation of homologues) but maintained between sister centromeres until anaphase II. Typically, MII errors are thought to result from the failure of sister chromatid separation. Also balanced PD phenomena, detachment of sister chromatids, have been observed in mature oocytes

and have been correlated to extended time in culture[70,71] and advanced female age.[72] This abnormality was recently observed also in fresh MII oocytes fixed shortly after ovum pick up (OPU) suggesting that balanced PD also occurs as a common mechanism. These oocytes, although genetically balanced, may be important contributors to embryo aneuploidy as they face, in the case of fertilization, the second meiotic division with a high chance of mis-segregation. Direct analysis of polar bodies by FISH and array-based technology have largely confirmed these theories on the origin of aneuploidies.

The parental origin of chromosome abnormalities is also of considerable interest as this may provide an insight into the mechanism by which they arise. Although, for numerical chromosomes aneuploidy a clear prevalence of maternal bias is known, for other common *de novo* structural rearrangement

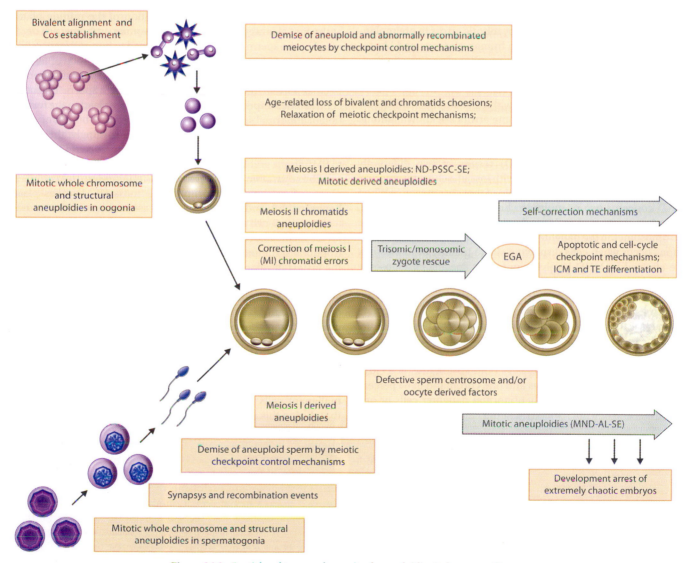

Figure 14.1: Spatial and temporal genesis of aneuploidies in human embryos

biomass of the embryo, with detrimental effects on further developmental potential. However, at the 8–12-cell stage, blastomeres retain totipotentiality, and the embryo can be biopsied successfully even when compacted. Moreover, the procedure together with the genetic testing, is compatible with a fresh transfer (within 5 days of culture).

The ideal number of cells to be removed is controversial and depend on embryo quality and on the specific genetic indication. In a recent prospective randomized trial,[103] it was shown that the biopsy of a single cell significantly lowers the efficiency of a PCR-based diagnosis, whereas the analytical efficiency of the FISH-PGD procedure remains similar. Moreover, it was demonstrated that the single blastomere removal is less invasive than two-cell removal particularly in embryos with poorer morphology. Day 3 embryo quality was shown to be the major predictor of blastocyst development. So depending on the embryo quality, the embryologist can determine how many cells to biopsy. For Mendelian disorders, a single cell biopsy on day 3 can be applied with an extraordinarily high accuracy.[8] However, this is not the case for aneuploidy screening in which mosaicism has a major impact.

Chromosome instability characterized by an elevated rate of gains or losses of complete chromosomes or segments per cell cycle resulting in cell-to-cell variability was shown to be extremely common in human preimplantation embryogenesis (called mosaicism). The first clinical applications of whole genome aneuploidy screening revealed as high as 65 percent frequency of mosaicism in preimplantation embryos with homogeneous abnormalities in only less than 8 percent.[104,105] This is true also for young, healthy couples with normal fertility.[58] In the abnormal embryos, not only mosaicism for whole chromosome aneuploidies (~83% of the embryos), but also frequent terminal segmental deletions, duplications or amplifications (~70% of the embryos) and uniparental disomies (~9% of the embryos) were frequently detected.[58] Almost half of the embryos analyzed in this study had no normal blastomeres at all, and only 9 percent were completely euploid.[58] It is thus clear that whereas a good proportion of mosaic postbiopsy embryo is correctly identified by a 2-cell analysis, a 1-cell biopsy cannot identify mosaicism. Furthermore the origin of aneuploidy (meiotic or mitotic) is impossible to be determined unless all blastomeres from the embryo are analyzed.

Theoretically, some mosaic embryos could change into a euploid status by means of apoptosis, overgrowth of euploid cells or displacement towards trophectoderm lineage (contributing to the development of extraembryonic tissues).[106] Therefore, the day-3 developmental stage (where the lowest rate of normal embryos and the highest rate of abnormal and mosaic embryos are present) seems not to be the most suitable timing for PGD-AS. The diagnostic accuracy is in fact very limited and error prone with a maximum risk of false positive and false negative when one blastomere is used to derive whole embryo chromosomal constitution and viability. Some authors have tried to draw from these important diagnostic information. A potential bias in the empirical calculations of these error rates is the fact that embryos with normal biopsy results are likely to be transferred

and withdrawn from further confirmatory investigations. This leads to an underestimate of the false-negative rate. From the theoretical model proposed by Los et al false-negative and false-positive rates can be calculated: 22.0 and 12.6 percent in case of a 1-cell biopsy and 14.2 and 6.0 percent in case of a 2-cell biopsy can be assumed.[107] Although several authors argue that in aneuploid embryos most part of the cells present with abnormalities and probably are not self-correcting PGD-AS on day 3 that will inevitably result in discarding potentially viable embryos.

Another major problem related to early stages biopsy is the paucity of material that is available, which might lead to an unreliable genetic diagnosis. If screening means to improve IVF outcomes, it is crucial that results are obtained using a sufficient amount of "sample" that reflects correctly the totality of embryo tested. Potentially, embryo biopsy at blastocyst stage obviates many of these problems. In this case, it is possible to remove several cells from the trophoblast layer without apparent detrimental effect. In addition, the inner cell mass that is destined to become the fetus is unlikely to be damaged, thereby reducing possible ethical concerns. Blastocyst biopsy normally takes place on day five or six after fertilization and is the last moment in which aneuploidy screening could be done. Little time is left for the genetic analysis so usually embryos have to be cryopreserved and transferred in subsequent cycle. However, the ET on unstimulated cycle can have a positive impact on endometrial receptivity. Although, normal euploid embryos display significantly higher blastocyst rates compared to chromosomally abnormal and mosaic ones and certain types of chromosomal abnormalities are negatively selected during preimplantation development,[108] a remarkable percentage of chromosomally abnormal embryos can develop normally to blastocyst stage. Among aneuploid embryos for autosomes, higher blastocyst rates were observed in trisomies than monosomies. In contrast, in embryos with sex chromosomes aneuploidy, similar blastocyst rates were observed between trisomies and monosomy X.[108,109] Single trisomies and mosaicism are the abnormalities exhibiting higher blastocyst rates, consistent with the most frequent chromosomal anomalies found in products from spontaneous abortions. Among mosaic embryos, those with two chromosomally abnormal cells on day 3 showed lower blastocyst developmental rates as compared to embryos with one normal euploid and one chromosomally abnormal cell.[108] Hence, the presumption of selection against aneuploid embryos occurring at the time of morula/blastocyst transition is only partially supported. Application of blastocyst biopsy has been hampered in the past by intrinsic difficulty related to prolonged embryo culture, technical difficulty related to trophoectoderm biopsy and the need of cryopreservation that could counteract the benefit derived from aneuploidy screening. Accordingly, few papers have been published addressing directly the chromosomal constitution of human blastocysts as ascertained by means of FISH or array-CGH.[110,111,142] The general message derived from these studies, although based on small numbers, was that the percentage of embryos exhibiting chromosomal mosaicism increases during *in vitro* preimplantation development at the blastocyst stage, whereas the percentage of abnormal cells per embryo decreases suggesting that mild mosaicism could be compatible with implantation and normal live birth.

The most recent analysis employing comprehensive chromosome screening (CCS) on TE leading to an overall abnormality estimated rate of about 40 percent with 37 years mean maternal age.[143] Aneuploidies involving almost all chromosomal groups were seen during the later stages of human preimplantation development. It is possible that the true aneuploidy rate is slightly higher than this figure, due to the inability of CGH to detect ploidy changes (e.g. triploidy, tetraploidy etc.). However, such abnormalities affect a small proportion (4%) of Day-3 embryos and the appearance of such cells is generally considered to be a hallmark of trophoblast differentiation and is probably not diagnostically or clinically relevant.[110]

Of major importance is the observation that a very high concordance rate (nearly 100%) between ICM and TE was shown using 24-chromosome microarray analysis.[112,143] This indicates that it should be possible to accurately assess the chromosome constitution of whole blastocyst by examining cells biopsied from the TE. This finding agrees with previous observations indicating that aneuploid and normal cells are evenly distributed in the TE and ICM in human blastocysts.[92]

The development of sequential, stage-specific media combined with ultra-stable low oxygen culture systems and the recent application of very efficient vitrification strategies might overcome this problem proposing blastocyst stage as an attracting and potentially optimal stage for genetic testing.[113-115] Another advantage of this strategy is that embryo blastocyst rate is certainly not hampered by previous biopsy procedures. Moreover, a limited number of embryos are competent to overcome the negative selection processes of EGA and compaction to reach the blastocyst stage resulting in a significant reduction of workload and cost minimization. In our opinion every PGS center should have at least a "no result rescue" program with the aim of reanalyze embryo without diagnosis at blastocyst stage and possibly to confirm the aneuploidy on trophoectoderm cells to exclude mosaicism and embryo self-correction.

However, it is yet unclear whether and to what extent *in vitro* environment may affect the chromosomal (in)stability in human embryo development. If this is the case, prolonged embryo exposure in culture could in principle worsen aneuploidy in blastocyst. Furthermore, *in vitro* culture might lead to more imprinting problems although this aspect has still to be determined and the supposed overall increased risk seems to be extremely low. Other limitation is that chromosome screening of blastocysts is challenging for some patients—with poor ovarian reserve or poor *in vitro* embryo development.

A brief listing on the potential advantages of performing biopsy at blastocyst stage for PGD-AS (with individual cryopreservation of biopsied embryos and transfer in subsequent cycle).
- Less embryos are biopsied, but the most robust ones.
- One obtains more than one cell—a clear advantage in any testing
- The issues of mosaicism are markedly reduced. (data are showing concordance between chromosomes in TE and ICM)

- There is no rush to perform diagnosing
- Transfer to a natural endometrium (possibly more receptive)
- Provides condition to transfer one embryo at a time, in natural cycle, until patient gets pregnant. Thus optimizing the IVF cycle and multiples are reduced.
- The molecular data are cleaner, clearer

In conclusion each stage presents with unique advantages and specific limits and in combination with analytic methods these has to be considered in clinical practice to fit PGD-AS strategies with genetic and infertility indications specific for each couple (**Table 14.1**).

Clinical Efficiency and Prevalence of PGD-AS to Date: Lack of Correlation

The first proposed clinical intent of PGD for chromosome abnormalities was as an alternative to prenatal diagnosis with the aim of reduce aneuploid offspring prevalence in patients undergoing IVF cycle. Although the prevention of trisomic conceptions is usually lumped together with the concept of improving ART outcome, it is an indication in itself. Theoretically employing an appropriate combination of centromeric probes on day 3 preimplantation embryo all viable aneuploidy of meiotic origin could be efficiently identified. A real statistical estimation of benefits is hampered by the low incidence of aneuploid delivery and by the need of a suitable control group. Preliminary results have shown that the observed rate of aneuploidy conceptions after conventional PGD-AS was significantly reduced to 0.5% compared to an expected 2.6 percent in IVF population providing convincing evidence of the reduced level of abnormal conceptions after PGD for aneuploidy.[116] However, trisomy 21 fetuses have been diagnosed with invasive PND and births of children with Down syndrome have been reported after PGD-AS.[117] Probably, these misdiagnosis arise as a consequence of failed hybridization during the FISH analysis. In the light of these evidence before PGS can be offered as an alternative to prenatal testing, misdiagnosis rate should be reduced and trials need to be performed to assess the sensitivity of PGS in detecting chromosomal problems in embryos and its effect on pregnancy rates.

As regard PGD-AS for improving IVF outcomes the most frequent population screened has been ARA with conventional strategy (FISH for a limited number of chromosomes on day 3 embryo), while for the other indications a paucity of date have been reported so far (ESHRE data collection).

First observational studies comparing cleavage-stage embryo biopsy or polar body approach with matched controls have shown an increased IVF outcomes after PGD-AS in ARA patients.[58,118-120] However, the design of these studies has varied concerning day of transfer, number of chromosomes and/or blastomeres analyzed and number of embryos transferred, as well as inclusion criteria. Moreover, the lack of randomization gives to these studies low evidence levels, making difficult to draw conclusions. Nevertheless, these data in conjunction with the attracting and convincing scientific hypothesis behind aneuploidy screening, had the effect of contributing to expand PGD-AS clinical application worldwide. However, recent more

Table 14.1: General aspects related to Day 0 and Day 1 PB biopsy, Day 3 blastomere biopsy and Day 5 trophectoderm biopsy

Colonna 1	1 PB	1 and 2 PB	Day 3	Day 5
Number of available embryos	All collected MII oocytes	Fertilized oocytes (about 70%)	Good quality day 3 embryos, generally >6 cell stage and <20% fragmentation (about 60% of fertilized oocytes)	Expanding and expanded blastocysts about 50% of day 3 embryos
Technical issues	Need of full maturity (assessed by spindle view); highest microenvironment sensitivity; biopsy is technically challenging and not routinely used worldwide; cryopreservation advisable to avoid oocyte aging; high workload	High microenvironment sensitivity; biopsy is technically challenging and not routinely used worldwide; high workload	Technically feasible and routinely used worldwide; allow fresh transfer; reduced microenvironment sensitivity; Reduced workload	Technically morel challenging and not routinely used worldwide; abundant material for reliable genetical testing; reduced microenvironment sensitivity; need of cryopreservation; need of high quality and efficient embryo culture system and cryopreservation strategy; reduced workload
Diagnostic efficiency (FISH and CGH)	FISH about 85% depending on operator; CGH: 90% About 90% of biopsied MII oocytes	FISH about 80%; CGH about 85% About 85% of fertilized oocytes	FISH about 85%;CGH about 90% about 90% of good quality day 3 embryos	FISH ~93%; CGH ~94% Almost all TE sampled
Information about the whole embryo chromosomal complement	Only I oocyte meiotic division; no male; no postzygotic; partial information about mitotic oogonia derived aneuploidies	I and II oocyte meiotic division, no paternal information; no postzygotic information	Maternal and paternal meiotic derived aneuploidies; relative information about mitotic aneuploidies and whole embryo chromosomal complement	Maternal and paternal meiotic derived aneuploidies; mitotic aneuploidies in TE cells; reduced chaotic mosaicism incidence; high concordance between TE and ICM
Legal, ethical and moral issues	No legal and ethical and religious problems, no embryo selection and discard (if needed) if fertilization is performed just on euploid oocytes. No Legal retriction worldwilde	Relative legal, ethical and religious issues because is performed prior to syngamy. No embryo selection and discard (if needed) only zygote	Possible legal, ethical and religious issues due to embryo selection and discarriage	Possible legal, ethical and religious issues due to embryo selection and discarding. Only extraembryonic cells sampled

recent studies using randomized control trials on conventional PGD-AS have not confirmed these initially promising findings and have shown inefficacy or even harmful effects. At present PGD-AS is one of the most debated application in reproductive medicine and genetics.

Regarding ARA patients, six randomized controlled trials (RCTs) have been published so far.[121-126] All have used cleavage-stage biopsy with FISH testing for a limited number of chromosomes, some concluding with no argument in favor of PGD-AS in terms of delivery rate per started cycle, while others have seen impaired outcomes with PGD-AS. Only one study used blastocyst biopsy with FISH analysis of TE cells but was stopped after just few tens of patients because a lack of benefit.[127]

In RIF patients, only one RCT has been published.[128] No significant differences in clinical pregnancies between PGD-AS and control groups were observed, but the trial included only 72 and 67 cycles respectively. Other two studies addressed the possibility that in young good prognosis patients PGD-AS could show a positive effect but failed in its intent.[129,130]

All together these RCTs provide sufficient evidence that conventional PGD-AS for ARA may not be an optimal procedure at least in improving delivery rate in IVF patients (per started cycle). As regard to other indications, such as RIF, RPL and SMF, there is a lack of data. However, relying on the same assumption and like the use of conventional PGD-AS for ARA, it would stand to reason that the lack of benefit in selecting embryos with an euploid complement would be equally inefficient if transposed to these other patients. This is an important message for those practicing reproductive medicine, since we may be over-manipulating the embryos in the IVF laboratories without practical evidence, and therefore increasing the total costs of an IVF cycle without significantly improving pregnancy outcomes. As a consequence various scientific society, ASRM, BFS and ESHRE have stated few years ago not to support the use of PGD-AS as it is currently practiced to improve the live birth rates.[131,132] As stated by the father of modern macroeconomics John Maynard Keynes "The difficulty lays not so much in developing new ideas as in escaping from old ones". Despite these findings, PGD-AS on day 3 embryos with conventional FISH analysis continued to be practiced currently worldwide. PGD-AS represents the largest part of all the preimplantation genetic testing-related procedures in USA and also in Europe and its application is continuously increasing.[8,9]

Another critical (but much less recognized) aspect of PGD-AS is its diagnostic value. Many patients who are not able to conceive using their own oocytes (due to cytoplasmic and chromosomal incompetence of the oocytes) may become easily pregnant when accepting donor oocytes. However, many of these patients may find it difficult to be convinced to switch to donor oocytes, unless there is a testing results that demonstrates "incompetency" of their oocytes/embryos. Since nonviable embryos are typically also chromosomally abnormal, PGD-AS testing (showing that most or all embryos are aneuploid) can be an important factor helping these patients to accept new approaches in their IVF treatment. However, we have to recognize, that there are cycle to cycle variations in both embryo developmental capacity (viability) and in the proportion of aneuploid embryos which may pose some practical challenge on how to use PGD-AS as diagnostic tool.[133]

For sure, at the time being there is a clear lack of correlation between scientific evidence and clinical practice. However, there is insufficient data to determine whether other strategies of PGD-AS are an effective intervention in IVF/ICSI for improving live birth rates. In this respect, new more appropriate approaches are encouraged to replace old ones and blastocyst stage embryo biopsy with the combination of novel diagnostic methods are certainly encouraging.

Pitfalls and Strategies, and Methodology to Improve the Outcomes

> "If the facts don't fit the theory, change the facts."
> —Albert Einstein

For the observed discrepancy between the theory and the practice, a number of reasons have been put forward, such as inappropriate inclusion criteria, team inexperience in embryo testing and culture, the insufficient number or wrong chromosomes tested and the harm caused by the biopsy procedure. *Prima face*, sample size reported are often too small or studies are prematurely terminated after very few observations. An important fact to be reported in order to support clinically relevant conclusions is the sample size analysis. So power analysis must be used to plan the sample size, which should always be fixed a priori based on a reasonable and justifiable expected difference. This critical aspect is often omitted or used incorrectly so that the study result is underpowered and inconclusive. Heterogeneity in inclusion criteria and inappropriate patient selection has hampered meta-analysis and comparison of results between different studies. More comprehensive and standardized inclusion criteria as well as detailed infertility work-up studies in the patients recruited could improve the scientific evidence and rule out nonembryonic causes in indications such as RIF or recurrent miscarriage.

Moreover several studies have reported very low blastocyst rate especially in the control group; a recent publication has shown the importance of embryo culture media in a PGD-AS program, suggesting that the laboratory expertise may significantly change the impact PGD-AS on clinical outcomes.[134] Another important issue is the limited number and the specific panel of chromosomes selected. Most of the quoted studies did not include chromosomes 15 and/or 22 in their analysis, highly associated with miscarriage with only one out of the nine studies including both chromosomes in the genetic screening. For instance, Meyer et al., who did not test their embryos for chromosome 15, reported a trisomy 15 miscarriage in the PGD-AS group.[119] This data analysis suggests justification for the varying outcomes different clinics have reported.

Although the lack of benefit is clear using conventional PGD-AS technique, these discrepancies partially explain differences between reports and point out that standardized methodology should be applied in further RCTs, before concluding whether or not PGD-AS benefits the candidate couples. In this sense, a set of guidelines has recently been proposed, including the validation of the assays and the participation in external quality schemes is very necessary.[135-137]

Conflicting results possibly reflect an incomplete understanding of important aspects of embryo biology, such as chromosomal mosaicism and nonequivalence of blastomeres on day 3 in determining embryo viability.[138,139] Biopsied cells may not represent the genetic make-up of the entire embryo and mosaic preimplantation embryos may be self-correcting. In this view, PGD-AS may lead to a reduction of the number of potentially viable embryos available for transfer in couples undergoing assisted reproduction.

For instance, an abnormal or mosaic biopsy reduces the limited mosaicism from the embryo but negatively affect its chance to be transferred. In contrast, a normal biopsy aggravates the mosaicism in the embryo and increases its chance for transfer. This leads to the paradoxical effect of an inverse relation between the developmental prospects of these embryos and their chances for transfer. It has also been demonstrated that aneuploidies present on day 3 postfertilization are often not found when the embryo is reanalyzed 2 days later on trophoectoderm.[106] Moreover, stem cell lines, derived from embryos classified as aneuploid on PGD, were karyotypically normal and none of the aneuploid lines presented the same anomaly as the original PGD analysis.[140] Similar results have been reported when human stem cells were derived from blastocyst-stage embryos diagnosed as aneuploid in PGD-AS on day 3. In this case, stem cell euploidy was not achieved through chromosome duplication, but originated from the mosaic embryo.[141] Finally, a significant positive correlation was observed between the total cell number and the percentage of normal cells in developing Day 5 and Day 8 human embryos cocultured for a further 72 h on an endometrial monolayer.[142]

Accordingly, some transferred mosaic diploid/aneuploid embryos can survive to term in a healthy state, suggesting that chromosomally normal blastomeres may display a proliferative advantage compared to abnormal cells, and therefore replace them during embryogenesis. So by not transferring an eight-cell embryo (diagnosed as aneuploid) we deprive it

120. Verlinsky Y, Tur-Kaspa I, Cieslak J, et al. Preimplantation testing for chromosomal disorders improves reproductive outcome of poor-prognosis IVF patients. Reprod Biomed Online 2005;11:219-25.

121. Staessen C, Platteau P, Van Assche E, Michiels A, Tournaye H, Camus M, Devroey P, Liebaers I, Van Steirteghem A. Comparison of blastocyst transfer with or without preimplantation genetic diagnosis for aneuploidy screening in couples with advanced maternal age: a prospective randomized controlled trial. Hum Reprod 2004;19:2849-58.

122. Mastenbroek S, Twisk M, van Echten-Arends J, Sikkema-Raddatz B, Korevaar JC, Verhoeve HR, Vogel NE, Arts EG, de Vries JW, Bossuyt PM, et al. *In vitro* fertilization with preimplantation genetic screening. N Engl J Med 2007;357:9-17.

123. Hardarson T, Hanson C, Lundin K, Hillensjö T, Nilsson L, Stevic J, Reismer E, Borg K, Wikland M, Bergh C. Preimplantation genetic screening in women of advanced maternal age caused a decrease in clinical pregnancy rate: a randomized controlled trial. Hum Reprod 2008;23:2806-12.

124. Stevens J, Wale P, Surrey ES, Schoolcraft WB. Is aneuploidy screening for patients aged 35 or over beneficial? A prospective randomized trial. Fertil Steril 2004;82:249.

125. Debrock S, Melotte C, Spiessens C, Peeraer K, Vanneste E, Meeuwis L, Meuleman C, Frijns JP, Vermeesch JR, D'Hooghe TM. Preimplantation genetic screening for aneuploidy of embryos after *in vitro* fertilization in women aged at least 35 years: a prospective randomized trial. Fertil Steril, 2009.

126. Schoolcraft WB, Katz-Jaffe MG, Stevens J, Rawlins M, Munne S. Preimplantation aneuploidy testing for infertile patients of advanced maternal age: a randomized prospective trial. Fertil Steril 2009;92:157-62.

127. Jansen RP, Bowman MC, de Boer KA, Leigh DA, Lieberman DB, McArthur SJ. What next for preimplantation genetic screening (PGS)? Experience with blastocyst biopsy and testing for aneuploidy. Hum Reprod 2008;23:1476-8.

128. Blockeel C, Schutyser V, De Vos A, Verpoest W, De Vos M, Staessen C, Haentjens P, Van der Elst J, Devroey P. Prospectively randomized controlled trial of PGS in IVF/ICSI patients with poor implantation. Reprod Biomed Online 2008;17:848-54.

129. Staessen C, Verpoest W, Donoso P, Haentjens P, Van der Elst J, Liebaers I, Devroey P. Preimplantation genetic screening does not improve delivery rate in women under the age of 36 following single-embryo transfer. Hum Reprod 2008;23:2818-25.

130. Meyer L, Klipstein S, Hazlett W, Nasta T, Mangan P, Karande VC. A prospective randomized controlled trial of preimplantation genetic screening in the 'good prognosis' patient. Fertil Steril 2009;91:1731-8.

131. Harper J, Coonen E, De Rycke M, Fiorentino F, Geraedts J, Goossens V, Harton G, Moutou C, Budak P, Renwick P, SenGupta S, Traeger-Synodinos J, Vesela K. What next for preimplantation genetic screening (PGS)? A position statement from the ESHRE PGD Consortium steering committee.

132. The practice committee of the Society of Assisted Reproductive Technology and the American Society of Reproductive Medicine. Preimplantation genetic testing: a practice committee opinion. Fertil Steril 2008;90:S136-S143.

133. Donoso P, Staessen C, Collins J, Verpoest W, Fatemi HM, Papanikolaou EG, Devroey P. Prognostic factors for delivery in patients undergoing repeated preimplantation genetic aneuploidy screening Fertil Steril 2010;94(6):2362-4.

134. Beyer CE, Osianlis T, Boekel K, Osborne E, Rombauts L, Catt J, Kralevski V, Aali BS, Gras L. Preimplantation genetic screening outcomes are associated with culture conditions. Hum Reprod 2009;24:1212-20.

135. Harton GL, Magli MC, Lundin K, Montag M, Lemmen J, Harper JC. ESHRE PGD Consortium/Embryology Special Interest Group—best practice guidelines for polar body and embryo biopsy for preimplantation genetic diagnosis/screening (PGD/PGS). Hum Reprod 2010 Oct 21. [Epub ahead of print].

136. Harton G, Braude P, Lashwood A, Schmutzler A, Traeger-Synodinos J, Wilton L, Harper JC. ESHRE PGD consortium best practice guidelines for organization of a PGD centre for PGD/preimplantation genetic screening. Hum Reprod 2010 Oct 21. [Epub ahead of print].

137. Harton GL, Harper JC, Coonen E, Pehlivan T, Vesela K, Wilton L. ESHRE PGD consortium best practice guidelines for fluorescence *in situ* hybridization-based PGD Hum Reprod. 2010 Oct 21. [Epub ahead of print].

138. Baart E, Van Opstal D, Los FJ, Fauser BCJM, Martini E. Fluorescence *in situ* hybridization analysis of two blastomeres from day-3 frozen-thawed embryos followed by analysis of the remaining embryo on day-5. Hum Reprod 2004;19:685-93.

139. Wong CC, Loewke KE, Bossert NL, Behr B, De Jonge CJ, Baer TM, Reijo Pera RA. Non-invasive imaging of human embryos before embryonic genome activation predicts development to the blastocyst stage. Nat Biotechnol 2010;28(10):1115-21. Epub 2010 Oct 3.

140. Peura T, Bosman A, Chami O, Jansen RP, Texlova K, Stojanov T. Karyotypically normal and abnormal human embryonic stem cell lines derived from PGD-analyzed embryos. Cloning Stem Cells 2008;10(2):203-16.

141. Lavon N, Narwani K, Golan-Lev T, Buehler N, Hill D, Benvenisty N. Derivation of euploid human embryonic stem cells from aneuploid embryos. Stem Cells 2008;26(7):1874-82. Epub 2008 May 1.

142. Santos MA, Teklenburg G, Macklon NS, Van Opstal D, Schuring-Blom GH, Krijtenburg PJ, de Vreeden-Elbertse J, Fauser BC, Baart EB. The fate of the mosaic embryo: chromosomal constitution and development of Day 4, 5 and 8 human embryos. Hum Reprod 2010;25(8):1916-26. Epub 2010 Jun 2.

143. Fragouli E, Katz-Jaffe M, Alfarawati S, Stevens J, Colls P, Goodall NN, Tormasi S, Gutierrez-Mateo C, Prates R, Schoolcraft WB, Munne S, Wells D. Comprehensive chromosome screening of polar bodies and blastocysts from couples experiencing repeated implantation failure. Fertil Steril 2010;94(3):875-87. Epub 2009 Jun 21.

144. Gutiérrez-Mateo C, Colls P, Sánchez-García J, Escudero T, Prates R, Ketterson K, Wells D, Munné S. Validation of micro-array comparative genomic hybridization for comprehensive chromosome analysis of embryos. Fertil Steril 2010 Oct 23. [Epub ahead of print].

145. Geraedts J, Collins J, Gianaroli L, Goossens V, Handyside A, Harper J, Montag M, Repping S, Schmutzler A. What next for preimplantation genetic screening? A polar body approach! Hum Reprod 2010;25(3):575-7. Epub 2009 Dec 23.

146. Schoolcraft WB, Fragouli E, Stevens J, Munne S, Katz-Jaffe MG, Wells D. Clinical application of comprehensive chromosomal screening at the blastocyst stage. Fertil Steril 2010;94(5):1700-6. Epub 2009 Nov 25.

Section III

Medical Management

15

Endocrinology of Male Infertility and Hormonal Intervention

Fnu Deepinder, Philip Kumanov

▮ INTRODUCTION

Infertility is defined by the World Health Organization (WHO) as the inability of a sexually active couple to achieve pregnancy despite unprotected intercourse for a period of greater than 12 months.[1] Approximately, 4–17 percent of human couples seek medical treatment for infertility and about 50 percent involve male factors.[2] Therefore, it can be accepted that about 7 percent of all men during their life confront with some disturbance of their fertility.[3] Although, the frequency of etiological factors varies among different reports, a specific cause remains un-explained in almost 1/3rd of the male individuals. This is a very heterogeneous group of idiopathic infertility. Only about 2 percent of infertile men have clinically significant diagnoses of endocrine disorders.[4]

Gonadotropin-releasing hormone (GnRH) is released in a pulsatile fashion, every 90 to 120 minutes, from neurons in the arcuate nucleus located in the mediobasal hypothalamus. GnRH enters the portal hypophyseal circulation to stimulate the anterior pituitary gland, which in turn, releases 2 gonadotropins: luteinizing hormone (LH) and follicle-stimulating hormone (FSH). Both are glycoproteins, with structure closely resembling those of thyrotropin stimulating hormone (TSH) and of human chorionic gonadotropin (hCG). LH stimulates the production of testosterone by Leydig cells, and FSH supports spermatogenesis. Androgens and estrogens inhibit gonadotropin secretion. Sertoli cells produce inhibin B which has negative feedback on FSH release.

Disorders Causing Infertility in Men

Hypogonadism

Male hypogonadism is defined as a clinical syndrome that results from failure of the testes to produce physiological levels of testosterone (androgen deficiency) and the normal number of spermatozoa due to disruption of one or more levels of the hypothalamic-pituitary-gonadal (HPG) axis.[5] Testosterone serum levels less than 300 ng/dL (10.4 nmol/liter), which according to some laboratories is the lower limit of the normal range for total testosterone level in healthy young men, are associated with clinical symptoms such as decreased libido, infertility, anemia, mood changes, small or shrinking testes, alterations in body hair distribution, decrease in lean muscle mass and bone density, increased body fat. However, it is recommended that the clinicians should use the lower limit of normal range of testosterone for healthy young adults established in their reference laboratory.[5]

Hypogonadism can be divided into 2 forms. Abnormalities at the testicular level cause primary gonadal failure, identified by low serum testosterone levels along with elevated LH and FSH (hypergonadotropic hypogonadism). Secondary or hypogonadotropic hypogonadism is defined by low testosterone levels associated with low or inappropriately normal LH and FSH serum levels because of central defects of the hypothalamus or pituitary.[4] Hypogonadism can be further separated into congenital and acquired forms.

Hypogonadotropic hypogonadism results from failure of the hypothalamus or pituitary to stimulate and maintain normal gonadal function.[6] Pituitary function may be affected in events of pituitary tumors, infarction, inflammatory and granulomatous diseases, surgery, and radiation. However, gonadotropin deficiency may also occur in the presence of otherwise normal pituitary function when the secretion or action of GnRH is altered: isolated hypogonadotropic hypogonadism (IHH).

Isolated hypogonadotropic hypogonadism is clinically defined as absent or incomplete puberty by the age of 18 years because of the low gonadotropin secretion. The GnRH deficiency can be due to impaired migration of the GnRH neurons to the hypothalamus during embryonic development, abnormal maturation or decreased survival of GnRH neurons, or resistance to the action of GnRH at the level of the pituitary. IHH can be either sporadic or familial. It may be inherited in an X-linked recessive, autosomal dominant or autosomal recessive mode. However, the genetics are not strictly mendelian. IHH may be due to mutations in more than one gene, as well as interactions between genes or between genes and environmental factors.[7] In males the prevalence is around 1 in 10,000. There are 2 forms of IHH depending on the presence or absence of the normal sense of smell: normosmic IHH and Kallmann syndrome.

Kallmann syndrome is the form of IHH associated with olfactory disturbances (hypo- or anosmia) due to the absence or hypoplasia of the olfactory bulbs and tract. The male preponderance of cases remains still unexplained. The olfactory and reproductive deficits are combined with various defects, including cryptorchidism, bimanual synkinesis (mirror movements), unilateral renal agenesis, craniofacial or dental abnormalities, syndactyly, sensorineural deafness.[8]

Hyperprolactinemia is another endocrine cause of secondary hypogonadism commonly seen in clinical practice. Prolactin is an anterior pituitary hormone which in excessive concentrations suppress the secretion of FSH and LH and/or impede their action on the gonads. Hyperprolactinemia can be caused by prolactinomas, pituitary tumors secreting both prolactin and growth hormone, processes causing pituitary stalk compression or section, empty sella syndrome, medications, primary hypothyroidism, chronic renal failure among other causes or may be idiopathic. Symptoms include depressed libido, erectile dysfunction, and infertility. Galactorrhea is rare in men.

Rare disorders include *isolated FSH deficiency* which may present with oligo- or azoospermia though such patients have normal virilization and normal testosterone and LH levels.[9] *Isolated LH deficiency (Pasqualini syndrome, fertile eunuch syndrome)* on the other hand leads to eunuchoid habitus, low testosterone levels, but normal maturation of germinal epithelium with Leydig cell atrophy on testicular biopsy. Serum levels of LH are low, but of FSH are normal.[3]

Other complex congenital syndrome associated with hypogonadotropic hypogonadism includes *Prader-Willi syndrome* where lack of GnRH secretion leads to LH and FSH deficiency. The hypogonadism in the very rare genetic disorders *Laurence-Moon syndrome* and *Bardet-Biedl syndrome* is not obligate.[3]

Hypergonadotropic Hypogonadism

This group includes different congenital and acquired disorders primarily affecting the gonads (**Table 15.1**). They result in testicular failure and infertility but some of them can cause only fertility disturbances without obvious signs of hypogonadism. Defects in androgen production, as well as conversion of testosterone to dihydrotestosterone due to deficiency of enzyme 5-alpha reductase, affect the phenotype and reproduction. A number of genetic disorders, such as Klinefelter syndrome and

Table 15.1: Disorders causing primary or hypergonadotropic hypogonadism

Klinefelter's syndrome (47, XXY)
XX male syndrome
47, XYY men
Gonadal dysgenesis
Noonan's syndrome
Defects in androgen biosynthesis
Bilateral anorchia (vanishing testes syndrome)
Acquired anorchy
Orchitis
Varicocele
Adult seminiferous tubule failure

Y-chromosome micro-deletions, have been implicated in spermatogenic failure.

Systemic diseases can affect the HPG axis causing hypogonadism and reproductive dysfunction.

Thyroid Disorders

Both hyper- and hypothyroidism may have an adverse impact on male fertility. Hyperthyroidism is known to cause elevation of sex hormone binding globulin (SHBG) and decline in semen quality especially in sperm motility.[10] In literature, hyperthyroid men has shown relative primary gonadal insufficiency that might be due to exaggerated SHBG levels and increased gonadotropin levels with copulsatility between LH and FSH, which was more pronounced than in healthy men.[11] Evidence is weak though about the possible deleterious effects of hypothyroidism on male reproductive system.[12]

Hormonal Excess

Androgen excess can induce a hypogonadal state by inhibiting gonadotropin production through negative feedback. The source of the androgen excess could be either endogenous production from adrenals or testes, or exogenous anabolic steroids. Deficiency of enzyme 21-hydoxylase is the most common cause of *congenital adrenal hyperplasia*. The excess of adrenal androgens in this condition may lead to precocious pseudopuberty and infertility. It can be diagnosed by high basal and ACTH stimulated plasma 17-alfa hydoxyprogesterone levels. Men with partial enzyme deficiency may remain undiagnosed until late in adulthood, though they are usually fertile. *Adrenal or testicular Leydig cell tumors* can also produce excess serum androgens and require radiological imaging for diagnosis.

Glucocorticoid excess (hypercortisolism) in *Cushing's syndrome* of either endogenous or exogenous etiology may also suppress LH secretion and testosterone biosynthesis resulting in testosterone deficiency and hypospermatogenesis.

Excess estrogen state can also produce secondary testicular failure by inhibiting pituitary gonadotropins. It can be derived from either estrogen secreting adrenal or testicular tumors or excess peripheral conversion of androgens to estrogens by aromatase enzyme in patients suffering from *chronic liver diseases or obesity*. Men with high estrogen levels may present with gynecomastia, erectile dysfunction and testicular atrophy.

Diabetes Mellitus and Metabolic Syndrome

Diabetes mellitus affects the reproductive function mainly through microangiopathy and neuropathy, which in turn lead to erectile dysfunction and ejaculate disturbances. Obesity as well as diabetes mellitus type 2 (DM 2) may cause hypogonadism and infertility. Both low and high body mass index (BMI) are associated with disturbances in spermatogenesis. In obesity, increased peripheral conversion of androgens to estrogens in excess peripheral adipose tissue suppresses the gonadotropin secretion. Another unfavorable effect of obesity may be the oxidative stress leading to impaired spermatogenesis.[13] Dyslipidemia also increases oxidative stress. Metabolic syndrome is not a separate disease by itself but a cluster of abnormalities, including visceral obesity, dyslipidemia, hypertension and impaired glucose metabolism or DM 2 with insulin resistance as the hypothesized underlying pathogenic mechanism. An association of metabolic syndrome with low testosterone and low SHBG serum levels is widely accepted, but the cause and effect relationship is still unclear. A negative correlation of total testosterone with insulin levels, insulin resistance and body mass index in young males with metabolic syndrome was reported.[14]

Disorders of Androgen Actions

Androgen insensitivity causes undermasculinization of various degrees in 46 XY individuals. The androgen receptor gene is located on the X-chromosome between Xq11 and Xq13. Androgen insensitivity syndromes result from defects in androgen receptor number or function. Androgen insensitivity may be complete or partial (incomplete). Complete androgen insensitivity syndrome (CAIS) (testicular feminization syndrome) is characterized by complete feminization of genetic males. Partial androgen insensitivity presents with great variations from normal male phenotype with infertility to individuals with genital ambiguity and gynecomastia.[15,16]

EVALUATION OF INFERTILE MAN FROM AN ENDOCRINOLOGIST'S PROSPECTIVE

For any infertile couple, evaluation begins with determining if the problem lies within the male or female partner, or both. If the female partner has regular menstrual cycles, patent fallopian tubes, normal FSH, LH, TSH, and prolactin levels, male factor infertility is the likely cause.[17] Like any other medical condition, work up starts with a detailed history. Attention should be paid to cryptorchidism and/or testicular torsion in childhood, pubertal development, sexually transmitted diseases, scrotal trauma, radiation exposure and any inguinal surgeries like hernia repairs. Physical examination should include arms span and its comparison with the body height, hair distribution, testicular size, and presence of gynecomastia or varicocele. Subnormal testicular volume indicates underdevelopment or regression of the seminiferous tubules.

Because of the circadian variations in secretion, serum samples for total testosterone determination should be obtained between 7:00 and 11:00 h AM.[18] About 2 percent of total testosterone in circulation is not bound. This is the free, biologically active fraction of testosterone. In order to determine free testosterone (free T) reliably, equilibrium dialysis or ultrafiltration techniques are required. These methods are complicated and not routinely recommended at present. However, a simple and reliable method for the clinical practice is the estimation of free T from the levels of total testosterone and SHBG by using a standard equation.[19] Calculated free T correlates well with free testosterone estimated by equilibrium dialysis.[18] In majority of cases free T shows good correlation with total testosterone. The measurement of free T should be considered when alterations in SHBG are expected. The serum total testosterone concentration

is not diagnostic of hypogonadism, as in obese patients or those with nephrotic syndrome, hyper- or hypothyroidism, chronic liver disease, or on therapy with anticonvulsants or steroids.[18]

Serum estradiol determination may be considered in select group of patients such as ones with Klinefelter's syndrome and in cases with gynecomastia.

Primary testicular failure presents with low testosterone and elevated FSH and LH serum levels whereas patients with selective spermatogenic failure have normal testosterone and LH, and only elevated FSH. In cases with low testosterone and low or inappropriately normal LH and FSH, it is important to determine prolactin, TSH and free thyroxine levels. These patients need brain imaging to determine cause of hypogonadotropic hypogonadism. Normal prolactin levels in men are usually less than 18 ng/dL (550 mIU/L). However, due to high assay variability, testing should be repeated if levels are elevated. If hyperprolactinemia is discovered, and secondary causes are ruled out or prolactin levels are above 150 ng/dL, a gadolinium enhanced MRI with special attention to the region of hypothalamus and pituitary is indicated for revealing of a prolactinoma or another space occupying process.

Both in complete and partial forms of androgen insensitivity serum testosterone and LH levels are usually elevated, but FSH may be normal or elevated. Estradiol is higher than in normal males. Failure of SHBG to decrease after testosterone administration confirms the androgen insensitivity. An hCG test demonstrating normal testosterone and dihydrotestosterone production can be used to distinguish partial androgen insensitivity syndrome from defects in testosterone biosynthesis and 5-alpha-reductase activity.[15,16] Karyotyping reveals 46 XY and is indicated especially in cases with ambiguous genitalia and bilateral inguinal hernias. Androgen receptor studies are helpful in cases with incomplete insensitivity.

Semen quality should be determined by analyzing semen samples obtained by masturbation after 2–7 days of abstinence. Semen volume, pH, sperm count, density, motility, morphology and viability are evaluated in accordance with WHO criteria.[20] It is important to obtain multiple semen samples to overcome tremendous variability in sperm parameters.

In men who are found to have azoospermia but normal testosterone, LH, and FSH levels and normal testes volume, obstructive disorders should be ruled out by measuring seminal levels of fructose and neutral alfa-glucosidase. The latter originates in the epididymis.[20] In case of azoospermia or severe oligospermia, normal testosterone and LH levels, but elevated FSH, primary spermatogenic failure should be considered. These patients should get testicular volume assessment, karyotyping and Yq microdeletion screening. Antisperm antibodies can be determined in oligospermic men who are found to have sperm agglutinations during semen analysis.[17]

Inhibin B is a direct product of Sertoli cells and its serum levels have been found to be better correlated to sperm parameters than FSH and thus may serve as a better marker of spermatogenesis.[21] Inhibin B levels can also be useful for monitoring the effects of gonadotropin therapy. However, inhibin B or FSH alone as well as the combination of both hormones cannot predict the finding of spermatozoa by testicular biopsy in patients with azoospermia who are candidates for ICSI-treatment.[3]

HORMONAL INTERVENTION IN MALE INFERTILITY

Adequate replacement therapy either with GnRH or LH and FSH can induce spermatogenesis in patients with hypogonadotropic hypogonadism. Maturation of the human sperm takes approximately 72 days,[22] so the treatment should last at least 3 months for the sperms to appear in the ejaculate. Usually a much longer period (up to 2 years or even more) is required, especially in congenital hypogonadotropic hypogonadism.

Gonadotropin Releasing Hormone

Physiological Principle

Gonadotropin releasing hormone (GnRH) stimulates anterior pituitary to secrete LH and FSH which in turn regulate testosterone production and spermatogenesis. It can thus be used in pulsatile fashion in men with hypogonadotropic hypogonadism caused by hypothalamic dysfunction but not in those having loss of pituitary function. It can also be used for induction of puberty.

Method

Gonadotropin releasing hormone (GnRH) is administered using portable pump in doses of 4–20 µg per pulse administered subcutaneously every 2 hours as pulsatile therapy. Doses are adjusted until serum testosterone reaches mid-normal levels. GnRH as nasal spray is used for treatment of cryptorchidim.

Evidence

Gonadotropin releasing hormone (GnRH) has been demonstrated to be quite effective in inducing androgenization and spermatogenesis in men with IHH.[23-25] It did not differ in efficacy in terms of spermatogenesis and pregnancy rates as compared to the gonadotropin therapy. In preliminary investigations involving infertile men who had cryptorchidism, GnRH analogs have been shown to improve spermatogenesis when used as an adjunct to orchidopexy.[26,27] On the basis of successful treatment of one single case Iwamoto et al concluded that GnRH analog buserelin in low-doses avoids pituitary down-regulation exerting stimulatory effect on it and therefore may be an effective and well-tolerated therapeutic option for patients with hypogonadotropic hypogonadism of hypothalamic origin.[28]

Drawbacks

Wearing of the portable pump is cumbersome and hence discouraging for patients. Formation of anti-GnRH antibodies in certain cases has also raised some concerns.[29] Furthermore, at present consensus exists that GnRH has no role as empiric therapy in idiopathic infertility.

Gonadotropins

Various urinary, purified, and recombinant forms of gonadotropins have been used including human chorion gonadotropin (hCG, with LH activity), human menopausal gonadotropin hMG (FSH analog), recombinant FSH and LH.

Mixed Gonadotropin Therapy

Physiological principle: In all forms of hypogonadism testosterone alone is sufficient for maturation and maintenance of secondary sex characteristics, libido, erectile function. In hypogonadotropic hypogonadism however the anterior pituitary hormones LH and FSH are required together to initiate and maintain spermatogenesis. A combined gonadotropin therapy can thus be used to treat hypogonadotropic infertility arising at the level of pituitary or hypothalamus including IHH, when treatment with GnRH is not desired or indicated. hCG is used as the source of LH activity to stimulate testosterone secretion by Leydig cells, whereas human menopausal gonadotropin (hMG) acts as FSH.[30] In recent years recombinant gonadotropins have been introduced in clinical practice.

Method: The therapy is started with hCG 1000–2500 IU 2 times/week subcutaneous or intramuscular; adjusting the dose to target mid-normal testosterone levels. Testosterone levels are measured 48 hrs after the hCG injection. Alternatively recombinant LH can be used. After a period of 8–12 weeks of hCG or recombinant human LH therapy highly purified hMG or recombinant human FSH is added at the doses of 150–225 IU 3 times/week subcutaneously.[17] The treatment continues until sperm appear in the ejaculate or pregnancy occurs respectively, but in some cases therapy may be required for 1–2 or more years.

As soon as in men with hypogonadotropic hypogonadism spermatogenesis is induced with combined gonadotropin treatment or with GnRH, it can be maintained qualitatively by hCG alone for long time, but the decreasing sperm counts indicate that FSH is necessary for maintenance of quantitatively normal spermatogenesis.[30]

Evidence: Several studies although not placebo controlled have shown induction of spermatogenesis and ability to induce pregnancy with use of mixed gonadotropin therapy[25,31,32] and it is presently the most widely used therapy for hypogonadotropic infertility. Testicular volumes of 8 ml or more and postpubertal onset of gonadotropin deficiency are more likely to respond than those with testicular volumes of less than 4 mL and prepubertal onset.[24] Nevertheless, this treatment is also indicated in cases with cryptorchidism or with small testicular volume.[23] According to a recent study men with a BMI < 30 kg/m[2] have a greater chance of achieving spermatogenesis than men with a BMI equal or greater than 30 kg/m[2].[6] Low BMI and advanced sexual maturity, especially large baseline mean testicular volume are predictors of a good response to combined therapy with recombinant human FSH and hCG.[6]

Drawbacks: Although spermatogenesis is induced in the majority of cases, some patients may not respond. For quantitatively normal spermatogenesis both gonadotropins are required. The treatments with gonadotropins and GnRH are expensive, therefore they should be introduced only when a desire for children is present or once to stimulate testicular function until inducement of spermatogenesis is achieved before switching to a long lasting substitution therapy with testosterone.[3]

Follicle-stimulating Hormone Monotherapy

Physiological principle: Follicle-stimulating hormone (FSH) has an established role in promoting spermatogenesis. It enhances the production of androgen-binding protein by Sertoli cells which are required to maintain high local concentration of testosterone in the seminiferous tubules thus supporting spermatogenesis.[33] However the role of FSH in the maintenance of spermatogenesis remains controversial.[30]

Method: Purified or recombinant human FSH is given at doses ranging from 50–300 IU administered subcutaneously 3 times weekly for over 3 months.

Evidence: Several randomized controlled trials have evaluated the efficacy of FSH in men with idiopathic infertility with mixed results.[34,35] In these studies, the gonadotrophic status of the patients was not well characterized. Although pregnancy outcomes were not reported in most of these studies, improvement in sperm parameters was noted in some when FSH was used at higher doses.[22,36] When used 50 days before ICSI, FSH has been shown to improve fertilization, implantation, and pregnancy rates in men with severe oligospermia.[37]

Drawbacks: Evidence is weak and the consensus is that FSH therapy alone has at the best little efficacy in treating idiopathic male infertility.

Androgen Therapy

Testosterone Therapy

Physiological principle: Although testosterone has contraceptive properties in men due to its negative feedback on hypothalamic-pituitary axis and thus inhibition of LH and FSH and spermatogenesis respectively, it has been tried to treat subfertile men with testosterone based on two rationales. Raising serum testosterone would improve epididymal maturation of spermatozoa; gonadotropins and sperm concentration respectively increase transiently upon sudden stopping of testosterone, the so-called "rebound effect".

Method: Male infertility is treated using testosterone undecanoate or mesterolone in doses of 120–240 mg/day and 75–150 mg/day respectively.

Evidence: Various meta-analyses have demonstrated no improvement in pregnancy outcomes with androgen therapy in idiopathic male infertility.[38,39]

Drawbacks: Published literature strongly discourages any role of testosterone monotherapy for men with idiopathic infertility.

Antiestrogen Therapy

Antiestrogen Monotherapy

Physiological principle: Antiestrogens indirectly stimulate the secretion of GnRH, FSH and LH by binding to estrogen receptors in the hypothalamus and pituitary thereby blocking estrogen feedback inhibition. The resultant increase of gonadotropin concentration is believed to improve the gametogenic function of the testes.

Method: The two most commonly used nonsteroidal antiestrogens are clomiphene citrate and tamoxifen. Clomiphene citrate is usually prescribed in doses of 12.5-50 mg per day either continuously or on a 25 days cycle with a 5 days rest period each month for 3–6 months. Tamoxifen is administered at a dosage of 10–20 mg daily over a period of 3–6 months.

Evidence: Cochrane meta-analysis of 10 randomized controlled trials with idiopathic infertility found no improvement in pregnancy rates with antiestrogen therapy.[40] Similarly another meta-analysis reported no significant change in pregnancy outcomes with clomiphene citrate or tamoxifen therapy of idiopathic infertile men (OR, 1.54; 95% CI: 0.99-2.40).[38] However, some studies demonstrated improvement in sperm count and sperm motility.[41] Hence empiric therapy for at least 3 months may have a beneficial effect on fertility status in subfertile men by improving semen parameters which may allow a downstaging of the required ART procedure, i.e. utilizing intrauterine insemination (IUI) instead of intracytoplasmic sperm injection (ICSI).

Drawbacks: Literature support remains inconclusive awaiting large randomized prospective trials of empiric therapy in idiopathic male infertility.

Tamoxifen and Testosterone Combination Therapy

Physiological principle: Tamoxifen has been shown to primarily increase sperm density without much improvement in other parameters such as sperm motility and morphology. One of the main reasons could be inferior androgenic environment in the reproductive tract of oligozoospermic men. This in turn may compromise epididymal maturation of the spermatozoa which can be theoretically overcome by supplementing tamoxifen treatment with testosterone.

Method: Tamoxifen and testosterone undecanoate are administered as 20 mg and 120 mg respectively in daily divided doses for 6 months.

Evidence: Treatment with tamoxifen and testosterone undecanoate improved sperm variables and led to a higher incidence of pregnancy in couples with subfertility related to idiopathic oligozoospermia.[42]

Drawbacks: Literature is scarce and primarily restricted to single group of investigators.

Tamoxifen and Kallikrein Combination Therapy

Physiological principle: While tamoxifen improves sperm count, kallikrein has been shown to improve sperm motility; hence a combination can hypothetically be useful in men with idiopathic oligoasthenozoospermia.

Method: Tamoxifen is administered as 20 mg/day along with 600 IU of kallikrein daily for 3 months.

Evidence: Improvement in both sperm count and motility with such a therapy has been demonstrated in few trials when used in idiopathic normogonadotropic men with oligoasthenospermia.[43]

Drawbacks: Pregnancy outcomes have not yet been studied and further studies are warranted to draw any inferences.

Therapy with Aromatase Inhibitors

Physiological Principle

Aromatase is a P450 cytochrome enzyme that converts androgens to estrogens. Aromatase inhibitors block its activity thereby reducing serum estradiol concentrations and its negative feedback on the hypothalamus and pituitary, resulting in elevated serum FSH levels which in turn, might improve spermatogenesis.[44] On the other hand, aromatase inhibitors lead to increase in testosterone which also might contribute to achievement of fertility.

Method

Two types of aromatase inhibitors are available, steroidal (e.g. testolactone) and nonsteroidal (letrozole and anastrozole). The latter is more effective in increasing testosterone to estrogen ratio and is less likely to cause interruption of the adrenal axis beyond aromatase inhibition. Testolactone is given in doses of 100–200 mg per day whereas anastrozole is used as 1 mg/day dosage and letrozole 2.5 mg daily orally for 4–6 months.

Evidence

In idiopathic oligozoospermic men studied in double blind randomized controlled fashion, testolactone therapy failed to show any improvement in semen parameters.[45] Normal spermatogenesis, proven by testis biopsy, was achieved with letrozole in one case with azoospermia and normal FSH serum levels.[44] Controlled studies evaluating efficacy of aromatase inhibitors on pregnancy outcomes are still lacking.

Drawbacks

Further investigation is needed before drawing any conclusions on the use of aromatase inhibitors in male infertility. Elevation of hepatic enzymes has been reported with both these drugs and hence caution is advised in those who have underlying liver disease.

Growth Hormone Therapy

Physiological Principle

Growth hormone (GH) acts on gonads directly or through hepatic secreted insulin-like growth factor-1 (IGF-1) and plays a significant role in sexual growth and differentiation, gonadal steroidogenesis and gametogenesis.[46]

Method

Recombinant GH is given for 12 weeks.

Evidence

Growth hormone (GH) therapy has shown mixed results in terms of improvement in sperm parameters and pregnancy rates when used in oligo- and asthenozoospermic men.[47,48] When used as an adjunct therapy in a small study of seven men with hypogonadotropic hypogonadism who failed gonadotropin therapy, GH has been demonstrated to help induce spermatogenesis.[49]

Drawbacks

Available literature is limited and further studies trying combination therapy of GH and gonadotropins for male infertility are awaited.

Oxytocin Therapy

Physiological Principle

Oxytocin has been shown to promote sperm progression through the reproductive tract by improving epididymal contractility. It can thus be used to increase sperm retrieval in men with oligozoospermia.

Method

Oxytocin is given as intravenous injections or intranasal just before ejaculation.

Evidence

Oxytocin therapy has failed to improve sperm output in severely oligozoospermic men.[50]

Drawbacks

This form of therapy lacks evidence in supporting any role in male infertility.

Endocrine Therapy for Hyperprolactinemia

Dopamine agonists are the primary therapy for both micro- and macro adenomas as well as for nontumorous hyperprolactinemia. Historically, bromocriptine (2.5–10.0 mg, maximal 30 mg a day) was the first effective medical therapy. Cabergoline, a nonergot dopamine agonist, is administered at a dosage of 0.25–1.0 mg twice per week. Both normalize prolactin levels, decrease tumor size and restore reproductive function. Cabergoline is better tolerated than bromocriptine. However there are some recent concerns of heart valvular defects with higher doses of cabergoline.[51]

Summary

Therapy for subfertile men generally falls under two categories: specific and empiric, depending upon the etiology. Endocrine evaluation of men presenting with infertility should aim at identifying candidates for specific therapy. For men who have hypogonadotropic hypogonadism due to hypothalamic lesions, both gonadotropin therapy and pulsatile GnRH are equally effective, while if the disorder is of pituitary origin, only gonadotropin therapy may restore fertility. However, idiopathic infertility which is a much more frequently encountered clinically problem responds poorly to empiric endocrine treatment. Recently several hormonal intervention studies have shown promise in management of idiopathic male infertility. Further trials with adequate sample size and study design are warranted before it can be put into routine clinical practice.

▮ REFERENCES

1. World Health Organization. WHO manual for the standardized investigation and diagnosis of infertile couple. Cambridge university press. Cambridge, UK, 200.
2. Gnoth C, Godehardt E, Frank-Herrmann P, Friol K, Tigges J, Freundl G. Definition and prevalence of subfertility and infertility. Hum Reprod 2005;20(5):1144-7.
3. Nieschlag E, Behre HM, Nieschlag S (Eds). Andrology, 3rd edition, Springer, Heidelberg, 2009.
4. Sigman M, Jarow JP. Endocrine evaluation of infertile men. Urology 1997;50(5):659-64.
5. Bhasin S, Cunningham GR, Hayes FJ, Matsumoto AM, Snyder PJ, Swerdloff RS, Montori VM. Testosterone therapy in adult men with androgen deficiency syndromes: an endocrine society clinical practice guideline. J Clin Endocrinol Metab 2006;91(6):1995-2010.
6. Warne DW, Decosterd G, Okada H, Yano Y, Koide N, Howles CM. A combined analysis of data to identify predictive factors for spermatogenesis in men with hypogonadotropic hypogonadism treated with recombinant human follicle-stimulating hormone and human chorionic gonadotropin Fertil Steril 2009;92(2):594-604.
7. Pitteloud N, Durrani S, Raivio T, Sykiotis GP: Complex genetics in idiopathic hypogonadotropic hypogonadis In: Quinton R (Ed). Kallmann Syndrome and hypogonadotropic hypogonadism Front Horm Res, Basel, Karger 2010;39.pp.142-53.
8. MacColl GS, Quinton R, Bülow HE. Biology of KAL 1 and its orthologs: implication for X-linked Kallmann syndrome and the search for novel candidate genes In: Quinton R (Ed). Kallmann Syndrome and hypogonadotropic hypogonadism Front Horm Res, Basel, Karger 2010;39.pp.62-77.
9. Al-Ansari AA, Khalil TH, Kelani Y, Mortimer CH. Isolated follicle-stimulating hormone deficiency in men: successful long-term gonadotropin therapy. Fertil Steril 1984;42(4):618-26.
10. Krassas GE, Pontikides N, Deligianni V, Miras K. A prospective controlled study of the impact of hyperthyroidism on reproductive function in males. J Clin Endocrinol Metab. 2002;87(8):3667-71.
11. Zähringer S, Tomova A, von Werder K, Brabant G, Kumanov P, Schopohl J. The influence of hyperthyroidism on the hypothalamic-pituitary-gonadal axis. Exp Clin Endocrinol Diabetes 2000;108:282-9.
12. Velázquez EM, Bellabarba Arata G. Effects of thyroid status on pituitary gonadotropin and testicular reserve in men. Arch Androl 1997;38(1):85-92.
13. Kasturi SS, Tannir J, Brannigan RE. The metabolic syndrome and male infertility. J Androl 2008;29:251-9.
14. Robeva R, Kirilov G, Tomova A, Kumanov PH. Low testosterone levels and unimpaired melatonin secretion in young males with metabolic syndrome. Andrologia 2006;38:216-20.
15. Balducci R, Ghirri P, Brown TR, Bradford S, Boldrini A, Boscherini B, Sciarra F, Toscano V. A clinician looks at androgen resistance. Steroids 1996;61(4):205-11.
16. Yong EL, Loy CJ, Sim KS. Androgen receptor gene and male infertility. Hum Reprod Update 2003;9(1):1-7.
17. Bhasin S. Approach to the infertile man. J Clin Endocrinol Metab 2007;92 (6):1995-2004.
18. Wang C, Nieschlag E, Swerdloff R, Behre HM, Hellstrom WJ, Gooren LJ, Kaufman JM, Legros JJ, Lunenfeld B, Morales A, Morley JE, Schulman C, Thompson IM, Weidner W, Wu FCW. Investigation, treatment, and monitoring of late-onset hypogonadism in males: ISA, ISSAM, EAU, EAA, and ASA recommendations. European Urology 2009;55:121-30.
19. Vermeulen A, Verdonck L, Kaufman JM. A critical evaluation of simple methods for the estimation of free testosterone in serum. J Clin Endocrinol Metab 1999;84:3666-72.
20. WHO laboratory manual for the examination and processing of human semen. 2010, 5th edition, WHO, Geneva.
21. Kumanov P, Nandipati K, Tomova A, Agarwal A. Inhibin B is a better marker of spermatogenesis than other hormones in the evaluation of male factor infertility. Fertil Steril 2006;86(2):332-8.
22. Paradisi R, Busacchi P, Seracchioli R, Porcu E, Venturoli S. Effects of high doses of recombinant human follicle-stimulating hormone in the treatment of male factor infertility: results of a pilot study. Fertil Steril 2006;86(3):728-31.
23. Büchter D, Behre HM, Kliesch S, Nieschlag E. Pulsatile GnRH or human chorionic gonadotropin/human menopausal gonadotropin as effective treatment for men with hypogonadotropic hypogonadism: a review of 42 cases. Eur J Endocrinol 1998;139(3):298-303.
24. Liu L, Banks SM, Barnes KM, Sherins RJ. Two-year comparison of testicular responses to pulsatile gonadotropin-releasing hormone and exogenous gonadotropins from the inception of therapy in men with isolated hypogonadotropic hypogonadism. J Clin Endocrinol Metab 1988;67(6):1140-5.
25. Kliesch S, Behre HM, Nieschlag E. High efficacy of gonadotropin or pulsatile gonadotropin-releasing hormone treatment in hypogonadotropic hypogonadal men. Eur J Endocrinol 1994;131(4):347-54.
26. Hadziselimovic F, Herzog B. Treatment with a luteinizing hormone-releasing hormone analogue after successful

orchiopexy markedly improves the chance of fertility later in life. J Urol 1997;158(3 Pt 2):1193-5.

27. Huff DS, Snyder HM 3rd, Rusnack SL, Zderic SA, Carr MC, Canning DA. Hormonal therapy for the subfertility of cryptorchidism. Horm Res 2001;55(1):38-40.

28. Iwamoto H, Yoshida A, Suzuki H, Tanaka M, Watanabe N, Nakamura T. A man with hypogonadotropic hypogonadism successfully treated with nasal administration of the low-dose gonadotropin-releasing hormone analog buserelin. Fertil Steril 2009;92(3):1169.e3.

29. Lindner J, McNeil LW, Marney S, Conway M, Rivier J, Vale W, Rabin D. Characterization of human anti-luteinizing hormone-releasing hormone (LRH) antibodies in the serum of a patient with isolated gonadotropin deficiency treated with synthetic LRH. J Clin Endocrinol Metab 1981;52(2):267-70.

30. Depenbusch M, von Eckardstein S, Simoni M, Nieschlag E. Maintenance of spermatogenesis in hypogonadotropic hypogonadal men with human chorionic gonadotropin alone. European Journal of Endocrinology 2002;147:617-24.

31. Burgués S, Calderón MD. Subcutaneous self-administration of highly purified follicle stimulating hormone and human chorionic gonadotrophin for the treatment of male hypogonadotrophic-hypogonadism. Spanish Collaborative Group on Male Hypogonadotropic Hypogonadism. Hum Reprod 1997;12(5):980-6.

32. Kung AW, Zhong YY, Lam KS, Wang C. Induction of spermatogenesis with gonadotrophins in Chinese men with hypogonadotrophic hypogonadism. Int J Androl 1994;17(5):241-7.

33. Dohle GR, van Roijen JH, Pierik FH, Vreeburg JT, Weber RF. Subtotal obstruction of the male reproductive tract. Urol Res 2003;31(1):22-4.

34. Matorras R, Pérez C, Corcóstegui B, Pijoan JI, Ramón O, Delgado P, Rodríguez-Escudero FJ. Treatment of the male with follicle-stimulating hormone in intrauterine insemination with husband's spermatozoa: a randomized study. Hum Reprod 1997;12(1):24-8.

35. Kamischke A, Behre HM, Bergmann M, Simoni M, Schäfer T, Nieschlag E. Recombinant human follicle-stimulating hormone for treatment of male idiopathic infertility: a randomized, double-blind, placebo-controlled, clinical trial. Hum Reprod 1998;13(3):596-603.

36. Foresta C, Bettella A, Merico M, Garolla A, Ferlin A, Rossato M. Use of recombinant human follicle-stimulating hormone in the treatment of male factor infertility. Fertil Steril 2002;77(2):238-44.

37. Ashkenazi J, Bar-Hava I, Farhi J, Levy T, Feldberg D, Orvieto R, Ben-Rafael Z. The role of purified follicle stimulating hormone therapy in the male partner before intracytoplasmic sperm injection. Fertil Steril 1999;72(4):670-3.

38. Liu PY, Handelsman DJ. The present and future state of hormonal treatment for male infertility. Hum Reprod Update 2003;9(1):9-23.

39. Kamischke A, Nieschlag E. Analysis of medical treatment of male infertility. Hum Reprod 1999;14 (Suppl 1):1-23.

40. Vandekerckhove P, Lilford R, Vail A, Hughes E. Clomiphene or tamoxifen for idiopathic oligo/asthenospermia Cochrane Database Syst Rev 2000;(2):CD000151.

41. Kadioglu TC, Köksal IT, Tunç M, Nane I, Tellaloglu S. Treatment of idiopathic and post varicocelectomy oligozoospermia with oral tamoxifen citrate. BJU Int 1999;83(6):646-8.

42. Adamopoulos DA, Pappa A, Billa E, Nicopoulou S, Koukkou E, Michopoulos J. Effectiveness of combined tamoxifen citrate and testosterone undecanoate treatment in men with idiopathic oligozoospermia. Fertil Steril 2003;80(4):914-20.

43. Maier U, Hienert G. Tamoxifen and kallikrein in therapy of oligoasthenozoospermia: results of a randomized study. Eur Urol 1990;17(3):223-5.

44. Patry G, Jarvi K, Grober ED, Lo KC. Use of the aromatase inhibitor letrozole to treat male infertility. Fertil Steril 2009;92: 2,829.

45. Clark R, Sherins RJ. Treatment of men with idiopathic oligozoospermic infertility using the aromatase inhibitor testolactone. Results of a double-blinded, randomized, placebo-controlled trial with crossover. J Androl 1989;10(3):240-7.

46. Hull KL, Harvey S. Growth hormone: roles in male reproduction. Endocrine 2000;13(3):243-50.

47. Lee KO, Ng SC, Lee PS, Bongso AT, Taylor EA, Lin TK, Ratnam SS. Effect of growth hormone therapy in men with severe idiopathic oligozoospermia. Eur J Endocrinol 1995;132(2):159-62.

48. Radicioni A, Paris E, Dondero F, Bonifacio V, Isidori A. Recombinant-growth hormone (rec-hGH) therapy in infertile men with idiopathic oligozoospermia. Acta Eur Fertil 1994;25(5):311-7.

49. Shoham Z, Conway GS, Ostergaard H, Lahlou N, Bouchard P, Jacobs HS. Cotreatment with growth hormone for induction of spermatogenesis in patients with hypogonadotropic hypogonadism. Fertil Steril 1992;57(5):1044-51.

50. Byrne MM, Rolf C, Depenbusch M, Cooper TG, Nieschlag E. Lack of effect of a single IV dose of oxytocin on sperm output in severely oligozoospermic men. Hum Reprod 2003;18(10):2098-2102.

51. Klibanski A. Clinical practice. Prolactinomas. N Engl J Med 2010;362(13):1219-26.

16

Infections in Male Infertility

Ralf Henkel

INTRODUCTION

About 7 percent of all men are confronted with fertility problems during their reproductive lifetime rendering male infertility a problem, which has an even higher prevalence than a 'common disease', diabetes mellitus, with an overall estimate of 2.8 percent in the year 2000 and 4.4 percent in 2030 (Nieschlag and Behre, 2000; Wild et al., 2004). Causes for male infertility can be different and apart from idiopathic infertility (28.4%) and varicocele (18.1%), male genital tract infections are the third single most (11.6%) cause of male infertility (Nieschlag and Behre, 1997). Other sources report a prevalence of male genital tract infections in non-selected men consulting for infertility of up to 35 percent or even up to 45 percent in patients with a history of urethral discharge as an unspecific indication of an infection (Bayasgalan et al., 2004; Henkel et al., 2007). Yet, seeing that infections are caused by microorganisms, infections are potentially correctable causes of male infertility. They can rationally be treated with anti-biotics and anti-inflammatories to relieve the consequences of the infection, obstruction of the excurrent genital ducts (Weidner et al., 1999).

In view of the fact that male genital tract infections are asymptomatic in many cases (Gonzales et al., 2004; Schuppe and Meinhardt, 2006; Kiessling et al., 2008), and that men do not readily consult a doctor as women do, it is difficult to detect the genital tract infection. Even more so as leukocytes frequently appear in ejaculates, even in those from fertile men (Wolff, 1995). Additionally, traditionally the presence of pathogens like *Neisseria gonorrhoeae* or *Chlamydia trachomatis* or the occurrence of elevated numbers (more than 10^3 bacteria/mL ejaculate = bacteriospermia) were regarded as signs of an active infection (Eneroth et al., 1978; WHO, 1999). However, the male reproductive tract, except for the urethra, is normally free of aerobic bacteria (Fowler and Kessler, 1983) and it is therefore extremely difficult, if not impossible, to obtain an ejaculate devoid of bacterial contamination (Purvis and Christiansen, 1993). Thus, it is not clear to what extend one can regard bacteria colonizing male reproductive tract as commensals and it is therefore not surprising that a high percentage of patients presenting with chronic symptomatic inflammations of the accessory sex glands do not have a bacteriospermia.

LEUKOCYTE PROBLEM

Generally the presence of leukocytes is indicative of infective processes and is recognized in andrological diagnostics by the WHO (1999, 2010). However, the seminal concentration leuko-cytes, although recommended by the WHO with a cut-off value for leukocytospermia of 10^6/mL, has repeatedly been questioned as being too high (Sharma et al., 2001; Punab et al., 2003; Henkel et al., 2005) as leukocytes are powerful producers of reactive oxygen species (ROS) that inflict damage to sperm functions and the DNA (Aitken et al., 1995; Alvarez et al., 2002a; Erenpreis et al., 2002). Others found that the detection of leukocytospermia is of no diagnostic value for the identification of men with actual micro-bial infections (Trum et al., 1998) and bacteria found in semen cultures were only contaminants from the genital tract as there was no humoral immunological response (Lackner et al., 2006). Independent from the presence of leukocytes, up to 50 percent of the cases of bacteriospermia are caused by contaminations (Cottell et al., 2000). Consequently, Kim and Goldstein (1999) as well as Punab et al. (2003) regard the presence of leukocytes as poor predictor for the presence of bacteria. On the other hand, Gdoura et al. (2008) recommended a new cut-off value of more than 0.275×10^6 leukocytes/mL to predict the presence of bacteria.

Thus, the clinical value of both leukocytospermia and bacte-riospermia are highly debated. While the WHO retained the cut-off for leukocytospermia in the latest edition of the labora-tory manual (WHO, 2010), the aforesaid might be reasons why the term bacteriospermia is not defined anymore.

IMPACT OF INFECTIONS ON MALE FERTILITY AND SPERM FERTILIZING CAPACITY

Depending on the site, infections and inflammations can seri-ously affect spermatogenesis and sperm transit during ejacu-lation as can be seen in clinical findings in cases of oligozoo-spermia, asthenozoospermia or azoospermia (Weidner et al., 2002; Schuppe et al., 2008). Chronic infections of the male genital tract including the accessory glands are often scarring and result in obstruction (Goluboff et al., 1995; Belmonte et al., 1998). Moreover, they can cause dysfunctional male accessory glands (Weidner et al., 1999) and significantly impair sperm functions

(Henkel and Schill, 1998; Sanocka-Maciejewska et al., 2005). These changes are triggered by direct action of the pathogens on spermatozoa and sperm functions (Monga and Roberts, 1994) or indirectly by inducing inflammatory processes in the seminal tract by activating leukocytes (Eggert-Kruse et al., 2007).

Sperm fertilizing capacity may directly be compromised by activated leukocytes infiltrating the infected organs and releasing high amounts of ROS and cytokines such as IL-6, IL-8 or TNF-α as inflammatory mediators (Comhaire et al., 1999; Henkel et al., 2005). Both, ROS and cytokines have been shown to be associated with the impairment of various sperm functions including the sperm DNA through oxidative stress (Köhn et al., 1998; Alvarez et al., 2002b; Kocak et al., 2002; Henkel et al., 2004; 2005; 2006). The mechanism by which this damage takes place involves oxidation of sperm membranes by means of lipid peroxidation as well as direct oxidation of the DNA (Aitken et al., 1989; Martinez et al., 2007).

Clinical reports indicate that infections and chronic inflammation may even impair testicular steroidogenesis and spermatogenesis resulting in temporary or permanent infertility (Adamopoulos et al., 1978; Baker, 1998). In animal experiments, local production of IL-1β and TNF-α has been reported to be responsible for a down-regulation of cholesterol transport protein, steroidogenic acute regulatory protein (StAR) and various enzymes of the steroid synthesis pathway (Hales et al., 1992; Lin et al., 1998). Furthermore, significant production of proinflammatory cytokines also activate the hypothalamic-pituitary-adrenal axis leading to an increased secretion of glucocorticoids (Imura et al., 1991), which, in turn, inhibit steroidogenesis via the hypothalamus and pituitary (Bambino and Hsueh, 1981). Thus, an infection mediated via lipopolysaccharides may inhibit Leydig cell function resulting in reduced testosterone synthesis as shown in an animal model (Gow et al., 2001).

■ INFECTIONS OF THE MALE UROGENITAL TRACT

Male urogenital tract infections can either be classified according to the kind of microorganism causing the infection or the location, namely the testis (orchitis), epididymis (epididymitis), prostate (prostatitis) or urethra (urethritis). The most prevalent pathogens are *Chlamydia trachomatis*, *Ureaplasma urealyticum*, *Neisseria gonorrhoeae*, *Mycoplasma hominis*, *Mycoplasma genitalium* or *Escherichia coli*. While the first pathogens are sexually transmitted, *E. coli* is regarded as the most common cause of nonsexually transmitted urogenital tract infection, particularly of epididymoorchitis or prostatitis where it is the cause of 65–80 percent of the cases (Pellati et al., 2008). Furthermore, viral infections like mumps virus, human papilloma virus (HPV), herpes simplex virus (HSV) and particularly human immunodeficiency virus (HIV) have also been associated with increased seminal leukocyte concentrations (Umapathy et al., 2001). The latter virus can infect the testes and male sex accessory glands (Le Tortorec et al., 2008).

Chlamydia trachomatis

Chlamydia trachomatis is worldwide one of the most frequently sexually transmitted bacterial pathogens accounting to an estimated 92 Mill. new urogenital infections per year (WHO, 2001).

Due to the high rate of asymptomatic presentations (approximately 70–80 percent of women and up to 50 percent of men) this number is rather underestimated (Gonzales et al., 2004). Since a high number of chlamydial infections remain undiagnosed, the pathogen can even be transferred to the newborn during delivery accounting for 25–50 percent of conjunctivitis and 10–20 percent of pneumonia in newborns, thus, posing an health risk on the offspring as well as enormous costs for diagnosis and treatment on countries health systems.

In men, *C. trachomatis* has been detected in the testis including Leydig cells (Villegas et al., 1991), the prostate (Kadar et al., 1995) and even epididymis and seminal vesicles (Bornman et al., 1998), thus causing orchitis, prostatitis, epididymitis and urethritis. Apart from the lesions triggered by the infection and its implications an acute inflammation can cause in the male genital tract, reports on the influence of *Chlamydia* infections on male fertility are inconsistent. While some authors (Ruijs et al., 1990; Habermann and Krause, 1999) found no significant association, most others have shown a direct negative influence of the chlamydial infection on male fertility (Kadar et al., 1995; Gallegos et al., 2008; Mazzoli et al., 2009). *In vitro* studies by Hosseinzadeh et al. (2000; 2003) even indicate that the pathogen directly causes changes in sperm proteins and premature cell death induced by lipopolysaccharides secreted by Chlamydiae.

Ureaplasma urealyticum

Ureaplasma urealyticum causes nongonococcal urethritis, pelvic inflammatory disease or infertility (Schiefer, 1998; Weidner et al., 1999). While the association between *Ureaplasma* infections and male infertility was discussed controversially in the past (Kjaergaard et al., 1997; Potts et al., 2000), a recent study (Wang et al., 2006) clearly showed these infections cause higher seminal viscosity, decreased sperm concentrations and lower pH. Additionally, Potts et al. (2000) revealed significantly increased seminal ROS levels and Reichart et al. (2000) higher levels of sperm DNA damage. The prevalence of male genital ureaplasma infections among infertile men varies considerably from 10–40 percent (Cottell et al., 2000).

Mycoplasma hominis, Mycoplasma genitalium

Both *M. hominis* and *M. genitalium* are significantly associated with genitourinary infections (Deguchi and Maeda, 2002; Andrade-Rocha, 2003). Frequencies of infection are with 10.8 percent for *M. hominis* and 5 percent for *M. genitalium*, respectively, lower than for other pathogens (Gdoura et al., 2007). Both species can attach to and penetrate human sperm plasma membrane (Taylor-Robinson, 2002; Diaz-Garcia et al., 2006), which might have a significant long-term impact on male fertility as well as on the onset of pregnancy and the health of the offspring. While the first may contribute to the distribution of the bacterium to the female to cause cervicitis and endometritis (Cohen et al., 2002) or an alteration of the plasma membrane affecting acrosome reaction (Köhn et al., 1998), the latter might particularly be caused by the sperm DNA damage triggered by the infection (Gallegos et al., 2008).

Neisseria gonorrhoeae

Neisseria gonorrhoeae are gram-negative, immotile cocci growing in pairs (diplococci). They cause the most common infectious disease in men leading to urethritis, prostatitis and epididymitis which in turn may impair male fertility. These bacteria have pili on their surface which facilitate attachment to other cells (Krause, 2008), which, in sperm, may bind to an asialoglycoprotein receptor that recognizes and binds lipopolysaccharides in gonococcal membranes (Harvey et al., 2000).

Even though its incidence has been declining in Western countries during the past decades, 150–400 new infections per 100,000 are still recorded in Europe per year (Krause, 2008). Presumably due to socioeconomic and behavioral factors, these numbers are much higher in third world and developing countries, with highest numbers in Sub-Saharan Africa and South and Southeast Asia (Avert.org, 2010).

Escherichia coli

Escherichia coli, a gram-negative bacterium, is responsible for most urogenital tract and male accessory gland infections (Weidner et al., H1999). In contrast to other pathogens *E. coli* has significant direct negative effects on sperm motility (Huwe et al., 1998) and acrosome reaction (Köhn et al., 1998). The latter might be due to morphological alterations, particularly on the acrosome and flagellum, seen after exposure of human sperm to the pathogen (Diemer et al., 2000a). *E. coli* directly interacts with the sperm plasma membrane (Sanchez et al, 1989) by means of bacterial pili (Diemer et al., 2003). More recently, Schulz et al. (2009) demonstrated two mechanisms by which the bacterium affects spermatozoa, the described direct interaction and by action of soluble factors that induce apoptosis and a breakdown in the mitochondrial membrane potential. Potential candidate substances causing these cellular reactions might be α-hemolysin and Shiga-like toxin as these have already been associated with sperm motility loss (Diemer et al., 2000b) and apoptosis in Hep-2 cells (Ching et al., 2002), respectively.

Viruses

A number of viruses are also able to infect all parts of the male genital system, e.g. the testes (mumps virus, HIV-1, epididymis (Coxsackie virus), seminal vesicle (cytomegalovirus), prostate (HPV, HSV, HIV-1) and the semen (e.g. HSV, HPV, HIV) (Dejucq and Jegou, 2001). Some of these viral infections are associated with poor semen and sperm quality (Umapathy et al., 2001; Kapranos et al., 2003).

The high number of more than 65 million HIV-infected patients that are seeking for assisted reproduction worldwide, however, demands not only proper diagnosis but also proper management and handling of the ART procedure in order not to infect the partner or the offspring. Apart from the risk of vertical transmission from a seropositive mother to her unborn child, problems arise from the fact that semen is a vector of viral propagation and sperm can bind and incorporate the virus via a CD-4 independent receptor and/or the HIV coreceptor CCR5

(Bandivdekar et al., 2003; Muciaccia et al., 2005). In addition, sperm can carry viral particles deriving from the testis or epididymis (Muciaccia et al., 2007; Le Tortorec and Dejucq-Rainsford, 2010). In view of the fact that seminal leukocytes shed different viral strains than those in the blood (Pillai et al., 2005), the question rises whether infected leukocytes and free virions contaminating the semen are of different origin and an infected testis might represent a special reservoir for the virus as this area is resistant to antiviral drugs due to the blood-testis barrier (Le Tortorec and Dejucq-Rainsford, 2010). Therefore, special care must be taken when separating sperm for assisted reproduction, particularly for ICSI.

■ MALE GENITAL TRACT INFECTIONS

Orchitis

An 'orchitis' is an inflammatory lesion of the testes associated with leukocytic exsudate inside and outside the seminiferous tubules and resulting in tubular damage (Weidner et al., 2002). It can be a reason for spermatogenic arrest and testicular atrophy resulting in low sperm concentration and poor sperm quality (Diemer and Desjardins, 1999; Weidner et al., 2002). Intratesticular obstruction as a result of an orchitis is the case in about 15 percent of obstructive azoospermia (Weidner et al., 2002).

As reported in a large study, the prevalence of an isolated orchitis is with 0.42 percent among testicular pathologies relatively low (Nistal and Paniagua, 1984). However, due to retrograde ascending infectious lesions a 'nonspecific' orchitis triggered by *Pneumococcus spec.*, *Salmonella spec.*, *Klebsiella spec.* or *Haemophilus influenzae* is in most cases associated with an epididymitis as epididymo-orchitis. The close vicinity of the different compartments as well as the ascending nature of the infections makes a distinction between inflammations, i.e. isolated epididymitis vs. epididymo-orchitis, very difficult in the clinical routine (Haidl et al., 2008).

Sexually transmitted bacteria like *C. trachomatis* and *N. gonorrhoeae* are the cause of the acute infection in men younger than 35 years, while *E. coli* is the predominant trigger in older men (Schuppe et al., 2008). On the other hand, an orchitis can also occur after hematogenous dissemination of pathogens like the Coxsackie-B or the mumps virus (Weidner et al., 2002) as a complication of a systemic viral infection. For instance, the mumps virus may affect the tests (mumps orchitis) in 20–30 percent (Bartak, 1973) and lead to infertility in 13 percent of the cases with unilateral and in 30–87 percent in patients with bilateral orchitis (Casella et al., 1997; Behrman et al., 2004). While bacterial infections as described above cause a 'nonspecific' orchitis, *Mycobacterium tuberculosis*, *M. leprae*, *Treponema pallidum* or *Brucella spec.* may cause a 'specific', predominantly granulomatous orchitis (Weidner et al., 2002).

Epididymitis

An epididymitis is an inflammation of the epididymis, which is most commonly caused by *C. trachomatis* and *N. gonorrhoeae* in sexually active men younger than 35 years. In contrast, *E. coli* is etiologically responsible for the disease in older men (Weidner et al., 1999; Ludwig, 2008). This group of patients is particularly at risk of having urethral strictures, bladder neck obstruction or benign prostate hyperplasia (BPH) resulting in increased voiding pressure to empty the bladder resulting in a reflux of contaminated urine into the excurrent genital ducts and subsequent infection (Chan and Schlegel, 2002).

In cases of acute infectious epididymitis, an involvement of the testicle due to ascending canalicular bacterial infections can represent a complication which may occur in up to 60 percent of affected patients as epididymo-orchitis (Ludwig, 2008). Although up to 35 percent of patients consulting for fertility problems present with male genital tract infections (Kopa et al, 2005; Henkel et al., 2007), data on the prevalence of epididymitis/ epididymo-orchitis vary considerably from 0.29 percent of all consultations (Collins et al., 1998) to 20% of all urologic admissions in an US Army setup (Vordermark, 1985).

Major problems for male fertility may arise particularly in patients with epididymitis as this disease appears to have a greater influence on semen quality and male fertility than an infection/inflammation of the prostate or seminal vesicle (Comhaire and Mahmoud, 2006). In addition, in quite a number of patients the diagnosis of chronic epididymitis is extremely difficult as these patients' health is not compromised and do not feel discomfort (Haidl et al., 2008). Due to a 'silent' nature of the infection/inflammation, epididymitis will only be diagnosed once these patients appear in an andrological clinic consulting for infertility. Eventually, inflammatory lesions of the epididymis can result in dysfunction of the organ and ultimately in obstructive azoospermia, which is the most common cause for this condition (Weidner et al., 2002).

Prostatitis

According to epidemiological studies, prostatitis is with prevalence of 4–11 percent the most common urological diagnosis in men younger than 50 years (Nickel et al., 2001), of which about 5–10 percent are of bacterial origin (Brunner et al., 1983). Even though many clinicians diagnose "prostatitis", it actually represents diverse clinical symptoms ranging from acute bacterial infection to chronic pelvic pain and should actually be referred to as "prostatitis syndrome" as patients present with a variety of urogenital, perineal and perianal complaints (Roberts et al., 1997; 1998).

In about 80 percent of acute bacterial prostatitis, *E. coli* can be identified as pathogen, while *Pseudomonas aeruginosa, Klebsiella* or Enterococci are the cause in the remaining patients (Lopez-Plaza and Bostwick, 1990). Nevertheless, there are major concerns differentiating the category II from category III prostatitis. Many of these patients have a history of recurrent urinary tract infections and are asymptomatic in noninfectious intervals. If the bacterial culture is positive for an established uropathogen like *E. coli* or *Klebsiella spec.*, the diagnosis is unproblematic (Nickel, 1998). However, in cases where enterococci or anaerobes are identified the detection might be false negative because the bacterial colonization of the prostate can be veiled as bacteria

can form microcolonies or aggregates, which are surrounded by a thick protective layer (Nickel et al., 1994; Nickel, 1998).

Urethritis

Urethritis is the infectious or noninfectious inflammation of the urethra. While noninfectious causes include injuries through traumas, masturbation, manipulation by the patient or medical treatments, acute infectious urethritis may be caused by known sexually transmitted uropathogens like *C. trachomatis, Mycoplasms* or *N. gonorrhoea* with incidences of 15–26, 10–21 and 0.4–18 percent, respectively. In addition, among the not sexually transmitted pathogens Enterobacteriaceae and staphylococci are causing the disease with frequencies between 20 and 31 percent (Ochsendorf, 2006). Chronic urethritis is a very rare condition which is why the prevalence is not known (Krieger et al., 1988). Normally, the infection remains localized to the urethra. However, ascension of gonococci may occur in about 1 percent of the infected patients causing epididymitis (Ochsendorf, 2006).

The impact of urethritis on male fertility is debatable, particularly since the inflammatory discharge present in the anterior urethra makes an ejaculate analysis impossible as the pus contaminates the ejaculate (Chambers, 1985) and both, direct effect of bacteria (Sanocka-Maciejewska et al., 2005; Schulz et al., 2009) and leukocytes (Henkel et al., 2005) demonstrated detrimental effects on sperm functions. On the other hand, obstruction due to urethral stricture or as a result of lesions in the area of the seminal colliculus may result in ejaculatory disturbances (Weidner et al., 2002).

■ MALE ACCESSORY GLAND INFECTION

According to definition, the male accessory glands comprise the prostate, seminal vesicles and the Cowper's glands. Considering that in Male Accessory Gland Infection (MAGI) these organs are commonly inflamed, clear distinctions between prostatitis, epididymitis or glandulitis vesiculitis cannot be made (Krause, 2008). General symptoms of male accessory gland infection (MAGI) are leukocytospermia ($\geq 10^6$ peroxidase-positive leukocytes/ml), elevated seminal levels of polymorphonuclear granulocyte elastase (≥ 230 ng/mL), ROS and cytokines (Depuydt et al., 1996; Kocak et al., 2002; Schiefer and von Graevenitz, 2006).

Due to the leukocyte infiltration seminal concentrations of proinflammatory cytokines like IL-6, IL-8 or TNF-α are elevated and sperm functions may be compromised by directly affecting sperm function and intensifying the level of oxidative stress, respectively (Aitken et al., 1998; Henkel et al., 2005; Fraczek et al., 2008). Additionally, the secretory functions of the accessory sex glands may be impaired, thus resulting in decreased seminal concentrations of citric acid, fructose, α-glucosidase, phosphatase and zinc (Cooper et al., 1990; Wolff et al., 1991; Krause, 2008).

In addition, there are concerns that patients presenting with MAGI are at a higher risk of developing sperm auto-antibodies due to the inflammatory processes compromising the immune barrier (Munoz et al., 1986; Bohring et al., 2001). Furthermore, like in orchitis or epididymitis, stenosis or obstruction of the excurrent ducts may occur.

CONCLUSION

To sum up it can be stated that male genital tract infections pose a significant health risk not only to the man, but also to his female partner and, depending on the circumstances, also to the offspring. Reasons for this are manifold and include factors like:

- The high proportion of asymptomatic cases
- The fact that men do not readily visit a doctor as women do and can therefore transmit the infection to the female
- The increased chance to genetic damage in the germ line of the offspring because of sperm DNA damage. If undetected at an early stage, male genital tract infections can cause irreversible serious fertility problems. However, seeing that infections are potentially curable as they are caused by microorganisms, the emphasis should be on a higher awareness of the subjects, male and female, of the consequences. Moreover, clinicians should have a better understanding of the pathophysiology of male infertility as well as the diagnostic and therapeutic options available.

BIBLIOGRAPHY

1. Adamopoulos DA, Lawrence DM, Vassilopoulos P. Pituitary-testicular interrelationships in mumps orchitis and other viral infections. Br Med J 1 (6121):1978;1177-80.
2. Aitken RJ, Buckingham DW, Brindle J, et al. Analysis of sperm movement in relation to the oxidative stress created by leukocytes in washed sperm preparations and seminal plasma. Hum Reprod 1995;10:2061-71.
3. Aitken RJ, Clarkson JS, Fishel S. Generation of reactive oxygen species, lipid peroxidation, and human sperm function. Biol Reprod 1989;41:183-97.
4. Aitken RJ, Gordon E, Harkiss D, et al. Relative impact of oxidative stress on the functional competence and genomic integrity of human spermatozoa. Biol Reprod 1998;59:1037-46.
5. Alvarez JG, Sharma RK, Ollero M, et al. Increased DNA damage in sperm from leukocytospermic semen samples as determined by the sperm chromatin structure assay. Fertil Steril 2002;78:319-29.
6. Alvarez JG, Sharma RK, Ollero M, et al. Increased DNA damage in sperm from leukocytospermic semen samples as determined by the sperm chromatin structure assay. Fertil Steril 2002a;78:319-29.
7. Andrade-Rocha FT. *Ureaplasma urealyticum* and *Mycoplasma hominis* in men attending for routine semen analysis. Prevalence, incidence by age and clinical settings, influence on sperm characteristics, relationship with the leukocyte count and clinical value. Urol Int 2003;71:377-81.
8. AVERT.org. STD Statistics Worldwide. Available at http://www.avert.org/stdstatisticsworldwide.htm. (accessed on 09 September 2010)
9. Baker HW. Reproductive effects of nontesticular illness. Endocrinol Metab Clin North Am 1998;27:831-850.
10. Bambino TH, Hsueh AJ. Direct inhibitory effect of glucocorticoids upon testicular luteinizing hormone receptor and steroidogenesis *in vivo* and *in vitro*. Endocrinology 1981;108:2142-8.
11. Bandivdekar AH, Velhal SM, Raghavan VP. Identification of CD4-independent HIV receptors on spermatozoa. Am J Reprod Immunol 2003;50:322-7.
12. Bartak V. sperm count, morphology and motility after unilateral mumps orchitis. J Reprod Fertil 1973;32:491-3.
13. Bayasgalan G, Naranbat D, Tsedmaa B, et al. Clinical patterns and major causes of infertility in Mongolia. J Obstet Gynecol Res 2004;30:386-93.
14. Behrman RE, Kliegman RM, Jenson HB. Nelson Textbook of Pediatrics, 17th edition, Philadelphia: Saunders; 2004.
15. Belmonte IG, Martin de Serrano MN. Partial obstruction of the seminal path, a frequent cause of oligozoospermia in men. Hum Reprod 1995;13:3402-5.
16. Bohring C, Krause E, Habermann B, et al. Isolation and identification of spermatozoa membrane antigens, recognized by antisperm antibodies and their possible role in immunological infertility disease. Mol Hum Reprod 2001;7:113-8.
17. Bornman MS, Ramuthaga TN, Mahomed MF, et al. *Chlamydia* infection in asymptomatic infertile men attending an andrology clinic. Arch Androl 1998;41:203-8.
18. Brunner H, Weidner W, Schiefer H-G. Studies on the role of *Ureaplasma urealyticum* and *Mycoplasma hominis* in prostatitis. J Infect Dis 1983;147:807-13.
19. Casella R, Leibundgut B, Lehman K, et al. Mumps orchitis: Report of a mini-epidemic. J Urol 1997;158:2158-61.
20. Chambers RM. The mechanism of infection in the urethra, prostate and epididymis. In: Keith LG, Berger GS, Edelmann DA (Eds). Infections in Reproductive Health. Common Infections. 1985; MTP Press, Lancaster, pp.283-96.
21. Chan PT, Schlegel PN. Inflammatory conditions of the male excurrent ductal system. Part II. J Androl 2002;23:461-9.
22. Ching JC, Jones NL, Ceponis PJ, et al. *Escherichia coli* shiga-like toxins induce apoptosis and cleavage of poly (ADP-ribose) polymerase via *in vitro* activation of caspases. Infect Immun 2002;70:4669-77.
23. Cohen CR, Manhart LE, Bukusi EA, et al. Association between *Mycoplasma genitalium* and acute endometritis. Lancet 2002;359:765-6.
24. Collins MM, Stafford RS, O'Leary MP, et al. How common is prostatitis? A national survey of physician visits. J Urol 1998;159: 1224-8.
25. Comhaire F, Mahmoud A. Infection/inflammation of the accessory sex glands. In: Schill W-B, Comhaire F, Hargreave TB (Eds). Andrology for the Clinician. 2006; Springer, Heidelberg, pp.72-74.
26. Comhaire FH, Mahmoud AM, Depuydt CE, et al. Mechanisms and effects of male genital tract infection on sperm quality and fertilizing potential: the andrologist's viewpoint. Hum Reprod Update 1999;5:393-8.
27. Cooper TG, Weidner W, Nieschlag E. The influence of inflammation of the human male genital tract on secretion of the seminal markers alpha-glucosidase, glycerophosphocholine, carnitine, fructose and citric acid. Int J Androl 1990;13:329-36.
28. Cottell E, Harrison RF, McCaffrey M, et al. Are seminal fluid microorganisms of significance or merely contaminants? Fertil Steril 2000;74:465-70.
29. Deguchi T, Maeda S. *Mycoplasma genitalium*: another important pathogen of non-gonococcal urethritis. J Urol 2002;167: 210-7.

30. Dejucq N, Jegou B. Viruses in the mammalian male genital tract and their effects on the reproductive system. Microbiol Mol Biol Rev 2001;65:208-31.

31. Depuydt CE, Bosmans E, Zalata A, et al. The relation between reactive oxygen species and cytokines in andrological patients with or without male accessory gland infection. J Androl 1996;17:699-707.

32. Diaz-Garcia FJ, Herrera-Mendoza AP, Giono-Cerezo S, et al. *Mycoplasma hominis* attaches to and locates intracellularly in human spermatozoa. Hum Reprod 2006;21:1591-8.

33. Diemer T, Desjardins C. Disorders of spermatogenesis. In: Knobil E, Neill JD (Eds). Encyclopedia of Reproduction. Vol. 4, Academic Press, San Diego 1999,pp.546-56.

34. Diemer T, Huwe P, Ludwig M, et al. Influence of autogenous leucocytes and *Escherichia coli* on sperm motility parameters *in vitro*. Andrologia 2003;35:100-5.

35. Diemer T, Huwe P, Michelmann HW, et al. *Escherichia coli*-induced alterations of human spermatozoa. An electron microscopy analysis. Int J Androl 2000a;23:178-86.

36. Diemer T, Ludwig M, Huwe P, et al. Influence of urogenital infection on sperm function. Curr Opin Urol 2000b;10:39-44.

37. Eggert-Kruse W, Kiefer I, Beck C, et al. Role for tumor necrosis factor alpha (TNF-alpha) and interleukin 1-beta (IL-1beta) determination in seminal plasma during infertility investigation. Fertil Steril 2007;87:810-23.

38. Eneroth P, Ljungh-Wadström Å, Moberg PJ, et al. Studies on the bacterial flora in semen from males in infertile relations. Int J Androl 1978;1:105-16.

39. Erenpreiss J, Hlevicka S, Zalkalns J, et al. Effect of leukocytospermia on sperm DNA integrity: a negative effect in abnormal semen samples. J Androl 2002;23:717-23.

40. Fowler JE Jr., Kessler R. Genital tract infection. In: Lipshultz LI, Howards SS (Eds). Infertility in the Male. Churchill Livingstone, New York, 1983,pp.283-98.

41. Fraczek M, Sanocka D, Kamieniczna M, et al. Proinflammatory cytokines as an intermediate factor enhancing lipid sperm membrane peroxidation in *in vitro* conditions. J Androl 2008;29: 85-92.

42. Gallegos G, Ramos B, Santiso R, et al. Sperm DNA fragmentation in infertile men with genitourinary infection by *Chlamydia trachomatis* and *Mycoplasma*. Fertil Steril 2008;90:328-34.

43. Gdoura R, Kchaou W, Chaari C, et al. *Ureaplasma urealyticum, Ureaplasma parvum, Mycoplasma hominis* and *Mycoplasma genitalium* infections and semen quality of infertile men. BMC Infect Dis 2007;7:129.

44. Gdoura R, Kchaou W, Znazen A, et al. Screening for bacterial pathogens in semen samples from infertile men with and without leukocytospermia. Andrologia 2008;40:209-18.

45. Goluboff ET, Stifelman MD, Fisch H. Ejaculatory duct obstruction in the infertile male. Urology 1995;45:925-31.

46. Gonzales GF, Munoz G, Sanchez R, et al. Update on the impact of *Chlamydia trachomatis* infection on male fertility. Andrologia. 2004;36:1-23.

47. Gow RM, O'Bryan MK, Canny BJ, et al. Differential effects of dexamethasone treatment on lipopolysaccharide-induced testicular inflammation and reproductive hormone inhibition in adult rats. J Endocrinol 2001;168:193-201.

48. Habermann B, Krause W. Altered sperm function or sperm antibodies are not associated with chlamydial antibodies in infertile men with leukocytospermia. J Eur Acad Dermatol Venerol 1999;12:25-9.

49. Haidl G, Allam JP, Schuppe HC. Chronic epididymitis: impact on semen parameters and therapeutic options. Andrologia 2008;40:92-6.

50. Hales DB, Xiong Y, Tur-Kaspa I. The role of cytokines in the regulation of Leydig cell P450c17 gene expression. J Steroid Biochem 1992;43:907-14.

51. Harvey HA, Porat N, Campbell CA, et al. Gonococcal lipooligosaccharide is a ligand for the asialoglycoprotein receptor on human sperm. Mol Microbiol 2000;36:1059-70.

52. Henkel R, Hajimohammad M, Stalf T, et al. Influence of deoxyribonucleic acid damage on fertilization and pregnancy. Fertil Steril 2004;81:965-72.

53. Henkel R, Kierspel E, Stalf T, et al. Effect of reactive oxygen species produced by spermatozoa and leukocytes on sperm functions in non-leukocytospermic patients. Fertil Steril 2005;83:635-42.

54. Henkel R, Ludwig M, Schuppe HC, et al. Chronic pelvic pain syndrome/chronic prostatitis affect the acrosome reaction in human spermatozoa. World J Urol 2006;24:39-44.

55. Henkel R, Maaß G, Jung A, et al. Age-related changes in seminal polymorphonuclear elastase in men with asymtomatic inflammation of the genital tract. Asian J Androl 2007;9:299-304.

56. Henkel R, Schill W-B. Sperm separation in patients with urogenital infections. Andrologia 1998;30 (Suppl. 1):91-7.

57. Hosseinzadeh S, Brewis IA, Pacey AA, et al. Coincubation of human spermatozoa with *Chlamydia trachomatis in vitro* causes increased tyrosine phosphorylation of sperm proteins. Infect Immun 2000;68:4872-6.

58. Hosseinzadeh S, Pacey AA, Eley A. *Chlamydia trachomatis*-induced death of human spermatozoa is caused primarily by lipopolysaccharide. J Med Microbiol 2003;52:193-200.

59. Huwe P, Diemer T, Ludwig M, et al. Influence of different uropathogenic microorganisms on human sperm motility parameters in an *in vitro* experiment. Andrologia 1998;30 (Suppl 1):55-9.

60. Imura H, Fukata J, Mori T. Cytokines and endocrine function: an interaction between the immune and neuroendocrine system. Clin Endocrinol 1991;35:107-15.

61. Kadar A, Bucsek M, Kardos M, et al. Detection of *Chlamydia trachomatis* in chronic prostatitis by *in situ* hybridization (preliminary methodological report). Orv Hetil 1995;136:659-62.

62. Kapranos N, Petrakou E, Anastasiadou C, et al. Detection of herpes simplex virus, cytomegalovirus, and Epstein-Barr virus in the semen of men attending an infertility clinic. Fertil Steril 2003;79 (Suppl 3):1566-70.

63. Kiessling AA, Desmarais BM, Yin HZ, et al. Detection and identification of bacterial DNA in semen. Fertil Steril 2008;90:1744-56.

64. Kim FY, Goldstein M. Antibacterial skin preparation decreases the incidence of false-positive semen culture results. J Urol 1999;161:819-21.

65. Kjaergaard N, Kristensen B, Hansen ES, et al. Microbiology of semen specimens from males attending a fertility clinic. APMIS 1997;105:566-70.

66. Kocak I, Yenisey C, Dündar M, et al. Relationship between seminal plasma interleukin-6 and tumor necrosis factor alpha levels with semen parameters in fertile and infertile men. Urol Res 2002;30:263-7.

67. Köhn FM, Erdmann I, Oeda T, et al. Influence of urogenital infections on sperm functions. Andrologia 1998;30(Suppl 1):73-80.

68. Kopa Z, Wenzel J, Papp GK, et al. Role of granulocyte elastase and interleukin-6 in the diagnosis of male genital tract inflammation. Andrologia 2005;37:188-94.

69. Krause W. Male accessory gland infection. Andrologia 2008;40:113-6.

70. Krieger JN, Hooton TM, Brust PJ, et al. Evaluation of chronic urethritis. Defining the role for endoscopic procedures. Arch Intern Med 1988;148:703-7.

71. Lackner JE, Herwig R, Schmidbauer J, et al. Correlation of leukocytospermia with clinical infection and the positive effect of antiinflammatory treatment on semen quality. Fertil Steril 2006;86:601-5.

72. Le Tortorec A, Dejucq-Rainsford N. HIV infection of the male genital tract - consequences for sexual transmission and reproduction. Int J Androl 2010;33:e98-e108.

73. Le Tortorec A, Le Grand R, Denis H, et al. Infection of semen-producing organs by SIV during the acute and chronic stages of the disease. PLoS ONE 2008;3:e1792.

74. Lin T, Wang D, Stocco DM. Interleukin-1 inhibits Leydig cell steroidogenesis without affecting steroidogenic acute regulatory protein messenger ribonucleic acid or protein levels. J Endocrinol 1998;156:461-7.

75. Lopez-Plaza I, Bostwick DG. Prostatitis. In: Bostwick DG (Ed). Pathology of the Prostate. New York, Churchill Livingstone 1990,pp.15-30.

76. Ludwig M. Diagnosis and therapy of acute prostatitis, epididymitis and orchitis. Andrologia 2008;40:76-80.

77. Martinez R, Proverbio F, Camejo MI. Sperm lipid peroxidation and pro-inflammatory cytokines. Asian J Androl 2007;9:102-7.

78. Mazzoli S, Cai T, Addonisio P, et al. *Chlamydia trachomatis* infection Is related to poor semen quality in young prostatitis patients. Eur Urol 2009 May 27. [Epub ahead of print].

79. Monga M, Roberts JA. Spermagglutination by bacteria: Receptor-specific interactions. J Androl 1994;15:151-6.

80. Muciaccia B, Corallini S, Vicini E, et al. HIV-1 viral DNA is present in ejaculated abnormal spermatozoa of seropositive subjects. Hum Reprod 2007;22:2868-78.

81. Muciaccia B, Padula F, Gandini L, et al. HIV-1 chemokine co-receptor CCR5 is expressed on the surface of human spermatozoa. AIDS 2005;19:1424-6.

82. Munoz MG, Jeremias J, Witkin SS. The 60 kDa heat shock protein in human semen: relationship with antibodies to spermatozoa and *Chlamydia trachomatis*. Hum Reprod 1986;11:2600-1.

83. Nickel JC, Costerton JW, McLean RJC, et al. Bacterial biofilms: influence on the pathogenesis, diagnosis and treatment of urinary tract infections. J Antimicrob Chemother 1994;33 (Suppl. A):31-41.

84. Nickel JC, Downey J, Hunter D, et al. Prevalence of prostatitis-like symptoms in a population based study using the National Institutes of Health chronic prostatitis symptom index. J Urol 2001;165:842-5.

85. Nickel JC. Prostatitis: myths and realities. Urology 1998;51:362-6.

86. Nieschlag E, Behre H. Andrology. Male Reproductive Health and Dysfunction 1997; Springer, Berlin.

87. Nieschlag E, Behre HM. Andrology. Male reproductive health and dysfunction. 2000; 2nd edition, Springer, Berlin Heidelberg New York.

88. Nistal M, Paniagua R. Testicular and Epididymal Pathology. Thieme, Stuttgart, New York, 1984.

89. Ochsendorf F. Urethritis, Sexually Transmitted Diseases (STD), Acquired Immunodeficiency Syndrome (AIDS). In: Schill W-B, Comhaire F, Hargreave TB (Eds). Andrology for the Clinician. Springer, Heidelberg 2006.pp.327-38.

90. Pellati D, Mylonakis I, Bertoloni G, et al. Genital tract infections and infertility. Eur J Obstet Gynecol Reprod Biol 2008;140:3-11.

91. Pillai SK, Good B, Pond SK, et al. Semen-specific genetic characterics of human immunodeficiency virus type 1 env. J Virol 2005;79:1734-42.

92. Potts JM, Sharma R, Pasqualotto F, et al. Association of *Ureaplasma urealyticum* with abnormal reactive oxygen species levels and absence of leukocytospermia. J Urol 2000;163:1775-8.

93. Punab M, Loivukene K, Kermes K, et al. The limit of leucocytospermia from the microbiological viewpoint. Andrologia 2003;35:271-8.

94. Purvis K, Christiansen E. Infection in the male reproductive tract. Impact, diagnosis and treatment in relation to male infertility. Int J Androl 1993;16:1-13.

95. Reichart M, Kahane I, Bartoov B. *In vivo* and *in vitro* impairment of human and ram sperm nuclear chromatin integrity by sexually transmitted *Ureaplasma urealyticum* infection. Biol Reprod 2000;63:1041-8.

96. Roberts RO, Lieber MM, Bostwick DG, et al. A review of clinical and pathological prostatitis syndromes. Urology 1997;49:809-21.

97. Roberts RO, Lieber MM, Rhodes T, et al. Prevalence of a physician-assigned diagnosis of prostatitis: the Olmsted County Study of Urinary Symptoms and Health Status Among Men. Urology 1998;51:578-84.

98. Ruijs GJ, Kauer FM, Jager S, et al. Is serology of any use when searching for correlations between *Chlamydia trachomatis* infection and male infertility? Fertil Steril 1990;53:131-6.

99. Sanchez R, Villagran E, Concha M, et al. Ultrastructural analysis of the attachment sites of *Escherichia coli* to the human spermatozoon after *in vitro* migration through estrogenic cervical mucus. Int J Fert 1989;34:363-7.

100. Sanocka-Maciejewska D, Ciupinska M, Kurpisz M. Bacterial infection and semen quality. J Reprod Immunol 2005;67:51-6.

101. Schiefer HG, von Graevenitz A. Clinical Microbiology. In: Schill W-B, Comhaire F, Hargreave TB (Eds). Andrology for the Clinician. Springer, Heidelberg 2006,pp.401-7.

102. Schiefer HG. Microbiology of male urethroadnexitis: diagnostic procedures and criteria for aetiologic classification. Andrologia 1998;30(Suppl 1):7-13.

103. Schulz M, Sanchez R, Soto L, et al. Effect of *Escherichia coli* and its soluble factors on mitochondrial membrane potential, phosphatidylserine translocation, viability, and motility of human spermatozoa. Fertil Steril 2009 Mar 24. [Epub ahead of print].

104. Schuppe HC, Meinhardt A, Allam JP, et al. Chronic orchitis: a neglected cause of male infertility? Andrologia. 2008;40:84-91.

105. Schuppe HC, Meinhardt A. Immunology of the testis and the excurrent ducts. In: W-B, Comhaire F, Hargreave TB (Eds). Andrology for the Clinician. Schill, Springer, Heidelberg 2006,pp.292-300.

106. Sharma RK, Pasqualotto AE, Nelson DR, et al. Relationship between seminal white blood cell counts and oxidative stress in men treated at an infertility clinic. J Androl 2001;22:575-83.

107. Taylor-Robinson D. *Mycoplasma genitalium* – an update. Int J STD AIDS 2002;13:145-51.

108. Trum JW, Mol BWJ, Pannekoek Y, et al. Value of detecting leuko-cytospermia in the diagnosis of genital tract infection in subfertile men. Fertil Steril 1998;70:315-9.

109. Umapathy E, Simbini T, Chipata T, et al. Sperm characteristics and accessory sex gland functions in HIV-infected men. Arch Androl 2001;46:153-8.

110. Villegas H, Pinon M, Shor V, et al. Electron microscopy of *Chlamydia trachomatis* infection of the male genital tract. Arch Androl 1991;27:117-26.

111. Vordermark JS. Acute epididymitis: experience with 123 cases. Mil Med 1985;150:27-30.

112. Wang Y, Liang CL, Wu JQ, et al. Do *Ureaplasma urealyticum* infections in the genital tract affect semen quality? Asian J Androl 2006;8:562-8.

113. Weidner W, Colpi GM, Hargreave TB, et al. EAU guidelines on male infertility. Eur Urol 2002;42:313-22.

114. Weidner W, Krause W, Ludwig M. Relevance of male accessory gland infection for subsequent fertility with special focus on prostatitis. Hum Reprod Update 1999;5:421-32.

115. Wild S, Roglic G, Green A, et al. Global prevalence of diabetes: estimates for the year 2000 and projections for 2030. Diabetes Care 2004;27:1047-53.

116. Wolff H, Bezold G, Zebhauser, M, et al. Impact of clinically silent inflammation on male genital tract organs as reflected by biochemical markers in semen. J Androl 1991;12:331-4.

117. Wolff H. The biologic significance of white blood cells in semen. Fertil Steril 1995;63:1143-57.

118. World Health Organization. Global prevalence and incidence of selected sexually transmitted diseases: overview and estimates. World Health Organization: Geneva, Switzerland, 2001.

119. World Health Organization: WHO Laboratory Manual for the Examination and Processing of Human Semen, 5th edn. World Health Organization, 2010.

120. World Health Organization: World Health Organization Laboratory Manual for Examination of Human Semen. Cambridge University Press, Cambridge, UK; 1999.

17

Psychological Aspects of Male Infertility

Tolou Adetipe, Nabil Aziz

INTRODUCTION

It is estimated that in Western Europe one in six couples experience infertility. Male factor infertility is encountered in approximately 50 percent of these couples. Given these figures, a significant number of men will avail themselves to investigations and treatments for infertility and in the process experiencing, with their partners, the anxieties associated with the uncertainties of the underlying pathology and the outcome of their treatment. Thus, the burden of infertility is not only physical and financial but also encompasses negative impact on the psychological and emotional wellbeing of individuals.

INDUCERS OF PSYCHOLOGICAL STRESS

The inability to become a parent gives rise to diverse outcomes and manifestations depending on the values of the immediate society, cultures and religious beliefs. The ability to procreate after one's self is a basic expectation of life particularly in people of reproductive age who are so inclined. That ability has been highly valued by different societies, cultures and religious beliefs as it suggests continuation of the human life form, a preservation of ideas, identities, norms and nuances that form the society, and so to say 'maintenance of status quo'.

On a personal level, the inability to procreate can create an atmosphere of increased stress and potentially can lead to psychiatric distress depending on the individual's internal coping mechanisms in relation to one's personality and availability of supportive social systems. It can impact on self-imagery, marital relationships, financial well-being, and relationships with family, friends and the greater society. The uncertainty as to positive outcomes and the potential chronicity of intervention and treatment also lends more to the psychological distress experienced. Infertility has been described as a major life stressor for people who identify having children as an essential part of life.[1]

Psychological support for the infertile male is poorly understood and practiced by healthcare providers. Bearing in mind that this may be the first occasion for the male in question to be actively seeking medical care, this can create a great amount of stress and therefore should be handled sensitively and adequately. According to Lipshultz,[2] 'male infertility is a common problem which continues undiagnosed or untreated with men poorly informed of potential treatments, embarrassed to consult with medical professionals or concerned about being labelled as 'infertile'.'

There is a paucity of research in psychological needs of the infertile male. However, there is more research available on the female partner or on couples undergoing assisted reproduction therapy. This may partly account for the lack of knowledge about the psychological needs of the infertile male as noted by Lipshultz.[2] This deficiency may also be rooted into the presumption that the female partner as the 'carrier' is a more important part of the process or it could simply be due to existing literature biased in favor of the female because of her willingness to participate in research.

The Relationship Between Emotional Stress and Male Fecundity

The relationship between emotional stress and male fecundity is yet to be objectively determined leaving many questions unresolved and many hypotheses untested. These include:

1. Is stress an additional risk factor of infertility in infertile men?
2. Is stress the only cause or risk factor in men with idiopathic infertility?
3. Hence, is the infertile male more at risk of stress as compared to the potentially fertile male partner of an infertile couple?
4. Is the potential stress generated through the process of investigation or treatment a negative prognostic risk factor?

Different studies have identified links between sperm quality and sperm concentration, erectile dysfunction and psychological stress.[3,4] If it is to be assumed that these factors were the sole contributory factor in the male infertility, the hypotheses that stress can be the sole contributory reason for male infertility is proven in the absence of other relevant pathology. This is however difficult to ascertain as infertility is often as a result of many mitigating factors involving both the male and the female. In addition, there are contradictory views reported in literature.[5] Limitations to interpretation of data from these studies include the lack of consensus in defining and measuring stress objectively.

As a reflection of the lack of clarity, different studies have identified all the above hypotheses as being true. Evidence for a relationship between stress on one hand and erectile dysfunction and sperm quality was derived from the observation that there was a reduction in sperm quality following a natural disaster in Japan and Lebanese civil war[3,4] with a return to normal sperm parameters after a certain time period. These studies, however, did not prove if there were any improvements in the sperm's ability to fertilize. In spite of this it can be argued from these studies that stress is an additional risk factor inducing infertility. Further studies by Clarke et al (1999) and Pook et al (2004)[6,7] have demonstrated the presence of changes in sperm motility and concentration in response to stress. Having corrected for male age, partner age, race, religion, educational level, employment status, prior pregnancy, duration of infertility, and prior paternity Smith et al (2009) identified an independent association of poor sexual function and quality of life score in male partners of couples with infertility but more so in the infertile males.[8]

Collodel et al (2008) suggested that stress in itself was a causative risk factor for male infertility not simply an association as identified by earlier studies.[9] This was demonstrated following an improvement in spermatogenic process (reduced incidence of sex chromosomes disomy and diploidy) after psychological support in the form of CRM (Conveyer of modulating radiance therapy), which was given in order to reduce stress during the study period. This has the potential to change the present perception of stress being an additional risk factor to that of a significant solitary factor in cases of idiopathic male infertility.

One study attempted to answer the question of whether infertile males are more adversely affected compared to fertile male partners of an infertile couples. In this study, Boivin et al (1998) demonstrated that men treated with the ICSI (Intracytoplasmic sperm injection) technique for male factor infertility had more distress particularly in the active stages of the treatment as compared to men who underwent standard IVF.[10] There was a high level of anticipatory anxiety in the 2 days preceding oocyte retrieval treatment. This would favor the hypotheses that infertile men experience more stress as compared to other male partners of couples with infertility and potentially during the active stages of treatment.

The processes of diagnosis of the condition and the treatment have been identified as factors increasing psychological stress. This may increase the prevalent underlying emotional stress associated with the couple's infertility. The impact of stress at this point in time must not be under estimated as it may lend itself to be a negative prognostic factor. The male who is already anxious, suspicious and worried about the inability as a couple to conceive, becomes increasingly anxious on the realization that this may be solely due to him. Prolonged treatment has also been identified to cause stress. Associations between prolonged ongoing treatment or failed treatment have been linked with increased male partner's stress.[11,12] Time frames have ranged from greater than 12 to 17 months. This could have a deleterious impact on sperm quantity and quality. Due to the increased stress at these time periods, care needs to be taken to identify those at particular risk of mental health disease as links between high neuroticism scores in men with idiopathic male infertility and depressive or anxiety disorders have also been recently identified.[13]

Psychological Manifestations of Male Infertility

The common psychological manifestations of male infertility that may need psychological support include:

Anger and guilt are experienced if the reason for impaired fertility was perceived to be due to self-inflicted reasons such as poor sexual health history, poor general health or exposure to fertility impairing conditions. This may also be experienced if there is a chance of passing on some form of genetic condition or disease to the offspring (ICSI couple are commonly counseled regarding the risk of forthcoming offspring being infertile).[14]

Depression and anxiety can result from reduced self-esteem, loss of potency, isolation and a sense of role failure which is sometimes seen in infertile males. Anxiety also increases in relation to the prolonged period of the investigations and/or treatment. The lack of timely appropriate tests will only lead to a heightened state of anxiety.[15] Equally, psychological stress can be caused by the diagnosis of a new potential chronic disease with reproductive dilemmas. Anxiety and stress could also result from the uncertainty of the outcome of assisted reproduction technologies (ART).

Depression has been known to occur if previously used psychological coping strategies by the male included distancing, avoidance and denial. Mental health intervention should be made available once it is noted that the infertile male is exhibiting a fragile mental state particularly if undergoing severe depression. This is characterized by loss of ability to function in daily life, extreme anxiety and entertainment of suicidal thoughts.

Marital strain is seen when there is a poor sense of self-worth (as a degree of personal failure may prevail) or personal or sexual inadequacy. It also occurs during treatment regimes when different psychological coping strategies employed by the male are different from those employed by his partner. Marital disharmony with potential for separation or extramarital relationships have been known to occur at this time.

Psychosomatic disorders and organic problems secondary to infertility-induced stress could result from a sense of personal and sexual inadequacy. This has been identified as being the common psychological manifestations of the infertile male in particular. This could also lead to a state of sexual dysfunction due to loss of control and the inherent hopelessness of the situation.

▮ MILESTONES AND PIVOTAL PERIODS

There are milestones during the periods of diagnosis, investigation and treatment when there can be increased psychological stress and need. Health professionals need to be aware and be sensitive and responsive to psychological needs expressed consciously and otherwise. Members of the team at the ART center ranging from receptionists to the medical team in charge need to be situation-aware and increasingly supportive at these pivotal periods. These range from the periods of diagnostic tests, therapeutic interventions and other events following reproductive therapy such as the first pregnancy scan or early signs of unsuccessful treatment. Men who may require long-term treatment or those with chronic or longstanding conditions are at increased psychological distress and are in need for support.[15] Even men with a pre-existent or longstanding condition, e.g. Klinefelter's syndrome, who have a level of prior engagement with health services, the chronicity and questionable prognosis of their fertility are still at increased risk of stress and a reduction in quality of life. The second pivotal time in male infertility treatment where psychological support is needed is when decisions regarding risks and impact of the economic costs of fertility treatment have to be made. This includes effects of costs of treatment, caring for multiple gestations, the possibility of preterm delivery, and the risk of genetic transmission of infertility (as seen in ICSI) or genetic condition. Finally, psychological support is needed by those men who may need to utilize certain treatment types, i.e. donor backup, donated gametes or embryos where issues of disclosure or nondisclosure feature highly.[14]

PSYCHOLOGICAL SUPPORT

Less than 20 percent of couples needing ART techniques will request psychological support at some point during their treatment.[16] Given the above milestones and description of different psychological needs, support can be offered in a timely likewise or preventative manner. The importance of psychological support to the woman has been described by different studies[17,18] whilst only few considered the male partner leading to a lack of robust evidence regarding psychological support to the male. As identified earlier, the importance of psychological support can not be under-emphasized as it may potentially improve both the present infertility and enhance ART outcome. Parents achieving pregnancy through IVF experience more stress during pregnancy than 'normal fertile' parents was also demonstrated. Increased risk of first trimester miscarriage has been linked with depression in the males and reduced ability to handle stress.[19] A large meta-analysis of studies spanning 20 years had demonstrated that psychological interventions had improved some patients' chances of becoming pregnant despite the absence of clinical effects on mental health measures more so in those not receiving ART.[20]

Psychological help should be in place for the male or the couple to handle potential successes, failures and potential complications of ART and its outcomes including the possibility of passing on genetic disorders to his offsprings. The need to stop treatment, when and how should be discussed. In those men who will go on to have permanent infertility, the terms of success may have to be redefined or goals readjusted.[14]

Various forms of therapy have been described to be helpful. These range from educational programmes, infertility counseling, and behavioral therapy to cognative behavioral therapy where thinking errors such as emotional reasoning are identified and monitored through the use of a thought record and challenged and corrected through the use of several techniques which include re-direction, emotion-focused coping and problem-focused coping.

Behavioral coping strategies which include goal adjustment, positive reappraisal, and the use of emotional support have been described as effective by Kraaij et al.[21] Use of active-confronting coping (letting out feelings, asking for other peoples' advice and obtaining social support) has also been described as effective by Schmidt et al.[22] The male is encouraged to re-evaluate the target goal with the intention of setting more achievable goals through behavior conditioning.

These coping strategies may be taught at the onset of the program with additional meetings planned if further needs arise. Denial, distancing, and avoidance which have been reported as the commonly used coping strategies by males can only add to increased stress on the long-term particularly in those who may go onto have a long course of investigations and treatment or may have or develop chronic conditions. So, men should be advised to avoid using these coping mechanisms as much as possible.

With adequate coping mechanisms in place, there have been studies to demonstrate that there are psychosomatic benefits to be derived such as reduced risk of sperm sex chromosomes disomies and diploidies.[9] These coping mechanisms may also help infertile men with known etiologies to deal with stress arising in other areas of their lives and which can be an additional risk factor for poor sperm quality.

Links between high neuroticism scores in men with idiopathic male infertility and depressive or anxiety disorders, which have been recently identified, only reinforce the need for psychological support.[13]

In summary, the effective support mechanisms that have been described in literature include:

Positive Reappraisal Coping Intervention

This is a self-help coping intervention, which could be developed as a generic, simple tool to be used at any time to help the male to cope with the stress of investigations and treatment. It manages rumination and intrusive thoughts.[23] It could be cheap to administer thereby cutting down on costs of implementation for the ART center.

Conveyer of Modulating Radiance Therapy

This form of light therapy has been found to be useful in improving spermatogenesis. Neuropsychomotor function is improved through short sessions involving the use of a radioelectric conveyer apparatus. It follows on the success of the use of light to treat seasonal affective disorder.

Cognitive coping strategies such as appraisal -oriented and active-coping methods have been suggested as being useful.[24] The thought processes behind any negative attitudes are identified and challenged. Thereafter he is encouraged to participate in activities that reinforce positive beliefs or attitudes. It can be administered as a computerized based system in order to reduce cost. User compliance is necessary as there is need for active patient participation for success to be achieved.

Pharmacotherapy has been used traditionally for treatment of erectile dysfunction. Certain medications such as sildenafil has been found to be useful for erectile dysfunction which may be stress related.

It has been suggested that the use of root powder of Witharia somnifera improves sperm quality in stress-related male infertility because of an increased serum concentration of anti-oxidants.[25] Acupuncture, reflexology, kinesiology, homeopathy, and naturopathy have been tried in certain centers. A recent study found no benefits with a reduction in pregnancy rates after the use of Complimentary and alternative medicine in the 1st 12 months.[26] Therefore, due to controversies involved with complimentary and alternative medicine caution is advised.

To offer the right intervention or treatment, an appropriate strategy has to be developed. Choosing the right strategy is partly dependant on the individual's personality type, degree of neuroticism, stage of treatment amongst other factors. Various tools exist to identify personality type and likelihood of the male developing depression. The nine-field assessment which has been found useful in the field of psychosomatic medicine may also be helpful in identifying stress type and potential beneficial therapies.[27] Cognitive coping strategies may be assessed by the use of cognitive emotion regulation questionnaire, which is a multidimensional questionnaire that identifies the individual's thoughts following a negative experience. The questionnaire, developed by Garnefski and Kraaij,[24] includes 36 items and is easy to administer. The ways of coping questionnaire (revised) was initially devised by Folkman and Lazarus to identify the coping processes (thoughts and acts) in a particular stressful situation rather than coping styles employed by individuals across the board.[21,22] It identifies the type of coping mechanism that includes confrontive, self-controling, escape-avoidance, seeking social support, and positive reappraisal. Marital well-being and adjustment to the threat of infertility should also be assessed. This can be done by a variety of tests one of which is Locke-Wallace marital adjustment test.

Signposting to self-help or support groups may be useful for those not ready to engage with the formal support structure available. This gives the male opportunities to liaise with available services at an acceptable pace of engagement.

SERVICE PROVISION

Developing a service geared in particular to providing psychological support to these men will be dependant on cost effectiveness, motivation of the ART center, involvement of the target group and financial implications. Given that most potential users of this service will be in full-time employment, the additional burden (temporal and financial) of attending more clinic visits simply for psychological support may not be particularly appealing. It also has to attract the men in question. It is known that women rather than men seek psychological counseling.[28] Principal reasons identified for men seeking help, were partner dissatisfaction, sexuality problems and female partner's depressive condition.

Hence, provision of a simple user-friendly tool for use by low to medium at-risk men identified by psychological profiling should be made available. This is important because a good percentage of men will fall into this category initially. In order to reduce cost and time implications, this could be done through the use of telephones rather than face-to-face counseling.[29]

The importance of provision of psychological support for the infertile male is being increasingly recognised. However, the uptake of this service may be poor initially but with increasing awareness of need and of service availability, the uptake will increase proving beneficial to patients and the ART centers alike. Of interest, it has been demonstrated that patients' awareness of the availability of psychosocial services was reassuring to the couple despite lack of use.[16]

Offer of support has traditionally been to the couple with emphasis on the female partner usually by a counsellor. Whether additional consultations for the male partner alone in order to fully identify needs and provide solutions are an extension of fertility services needs further clarification. The caregiver may also need specialized knowledge in order to adequately deal with concerns. This enables the man to put down the 'mask' he may have had to put on in order to look in control of the situation and reinforce confidence in his partner. The clinical team should be better equipped to understand the emotional and psychological stress involved and be able to provide support sensitively. In our view, the clinical team's attention should not be solely to achieve a 'live birth' or 'child' but should exercise care to discuss all acceptable routes of ART regardless of outcome. The team should be able to support and prepare patients for both successes and failures of the ART therapy. Time and space should be available to allow men express themselves at their own pace. This should enhance patients' response to medical advice as they feel better understood by the entire team.

In summary, infertility can create a reduction in quality of life whilst impacting self-esteem, social standing in the community and relationship with others. Due to the chronic nature of some etiologies, the inherent coping mechanisms in place may be inadequate. Psychological help should be in place for the male or couple to handle potential successes, failures and potential complications of assisted reproductive techniques and outcomes, the possibility of passing on genetic disorders to his offsprings. The need to stop treatment when and how; should be discussed. In those who will go on to have definitive infertility, success may have to be redefined or goals readjusted. Little is known about the psychologies of those men who have definitive causes of infertility and therefore needs more research.

CONCLUSION

Psychological support provided to the infertile male will enable him cope with his condition, potential chronicity of underlying etiology. It also protects and maybe enhance his relationship with spouse and the larger social community, preparing him for potential complications and the risk of passing on potential genetic medical conditions to his biological off-springs while potentially improving outcomes of his fertility treatment, psychological support should have a positive impact on the personal quality of life and improving overall patient satisfaction.

REFERENCES

1. Campagne DM. Should fertilization treatment start with reducing stress? Hum Reprod 2006;21:1651-8.
2. Lipshultz L. Addressing male reproductive issues: the Reproductive Health Council of the American Foundation for Urologic disease. Family Building (Resolve) 2003;3(1):21.

3. Abu-Musa AA, Nassar AH, Hannoun AB, Usta IM. Effect of the Lebanese civil war on sperm parameters. Fertil Steril 2007;88:1579-82.

4. Fukuda M, Fukuda K, Shimizu T, Yomura W, Shimizu S. Kobe earthquake and reduced sperm motility. Hum Reprod 1996;11:1244-6.

5. Said MT. Emotional stress and male infertility. Indian J Med Res 2008;128:228-30.

6. Clarke RN, Klock SC, Geoghegan A, Travossos DE. Relationship between psychological stress and semen quality among *in-vitro* fertilization patients. Hum Reprod 1999;14:753-8.

7. Pook M, Tuschen-Caffier B, Krause W. Infertility a risk factor for impaired male infertility? Hum Reprod 2004;19:954-9.

8. Smith JF, et al. Sexual Marital and Social impact of a man's perceived infertility diagnosis. J Sex Med 2009;6:2505-15.

9. Collodel G, Moretti E, Fontani V, et al. Effect of emotional stress on sperm quality. Indian J Med Res 2008;128:254-61.

10. Boivin J, Shoog-Svanberg A, Andersson L, Hjelmstedt A, Bergh T, Collins A. Distresss levels in men undergoing intracytoplasmic sperm injection versus *in-vitro* fertilization. Hum Reprod 1998; 13:1403-6.

11. Pook M, Krause W. The impact of treatment experiences on the course of infertility distress in male patients. Hum Reprod 2005;20:825-8.

12. Peronace LA, Boivin J, Schmidt L. Patterns of suffering and social interactions in infertile men: 12 months after unsuccessful treatment. J of Psychosom Obstet and Gynaecol 2007;28:104-14.

13. Volgsten H, Ekselius L, Poroma IS, Svanberg AS. Personality traits associated with depressive and anxiety disorders in fertile women and men undergoing *in vitro* fertilization treatment. Acta Obstet Gynecol Scand 2010;89:27-34.

14. Applegarth LD. Psychological issues of infertility and assisted reproductive technology Chapt 30 Infertility in the a male, 4th edn Larry I Lipshultz, Stuart S. Howards and Craig S Niederberger Cambridge University Press, 2009.

15. Bhasin S. Approach to the infertile man. J Clin Endocrinol Meta 2007;6:1995-2004.

16. Boivin J, Scanlon L, Walker SM. Why are infertile couples not using psychosocial counseling? Hum Reprod 1999;14:1384-91.

17. Lund R, Sejbaek CS, Christensen U, Schmidt L. The impact of social relations on the incidence of depressive symptoms among infertile men and women. Hum Reprod 2009;24:2810-20.

18. Wischmann T, Scherg H, Strowitzki Th, Verres R. Psychosocial characteristics of women and men attending infertility counselling. Hum Reprod 2009;24:378-85.

19. Zorn B, Auger J, Velikonja V, Kolbezen M, Meden-Vrtovec H. Psychological factors in male partners of infertile couple: relationship with semen quality and early miscarriage. Int J Androl 2008;6:557-64.

20. Hammerli K, Znoj H, Barth J. The efficacy of psychological interventions for infertile patients: a meta-analysis examining mental health and pregnancy rate. Hum Reprod Update 2009;15:279-95.

21. Kraaij V, Garnefski N, Schroevers MJ. Coping, Goal Adjustment, Positive and Negative Affect in Definitive Infertility. J Health Psychol 2009;14:18-26.

22. Schmidt L. Social and psychological consequences of infertility and assisted reproduction – what are the research priorities? Hum Fertil 2009;12:14-20.

23. Lancastle D, Boivin J. A feasibility study of a brief coping intervention (PCRI) for the waiting period before a pregnancy test during fertility treatment. Hum Reprod 2008;23:2299-307.

24. Kraaij V, Garnefski N, Vlietstra A. Cognitive coping and depressive symptoms in definitive infertility: a prospective study. J Psychom Obstet and Gynaecol 2008;29:9-16.

25. Mahdi AA, et al. Withania somnifera improves semen quality in stress-related male fertility. Evid based Complement Alternat Med, 2009.

26. Boivin J, Schmidt L. Use of complementary and alternative medicines associated with a 30% lower ongoing pregnancy/ live birth rate during 12 months of fertility treatment. Hum Reprod 2009;24:1626-31.

27. Lal M. Psychomatic approaches to obstetrics, gynecology and andrology- a review. J Obstet Gynaecol 2009;29:1-12.

28. Wischmann T, Scherg H, Strowitzki T, Verres R. Psychosocial characteristics of women and men attending infertility counseling. Hum Reprod 2009;24:378-85.

29. Wischmann T. Implications of psychosocial support in infertility-a critical appraisal. J Psychosom Obstet Gynaecol 2008;29:83-90.

18

Surgical Management of Genital Tract Obstruction

Edmund Y Ko, Edmund Sabanegh

■ INTRODUCTION

Male factor infertility is present in 50 percent of infertile couples.[1] Up to 12 percent of men with primary infertility will have genital duct obstruction, a condition which is potentially reversible with surgical reconstruction.[2] Etiologies include congenital, inflammatory, traumatic, iatrogenic, and idiopathic obstruction.

Vasectomy is one of the most common iatrogenic causes of genital trace obstruction. Approximately half a million vasectomies are performed each year making it one of the most commonly performed urologic procedures in the United States.[3] At least 5 percent of males will ultimately desire to undergo vasectomy reversal for various reasons.[4]

This chapter will focus on the surgical approaches to male genital tract obstruction along with their outcomes. We will briefly discuss anatomy, physiology, and the pathology of obstruction.

■ ANATOMY AND PHYSIOLOGY OF THE GENITAL TRACT

A thorough knowledge of anatomy and physiology of the male genital tract is crucial to understanding the different procedures required to restore patency to an obstructed ductal system.

The average testis in a healthy male measures 15–25 mL in volume and 4.5–5.0 centimeters in longitudinal length.[5] The testicular parenchyma is surrounded by a dense capsule made up of three layers (outer to inner):
1. Visceral tunica vaginalis
2. Tunica albuginea
3. Tunica vasculosa.

Septae divide each testis into compartments containing 600–1200 highly coiled seminiferous tubules that span approximately 250 meters when fully stretched out.[6]

The testes provide the important functions of spermatogenesis and hormone production. Spermatogenesis occurs in the seminiferous tubules of the testes taking approximately 64 days to complete.[7] Sertoli cells support spermatogenesis under the stimulation of follicle stimulating hormone (FSH) and influence of Leydig cell testosterone, which is stimulated by luteinizing hormone (LH). Tight junctions between the Sertoli cells form the blood-testis barrier creating an immunologically privileged location within the testis.

Spermatogenesis starts in the basal compartment and progresses towards the adluminal compartment in the seminiferous tubules. Spermatogonia (2n = 46 chromosomes) undergo mitosis and become spermatocytes (2n) near the periphery of the seminiferous tubules. After undergoing meiosis, the spermatocytes become spermatids (1n = 23 chromosomes). The spermatids undergo spermiogenesis and become spermatozoa (1n). The spermatozoa are released into the lumen of the seminiferous tubules, pass through the rete testis, efferent ductules, and enter into the proximal epididymal tubules. An estimated 70 million spermatozoa are produced daily.[8]

The epididymis is a single 3 meter convoluted thin walled tubule that is wound together forming a 4–5 centimeter structure located posterolateral to each testicle. The spermatozoa mature as they travel from the caput to the cauda epididymis. A thick muscular wall delineating the proximal vas deferens invests the tubule at the termination of the cauda epididymis.

The epididymis provides four important functions for spermatozoa:
1. Maturation
2. Transport
3. Concentration
4. Storage

Although it is a critical process, the exact mechanism by which maturation occurs is unknown. Progressive fertilizing capacity and motility increase dramatically from sperm harvested from the distal versus the proximal epididymis.[9-12] Fertility chances also increase with longer transit lengths through the epididymis after vasoepididymostomy. The average transit time through the human epididymis is 2–6 days.[13] The cauda epididymis functions as a sperm storage area and does not have a large impact on sperm development.

Sympathetic nervous system mediated smooth muscle contractions propel sperm toward the ampulla of the vas. After leaving the testicle, the vas deferens travels with the spermatic cord along the inguinal canal, posterior to the testicular vessels, and through the external and internal inguinal rings. Once the vas deferens enters the retroperitoneum, it diverges medially away from the testicular vessels and crosses anterior to the ureter and posterior to the medial umbilical ligament (inferior epigastric artery) toward the prostate. It dilates to become the ampulla and joins the seminal vesicle (SV) in the retrovesical space. The

if additional mobilization of the distal vas deferens is necessary. These incisions will measure one to two centimeters in length to allow the delivery of the proximal and distal segments for a VV. A longer incision may be utilized to deliver the testicle into the operative field if there is a particularly long vasal defect or a VE is required.

The vas, along with its vascular pedicle, is dissected free from surrounding adventitia. Meticulous hemostasis is maintained with microsurgical bipolar electrocautery or disposable battery-operated thermal cautery unit to minimize injury to the surrounding delicate structures. After the vasa have been adequately mobilized proximal and distal to the site of obstruction, the vascular pedicle is ligated using 6-0 nylon suture approximately 1 mm from the site of planned vasal transsection. The length of mobilized vas should be adequate to allow the freshly cut ends to overlap each other to ensure a tension free anastomosis. A 6-0 nylon holding suture is placed 2 cm from the planned site of transsection into the periadventitial tissue of each vasal end to maintain control of each structure (**Fig. 18.1**). Alternatively, some surgeons prefer using vas clamps to maintain control of the vasa.

The vas is then transected at the site of normal healthy tissue to avoid early post-operative luminal stenosis. This can be performed with microscope magnification or through the groove of nerve holding forceps (ASSI.NHF-2.5, Accurate Surgical and Scientific Instruments, Westbury, NY) to ensure a straight cut end (**Fig. 18.2**). After the vas has been transected, the cut ends are inspected and gently dilated with the tips of fine microsurgical forceps. Dilation can be performed with lacrimal duct probes but these instruments can tear and traumatize the delicate vas lumen.

Fluid is expressed from the proximal vas and collected onto a glass slide. Light microscopy is performed to determine the presence of viable whole sperm or sperm fragments. The presence of sperm is associated with the best prognosis for future fertility.[32] Copious clear fluid without any spermatozoa also points toward a good outcome.[30] VV can be performed if these findings are present. If the fluid is thick, pasty, and lacks the presence of sperm, VE should be highly considered.

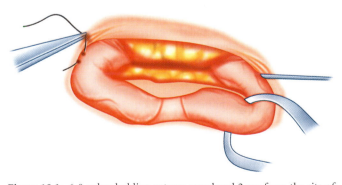

Figure 18.1: 6-0 nylon holding sutures are placed 2 cm from the site of planned vasovasostomy to keep the proximal and distal ends of the vas deferens in the operative field

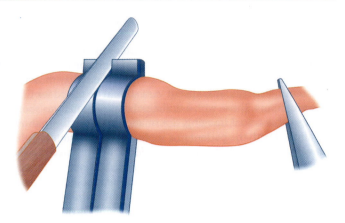

Figure 18.2: A fresh scalpel is used to transect the distal end of the vas deferens at a healthy site through the groove of a nerve holding forceps to ensure a straight cut end

■ VASOVASOSTOMY

The two most commonly accepted techniques for VV are:
1. Modified 1-layer.
2. Multilayer anastomosis.

When performed by an experienced surgeon, both of these techniques have equivalent outcomes with regard to patency and pregnancy rates.[30] The one-layer technique is useful for performing the anastomosis in the straight portion of the vasa when there is minimal size discrepancy between the proximal and distal ends. Alternatively, the multilayer technique assures great precision in luminal approximation, especially when there is a significant size discrepancy between the luminal diameters.

Surgical Technique

Modified One-layer Vasovasostomy

The one-layer VV was initially described and popularized by Schmidt in 1978 and later modified.[33] Some surgeons prefer this method over the multilayer technique because it is simpler, uses fewer sutures, and requires less microsurgical skill. It can be performed with either loupe or microscope magnification.

First, a full-thickness 9-0 or 10-0 nylon suture is placed through the posterior wall (6-o'clock) of the vas deferens. On the proximal end, the suture sequentially passes through the serosa, muscularis, and the edge of the mucosa. The reverse is performed on the distal end. It is important to incorporate only a small mucosal edge into the suture to prevent luminal compression and obstruction. Two additional full-thickness sutures are then placed on either side of the first suture at 4- and 8-o'clock to reapproximate the posterior wall of the vas deferens (**Fig. 18.3**). Three full-thickness sutures are placed at the 10- 12-, and 2-o'clock positions to reapproximate the anterior wall of the vas deferens (**Fig. 18.4**). The sutures are tied securely to approximate the tissue. Additional 9-0 nylon sutures are then placed to reapproximate the muscularis and adventitia between the previously tied sutures to complete the anastomosis (**Fig. 18.5**).

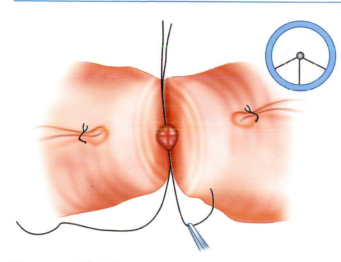

Figure 18.3: Full thickness nylon sutures are passed through the posterior wall of the vas deferens at the 4-, 6-, and 8-o'clock positions

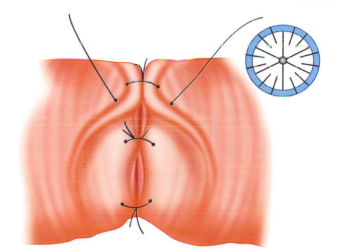

Figure 18.5: Additional sutures are placed in the muscularis and adventitia between the previously placed full thickness sutures to complete the anastomosis

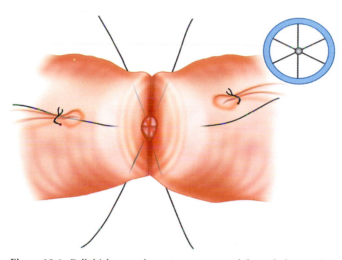

Figure 18.4: Full thickness nylon sutures are passed through the anterior wall of the vas deferens at the 10-, 12-, and 2-o'clock positions

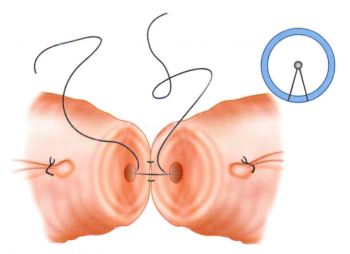

Figure 18.6: After the anastomosis is stabilized with two posterior nylon sutures, a double-armed 10-0 nylon suture is passed through the mucosa of the vas deferens the 6-o'clock location

Multilayer Vasovasostomy

Silber initially described the multilayer VV as a two-layer procedure in 1976 and subsequently modified, popularized, and refined into the multilayer technique in 1977.[34,35] Three separate layers are reapproximated:

- Luminal
- Seromuscular
- Periadventitial.

An operating microscope is required to ensure the precise placement of sutures and should be performed by an appropriately trained surgeon.

The two ends of the vas are exposed and prepared as previously described. Two 9-0 nylon sutures are placed at the 5- and

7-o'clock location through the seromuscular layers of the proximal and distal vasal ends to stabilize the anastomosis. The first luminal suture is then passed and tied at the 6-o'clock location inside to out through the mucosal edges of each vasal end with a double-armed 10-0 nylon suture (**Fig. 18.6**). The next two sutures are placed adjacent to the posterior suture at the 5- and 7-o'clock positions and tied. Three to five additional luminal sutures are passed circumferentially at equally spaced distances (1-, 3-, 9-, 11-, 12-o'clock) and left untied until all of the sutures have been placed (**Fig. 18.7**). Sutures should be placed at equally spaced intervals to carefully align the dilated proximal vas lumen to the smaller distal vas lumen. This prevents mucosal bunching, which can interfere with mucosal apposition and cause luminal obstruction.

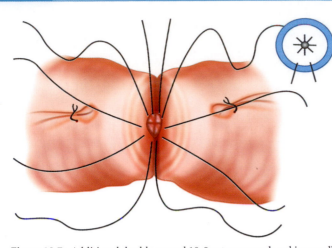

Figure 18.7: Additional double-armed 10-0 sutures are placed in equally spaced intervals around the mucosa to carefully align the proximal and distal vasal lumen

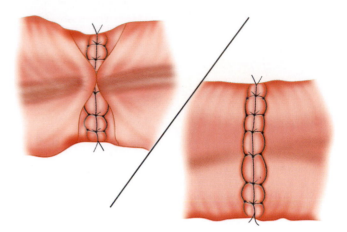

Figure 18.9: Reapproximation of periadventitial (third) layer

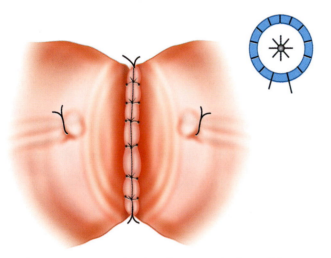

Figure 18.8: Reapproximation of seromuscular (second) layer

The seromuscular (second) layer is then reapproximated with 9-0 nylon at equally spaced intervals around the anastomosis (9-, 3-, 11-, 1-, and 12-o'clock) (**Fig. 18.8**). The periadventitial (third) layer is then reapproximated over the muscularis layer with interrupted 9-0 sutures to complete the anastomosis (**Fig. 18.9**).

Complex Vasal Reconstruction

Special reconstructive approaches are required if the obstruction point is outside of the scrotum or when a solitary functioning testis has an absent or inoperable ductal system in conjunction with a poorly functioning contralateral testis with normal ductal anatomy.

Obstruction of the extrascrotal vas deferens is most commonly caused by vasal injury sustained during pediatric inguinal hernia

repairs.[36] Up to 27 percent of subfertile males with a prior childhood history of inguinal hernia repair have unilateral iatrogenic vasal obstruction.[37] The vas can also be injured during retroperitoneal surgeries (i.e. undescended intra-abdominal testis). Pediatric iatrogenic vas deferens injuries are usually diagnosed years later presenting as infertility at reproductive age. Inguinal vasal obstruction should be suspected in any infertile male with prior history of childhood inguinal hernia repair.

There are also reports of vasal obstruction attributed to laparoscopic and open hernia repairs with mesh in adults.[38,39] Synthetic mesh placed during inguinal hernia repair stimulates an inflammatory response that can compromise the vasal lumen resulting in luminal narrowing or complete obstruction.[40,41] If the contralateral testis is unobstructed and functioning normally a patient may have normal fertility and never be diagnosed with unilateral vasal obstruction.

Physical examination of these patients may demonstrate a normally sized testis, full and firm epididymis, and a thickened vas deferens with a prominent convoluted portion on the ipsilateral side. Vasography can confirm the diagnosis, demonstrating a dilated vas deferens with contrast material reaching to and stopping at the inguinal canal near the internal ring or in the retroperitoneum. Patients with bilateral vasal obstruction or a contralateral hypofunctioning testis are candidates for inguinal or retroperitoneal vasal repair. If primary reanastomosis cannot be performed due to severe damage to or absence of the vas, a crossover procedure can be considered.

Testis biopsy is indicated to confirm active spermatogenesis in a normally sized testicle at the time of surgical correction. A high inguinal incision parallel to the inguinal ligament at the level of the internal ring will allow for adequate exposure of the inguinal vas deferens and isolation of the testicular (proximal) segment. A thin fibrous strip of scar tissue may connect the testicular and abdominal (distal) vasal segments in the absence of mesh or if the vas was injured during a pediatric hernia repair (**Fig. 18.10**). Care is taken to avoid avulsing this thin strip, which

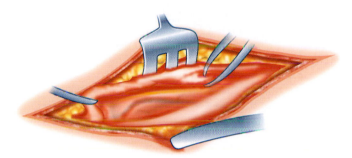

Figure 18.10: Thin fibrous strip connecting proximal to distal end of inguinal vas deferens

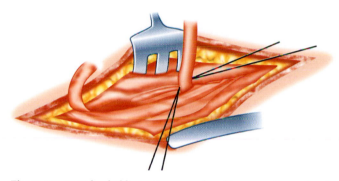

Figure 18.11: Nylon holding sutures are placed to secure the vasal ends for reanastomosis

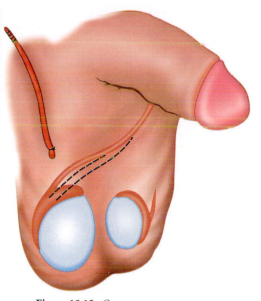

Figure 18.12: Crossover vasovasostomy

may make finding the proximal end more difficult. The distal segment of the vas is usually found just below the level of the internal inguinal ring.

The scar tissue is excised and the ends are cut back to healthy vasal tissue. If mesh was used for the previous hernia repair, the vas deferens may be densely adhered to the floor of the inguinal canal or encased in a fibrotic mass of tissue. Separation from the inflammatory mass may risk injury to the vas deferens. It may be necessary to extend the incision, enter the retroperitoneum, and free the vas deferens away from the mesh. 6-0 stay sutures are placed to secure the vasal ends at the skin level for reanastomosis (**Fig. 18.11**). Expressed fluid is examined microscopically as previously described. However, the patient must understand that delayed VE may be required 3–6 months postoperatively if azoospermia persists.

Inguinal vasovasostomies are complicated by the dense fibrotic reaction encasing the vas deferens making adequate mobilization difficult. Laparoscopy has been used to mobilize additional vasal length for a tension free inguinal anastomosis.[42] Despite the complicated nature of this approach, inguinal reconstructions have comparable patency and pregnancy rates to scrotal vasovasostomies.[43]

A crossover VV can be considered in patients whose ipsilateral vas is damaged beyond repair or if they have a normal contralateral vas deferens but the associated testicle is atrophic, a situation that occurs in 6 percent of azoospermic patients.[44]

The abdominal end of the normal vas deferens from the atrophic testis is mobilized with its vascular pedicle and brought through an opening in the scrotal raphe to be anastomosed to the testicular vas deferens or epididymis of the normal contralateral testicle (**Fig. 18.12**). Different series in the literature report moderate success rates with this technique.[45,46] An early report on crossover vasoepididymostomies demonstrated mean sperm concentrations to be greater than 15 million/mL in 89 percent of patients.[47]

Repeat VV patients present a special challenge to the surgeon. They oftentimes have a marked desmoplastic reaction around the vasa, a shorter usable length from prior resection and reconstruction, as well as a higher likelihood of secondary epididymal obstruction. Three to four additional centimeters can be obtained by extending the vertical scrotal incision up to the lower inguinal region to dissect the vas up to the inguinal canal. In patients undergoing repeat vasovasostomies, up to 73 percent require a VE on at least one side when compared to those undergoing their first procedure.[19,30]

Vasovasostomy Outcomes

The VV success rates can be influenced by perioperative factors including surgeon experience, time of obstruction, prior surgeries, intraoperative findings, and partner age. Outcomes can be defined with patency rates or pregnancy rates.

Time of obstruction is an important factor that has a direct effect on surgical success with increased time of obstruction resulting in decreasing surgical success[30,48] (**Table 18.1**).

Prior history of failed reversal was found to have an insignificant impact on the outcomes of repeat procedures. Patency as well as pregnancy rates were comparable to initial reversal rates when accounting for total time of obstruction.[19]

Table 18.1: Vasovasostomy outcomes[30]

Obstructive interval (years)	Patency rates (%)	Pregnancy rates (%)
< 3	97	76
3-8	88	53
9-14	79	44
≥ 14	71	30

Fluid expressed from the vas deferens also impacts postoperative outcome 94 percent of patients with clear fluid and motile sperm expressed from the proximal vas deferens had return of sperm on their ejaculate on postoperative semen analysis. This is compared to 60 percent of patients without the presence of sperm in the fluid.[30] In intraoperative samples without the presence of sperm, the best outcomes were seen in those with abundant clear fluid.

Female partner age is an important nonsurgical factor that impacts pregnancy outcomes after reversal. In partners under 30 years old, the pregnancy rate has been reported to be 64 percent, dropping precipitously to 28 percent in females over 40 years old.[26] For women under 35 years of age, the pregnancy rates are better in VV when compared to intracytoplasmic sperm injection (ICSI). After the age of,[35] the pregnancy success rates decline for both VV and ICSI. However, studies have demonstrated good pregnancy rates in female partners over 35 years of age.[49,50]

Reported surgical outcomes are difficult to compare across institutions due to the lack of defined obstructive intervals, variations in the surgical pathways to choosing VV versus VE, and the existence of female factor infertility. Despite these factors, microsurgical VV (single- or multi-layer technique) has demonstrated superior results when compared to surgical reconstruction performed without the aid of magnification.[30,48,51] Overall patency rates range from 38–96 percent with pregnancy rates ranging from 19–76 percent.[52]

◼ VASOEPIDIDYMOSTOMY

If sperm is found on testicular biopsy and the vas deferens is patent, the obstruction is located between the two structures. Obstruction proximal to the vas deferens occurs most commonly in the epididymis and is usually correctable with surgery. Rarely, obstruction will occur at the rete testis or the efferent ducts, otherwise known as "empty epididymis syndrome", a situation that is usually not amenable to surgical reconstruction.[53] VE should be considered if the fluid expressed from the proximal vas is thick, pasty, and lacks the presence of sperm.

Surgical Technique

The testicle is delivered into the operative field by extending the vertical incision. The epididymis is examined carefully under microscopic magnification. The point of obstruction is identified by the dramatic transition from flat to distended tubules.

A blue-brown lipofuschin discoloration may demarcate the area of obstruction beneath the epididymal tunic. This represents an area of sperm breakdown and extravasation.

A one-centimeter window is made in the epididymal tunic with curved microscissors allowing examination of multiple epididymal tubules. The fluid within the epididymal tubule is examined to confirm the area of obstruction. Exploration is carried out in a systematic manner starting at the cauda and moving towards the caput. Examination is continued until morphologically normal motile or non-motile sperm are identified. A single dilated loop is then isolated from the rest of the tubules and opened depending on the anastomotic technique.

End-to-end Vasoepididymostomy

The first true microsurgical approach to end-to-end vasoepididymal reconstruction was described in the 1970's.[54] The end of the epididymis is transected proximal to the obstruction point. This is identified by the free flow of sperm from a single epididymal tubule. The vasoepididymal anastomosis is started by placing 9-0 nylon sutures in the seromuscular layer of the distal cut end of the vas deferens and the epididymal tunica at 5- and 7-o'clock locations to stabilize the posterior anastomosis (**Fig. 18.13**). Four double-armed 10-0 nylon sutures are then placed in 4 quadrants to approximate the mucosal edges of the two structures without tying the sutures until all sutures have been positioned. Interrupted 9-0 nylon sutures are then placed to complete the closure between the vasal seromuscular and epididymal tunical layers.

End-to-side Vasoepididymostomy

The end-to-side VE offers advantages over the end-to-end reconstruction include reduced bleeding since resection of the epididymis is not required and more precise identification of the proximal tubular lumen since multiple loops are not cut

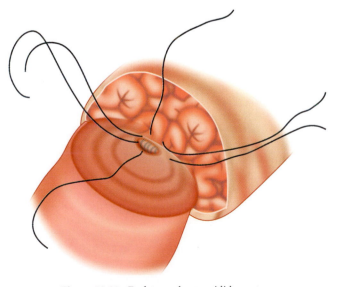

Figure 18.13: End-to-end vasoepididymostomy

with this approach.[55,56] After identifying a patent epididymal tubule, a microknife is employed to make a one-millimeter incision on the side of the tubule. The fluid is then examined under light microscopy to confirm the presence of sperm. A 10-0 nylon suture is placed outside-in on the lateral cut mucosal edge of the epididymal tubule as an identification suture to facilitate the anastomosis. 9-0 nylon suture is then placed at the 5- and 7-o'clock location to secure and stabilize the vasal seromuscular layer to the epididymal tunic. Three to four 10-0 nylon sutures are then placed in the corresponding quadrants between the epididymal and vasal mucosal edges (**Fig. 18.14**). 9-0 nylon sutures are placed in the vasal seromuscular and epididymal tunical layers as previously described. Additional 9-0 nylon sutures are placed away from the anastomotic site to anchor the vas deferens to the parietal layer of the tunica vaginalis and to facilitate a tension free anastomosis.

End-to-side Intussusception Vasoepididymostomy

Intussusception VE is the latest major technical modification to the end-to-side approach, first described by Berger in the 1990's, with recent technical updates involving triangular suture placement and tubular intussusception or tubular invagination.[57-59] The major difference from the originally described end-to-side technique is the placement of sutures prior to opening the lumen of the epididymal tubule and the loop is drawn into the end of the vasal lumen with the previously placed sutures rather than approximated to it. This technique simplifies and minimizes microsuture placement.

A small window is opened in the epididymal tunic and dilated tubules are identified as previously described. Once an appropriate tubule is identified, it is dissected free from the surrounding tissue to allow maximal mobility for intussusception

into the vasal segment. The distal end of the vas deferens is secured to the epididymal tunic with 9-0 nylon at the 5- and 7-o'clock positions. Three double-armed 10-0 nylon sutures are placed in a triangular configuration into the tissue around the site of planned entry into the dilated epididymal tubule (**Fig. 18.15**). The tubule is opened between the sutures and once the presence of sperm is confirmed, the sutures are passed inside-out through corresponding locations on the distal vasal segment and tied (**Fig. 18.16**), thereby invaginating the epididymal loop into the vasal lumen (**Fig. 18.17**). Additional 9-0 nylon sutures are then

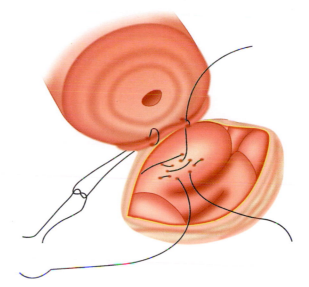

Figure 18.15: End-to-side intussuscepted vasoepididymostomy. Triangular placement of nylon sutures in a single epididymal tubule

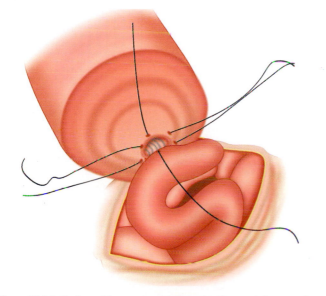

Figure 18.14: End-to-side anastomosis between the vas deferens and a single epididymal tubule

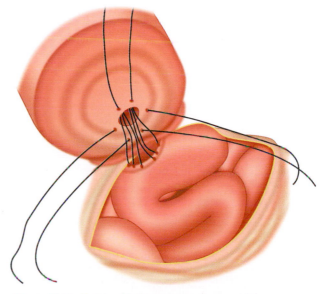

Figure 18.16: End-to-side intussuscepted vasoepididymostomy. Sutures are passed through the corresponding locations on the vas deferens

placed to secure the vasal seromuscular layer to the epididymal tunic and anchor the anastomosis as previously described.

Vasoepididymostomy Outcomes

There are many factors that can affect VE outcomes, many of which are similar to VV outcomes. In addition, the level of epididymal obstruction is also a factor. While VVs may demonstrate patency several weeks after surgery, VE patients may not have any sperm in the ejaculate until 3–6 months postoperatively and even longer in some cases. VEs are therefore not considered failures until at least 12 months after the postoperative period.[60,61] Overall patency outcomes have been reported to be between 39–92 percent, with pregnancy outcomes ranging from 4–56 percent[52,62-64] (**Table 18.2**).

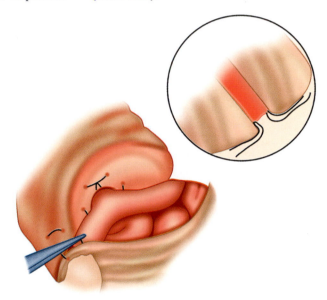

Figure 18.17: Completed end-to-side intussuscepted vasoepididymostomy

SURGICAL MANAGEMENT OF EJACULATORY DUCT OBSTRUCTION

There are several treatment options available for the treatment of ejaculatory duct obstruction. For men with partial obstruction and oligospermia, intrauterine insemination or *in vitro* fertilization (IVF) can be attempted depending on the semen analysis. For those with complete obstruction, epididymal or testicular sperm extraction combined with IVF techniques can be employed.

Transurethral resection of the ejaculatory ducts (TURED) may restore patency. With the patient in lithotomy position under anesthesia, vasography or TRUS-guided seminal vesiculography can be carried out with methylene blue mixed with contrast. Resection is carried out transurethrally with a standard 24 French resectoscope with a small electrocautery loop using cutting current. The proximal verumontanum is resected along with the ejaculatory ducts (**Fig. 18.18**). Resection must be continued until the site of obstruction is cleared if a calculus or ductal stenosis is the cause. Clearance may be confirmed with visualization of dye efflux from the ducts. Minimal coagulation is used to prevent ductal stricture. A foley catheter is placed for 24 hours.

Between 33–90 percent of men with experience improvement of semen parameters and between 9–43 percent of couples will achieve a natural pregnancy after TURED.[65] The greatest improvement in semen parameters have been reported in men with midline ejaculatory duct cysts and dilated seminal vesicles.[66]

SURGICAL COMPLICATIONS

Potential complications of reconstructive surgery include bleeding, infection, testicular devascularization, restenosis of anastomosis, prolonged operative time, and anesthesic complications. Meticulous hemostasis is essential throughout the entirety of the procedure. Unrecognized bleeding can result

Table 18.2: Vasoepididymostomy outcomes[52,62-64]

Author	Year	Number of patients	Anastomosis type	Patency rates (%)	Pregnancy rates (%)
Dublin	1985	46	End-to-end	39	13
Silbera	1989	139	End-to-end	78	56
Dewire	1995	137	End-to-side	79	50
Berger	1998	12	Intussusception	92	Not reported
Marmar	2000	9	Intussusception	78	22
Chan	2005	68	Intussusception	84	40
Schiff	2005	153	End-to-end End-to-side 2-suture intussusception 3-suture intussusception	73 74 80 84	20 40 44 46
Ho	2009	23	Intussusception	57	32
Zhang	2009	49	2-suture intussusception	71	26
Kumar	2010	24	2-suture intussusception	48	4

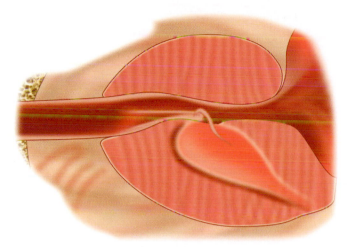

Figure 18.18: Sagittal view of transurethral resection of ejaculatory duct (TURED)

in postoperative hematoma formation potentially leading to disruption of the delicate anastomosis and significant swelling and pain. Most hematomas are small and will resolve on their own with conservative management.

Testicular ischemia and atrophy can result if the testicular artery is injured. This can rarely occur if the testicular vasculature has been previously compromised during vasectomy, hernia repair, varicocele repair, or orchidopexy. Intraoperative Doppler ultrasound is recommended to identify the testicular artery apart from the vas deferens if previous inguinal surgery has been performed.

The risks of venous thromboembolism, pressure induced tissue necrosis, and alopecia are present given the prolonged period of immobilization to complete the procedure. Prolonged operative times can be seen in complex reconstructions and redo procedures involving significant scar tissue from previous operations. All patients should have sequential compression stockings for prophylaxis and pressure points padded adequately as previously discussed.

Other Vasovasostomy Anastomotic Techniques and Considerations

During the last two decades, alternative methods or modifications of current methods for VV and VE have been researched in hopes of simplifying the procedure and reducing operative time.

Microscopic reversal approaches have been accepted to be superior to macroscopic approaches, although some surgeons have demonstrated satisfactory outcomes using loupe assisted techniques with shorter operative times.[67] Macrosurgical single layer reversals demonstrate patency rates of 70–80 percent and pregnancy rates of 20–40 percent compared to microsurgical reversal patency rates of 85–90 percent and pregnancy rates of 50–70 percent.[68,69] Proponents of the macroscopic technique encourage this technique because of shorter operative times, lack of need for microscope, and less expensive instruments,

although they reserve this approach for simple, straightforward vasectomy reversals only.

Fibrin glue assisted VV has also been described as a viable modification in a single human study.[70] Patients underwent a fibrin glue assisted microsurgical 3-suture VV with significantly shorter operative times when compared to standard microsurgical 1- or 2-layer techniques with the same microsurgeon. Patency rates were 93 percent in this small series although follow-up was short. Therefore, the rate of delayed scarring or obstruction is unknown microsurgical skills are still required to place the three sutures prior to application of fibrin glue. To date there have been no long term or validated studies comparing this technique to the standard microsurgical VV.

Robot-assisted VV has also been reported as a viable approach in humans.[71,72] Proposed benefits of this technique include shorter training period and learning curve, improved surgeon ergonomics and comfort, improved surgical precision, shorter operative times, as well as elimination of physiologic tremors. Negatives to this approach include decreased magnification, lack of tactile feedback with the risk of breaking sutures and damaging delicate tissues, and increased cost in an elective procedure. Current standard robotic optics allow for 10–15X magnification when compared to 20–25X magnification with a surgical microscope. Newer advanced digital camera technology will soon allow magnification up to 250X.[73] Further evaluation of this technology is needed to assess its potential applications in microsurgical procedures.

SUMMARY

Technological advances as well as methodological improvements have allowed surgeons to restore patency in patients with genital tract obstruction. Outcomes continue to be dependent on surgeon experience as well as the chosen surgical approaches. Newer technologies currently being tested attempt to improve operative time as well as precision of surgery, but with small cohorts and short postoperative follow-up remain experimental compared to the gold standard microscopic approaches. The surgeon performing surgery for genital tract obstruction must be versatile in the different approaches used to obtain patency.

REFERENCES

1. Thonneau P, Bujan L, Multigner L, Mieusset R. Occupational heat exposure and male fertility: A review. Hum Reprod 1998;13:2122-5.
2. Jarrow JP, Espeland MA, Lipshultz LI. Evaluation of the azoospermic patient. J Urol 1989;142:62-5.
3. Magnani RJ, Haws JM, Morgan GT, Gargiullo PM, Pollack AE, Koonin LM. Vasectomy in the United States, 1991 and 1995. Am J Public Health 1999;89:92-4.
4. Sandlow JI, Nagler HM. Vasectomy and vasectomy reversal: important issues. Preface. Urol Clin North Am 2009;38:13-4.
5. Prader A. Testicular size: Assessment and clinical importance. Triangle 1966;7:240-3.
6. Lennox B, Ahmad KN. The total length of tubules in the human testis. J Anat 1970;107:191.

7. Clermont Y. Kinetics of spermatogenesis in mammals: Seminiferous epithelium cycle and spermatogonial renewal. Physiol Rev 1972;52:198-236.

8. Amann RP, Howards SS. Daily spermatozoal production and epididymal spermatozoal reserves of the human male. J Urol 1980;124:211-5.

9. Hinrichsen MJ, Blaquier JA. Evidence supporting the existence of sperm maturation in the human epididymis. J Reprod Fertil 1980;60:291-4.

10. Lacham O, Trounson A. Fertilizing capacity of epidi ymal and testicular spermatozoa microinjected under the zona pellucida of the mouse oocyte. Mol Reprod Dev 1991;29:85-93.

11. Silber SJ. Apparent fertility of human spermatozoa from the caput epididymidis. J Androl 1989;10:263-9.

12. Schlegel PN, Goldstein M. Microsurgical vasoepididymostomy: refinements and results. J Urol 1993;150:1165-8.

13. Johnson L, Varner DD. Effect of daily spermatozoan production but not age on transit time of spermatozoa through the human epididymis. Biol Reprod 1988;39:812-7.

14. Schlegel PN, Shin D, Goldstein M. Urogenital anomalies in men with congenital absence of the vas deferens. J Urol 1996;155:1644-8.

15. Ferlin A, Raicu F, Gatta V, Zuccarello D, Palka G, Foresta C. Male infertility: role of genetic background. Reprod Biomed Online 2007;14:734-45.

16. Practice Committee of American Society for Reproductive Medicine in collaboration with Society for Male Reproduction and Urology. Evaluation of the azoospermic male. Fertil Steril 2008;90:S74-77.

17. Paavonen J, Eggert-Kruse W. Chlamydia trachomatis: impact on human reproduction. Hum Reprod Update 1999;5:433-47.

18. Hopps CV, Goldstein M. Microsurgical reconstruction of iatrogenic injuries to the epididymis from hydrocelectomy. J Urol 2006;176:2077-9.

19. Hernandez J, Sabanegh ES. Repeat vasectomy reversal after initial failure: overall results and predictors for success. J Urol 1999;161:1153-6.

20. Mayersak JS. Urogenital sinus-ejaculatory duct cyst: a case report with a proposed clinical classification and review of the literature. J Urol 1989;142:1330-2.

21. Meachum RB, Hellerstein DK, Lipschultz LI. Evaluation and treatment of ejaculatory duct obstruction in the infertile male. Fertil Steril 1993;59:393-7.

22. Jarow JP, Budin RE, Dym M, Zirkin BR, Noren S, Marshall FF. Quantitative pathologic changes in the human testis after vasectomy. A controlled study. N Engl J Med 1985;313:1252-6.

23. Hadley MA, Dym M. Spermatogenesis in the vasectomized monkey: quantitative analysis. Anat Rec 1983;205:381-6.

24. Shiraishi K, Naito K, Yoshida K. Vasectomy impairs spermatogenesis through germ cell apoptosis mediated by p53-Bax pathway in rat. J Urol 2001;166:1565-71.

25. Chawla A, O'Brien J, Lisi M, Zini A, Jarvi K. Should all urologists performing vasectomy reversals be able to perform vasoepididymostomies if required? J Urol 2004;172:1048-50.

26. Fuchs EF, Burt RA. Vasectomy reversal performed 15 years or more after vasectomy: correlation of pregnancy outcome with partner age and with pregnancy results of in vitro fertilization with intracytoplasmic sperm injection. Fertil Steril 2002;77:516-9.

27. Parekattil SJ, Kuang W, Agarwal A, Thomas AJ. Model to predict if a vasoepididymostomy will be required for vasectomy reversal. J Urol 2005;173:1681-4.

28. Parekattil SJ, Kuang W, Kolettis PN, Pasqualotto FF, Teloken P, Teloken C, Nangia AK, Daitch JA, Niederberger C, Thomas AJ Jr. Multi-institutional validation of vasectomy reversal predictor. J Urol 2006;175:247-9.

29. Fox M. Vasectomy reversal—microsurgery for best results. Br J Urol 1994;73:449-53.

30. Belker AM, Thomas AJ, Jr. Fuchs EF, Konnak JW, Sharlip ID. Results of 1469 microsurgical vasectomy reversals by the Vasovasostomy Study Group. J Urol 1991;14:505-11.

31. Fischer MA, Grantmyre JE. Comparison of modified one- and two-layer microsurgical vasovasostomy. BJU Int 2000;85:1085-8.

32. Lipschultz LI, Rumohr JA, Bennett RC. Techniques for vasectomy reversal. Urol Clin North Am 2009;36:375-82.

33. Schmidt SS. Vasovasostomy. Urol Clin North Am 1978;5:585-92.

34. Silber SJ. Microscopic technique for reversal of vasectomy. Surg Gynecol Obstet 1976;143:631.

35. Silber SJ. Microscopic vasectomy reversal. Fertil Steril 1977;28:1191-1202.

36. Matsuda T. Diagnosis and treatment of post-herniorrhaphy vas deferens obstruction. Int J Urol 2000;7:S35-38.

37. Matsuda T, Horii Y, Yoshida O. Unilateral obstruction of the vas deferens caused by childhood inguinal herniorrhaphy in male infertility patients. Fertil Steril 1992;58:609-13.

38. Ridgeway PF, Shah J, Darzi AW. Male genital tract injuries after contemporary inguinal hernia repair. BJU Int 2002;90:262-76.

39. Shin D, Lipshultz LI, Goldstein M, Barmé GA, Fuchs EF, Nagler HM, McCallum SW, Niederberger CS, Schoor RA, Brugh VM 3rd, Honig SC. Herniorrhaphy with polypropylene mesh causing inguinal vasal obstruction: a preventable cause of obstructive azoospermia. Ann Surg 2005;241:553-8.

40. Meachum RB. Potential for vasal occlusion among men after hernia repair using mesh. J Androl 2002;23:759-61.

41. Berndsen FH, Bjursten LM, Simanaitis M, Montgomery A. Does mesh implantation affect the spermatic cord structures after inguinal hernia surgery? An experimental study in rats. Eur Surg Res 2004;36:318-22.

42. Kim A, Shin D, Martin TV, Honig SC. Laparoscopic mobilization of the retroperitoneal vas deferens for microscopic inguinal vasovasostomy. J Urol 2004;172:1948-9.

43. Matsuda T, Muguruma K, Hiura Y, Okuno H, Shichiri Y, Yoshida O. Seminal tract obstruction caused by childhood inguinal herniorrhaphy: results of microsurgical reanastomosis. J Urol 1998;159:837-40.

44. Hendry WF, Parslow JM, Stedronska J. Exploratory scrototomy in 168 azoospermic males. Br J Urol 1983;55:785-91.

45. Lizza EF, Marmar JL, Schmidt SS, Lanasa JA Jr, Sharlip ID, Thomas AJ, Belker AM, Nagler HM. Transseptal crossed vasovasostomy. J Urol 1985;134:1131-2.

46. Hamidinia A. Transvasovasostomy - an alternative operation for obstructive azoospermia. J Urol 1988;140:1545-8.

47. Sabanegh E, Thomas AJ. Effectiveness of crossover transseptal vasoepididymostomy intreating complex obstructive azoospermia. Fertil Steril 1995;63:392-5.

48. Holman CD, Wisniewski ZS, Semmens JB, Rouse IL, Bass AJ. Population based outcomes after 28,246 in-hospital

vasectomies and 1,902 vasovasostomies in Western Australia. BJU Int 2000;86:1043-9.

49. Kolettis PN, Sabanegh ES, Nalesnik JG, D'Amico AM, Box LC, Burns JR. Pregnancy outcomes after vasectomy reversal for female partners 35 years old or older. J Urol 2003; 169:2250-2.

50. Gerrard ER, Sandlow JI, Oster RA, Burns JR, Box LC, Kolettis PN. Effect of female partner age on pregnancy rates after vasectomy reversal. Fertil Steril 2007;87:1340-4.

51. Nagler HM, Rotman M. Predictive parameters for microsurgical reconstruction. Urol Clin North Am 2002;29:913-9.

52. Sabanegh ES, Thomas AJ. Microsurgical treatment of male infertility. In: Lipschultz LI, Howards SS, Niederberger CS, (Eds). Infertility in the male. 4th edn. Cambridge. Cambridge University Press; 2009.

53. Hendry WF. The long-term results of surgery for obstructive azoospermia. Br J Urol 1981;53:664-8.

54. Silber SJ. Microscopic vasoepididymostomy: specific microanastomosis to the epididymal tubule. Fertil Steril 1978;30:565-71.

55. Fogdestam I, Fall M, Nilsson S. Microsurgical epididymovasostomy in the treatment of occlusive azoospermia. Fertil Steril 1986;46:925-9.

56. Thomas AJ. Vasoepididymostomy. Urol Clin North Am 1987;14: 527-38.

57. Berger RE. Triangulation end-to-side vasoepididymostomy. J Urol 1998;159:1951-3.

58. Marmar JL. Modified vasoepididymostomy with simultaneous double needle placement, tubulotomy and tubular invagination. J Urol 2000;163:483-6.

59. Chan PT, Li PS, Goldstein M. Microsurgical vasoepididymostomy: a prospective randomized study of 3 intussusception techniques in rats. J Urol 2003;169:1924-9.

60. Schoysman R. Vasoepididymostomy – a survey of techniques and results with considerations of delay of appearance of spermatozoa after surgery. Acta Eur Fertil 1990;21:239-45.

61. Jarow JP, Sigman M, Buch JP, Oates RD. Delayed appearance of sperm after end-to-side vasoepididymostomy. J Urol 1995;153:1156-8.

62. Ho KL, Wong MH, Tam PC. Microsurgical vasoepididymostomy for obstructive azoospermia. Hong King Med J 2009;15:452-7.

63. Zhang GX, Bai WJ, Xu KX, Wang XF, Zhu JC. Clinical observation of loupe-assisted intussusception vasoepididymostomy in the treatment of obstructive azoospermia (analysis of 49 case reports). Asian J Androl 2009;11:193-9.

64. Kumar R, Mukherjee S, Gupta NP. Intussusception vasoepididymostomy with longitudinal suture placement for idiopathic obstructive azoospermia. J Urol 2010;183:1489-92.

65. Chudnovsky A, Brugh VM. Management of ejaculatory duct obstruction. In: Lipschultz LI, Howards SS, Niederberger CS, (Eds). Infertility in the male. 4th edn. Cambridge. Cambridge University Press; 2009.

66. Kadioglu A, Cayan S, Tefekli A, Orhan I, Engin G, Turek PJ. Does response to treatment of ejaculatory duct obstruction in infertile men vary with pathology? Fertil Steril 2001;76:138-42.

67. Hsieh ML, Huang HC, Chen Y, Huang ST, Chang PL. Loupe-assisted vs microsurgical technique for modified one-layer vasovasostomy: is the microsurgery really better? BJU Int 2005;96:864-6.

68. Belker AM. Microsurgical vasectomy reversal. In: Lytton B, Catalona WJ, Lipshultz LI, McGuire EJ, (Eds). Advances in urology. Chicago: Year Book Medical 1988.pp.193-230.

69. Jee SH, Hong YK. One-layer vasovasostomy: microsurgical versus loupe-assisted. Fertil Steril. Forthcoming 2010.p.12.

70. Ho KL, Witte MN, Bird ET, Hakim S. Fibrin glue assisted 3-suture vasovasostomy. J Urol 2005;174:1360-3.

71. Fleming C. Robot-assisted vasovasostomy. Urol Clin North Am 2004;31:769-72.

72. Parekattil SJ, Atalah HN, Cohen MS. Video technique for human robot-assisted microsurgical vasovasostomy. J Endourol 2010;24:511-4.

73. Parekattil SJ, Cohen MS. Robotic surgery in male infertility and chronic orchialgia. Curr Opin Urol 2010;20:75-9.

CHAPTER

19

Varicocele Surgery in Modern Practice

Fábio Firmbach Pasqualotto, Giovana Cobalchini, Eleonora Bedin Pasqualotto

INTRODUCTION

Varicoceles are present in 15 percent of the normal male population and in approximately 40 percent of men presenting with infertility. The preponderance of experimental data from clinical and animal models demonstrates a deleterious effect of varicoceles on spermatogenesis. The American Urological Association and American Society of Reproductive Medicine jointly convened Best Policy Practice Groups for Male Infertility and recently stated, "Varicocele repairs may be considered the primary treatment option when a man with a varicocele has suboptimal semen quality and a normal female partner." They considered percutaneous embolization and surgery for varicocele treatment, and noted that most experts performed inguinal or subinguinal microsurgical repairs to maximize preservation of preservation of arterial and lymphatic vessels while reducing the chances of persistence or recurrence. This review offers recommendations regarding the role of varicocele surgery in the era of assisted reproductive techniques.

In 1955, Tulloch reported that ligation of the spermatic vessels cured a 27-year-old azoospermic male with bilateral varicoceles.[1] Within 3 months of the surgery, spermatozoa had returned to the seminal fluid, and within 9 months the patient's wife became pregnant. Tulloch's account sparked a renewed interest in the surgical correction of varicoceles, but this interest would not be long-lasting. Uncertain of the value of treating varicoceles for infertility, Baker et al reviewed a series of 651 subfertile couples in which the man had a varicocele.[2] They detected no improvement in pregnancy rates in couples where the man had undergone varicocele ligation and concluded that testicular vein ligation is not effective in improving fertility. They declared that the "onus is now on proponents of the treatment of varicoceles in infertile men by operation or other techniques to prove their case." The debate has since raged, and countless studies and reviews have been published on this topic, few of which have succeeded in bringing clarity to the controversy. In the past decade, several controlled studies involving modern techniques of diagnosis and treatment have been published on this subject.

For this review, we used the level of evidence accordingly:
- Experimental and observational studies (high quality-without heterogeneity)
- Experimental and observational studies (low quality–with heterogeneity)
- Series of cases
- Expert consensus, "proof of principles".

INCIDENCE

Varicocele remains an enigma in the treatment of male infertility.[3-7] Despite over 30 years of evidence that the repair of varicoceles results in improved fertility, the retrospective nature of most of these reports has led to controversy regarding the utility of treatment.[8-10] The enigma of the varicocele, although a source of frustration for clinicians, has been a siren call for researchers as attested to by the substantial, if flawed body of literature on the topic.

Evaluation of a patient with a varicocele should include a careful medical and reproductive history, a physical examination and at least two semen analyses.[11,12] The physical examination should be performed with the patient in both the recumbent and upright positions. It is considered a subclinical varicocele when detected only with the ultrasound, Grade I, palpable with Valsalva, Grade II, palpable without Valsalva, and Grade III, easily observed (**Fig. 19.1**).

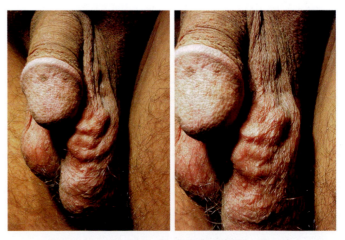

Figure 19.1: Example of a clinical grade III varicocele

Imaging studies are not indicated for the standard evaluation unless the physical exam is inconclusive.[11] Therefore, when a suspected varicocele is not clearly palpable, the scrotum should be examined while the patient performs a Valsalva maneuver in a standing position.

The incidence of varicocele varies according to age with the following distribution: 2–6 years, 0.79 percent; 7–10 years, 0.96 percent; 11–14 years, 7.8 percent and 15–19 years, 14.1 percent [GR-A].[13] After the twenties, it's incidence varies from 10–25 percent [GR-C].[14] In the elderly, (median of 60 years), varicocele is present in up to 42.9 percent of the population.[15] Up to now, there are no prospective, randomized controlled studies to demonstrate a relationship between varicocele and hormonal abnormalities.

The incidence of varicocele is about 20 percent in the general population rising to almost 40 percent in infertile men [GR-B].[16] In men with secondary infertility, the prevalence of varicocele may be as high as 80 percent,[17,18] although in one study the prevalence of varicocele in men with primary and secondary infertility was no different (45 and 44%, respectively).[19] These observations suggest that the presence of a varicocele can cause a progressive decline in fertility but also that a significant proportion of men with a varicocele (75%) are fertile. However, it is important to realize that there is some variability in the reported prevalence of varicoceles in populations of fertile and infertile men.[20] Much of this may have to do with the interphysician variability in establishing the clinical diagnosis of the varicocele and in the notable increase in prevalence of varicocele with age.[20,21] Also, an inverse correlation seems to exist between body mass index (BMI) and the incidence of varicocele [GR-B].[22]

But the main question remains: are all adult varicoceles alike? Are varicoceles in a 25-year-old man the same as those in a 55-year-old man? A recent article addressed this very important question. The authors reviewed 581 consecutive nonazoospermic men presenting with a clinical varicocele and infertility, dividing them into two groups, 115 men aged 40 years and over and 466 men younger than 40 years of age.[23] The authors compared preoperative clinical parameters and outcome measures including semen analysis, pregnancy rate and ART utilization rate. The proportion of men with secondary infertility was significantly higher in the group of men aged 40 years and older as was partner age. More importantly, they found no significant differences in mean improvement in sperm parameters, assisted reproductive technology (ART) utilization or pregnancy rates after varicocelectomy in the older group compared with the younger group. They also compared the spontaneous pregnancy rate in couples with advanced paternal age (40 years or older) who underwent varicocelectomy to an age-matched control group who did not undergo surgery. The authors concluded that paternal age may not adversely affect pregnancy outcome after varicocelectomy, supporting the practice of surgical management in older men with clinical varicocele and infertility.

The reason for this discrepancy remains unknown, although it is postulated that the cause of infertility is related to both temperature and time.[11,12,24] The blood supply to the testes, as well as the resulting counter current heat exchange, results in cooler intratesticular temperatures than body temperatures.[9,10]

Disruption of this system can result in hyperthermia of the testes. As the left side drains into a system with higher resistance, small venules may persist or open during embryogenesis. Testicular blood flow remains low before puberty, and therefore these veins do not become clinically apparent until adolescence when testicular blood flow increases, which explains the appearance of most varicoceles around puberty.

Men with varicocele who have intense physical activity regularly 4–5 time a week, lasting from 2–4 hours/day over a period of 4 years have a decrease in semen parameters [GR-A].[25] Also, the presence of varicocele in first degree relatives is more frequent than in the general population [GR-B].[26]

▋VARICOCELE: REASON FOR INFERTILITY

The true effect of varicocele on male fertility potential is not known. Numerous studies have demonstrated an association between varicocele and reduced male fertility potential (e.g. poor semen parameters, infertility). However, most varicocele studies involve highly selected populations (e.g. infertile men) and rarely examine unselected men, representing an important reason for the difficulty in relating varicoceles with male fertility. Moreover, the lack of reliable end-points for measuring fertility represents another challenge in relating varicoceles with male infertility.

Conventional semen parameters (sperm concentration, motility, and morphology) are generally monitored in varicocele studies, but these parameters exhibit a high degree of biological variability and are of modest value in predicting male fertility potential.[27] Pregnancy is also of limited value in assessing the influence of varicocele on male fertility potential because this outcome is heavily influenced by female factors.[28]

Varicocele remain the most common cause of male infertility, although the literature shows conflicting data as well as the conclusions obtained throughout studies with low level of evidence or inadequate trials. The World Health Organization (WHO) observational study involving 9,034 men, verified that 25.6 percent of patients with abnormal semen analysis have varicocele and in these men there is a significant decrease in the ipsilateral testicle volume compared to the contralateral testicle. This decrease in testicular volume does not happen in men with infertility without varicocele [GR-B].[20]

It has been demonstrated that testicular atrophy may be associated with an adverse effect of varicocele on male fertility.[29-32] In men with a left varicocele, mean left testicular volume is less than right testicular volume.[30-32] However, the relationship between varicocele grade and the degree of testicular atrophy is less clear. The impact of testicular atrophy on male fertility remains to be established, although most studies indicate that atrophy is associated with reduced sperm parameters. Studies have reported that in men with left varicocele, those with testicular atrophy have poorer sperm parameters than do men without atrophy. Similarly, in adolescents, a volume differential greater than 10 percent between the normal and affected testis correlates with a significantly decreased sperm concentration and total motile sperm count. However, loss of testicular volume is not clearly associated with loss of fertility.[30]

The influence of varicocele on sperm parameters has not been established conclusively. In studies of infertile men, varicoceles have been associated with abnormal sperm parameters. It has been observed that the majority of semen samples from infertile men with varicocele have poorer sperm parameters (lower sperm counts, increased numbers of spermatozoa with abnormal forms, and decreased sperm motility) than those of fertile men. However, the "stress pattern" described by MacLeod (i.e., increased proportions of sperm with tapered heads and immature forms) is not a specific marker for varicocele and, therefore, is not diagnostic of this condition.[33,34] Although studies on the prevalence of varicocele in men with primary and secondary infertility suggest that the presence of a varicocele may cause a progressive decline in fertility, this has not been confirmed by prospective studies. Pasqualotto et al demonstrated a clear correlation between semen quality and clinical varicocele in men with infertility.[35] The authors showed that semen quality from men without infertility but with the presence of clinical varicocele did not differ from men without clinical varicocele.

Few studies in the past 3 years have assessed the impact of varicocele repair on serum testosterone levels. Although the impact of varicocele on testosterone production is not well understood and the utility of varicocelectomy to prevent or reduce deterioration in Leydig cell function remains unproven, recent data suggest an adverse effect of varicocele and possible benefit of repair. Further human clinical studies are warranted to better define these relationships.[36,37]

■ SURGICAL VS EMBOLIZATION APPROACH

The aim of varicocele repair is to occlude the spermatic veins to prevent venous reflux. Varicocele may be treated with many different modalities, including radiologic, laparoscopic, and open surgical approaches. The best treatment modality for varicocele in infertile men should include higher seminal improvement and spontaneous pregnancy rates with lower rates of complications such as recurrence or persistence, hydrocele formation, and testicular atrophy. Therefore, the ideal technique should aim for ligation of all internal and external spermatic veins with preservation of spermatic arteries and lymphatics.

This may be accomplished with open surgery, microsurgical or laparoscopic ligation of the internal spermatic veins, or by introducing sclerosing agents or embolization devices into the spermatic veins. The treating physician's experience and expertise, together with the option available, should determine the choice of varicocele treatment. There are two approaches to varicocele repair: surgery and percutaneous embolization.[11,12] Surgical repair of a varicocele may be accomplished by various open surgical methods, including retroperitoneal, inguinal and subinguinal approaches, or by laparoscopy.[38,39] Even though none of these methods have been proven to be superior to the others in its ability to improve fertility, several studies have shown that microsurgical inguinal or subinguinal techniques have significantly better results in terms of sperm motility improvement, pregnancy rate, recurrence, and complications

than those of the traditional surgical approaches of high ligation or of laparoscopy.

Marmar et al[40] introduced the subinguinal microsurgical varicocelectomy with ligation, and Goldstein et al[41] modified the microsurgical technique with delivery of the testis in search of scrotal collaterals including the gubernacular veins.

The percutaneous embolization is done through the occlusion of the internal spermatic vein [GR-A].[42] There are no studies proving one method is superior to another regarding fertility improvement, however, differences in the complication and recurrence rates have been described [GR-A].[43]

Subinguinal varicocelectomy with optical magnification increases the probability of arterial and lymphatic preservation, significantly decreasing the risks of recurrence and postoperative complication in relation to laparoscopy and surgeries without magnification [GR-A][43] [GR-C][44] [GR-D].[45] In fact, there are two approaches to increase the magnification: loupe and operative microscope. While the use of loupe increases few time the magnification, experienced surgeons use the microscope in order to recognize and avoid unnecessary injuries to the vas deferens, lymphatics and arteries. On the other hand, there have been no prospective, randomized studies of microsurgical varicocelectomy versus no treatment.

Percutaneous embolization is associated with higher recurrence rates, even higher than the conventional surgical approaches, without taken into account the complications related to the percutaneous embolization method itself [GR-A].[46] Patients with bilateral clinical varicoceles should be considered for bilateral varicocelectomy [GR-A].[47]

A recent meta-analysis evaluated 36 studies reporting postoperative spontaneous pregnancy rates and/or complication rates after varicocele repair using various techniques in infertile men with palpable unilateral or bilateral varicocele.[49] Overall spontaneous pregnancy rates were 37.69 percent in the Palomo technique group, 41.97 percent in the microsurgical varicocelectomy group, 30.07 percent in the laparoscopic varicocelectomy group, 33.2 percent in the radiologic embolization, and 36 percent in the macroscopic inguinal (Ivanissevich) varicocelectomy group, revealing significant differences among the techniques. Overall recurrence rates were 14.97 percent in the Palomo group, 1.05 percent in the microsurgical varicocelectomy group, 4.3 percent in the laparoscopic varicocelectomy group, 12.7 percent in the radiologic embolization, and 2.63 percent in the macroscopic inguinal (Ivanissevich) or subinguinal varicocelectomy group, demonstrating significant difference among the techniques. Overall hydrocele formation rates were 8.24 percent in the Palomo technique group, 0.44 percent in the microsurgical varicocelectomy group, 2.84 percent in the laparoscopic varicocelectomy, and 7.3 percent in the macroscopic inguinal (Ivanissevich) or subinguinal varicocelectomy group, showing, again, significant difference among the techniques. Therefore, the authors concluded in this meta-analysis that the microsurgical varicocelectomy technique has higher spontaneous pregnancy rates and lower postoperative recurrence and hydrocele formation than conventional varicocelectomy techniques in infertile men. However, prospective, randomized, and comparative studies with large number of patients are needed to compare the efficacy of microsurgical varicocelectomy with that of other treatment modalities in infertile men with varicocele.

AZOOSPERMIA AND VARICOCELE

A varicocele repair may be considered for men with azoospermia who have a palpable varicocele. Therefore, azoospermic patients with Germ cell aplasia in a single large testis biopsy may have an improvement in semen quality following varicocelectomy. Due to the possibility of their relapsing into azoospermia after an initial improvement in semen quality following varicocelectomy, patients should be informed of the possibility of sperm cryopreservation. In azoospermic patients, the surgical treatment of varicocele may promote spermatogenesis, avoiding the need to obtain sperm from the testicle for assisted reproduction [GR-A].[49-52]

It is of utmost importance to consider the genetics before repairing a clinical varicocele in cases of azoospermia. Patients with varicocele and azoospermia and with abnormal kariotype or Y-microdeletion most probably does not benefit from the surgical procedure.

A recent meta-analysis evaluating a total of 233 patients was performed. After varicocele repair 91 (39.1%) patients had motile sperm in the ejaculate and 14 spontaneous pregnancies were reported. Success rates in patients with maturation arrest (42.1%) or hypospermatogenesis (54.5%) were significantly higher than in those with Sertoli-cell-only (11.3%, p <0.001 in both groups). Patients with late maturation arrest had a higher probability of success (45.8%) than those with early maturation arrest (0%, p = 0.007). Therefore, the authors concluded that infertile men with nonobstructive azoospermia can have improvement in semen analysis and achieve spontaneous pregnancy after repair of clinical varicoceles. This meta-analysis demonstrates that men with late maturation arrest and hypospermatogenesis have a higher probability of success and, therefore, histopathology should be considered before varicocele repair in men with nonobstructive azoospermia.[52]

IMPROVEMENT IN SEMEN PARAMETERS AFTER VARICOCELECTOMY: IS THERE AN IMPROVEMENT WITH ASSISTED FERTILIZATION?

Varicocele repair, intrauterine insemination (IUI) and *in vitro* fertilization/intracytoplasmic sperm injection (IVF/ICSI) are options for the management of couples with male factor infertility associated with a varicocele.[53,54] The decision as to which method of management to use is influenced by many factors. Most importantly, varicocele repair has the potential to reverse a pathological condition and effect a permanent cure for infertility, as opposed to IUI or the assisted reproduction techniques (ART) required for each attempt at pregnancy.[54] Other factors to be considered are age of the female partner, the unknown long-term health effects of IVF and ICSI on the offspring resulting from these techniques, and the possibly greater cost-effectiveness of

varicocele treatment than of IVF with or without ICSI.[55] Finally, failure to treat a varicocele may result in a progressive decline in semen parameters, further reducing a man's chances for future fertility.

There are few studies with level A evidence evaluating outcomes following varicocelectomy. Further, there are no standard patterns in the selection methods, diagnosis, forms of treatment and variables evaluated.

One randomized study demonstrated that there is an improvement in semen quality in 50 percent of the cases [GR-A].[54] A meta-analysis of clinical randomized studies demonstrated that surgery or embolization treatment for varicocele in men with infertility does not increase the chance of natural pregnancy [GR-A],[56] however, there are several criticisms regarding the selection of the studies included in this article [GR-A].[59] Another recent meta-analysis demonstrated that after varicocelectomy the chances of natural pregnancy increased 2.8 times comparing to patients without any type of treatment or with clinical treatment [GR-A].[58]

Testicular size, grade of varicocele, seminal parameters and hormonal levels may be considered as prognostic parameters for men with varicocele [GR-D].[59] However, it is not possible to draw conclusions as to which parameters are predictive as treatment outcomes [GR-B],[14] [GR-A].[60,61] Recently, it was demonstrated that, besides an improvement in semen parameters, the DNA fragmentation may decrease following the varicocele repair.[62]

Although a large body of literature suggests improved semen parameters and fertility following varicocelectomy, some investigators have challenged the benefit of these procedures because these are case controlled studies rather than prospective randomized trials.[63] In fact, even though the preponderance of adult studies supports a favorable effect of varicocelectomy on male fertility potential, most of these studies are uncontrolled. The statistical evaluation of these data is the subject of an ongoing debate and the fertility outcomes of varicocele repair have been described in numerous published studies.[35,64] Most of these studies lack adequate numbers of patients, randomization and/or controls, and it is not possible therefore to reach a clear conclusion on the fertility outcome.[56]

Several recent reviews have critically examined the results of randomized, controlled trials of varicocelectomy. Recently, Evers and Collins reported a meta-analysis including 7 prospective randomized trials that evaluated varicocelectomy and pregnancy outcomes.[56] They claimed that there was insufficient evidence to conclude that treatment of clinical varicocele improved the likelihood of conception for couples with male infertility. They stated that the routine treatment of the male partner of subfertile couples was unadvisable. This conclusion is regrettable because the data in the meta-analysis were questionable. Specifically, several patients in the study groups had normal semen analysis. Of the 7 studies, 4 included men with subclinical varicoceles. Two of the studies had questionable data for the outcome of controls, including one with an accumulative pregnancy rate for controls of 47 percent, whereas the other had a 24.5 percent pregnancy rate with counseling of controls that actually included optimization of female reproductive functions.[56] The pregnancy rates for controls among the remaining studies in the meta-analysis ranged between 4.5 and 10 percent. Finally, the varicocele treatment did not include microsurgical procedures as suggested by the Best Practice Study Groups, and there was limited follow up information concerning recurrences with either high ligation or embolization.[11]

A Cochrane review identified five randomized controlled trials that examined the outcomes in couples with male factor infertility and varicoceles and concluded that they did not show sufficient evidence regarding the treatment of varicoceles to warrant their repair.[65] However, these studies were chosen for this review only because of their status as randomized clinical trials; no evaluation of the methods was performed. A review of these trials shows that one examined only subclinical varicoceles, and three others exhibited methodological problems including the use of embolization, high pregnancy rates in untreated couples (25% in a one-year period), and inherent selection bias in the study (many couples opted to pursue assisted reproductive technology rather than enter the study).

Although few randomized controlled trials show the benefit of treating varicocele-related infertility, many non-randomized studies support this concept.[65] Numerous studies, most of them retrospective, were reviewed and the following conclusions drawn. Most participants showed improvement in postoperative sperm density and motility. The natural pregnancy rates varied, but the overall average was 37 percent, a clearly higher figure than any reported for non-treatment. Although many of these studies suffer from the flaws of nonrandomized trials, these results would be difficult to explain on the basis of chance alone.

■ VARICOCELE IN THE ADOLESCENT

An important consideration for varicocele management is patient age. Pediatric or adolescent varicocele is a different disease entity from adult varicocele, with its own diagnostic and therapeutic considerations. The main challenge in the management of a varicocele in adolescents is to establish criteria for the indications of treatment, in other words, to identify which of the patients will be benefit from surgery.

Adolescent males who have unilateral or bilateral varicoceles and objective evidence of reduced testicular size ipsilateral to the varicocele should be considered candidates for varicocele repair.[7,11,66,67] If objective evidence of reduced testis size is not present, adolescents with varicoceles should be followed up with annual objective measurements of testis size and/or semen analysis in order to detect the earliest sign of varicocele-related testicular injury.[11,12] Varicocele repair should be offered at the first detection of testicular or semen abnormality.

In the adolescent population, the hypotrophy rate caused by varicocele is 9 percent, and should be always related to the child/adolescent development according to the Tanner Kass classification (GR-D).[68]

Most studies of adolescents with varicocele indicate that varicocelectomy has a beneficial effect on testicular function and/or male fertility potential. In general, surgery is indicated in boys with testicular atrophy and/or abnormal semen parameters. Controlled studies indicate that at follow-up evaluation (1–15 years), varicocelectomy is associated with higher sperm parameters and higher testicular volumes than that of observation. Moreover, microsurgical repair has been associated with better outcomes (testicular growth, complication rate) than that of nonmicrosurgical varicocelectomy in adolescents.[48,54] As such, the data indicate that varicocelectomy is recommended in adolescents with varicocele and abnormal sperm parameters and/or testicular atrophy.

In adults, the grade of varicocele is related to the testicular volume: the presence of varicocele grade I have low impact in testicular volume, grade II is related to unilateral atrophy and grade III with bilateral abnormalities [GR-D].[67] Despite that, the grade of varicocele is not related to the presence or gravity of testicular disproportion in adolescents [GR-C].[69]

The criteria for definition of testicular hypotrophy include:
- Difference in both testicular sizes between 10–25 percent [GR-C].[70]
- The absolute difference between both testicles between 2–3 mL [GR-D].[70]

Scrotal pain appears to be not common in adolescents with varicocele, with an incidence of 2–4 percent [GR-D].[71] There are no studies evaluating the indications for varicocelectomy in these cases.

The same techniques for varicocele repair in adults are routinely used in the adolescents [GR-C].[71]

The improvement in sperm motility following varicocelectomy is higher in adolescents compared to adults [GR-C][72] and the increase in testicular size of the affected testis occurs in between 50 to 90 percent of the cases [GR-C].[71]

In the presence of bilateral normal testicular development and absence of symptoms, there is no evidence to support the benefits of varicocele repair. These adolescents must be followed annually with physical exam, ultrasound and semen analysis, whenever possible [GR-D].[71] In cases of testicular hypotrophy and/or abnormalities in the semen, surgical repair of the varicocele should be considered. Adolescents with varicoceles represent a large and heterogeneous group. This patient population has rapidly changing hormonal levels and may present at different stages of physical and pubertal development. A standard approach to these patients may not be possible. An individualized approach in which all parameters, including physical findings, percentage asymmetry, and abnormal ultrasound parameters, may be considered and should be used as part of an overall clinical decision.[73] Currently, there are no parameters that can predict impairment of fertility in adulthood for these patients. The ideal clinical follow-up protocol as well as the indications for surgical intervention and the optimal choice for the operative approach continue to be debated.[73]

BENEFIT OF SURGERY FOR COUPLES WITH A CLEAR INDICATION OF ASSISTED FERTILIZATION

There is a benefit of surgery for couples with a clear Indication of assisted fertilization.

Some studies indicate that IVF/ICSI seem to be no more effective than varicocelectomy, but more expensive than the surgical procedure.[74,75] In their meta-analysis, Penson et al reported that the probability of a live birth after varicocelectomy was 29.7 percent (with 1% having twins) as compared to 25.4 percent after IVF/ICSI (with a multiple gestation rate of 39%).[75] In a separate study Schlegel reported that the cost per baby delivered with IVF/ICSI was $89, 091 as compared to $26, 268 after varicocelectomy.[74] Thus, varicocele surgery seems desirable for selected varicocele cases.

The surgical approach of the varicocele may be capable to avoid the need of assisted reproduction, even reducing the treatment complexity grade when indicated [GR-D].[53,54] In azoospermic patients, the surgical treatment of varicocele may promote spermatogenesis, avoiding the need to obtain sperm from the testicle for assisted reproduction [GR-C].[49-52]

Patients should be evaluated after varicocele treatment for persistence or recurrence of the varicocele. If the varicocele persists or recurs, internal spermatic venography may be performed to identify the site of persistent venous reflux. Either surgical ligation or percutaneous embolization of the refluxing veins may be used. Semen analysis should be performed after varicocele treatment at about three-month intervals for at least one year or until pregnancy is achieved. IUI or ART should be considered for couples in which infertility persists after anatomically successful varicocele repair.[11,12]

Agarwal et al analyzed 17 studies reporting outcomes of microsurgical varicocelectomy a high ligation series for varicocele treatment in infertile men, and they demonstrated that surgical varicocelectomy significantly improves semen parameters in infertile men with palpable varicocele and abnormal semen analysis.[76] There has always been a problem defining the exact sub-group that would indeed benefit from varicocele surgery. Attempts have been made using the patient age, semen report, varicocele grade, hormone profile GnRH stimulation test, testicular histology, etc but most have failed to provide clear results.[11] Faced with this dilemma, the guidelines proposed by the American Urology Association and the American Society of Reproductive Medicine seem to be the most prudent evidence based medicine that should be followed.[11] These guidelines suggest that varicocelectomy should be offered only to men who are infertile, have a normal or correctable disease in the partner, have a clinically palpable varicocele and have a consistent abnormality in their semen analysis or sperm functions. In addition, it is advisable to obtain several semen tests over a period of time to confirm the abnormality before proceeding with surgery. The AUA guidelines are applicable to the majority of patients that present with a varicocele. However, the patient with azoospermia and a clinically palpable varicocele continues to be a problem in clinical decision making.

CONCLUSION

Despite the absence of definitive studies on the fertility outcome of varicocele repair, varicocele treatment should be considered as a choice for appropriate infertile couples because varicocele repair has been proven to improve semen parameters in most men. Varicocele treatment may improve fertility and the risks of varicocele treatment are small. Epidemiological data and observations on the pathogenic mechanisms leave no reasonable doubt on the association between varicocele and male reproductive failure.

Varicoceles continue to stimulate controversy among reproductive experts. Despite conflicting evidence from both randomized and nonrandomized trials, clinical experience still favors the surgical treatment of clinical varicoceles in men with infertility. Considering economical, ethical and evidence-based arguments, varicocele treatment should be offered to selected subfertile patients. However, it is incumbent on fertility specialists to design and recruit participants (or patients) in randomized, properly controlled trials to reach a definitive conclusion.

In addition, several recent publications indicate that treatment of adolescents may prevent sperm deterioration from occurring later in life These publications may encourage early diagnosis and (nonsurgical) treatment of varicocele at school age.

REFERENCES

1. Tulloch WS. Varicocele in subfertility; results of treatment. BMJ 1955;2:356-8.
2. Baker HW, Burger HG, de Kretser DM, Hudson B, Rennie GC, Straffon WG. Testicular vein ligation and fertility in men with varicoceles. Br Med J (Clin Res Ed) 1985;291:1678-80.
3. Noske HD, Weidner W. Varicocele a historical perspective. World J Urol 1999;17:151-7.
4. Galarneau GJ, Nagler HM. Cost-effective infertility therapies in the '90s: To treat or to cure? Contemporary Urology 1999;11:32-45.
5. World Health Organization. The influence of varicocele on parameters of fertility in a large group of men presenting to infertility clinics. Fertil Steril 1992;57:1289-93.
6. Steeno O, Knops J, Declerck L, Adimoelja A, Van de Voorde H. Prevention of fertility disorders by detection and treatment of varicocele at school and college age. Andrologia 1976;8:47-53.
7. Kursh ED. What is the incidence of varicocele in a fertile population? Fertil Steril 1987;48:510-1.
8. Pryor JL, Howards SS, Varicocele. Urol Clin North Am 1987;14:499-513.
9. Nagler HM, Grotas AB. Varicocele. In: Lipshultz LI, Howards SS, Niederberger CS (Eds), 4th edn. Infertility in the Male. Cambridge University Press, 2010.
10. Zini A, Girardi SK, Goldstein M. Varicocele. In: Hellstrom WJG, (Ed). Male Infertility and Sexual Dysfunction. New York, Springer-Verlag 1997.pp.201-18.
11. Jarow J, Sharlip ID, Belker AM, Lipshultz LY, Sigman M, Thomas AJ Jr, et al. Best practice policies for male infertility. J Urol 2002;167:2133-44.
12. Weidner W, Colpi GM, Hargreave TB, Papp GK, Pomerol JM. EAU guidelines on male infertility. Eur Urol 2002;42:313-22.

13. Akbay E, Cayan S, Doruk E, Duce MN, Bozlu M. The prevalence of varicocele and varicocele-related testicular atrophy in Turkish children and adolescentes. BJU Int 2000;86:490-3.

14. Callam MJ. Epidemiology of varicoses veins. BJU Int 1994;81:167-73.

15. Canales BK, Zapzalka DM, Ercole CJ, Carey P, Haus E, Aeppli D, Pryor JL. Prevalence and effect of varicoceles in an elderly population. Urology 2005;66:627-31.

16. Magdar I, Weissemberg R, Lunenfeld B, Karasik A, Goldwasser B. Controlled trial of high spermatic vein ligation for varicocele in infertile men. Fertil Steril 1995;63:120-4.

17. Gorelick JI, Goldstein M. Loss of fertility in men with varicocele. Fertil Steril 1993;59:613-6.

18. Witt MA, Lipshultz LI. Varicocele: a progressive or static lesion? Urology 1993;42:541-3.

19. Jarow JP, Coburn M, Sigman M. Incidence of varicoceles in men with primary and secondary infertility. Urology 1996;47:73-6.

20. World Health Organization. The influence of varicocele on parameters of fertility in a large group of men presenting to infertility clinics. Fertility and Sterility 1992;57(6):1289-93.

21. Levinger U, Gornish M, Gat Y, Bachar GN. Is varicocele prevalence increasing with age? Andrologia 2007;39:77-80.

22. Handel LN, Shetty R, Sigman M. The relationship between varicoceles and obesity. J Urol 2006;176:2138-40.

23. Zini A, Boman J, Jarvi K, et al. Varicocelectomy for infertile couples with advanced paternal age. Urology 2008;72:109-13.

24. Pasqualotto FF, Lucon AM, Góes PM, Hallak J, Pasqualotto EB, Arap S. The effect of varicocelectomy on serum hormonal levels in infertile men with clinical varicoceles. Fertil Steril 2003;80:S29.

25. Luigi L, Gentile V, Pigozzi F, Parisi A, Giannetti D, Romanelli F. Physical activity as a possible aggravating factor for athletes with varicocele: impact on the semen profile. Human Reproduction 2001;16:1180-4.

26. Buschi AJ, Harrison RB, Norman A, et al. Distended left renal vein: CT/sonographic normal variant. AJR Am J Roentgenol 1980;135:339-42.

27. Guzick DS, Overstreet JW, Factor-Litvak P, et al. Sperm morphology, motility, and concentration in fertile and infertile men. N Engl J Med 2001;345:1388-93.

28. Pasqualotto FF. Relação do estresse oxidativo, características seminais e diagnósticos clínicos em homens submetidos à investigação infertilidade masculina. Tese de Doutorado apresentada à Faculdade de Medicina da Universidade de São Paulo, 2002, São Paulo, Brazil.

29. Lipshultz LI, Corriere JN Jr. Progressive testicular atrophy in the varicocele patient. J Urol 1977;117:175-6.

30. Pinto KJ, Kroovand RL, Jarow JP. Varicocele related testicular atrophy and its predictive effect upon fertility. J Urol 1994;152(2 Pt 2):788-90.

31. Sigman M, Jarow JP. Ipsilateral testicular hypotrophy is associated with decreased sperm counts in infertile men with varicoceles. J Urol 1997;158:605-7.

32. Zini A, Buckspan M, Berardinucci D, Jarvi K. The influence of clinical and subclinical varicocele on testicular volume. Fertil Steril 1997;68:671-4.

33. MacLeod J. Seminal cytology in the presence of varicocele. Fertil Steril 1965;16:735-57.

34. Ayodeji O, Baker HW. Is there a specific abnormality of sperm morphology in men with varicoceles? Fertil Steril 1986;45:839-42.

35. Pasqualotto FF, Lucon AM, de Goes PM, et al. Semen profile, testicular volume, and hormonal levels in infertile patients with varicocele compared with fertile men with and without varicocele. Fertil Steril 2005;83:74-7.

36. Tanrikut C, Goldstein M. Varicocele repair for the treatment of androgen deficiency. Curr Opin Urol 2010;20:500-2.

37. Zohdy W, Ghazi S, Arafa M. Impact of varicocelectomy on gonadal and erectile functions in men with hypogonadism and infertility. J Sex Med 2010 Aug 16. [Epub ahead of print].

38. Raman JD, Walmsley K, Goldstein M. Inheritance of varicoceles. Urology 2005;65:1186-9.

39. Nistal M, Gonzalez-Peramato P, Serrano A, Regadera J. Physiopathology of the infertile testicle. Etiopathogenesis of varicocele. Arch Esp Urol 2004;57:883-904.

40. Marmar JL, Kim Y. Subinguinal microsurgical varicocelectomy: a technical critique and statistical analysis of semen and pregnancy data. J Urol 1994;152:1127-32.

41. Goldstein M, Gilbert BR, Dicker AP, Dwosh J, Gnecco C. Microsurgical inguinal varicocelectomy with delivery of the testis: an artery and lymphatic sparing technique. J Urol 1992;148:1808-11.

42. Gat Y, Bachar GN, Everaert K, Levinger U, Gornish M. Induction of spermatogenesis in azoospermic men after internal spermatic vein embolization for the treatment of varicocele. Hum Reprod 2005;20:1013-7.

43. Al-Kandari AM, Shabaan H, Ibrahim HM, Elshebiny YN. Shokeir AA. Comparison of outcomes of different varicocelectomy techniques: open inguinal, laparoscopic, and subinguinal microscopic varicocelectomy: a randomized clinical trial. Urology 2007;69:417-20.

44. Yavetz H, Levy R, Papo J, Yogev L, Paz G, Jaffa AJ, Homonnai ZT. Efficacy of varicocele embolization versus ligation of the left internal spermatic vein for improvement of sperm quality. Int J Androl 1992;15:338-44.

45. Nieschlag E, Behre HM, Schlingheider A, Nashan D, Pohl J, Fischedick AR. Surgical ligation vs angiographic embolization of the vena spermatica: a prospective randomized study for the treatment of varicocele-related infertility. Andrologia 1993;25:233-7.

46. Shlansky-Goldberg RD, Van Arsdalen KN, Rutter CM, Soulen MC, Haskal ZJ, Baum RA, Redd DC, Cope C, Pentecost MJ. Percutaneous varicocele embolization versus surgical ligation for the treatment of infertility: changes in seminal parameters and pregnancy outcomes. J Vasc Interv Radiol 1997;8:759-67.

47. Libman J, Jarvi K, Lo K, Zini A. Beneficial effect of microsurgical varicocelectomy is superior for men with bilateral versus unilateral repair. J Urol 2006;176:2602-5.

48. Çayan S, Shavakhabov S, Kadioglu A. Treatment of palpable varicocele in infertile men: a meta-analysis to define the best technique. J Androl 2009;30(1):33-40.

49. Pasqualotto FF, Lucon AM, Hallak J, Goes PM, Saldanha LB, Arap S. Induction of spermatogenesis in azoospermic men undergoing varicocele repair. Hum Reproduction 2003;18:108-12.

50. Schlegel PN, Kaufmann J. Role of varicocelectomy in men with nonobstructive azoospermia. Fertil Steril 2004;81:1585-8.

51. Pasqualotto FF, Sobreiro BP, Hallak J, Pasqualotto EB, Lucon AM. Induction of spermatogenesis in azoospermic men after varicocelectomy repair: an update. Fertil Steril 2006;85:635-9.

52. Weedin JW, Khera M, Lipshultz LI. Varicocele repair in patients with nonobstructive azoospermia: a meta-analysis. J Urol 2010;183:2309-15.

53. Daitch JA, Bedaiwy MA, Pasqualotto EB, Hendin BN, Hallak J, Falcone T, et al. Varicocelectomy improves intrauterine insemination success rates among men with varicocele. J Urol 2001;165:1510-3.

54. Çayan S, Erdemir F, Ozbey I, Turek P, Kadioglu A, Tellaloglu S. Can varicocelectomy significantly change the way couples use assisted reproductive technologies? J Urol 2002;167:1749-52.

55. Penson DF, Paltiel DA, Kramholz HM, Palter S. The cost effectiveness of treatment for varicocele related infertility. J Urol 2002;168:2490-4.

56. Evers JL, Collins JA. Surgery or embolisation in subfertile men: The Cochrane Library, Issue 2007.p.1.

57. Ficarra V, Cerruto MA, Liguori G, Mazzoni G, Minucci S, Tracia A, Gentile V. Treatment of varicocele in subfertile men: The Cochrane Review a contrary opinion. Eur Urol 2006;49(2): 217-9.

58. Marmar JL, Agarwal A, Prabakaran S, Agarwal R, Short RA, Benoff S, Thomas AJ Jr. Reassessing the value of varicocelectomy as a treatment for male subfertility with a new meta-analysis. Fertil Steril 2007.p.13.

59. Fretz PC, Sandlow JI. Varicocele: current concepts in pathophysiology, diagnosis, and treatment. Urol Clin N Am 2002;29: 921-37.

60. Krause W, Muller HH, Schafer H, Weidner W. Does treatment of varicocele improve male fertility? results of the, Deutsche Varikozelenstudie, a multicentre study of 14 collaborating centres. Andrologia 2002;34(3):164-71.

61. Grasso M, Lania C, Castelli M, Galli L, Franzoso F, Rigatti P. Low-grade left varicocele in patients over 30 years old: the effect of spermatic vein ligation on fertility. BJU Int 2000;85(3):305-7.

62. Smit M, Romijn JC, Wildhagen MF, Veldhoven JL, Weber RF, Dohle GR. Decreased sperm DNA fragmentation after surgical varicocelectomy is associated with increased pregnancy rate. J Urol 2010;83:270-4.

63. Benoff S, Gilbert BR. Varicocele and male infertility: Part I Preface. Hum Reprod Update 2001;7:47-54.

64. Al-Kandari AM, Shabaan H, Ibrahim HM, Elshebiny YN, Shokeir AA. Comparison of outcomes of different varicocelectomy techniques: open inguinal, laparoscopic, and subinguinal microscopic varicocelectomy: a randomized clinical trial. Urology 2007;69:417-20.

65. Evers JL, Collin JA, Vandekerckhove P. Surgery or embolisation for varicocele in subfertile men. Cochrane Database Syst Rev 2001;1:CD0000479.

66. Madgar I, Weissenberg R, Lunenfeld B, Karasik A, Goldwasser B. Controlled trial of high spermatic vein ligation for varicocele in infertile men. Fertil Steril 1995;63:120-4.

67. Laven JS, Haans LC, Malli WP, Te Velde ER, Wensing CJ, Eimers JM. Effects of varicocele treatment in adolescents: a randomized study. Fertil Steril 1992;58:756-62.

68. Kass EJ, Stork BR, Steinert BW. Varicocele in adolescence induces left and right testicular volume loss. BJU International 2001;87(6):499-501.

69. Alukal JP, Zurakowski D, Atala A, et al. Testicular hypotrophy does not correlate with grade of adolescent varicocele. J Urol 2005;174(6):2367-70.

70. Podesta ML, Gottlieb S, Medel R, Ropelato G, Bergada C, Quesada E. Hormonal parameters and testicular volume in children and adolescents with unilateral varicocele: preoperative and postoperative findings. J Urol 1994;152:794-7.

71. Diamond D. Adolescente varicocele. Curr Opin Urol 2007;17(4): 263-7.

72. Ku JH, Kim SW, Park K, Paick JS. Benefits of microsurgical repair of adolescent varicocele: comparison of semen parameters in fertile and infertile adults with varicocele. Urology 2005;65:554-8.

73. Glassberg KI, Korets R. Update on the management of adolescent varicocele. F1000 Med Rep 2010;2:25.

74. Schlegel PN. Is assisted reproduction the optimal treatment for varicocele-associated male infertility? A cost-effectiveness analysis. Urology 1997;49:83-90.

75. Penson DF, Paltiel DA, Kramholz HM, Palter S. The cost effectiveness of treatment for varicocele related infertility. J Urol 2002;168:2490-4.

76. Agarwal A, Deepinder F, Cocuzza M, Agarwal R, Shart RA, Sabanegh E, Marmar JL. Efficacy of varicocelectomy in improving semen parameters: new meta-analytic approach. Urology 2007;70:532-8.

The literature reports a high SRR with MESA with rates over 90 percent.[16] The rates of complication are acceptably low and minor. The significant drawbacks of MESA are the added expense associated with the increased anesthetic requirement, the need for an open approach, and the need for an operating microscope. As is the case with PESA, MESA is not suitable for men with NOA.

Testis

Testicular Sperm Aspiration

There are a variety of techniques for testicular sperm aspiration (TESA) to include fine needle aspiration (FNA), large needle cutting (or "coarse") biopsy (LNCB), and large needle aspiration biopsy (LNAB). Percutaneous methods have the advantage of decreased anesthetic requirements and operative time and, therefore, less expense as compared to the open testicular techniques. Unlike the epididymal approaches, the percutaneous testis procedures are suitable for men with NOA, but SRR vary (see below). It is helpful to conceive of these methods as having two main objectives, the first being diagnostic (i.e. provide information in anticipation of future intervention) and the second being therapeutic (provide sperm in preparation for IVF/ICSI). FNA can be diagnostic or therapeutic depending on the quantity of the sperm retrieved and the intent of the operation. FNA does not provide material suitable for histopathologic analysis. LNCB and LNAB both provide tissue adequate for histology and may provide adequate sperm for IVF/ICSI depending on the robustness of the sample and the underlying pathology.

The percutaneous testicular sperm retrieval methods all begin with the surgeon orienting and fixing the selected testis in the scrotum in an appropriately anesthetized and prepped patient. Spermatic cord block and skin anesthesia are adequate for FNA and LNAB while men undergoing LNCB may require sedation. For FNA the surgeon inserts a small bore needle (typically 20–23 gauge) into the testicular parenchyma. Negative pressure is then applied to the syringe while the surgeon gently passes the needle through the testicular parenchyma in varying directions (**Fig. 20.1**). A syringe holder, such as the Cameco, can facilitate the procedure. The tubing is clamped before the needle is removed from the tissue and the resulting aspirate is evaluated. The procedure may be repeated. The technique for LNAB is similar to FNA except a larger bore needle (typically 18–22 gauge) is used. LNCB uses a 14–18 gauge stand alone biopsy needle (such as the Tru-Cut biopsy needle) or a similar sized biopsy needle incorporated into a biopsy gun (such as that used for prostate needle biopsy). A small skin incision may facilitate passage of the needle. The surgeon advances the needle up to or into the testicular parenchymal and then performs the biopsy. The procedure is repeated as needed to obtain adequate samples.

As would be expected, the TESA SRR for men with OA is high (90%) and therefore the discussion herein will be tailored towards men with NOA.[17] The impact of testis histology and the random sampling obtained by needle biopsy explain both the variability in published SRR for TESA and the lower overall SRR achieved with TESA as compared to open testis biopsy. Hauser et al. 2006 reported a FNA SRR of 24.1 versus 62.1 percent in NOA men who underwent FNA immediately followed by open testicular biopsies.[18] Turek et al. reported SRR 47 percent in NOA men who underwent multiple FNA of the testes to procedure a diagnostic map of spermatogenesis. Notably of the NOA men with sperm found on FNA that elected to proceed to sperm harvest, Turek reported subsequent sperm retrieval for ICSI was successful in 93 percent.[19] Houwen et al. and Vicari et al. report similarly high SRR with TESA in NOA men 45.9 and 47.3 percent respectively.[17,20] For comparison, much lower overall SRR rates were reported by Mercan et al. Ezeh et al. and El-Haggar et al. at 14, 14 and 10 percent respectively.[21-23] The impact of histology on SRR is supported by these studies as higher TESA SRR rates reported for hypospermatogenesis as compared to maturation arrest and Sertoli cell only.

Pain necessitating sedation during the procedure and post-procedure hematoma have been reported more frequently for LNCB than FNA or LNAB techniques, but overall the rate of complications is acceptably low and minor with all TESA methods.[24] Patients should be counseled that repeat or additional procedures may be necessary after successful TESA as less tissue and therefore typically fewer sperm are obtained as compared to an open biopsy. Generally this limitation is offset by the low rate of complication, relative ease, and decreased expense of TESA versus open procedures.

Testicular Sperm Extraction

Open testicular sperm extraction (TESE) for NOA has good overall SRR with typical rates between 40–50 percent. SRR are influenced by underlying testicular histology and a variety of procedures meet the definition of testicular sperm extraction—both of which complicate the comparison of outcomes among published reports. Commonly practiced variations for testicular sperm extraction include unilateral versus bilateral biopsies, single versus multiple biopsies, surgery with and without optical magnification, and selection of tubules based on their appearance under optical magnification versus random sampling. During the following discussion cTESE will refer to conventional testicular sperm extraction wherein the seminiferous tubules are sampled randomly. The mTESE will refer to microscopic testicular sperm extraction wherein tubules are sampled based on their appearance under optical magnification. Notably there is only one trial wherein outcomes from cTESE and mTESE were randomized and compared. The balance of the remaining published reports examined case series or compared outcomes with patients serving as their own controls. Nevertheless, some useful conclusions can be drawn from the published data.

All TESE techniques begin with a properly anesthetized and prepped patient. While a limited biopsy may be done with local and locoregional anesthetic, more extensive procedures typically require a regional or general anesthesia. The scrotum and tunica vaginalis are opened as previous described. For unilateral single site cTESE the tunica albuginea is inspected, a small incision is made through an avascular plane, the testis is gentle squeezed and the extruded tubules sharply removed and sent for analysis. Hemostasis is obtained and the tunica albuginea is closed with fine suture. The procedure may be repeated on the contralateral side. The premise for single biopsy cTESE is that given the heterogeneity in spermatogenesis in many men with NOA, the relatively larger amount of tissue is more likely to detect mature sperm. There is no proscribed area of the testis for single site cTESE however the anterior midline surface in the mid to upper half of the testis is frequently selected. Optical magnification may aid with hemostasis and tunical closure.

Unilateral or bilateral multiple site cTESE presumes that smaller samples from a variety of areas of the testis are more likely to reveal areas of active sperm production than one large sample. The initial surgical approach is described above except several, typically two to four, small incisions are made through avascular planes overlying the upper, mid, and lower poles of the testis. Smaller samples are removed and assessed for sperm production and/or sent for histopathology. The procedure may be repeated on the contralateral testicle. Hemostasis is obtained and the tunica is closed with fine suture.

The mTESE presumes that active spermatogenesis can be detected based on the appearance of the seminiferous tubules. After appropriate prepping and draping, the testis is delivered and the tunica vaginalis is opened. An avascular plane near the midline is selected and an equatorial incision is made to expose a broad swath of tubules. Optical magnification is used to select engorged, opalescent appearing tubules which are then removed and assessed for sperm production (**Fig. 20.2**). Gentle traction on the cut edges of the tunica will open the testicular parenchyma along a natural plane of cleavage and expose down to the mediastinum testis. The lobules can likewise be peeled apart with

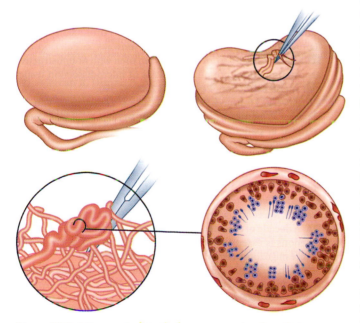

Figure 20.2: Microsurgical testicular sperm extraction. A transverse, near circumferential incision is made through the tunica at the midpole of the testis while taking care to minimize disruption of the subtunical vessels. Gentle traction will separate the lobules of the parenchyma along natural cleavage planes. Optical magnification is used to select engorged appearing seminiferous tubules for harvest

gentle traction allowing the surgeon to inspect a large area of the parenchyma. Hemostasis is obtained and the tunica is closed with fine suture.

OUTCOMES

Mean SRR for TESE is 49.5 percent with a range of 16.7–86.6 percent.[25] This variation is influenced by a variety of factors to include impact of histopathology, difference in TESE techniques and inclusion of men with previous successful sperm retrieval or unappreciated OA. The published data favors multiple biopsies cTESE over single biopsy cTESE and is highlighted by the following studies. In 1999, Amer et al. compared the outcomes of single versus multiple biopsy cTESE in 316 NOA men and found a significantly greater SRR with multiple biopsy (49%) versus single biopsy (37.5%).[26] Hauser et al. performed bilateral cTESE with three predetermined biopsy sites in each testis in 29 men with NOA and reported SRR rates of 28.6, 17.9, and 53.6 percent when only one, two, or all three sites were considered.[27] A notable outlier is Fahmy et al. who performed immediate single large bilateral cTESE versus multiple bilateral cTESE in a group of NOA men who had no sperm found on initial small cTESE. SRR (defined as the presence of spermatozoa or late spermatids) were comparable between the two groups at 29.5 and 26.7 percent for groups 1 and 2 respectively.[28] The strategy for allocating patients and selecting the additional biopsy sites was not described in the abstract, however, the authors did report that equal amounts of tissue (250–500 mg) were removed with both techniques.

Comparison of published SRR with cTESE versus mTESE reveals better SRR with mTESE. In 2000, Amer et al. reported SRR of 30 versus 47 percent in 100 NOA men with identical histopathology in both testes who underwent cTESE on one side and mTESE on the other.[29] Okada et al. published SRR of 16.7 percent for cTESE compared to 44.6 percent for mTESE in a series of NOA men and noted that success was influenced by histopathology with mTESE yielding the highest SRR in hypospermatogenesis (100%) followed by maturation arrest (75%) and Sertoli cell only (33.9%).[4] In 2007 Ramasamy et al. published a series of 176 NOA men who underwent salvage mTESE. SRR were 56 and 51 percent for men who had undergone 1 and 2 previous negative biopsies respectively and 45 percent in the 20 men who had failed previous cTESE.[30] Tsujimura et al. reported an overall SSR of 44 percent in 134 NOA men who underwent mTESE which included a SSR of 47.8 percent for salvage mTESE after bilateral single site cTESE and 33.3 percent for salvage mTESE after bilateral multiple site cTESE.[31] These studies confirm a role for mTESE in NOA men who have failed previous attempts at sperm retrieval.

Colpi et al. reported results of a trial in which 154 NOA men were allocated by means of their operative date to undergo mTESE versus single biopsy cTESE with both groups proceeding to contralateral single biopsy cTESE if no sperm were detected within 10 minutes. Histopathology was determined for all testes. One hundred ninety four testicles were sampled, 78 by mTESE and 117 by cTESE, and subsequently categorized into one of 48 potential blocks based on testicular volume, FSH, and histopathology. Data was then randomized by pairing mTESE testis

Section V

Intrauterine Insemination

Intrauterine Insemination in the Era of Assisted Reproduction

Hassan N Sallam, Botros RMB Rizk

■ INTRODUCTION

Artificial insemination is the oldest and simplest method of assisted conception. It entails the deposition of the husband's semen inside the female genital tract of the wife. Three types of artificial insemination must be distinguished:

Intravaginal Insemination

Here, the native (unprocessed) semen sample is deposited inside the vagina using a suitable cannula. This technique is only of help in cases where the sperm cannot be deposited inside the vagina through sexual intercourse, e.g. in cases of dyspareunia on the part of the wife or impotence on the part of the husband.

Intracervical Insemination

Here, the native (unprocessed) semen sample is deposited in the cervical mucus using a suitable cannula in order to improve the chances of pregnancy. As in the case of intravaginal insemination, intracevical insemination does not increases the chances of pregnancy above natural coitus and is only of value in cases of impotence or when physical disability prevents normal sexual intercourse.

Intrauterine Insemination of Processed Semen

As mentioned previously, the success of *in vitro* fertilization has led to a better understanding of the *in vivo* fertilization procedures. Intrauterine insemination of native (unprocessed) semen, practiced before the era of IVF, did not result in improving the pregnancy rate and usually resulted in painful contractions and expulsion of the semen outside the uterus. This is because the native semen contains prostaglandins and other prostatic and seminal plasma constituents which have to be removed before the spermatozoa reach the uterine cavity. The success of IVF has led to a better understanding of fertilization *in vivo*. Intrauterine insemination should therefore be carried out after processing the semen sample, i.e. separating the spermatozoa from the seminal plasma and resuspending them in a culture medium similar to the fallopian tube environment.

■ INDICATIONS

Intrauterine insemination (IUI) is used for the treatment of infertility in the following clinical conditions (**Fig. 21.1** and **Flow chart 21.1**):

Male Factor Infertility

Here, the postcoital test is negative due to oligo, terato and/or asthenospermia. The cervical mucus is good (score 8 or more) but no or very few spermatozoa are found in the cervical mucus.

Cervical Factor Infertility

Here, the post-coital test is negative despite the presence of repeatedly normal seminal fluid analyzes. The problem lies in the cervical mucus and the cervical score is less than 8.

Unexplained Infertility

Here, the postcoital test is positive and intrauterine insemination is performed to increase the chances of pregnancy by increasing the number of spermatozoa reaching the ampullary end of the fallopian tube. This is usually accompanied by controlled ovarian hyperstimulation (COH) to increase the number of ovarian follicles.

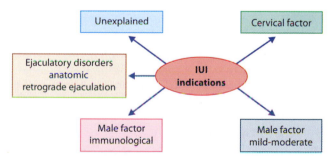

Figure 21.1: IUI first line treatment. Modified with permission from Sallam HN, Rizk B. Intrauterine Insemination. *Source*: In: Rizk B, Sallan HN (Eds). Clinical Infertility and *In Vitro* Fertilization. New Delhi: Jaypee Brothers Medical Publishers, 2012. Chapter 28, 236

Flow chart 21.1: Algorithm for male subfertility treatment. Modified with permission from Ombelet W. IVF for the developing countries. 30 years of IVF, Second Alexandria Forum for Women's Health. Alexandria, Egypt. March 2008

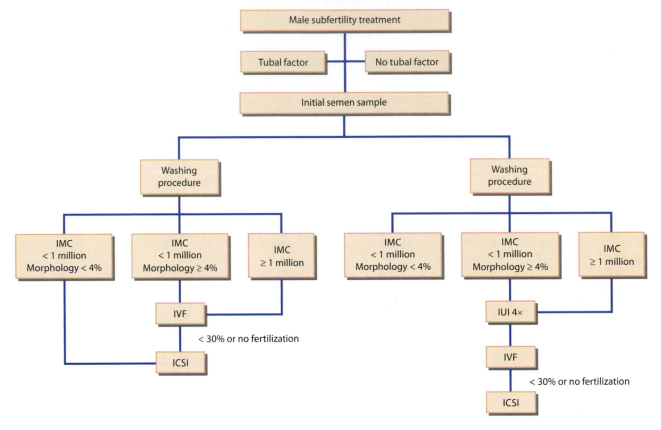

STIMULATION PROTOCOLS

Although IUI can be performed in a spontaneous (non-stimulated) cycle, most workers in the field prefer to perform it during a stimulated cycle to increase the chances of pregnancy (**Figs 21.2 to 21.7**). Many stimulation protocols have been used but the most common are the following:

Clomiphene Citrate

In this protocol, clomiphene citrate 50–200 mg/day are given orally and started on day 1, 2, 3 or 5 of the menstrual cycle. Multiple follicular development occurs in 30–40 percent of the patients (Sallam et al., 1983).

Human Menopausal Gonadotrophin

In this protocol, 2–3 HMG ampoules are administered by intramuscular injection starting on day 5 of the cycle. The response is monitored with ultrasound scanning of the ovarian follicles and the dose is adjusted accordingly. Multiple follicular development

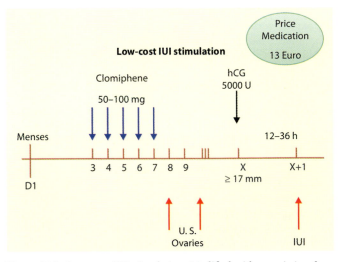

Figure 21.2: Low cost IUI stimulation. Modified with permission from Ombelet W. IVF for the developing countries. 30 years of IVF, Second Alexandria Forum for Women's Health. Alexandria, Egypt. March 2008

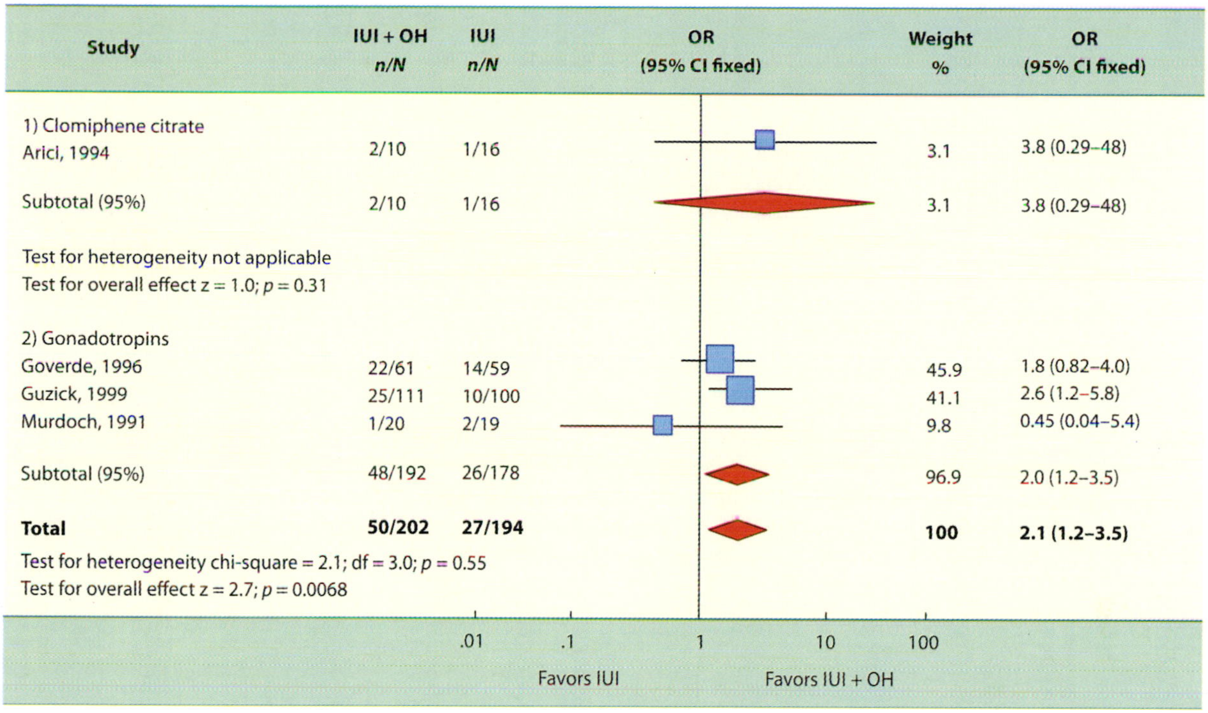

Study	IUI + OH n/N	IUI n/N	OR (95% CI fixed)	Weight %	OR (95% CI fixed)
1) Clomiphene citrate					
Arici, 1994	2/10	1/16		3.1	3.8 (0.29–48)
Subtotal (95%)	2/10	1/16		3.1	3.8 (0.29–48)
Test for heterogeneity not applicable					
Test for overall effect z = 1.0; p = 0.31					
2) Gonadotropins					
Goverde, 1996	22/61	14/59		45.9	1.8 (0.82–4.0)
Guzick, 1999	25/111	10/100		41.1	2.6 (1.2–5.8)
Murdoch, 1991	1/20	2/19		9.8	0.45 (0.04–5.4)
Subtotal (95%)	48/192	26/178		96.9	2.0 (1.2–3.5)
Total	**50/202**	**27/194**		**100**	**2.1 (1.2–3.5)**
Test for heterogeneity chi-square = 2.1; df = 3.0; p = 0.55					
Test for overall effect z = 2.7; p = 0.0068					

.01   .1   1   10   100

Favors IUI   Favors IUI + OH

Figure 21.3: IUI in natural cycle versus IUI in stimulated cycles. Outcome: live birth rate per couple. Modified with permission from Veltman-Verhulst S, Cohlen BJ, Hughes E, Heineman MJ. Intrauterine insemination for unexplained subfertility. Cochrane Database of Systematic Reviews 2006;4:CD001838

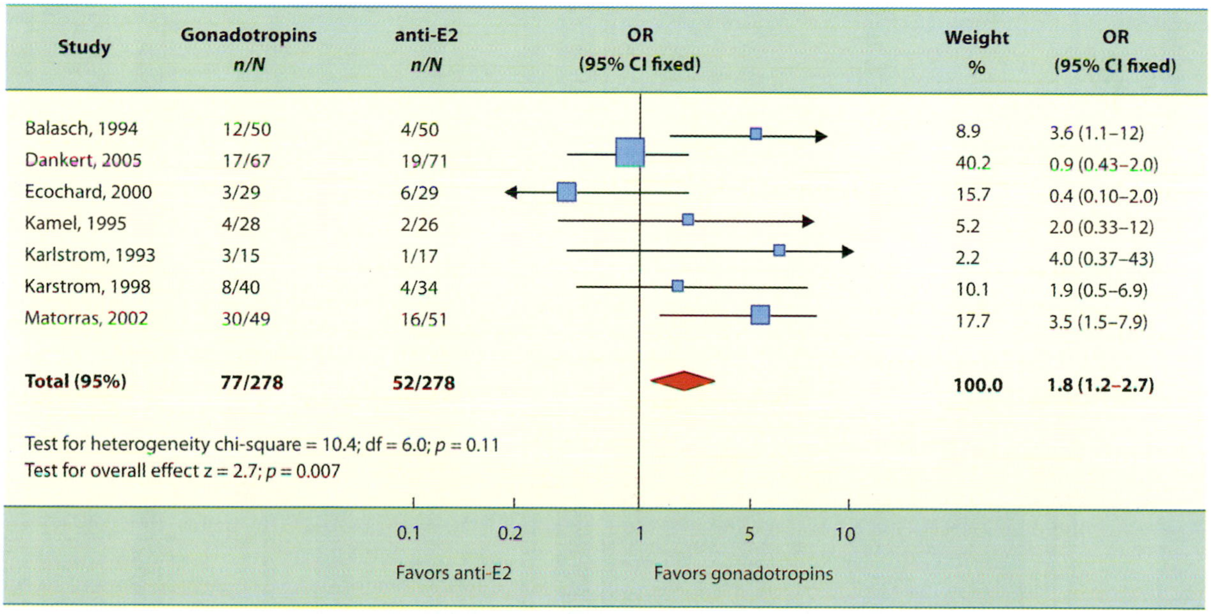

Study	Gonadotropins n/N	anti-E2 n/N	OR (95% CI fixed)	Weight %	OR (95% CI fixed)
Balasch, 1994	12/50	4/50		8.9	3.6 (1.1–12)
Dankert, 2005	17/67	19/71		40.2	0.9 (0.43–2.0)
Ecochard, 2000	3/29	6/29		15.7	0.4 (0.10–2.0)
Kamel, 1995	4/28	2/26		5.2	2.0 (0.33–12)
Karlstrom, 1993	3/15	1/17		2.2	4.0 (0.37–43)
Karstrom, 1998	8/40	4/34		10.1	1.9 (0.5–6.9)
Matorras, 2002	30/49	16/51		17.7	3.5 (1.5–7.9)
Total (95%)	**77/278**	**52/278**		**100.0**	**1.8 (1.2–2.7)**
Test for heterogeneity chi-square = 10.4; df = 6.0; p = 0.11					
Test for overall effect z = 2.7; p = 0.007					

0.1   0.2   1   5   10

Favors anti-E2   Favors gonadotropins

Figure 21.4: Antiestrogens versus gonadotropins combined with intrauterine insemination. Outcome: pregnancy rate per couple. Modified with permission from Cantineau AE, Cohlen BJ, Heineman MJ. Ovarian stimulation protocols (antiestrogens, gonadotrophins with and without GnRH agonists/antagonists) for intrauterine insemination (IUI) in women with subfertility. Cochrane Database Systematic Reviews 2007;2:CD005356

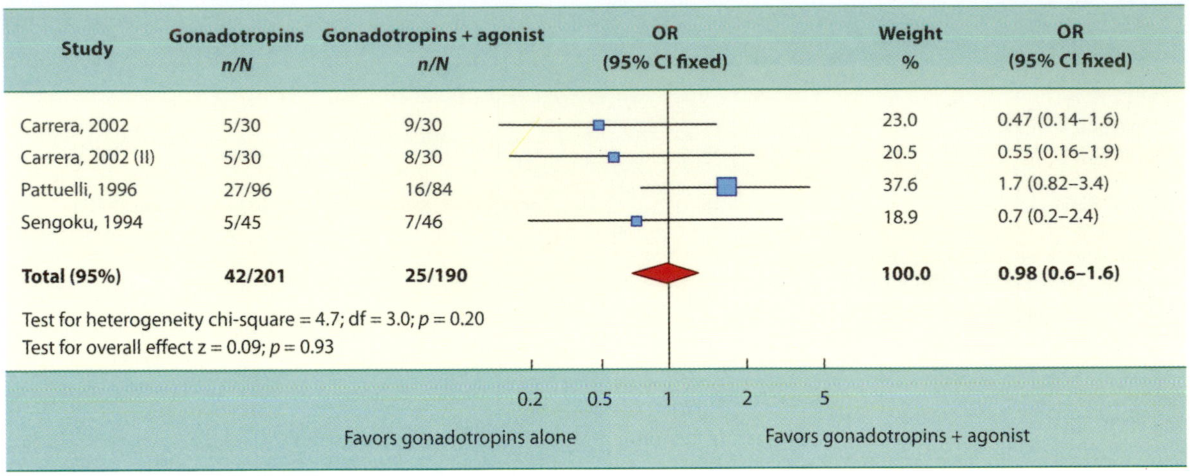

Study	Gonadotropins n/N	Gonadotropins + agonist n/N	OR (95% CI fixed)	Weight %	OR (95% CI fixed)
Carrera, 2002	5/30	9/30		23.0	0.47 (0.14–1.6)
Carrera, 2002 (II)	5/30	8/30		20.5	0.55 (0.16–1.9)
Pattuelli, 1996	27/96	16/84		37.6	1.7 (0.82–3.4)
Sengoku, 1994	5/45	7/46		18.9	0.7 (0.2–2.4)
Total (95%)	**42/201**	**25/190**		**100.0**	**0.98 (0.6–1.6)**

Test for heterogeneity chi-square = 4.7; df = 3.0; p = 0.20
Test for overall effect z = 0.09; p = 0.93

0.2 0.5 1 2 5
Favors gonadotropins alone | Favors gonadotropins + agonist

Figure 21.5: Gonadotropins alone versus gonadotropins with GnRH agonist. Outcome: pregnancy rate per couple. Modified with permission from Cantineau AE, Cohlen BJ, Heineman MJ. Ovarian stimulation protocols (antiestrogens, gonadotrophins with and without GnRH agonists/antagonists) for intrauterine insemination (IUI) in women with subfertility. Cochrane Database Systematic Reviews 2007;2:CD005356

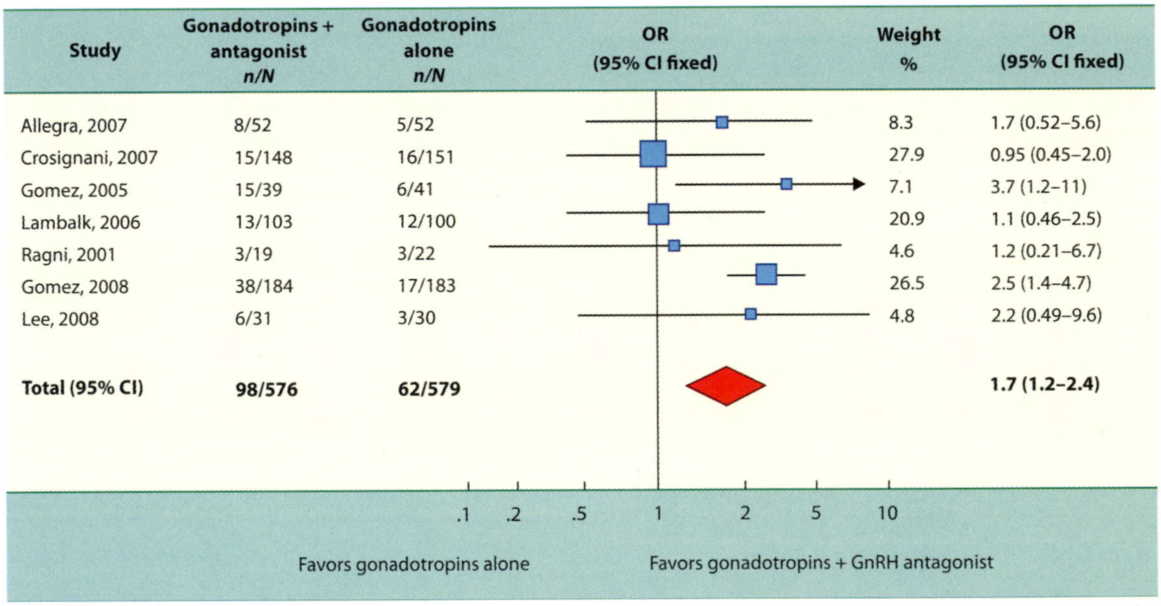

Study	Gonadotropins + antagonist n/N	Gonadotropins alone n/N	OR (95% CI fixed)	Weight %	OR (95% CI fixed)
Allegra, 2007	8/52	5/52		8.3	1.7 (0.52–5.6)
Crosignani, 2007	15/148	16/151		27.9	0.95 (0.45–2.0)
Gomez, 2005	15/39	6/41		7.1	3.7 (1.2–11)
Lambalk, 2006	13/103	12/100		20.9	1.1 (0.46–2.5)
Ragni, 2001	3/19	3/22		4.6	1.2 (0.21–6.7)
Gomez, 2008	38/184	17/183		26.5	2.5 (1.4–4.7)
Lee, 2008	6/31	3/30		4.8	2.2 (0.49–9.6)
Total (95% CI)	**98/576**	**62/579**			**1.7 (1.2–2.4)**

.1 .2 .5 1 2 5 10
Favors gonadotropins alone | Favors gonadotropins + GnRH antagonist

Figure 21.6: Gonadotropins alone versus gonadotropins with GnRH antagonist. Outcome: ongoing pregnancy rate per couple. Modified with permission from Cohlen BJ, Cantineau AE. Mild ovarian hyperstimulation in combination with intrauterine insemination. In: Aboulghar M, Rizk B (Eds). Ovarian Stimulation. Cambridge: Cambridge University Press, 2011. Chapter 3, 30

occurs in most of the patients. HCG is administered when the response is optimum, i.e. when the leading follicle reaches 18 mm in diameter (Sallam et al., 1982).

Down Regulation Protocols

In these protocols, short acting GnRH analogues are administered by the subcutaneous or intranasal routes before starting the HMG injections. Alternatively, a long acting GnRH analogue is administered intramuscularly before starting HMG. These protocols are too complicated for IUI and are usually used in *in vitro* fertilization or intracytoplasmic sperm injection as described in chapter 17.

■ SEMEN PROCESSING

As mentioned before, native semen cannot be injected directly inside the uterine cavity. This usually produced painful

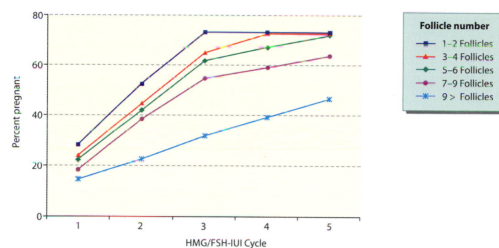

Figure 21.7: Cumulative pregnancy rate in relation to number of preovulatory follicles 10 mm or larger for first five cycles of hMG or FSH-IUI. Modified with permission from Dickey R. In: Rizk B, Garcia-Velasco JA, Sallam HN, Makrigiannakis A (Eds). Infertility and Assisted Reproduction. Cambridge: Cambridge University Press, 2008. Chapter 28, 262

contractions expelling the semen outside the uterus. The native semen must therefore be processed first in order to separate the spermatozoa from the seminal plasma. This can be carried out by one of the following methods (Mortimer, 1991):[1-8]

Swim up Method

In this method, the semen is overlayed with an equal amount of culture medium in a sterile test tube. This culture medium is a balanced salt solution occasionally enriched by amino acids with a pH of 7.4 and an osmolarity of 280 mOsm/L. The test tube is left in the incubator for 30–60 minutes. Healthy spermatozoa migrate upwards from the native semen to the culture medium. The supernatant, containing these healthy spermatozoa, is then removed and centrifuged in a new test tube at 600 g for 5–10 minutes. The pellet is then resuspended in 0.5–1 mL and this is used for the insemination.

Percoll Gradients

In this method, Percoll, a silica-like substance is used to filter the healthy spermatozoa. Percoll is mixed with the culture medium in different concentrations and these are layered with the most concentrated fraction placed in the bottom of the tube, e.g. 60, 70, 80 and 90 percent. The semen is then deposited on top of the Percoll and the tube is centrifuged for about 30 minutes. In this case, the healthy spermatozoa capable of penetrating the higher concentrations of Percoll are deposited at the bottom of the tube. This pellet is then removed and resuspended in 0.5–1 mL of culture medium and this is used for the insemination. If the concentration of the semen permits, the pellet can be used for a swim up step before its final preparation. Mini-Percoll gradients are sometimes used if the concentration of the semen is low. In this case, 2 layers only are used (e.g. 40 and 80%). Other substances have been used to prepare similar gradient methods (e.g. Ficoll, Nicodenz, etc.).

Sperm Washing

This simple method can only be used when the semen is normal or when the only problem is oligospermia. In these cases, the semen is mixed with an excess volume of culture medium (e.g. 2–3 times) and the mixture is centrifuged. The pellet is then resuspended in 0.5–1 mL and this is used for the insemination. This method has the disadvantages of retaining dead spermatozoa and other debris. These produce unwanted reactive oxygen species (ROS) which in turn induce peroxidation of the sperm plasma membrane phospholipids impairing sperm function (Aitken and Clarkson, 1988).

Problem Samples

Increased viscosity of the semen may be treated by passing the sample into needles of decreasing diameters or by the addition of a proteolytic enzyme (e.g. chemotrypsin). In cases of athenospermia, sperm motility can be increased by adding caffeine, pentoxifyllin or 2-deoxy-adenosine (2DA) (Tesarik et al., 1992).

■ TIMING OF INSEMINATION

Insemination should be carried out during the maximum fertile period of the wife. Many methods have been described to determine the maximum fertile period and these are detailed in chapters 7 and 22. However, the two practical and most commonly used methods rare the following:

Serial Measurement of Beta

HCG in urine, serum or saliva. This can be determined using immuno-assay techniques, however, simpler dip-stick methods are now available. These depend on changing their color or giving a similar signal once the concentration of beta-HCG reaches a certain threshold. This method is suitable if insemination is performed during a spontaneous (unstimulated) cycle or in patients receiving clomiphene citrate.

Serial Ultrasound Scanning of the Follicles

This is described in chapter 22. The patients are serially examined by abdominal or vaginal sonography to visualize the developing follicles. The maximum fertile period starts when the leading follicle reaches 18 mm in diameter (Marinho et al, 1982; Sallam, 1983). This method is suitable in spontaneous cycles as well as cycles stimulated with clomiphene citrate or HMG.

TECHNIQUE

With the patient in the lithotomy position, the cervix is exposed using a suitable speculum. The cervix can be stabilized in position using a vulsellum. After cleaning the cervix with a cotton swab, the processed semen is slowly deposited inside the uterine cavity using a plastic cannula attached to a 1 mL plastic syringe. Different cannulas and various insemination devices have been described but none has shown its particular superiority. The insemination is carried out once or twice during the same cycle on successive or alternate days. A recent study showed that performing IUI on two successive days significant increases the pregnancy rate (Ragni et al, 1999).

RESULTS

In a recent meta-analysis of 22 studies including 5214 treatment cycles, Hughes found that the mean fecundity rate (i.e. the percentage of patients pregnant after one cycle of treatment) was 9.8 percent. The fecundity rate was 6 percent in unstimulated cycles, 7 percent in patients receiving clomiphene citrate and 15 percent in patients stimulated with HMG. The study also found that IUI alone or HMG alone resulted in a 2-fold increase in the pregnancy rate compared to natural intercourse and that the combination of both HMG and IUI resulted in a 5-fold increase in the pregnancy rate.

REFERENCES

1. Aitken RJ, Clarkson JS. Significance of reactive oxygen species and antioxidants in defining the efficacy of sperm preparation techniques. J Androl 1988;9:367.
2. Hughes EG. The effectiveness of ovulation induction and intrauterine insemination in the treatment of persistent infertility: a meta-analysis. Hum Reprod 1997;9:1865.
3. Marinho AO, Sallam HN, Campbell S, et al. Real time pelvic ultrasonography during the periovulatory period of patients attending an AID clinic. Fertil Steril 1982;37:633.
4. Mortimer D. Sperm preparation techniques and iatrogenic failures of *in vitro* fertilization. Hum Reprod 1991;6:173.
5. Ragni G, Maggioni P, Guermandi E. Efficacy of double insemination in controlled ovarian hyperstimulation cycles. Fertil Steril 1999;72:619.
6. Sallam RN, Marinho AO, Campbell S, et al. Monitoring gonadotrophin therapy with real-time ultrasound scanning of ovarian follicles. Br J Obstet Gynaecol 1982;89:155.
7. Sallam HN. Biophysical and biochemical approaches to ovarian function. PhD thesis, University of London, 1983.
8. Tesarik J, Thebault A, Testart J. Effect of pentoxifyllin on sperm movement characteristics in normozoospermic and asthenozoospermic specimens. Hum Reprod 1992;7:1257.

22

Ovarian Stimulation for Intrauterine Insemination

Sudha Ranganathan, Botros RMB Rizk

INTRODUCTION

Although the concept of artificial insemination was first introduced 200 years ago by John Hunter,[1] it was only after the success and better understanding of *in vitro fertilization* (IVF) in the 1980s that the procedure became very popular. In the beginning, intrauterine insemination (IUI) was performed using unprocessed semen, which was associated with painful uterine contractions and expulsion of semen without increasing pregnancy rate. The current trend is to employ sperm preparation techniques applied in IVF for IUI in either natural or stimulated cycles.

The main indications for IUI are male factor infertility, cervical factor infertility, ovulation dysfunction, mild or minimal endometriosis, and unexplained infertility. The rationale of combining ovarian stimulation and IUI is to increase the number of available oocytes and the density of healthy motile sperms close to each other around the time of fertilization, enhancing the probability of conception. The use of ovarian hyper stimulation may also correct subtle cycle disorders and allows for optimal timing of the insemination. In this chapter, we analyzed the ovarian stimulation used in IUI protocols.

NATURAL VERSUS STIMULATED CYCLES

The success of IUI depends on the type of infertility, whether it is done in stimulated or natural cycles, and the type of drugs used for ovarian stimulation (**Figs 22.1 to 22.8**). Cohlen et al. (1998) found that in couples with male subfertility, IUI + COH (controlled ovarian hyperstimulation) with gonadotropins led to higher conception rate when the total motile sperm (TMS) count is $> 10 \times 10^2$. They found no significant difference in conception rate if clomiphene citrate (CC) is used for COH or when TMC $< 10 \times 10^6$.[2] NICE guidelines (National Institute of clinical excellence-2004 guidelines) recommend IUI without ovarian stimulation to manage male factor fertility problems (as it is no more clinically effective than unstimulated IUI and has the risk of multiple pregnancy) and IUI + COH to manage minimal or mild endometriosis, as it is uncertain whether or not unstimulated IUI may also be beneficial.[3]

Many randomized trials among couples with unexplained infertility have reported that IUI in stimulated cycles improves probability of conception compared to natural cycles (OR 2.0,

95% CI 2-3.5) or with ovulation induction alone (**Fig. 22.1**).[4-8] To obtain an additional pregnancy it has been estimated that 40 cycles with empiric clomiphene therapy or 37 cycles of IUI without stimulation would be needed when compared with COH + IUI.[9] In conclusion, IUI in natural cycles could be beneficial in mild male factor infertility and cervical hostility, as the pregnancy rate is not compromised and has a lower risk of multiple pregnancy and ovarian hyperstimulation syndrome: For unexplained infertility and mild endometriosis, IUI + COH is recommended as it clearly improves the conception rate.

OVARIAN STIMULATION PROTOCOLS

In contrast to ovulation induction in oligo or an-ovulatory women, which aims at mono-follicular development, super ovulation (SO) or controlled ovarian hyperstimulation (COH) is aimed at development and maturation of multiple follicles in already ovulating women to enhance overall cycle fecundity. There is no universally agreed protocol or guidelines for COH with IUI. However, many consider the duration and type of infertility, age of the couple, response of individual patient to different drug regimen, and the risk and cost in deciding the drugs and dosages to individual couples.

The fertility medications most commonly used in stimulation protocols for IUI are the following:

Antiestrogens

Clomiphene citrate (CC) is the most commonly used oral drug in dosages ranging from 50–250 mg daily for five days given on day 2-6 of cycle in Europe and day 5-9 of cycle in the United States. It is a non-steroidal selective estrogen receptor modulator which competitively blocks the hypothalamic estrogen receptors signaling hypoestrogenic state. This leads to an increase in endogenous gonadotropin secretion and subsequent ovulation induction. It does not need extensive monitoring and is associated with lower risks of OHSS and multiple pregnancy when compared to gonadotropins.[10] Convenience, low cost and relative safety of the drug makes it a popular option. In a large Cochrane review (2007), Cantineau and Cohlen analyzed 43 randomized controlled trials, comparing different ovarian stimulation protocols followed by IUI. They pooled seven studies comparing

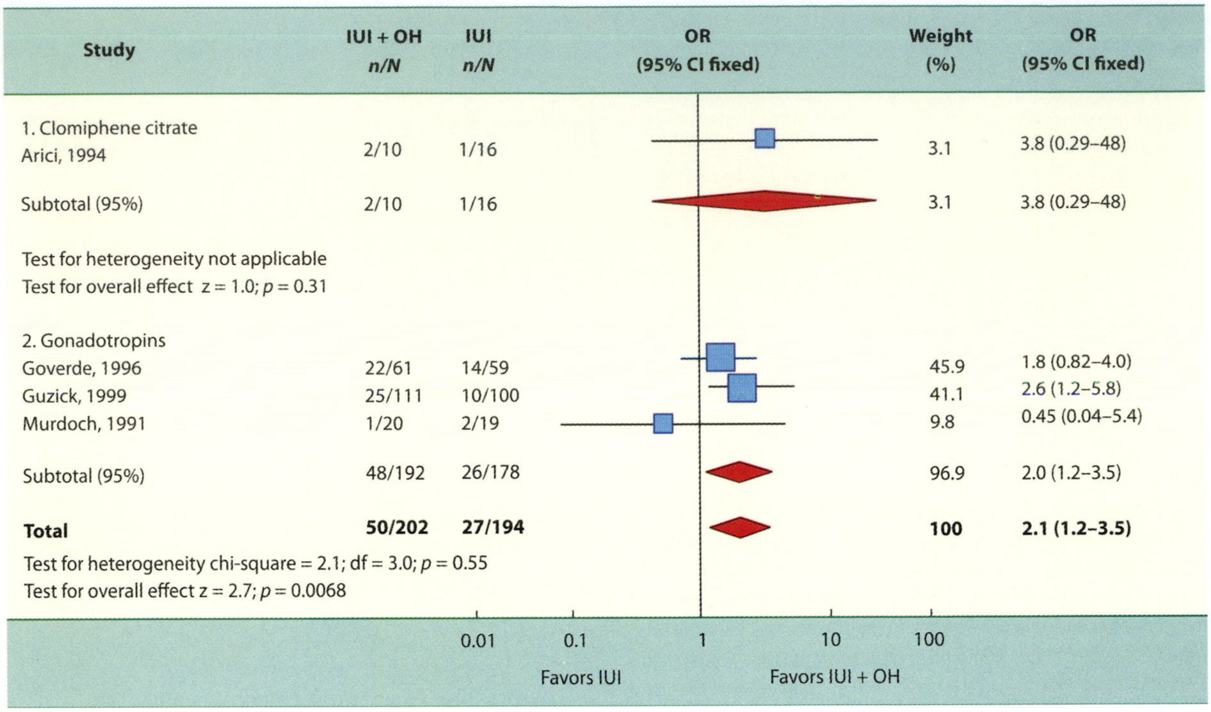

Study	IUI + OH n/N	IUI n/N	OR (95% CI fixed)	Weight (%)	OR (95% CI fixed)
1. Clomiphene citrate					
Arici, 1994	2/10	1/16		3.1	3.8 (0.29–48)
Subtotal (95%)	2/10	1/16		3.1	3.8 (0.29–48)
Test for heterogeneity not applicable					
Test for overall effect z = 1.0; p = 0.31					
2. Gonadotropins					
Goverde, 1996	22/61	14/59		45.9	1.8 (0.82–4.0)
Guzick, 1999	25/111	10/100		41.1	2.6 (1.2–5.8)
Murdoch, 1991	1/20	2/19		9.8	0.45 (0.04–5.4)
Subtotal (95%)	48/192	26/178		96.9	2.0 (1.2–3.5)
Total	**50/202**	**27/194**		**100**	**2.1 (1.2–3.5)**
Test for heterogeneity chi-square = 2.1; df = 3.0; p = 0.55					
Test for overall effect z = 2.7; p = 0.0068					

0.01   0.1   1   10   100

Favors IUI   Favors IUI + OH

Figure 22.1: IUI in natural cycle versus IUI in stimulated cycles. Outcome: live birth rate per couple. *Source*: Modified with permission from Veltman-Verhulst S, Cohlen BJ, Hughes E, Heineman M. Intra-uterine insemination for unexplained subfertility. Cochrane Database of Systematic Reviews 2006;4:CD001838

gonadotropins with antiestrogens and found significantly higher pregnancy rates without affecting adverse outcomes with gonadotropins (or 1.8, 95% CI 1.2 to 2.7) (**Fig. 22.2**). They concluded that antiestrogens, although less effective than gonadotropins, appear to be the most cost effective and less invasive in IUI programs.[11]

Reported adverse effects with CC are: hot flashes, visual disturbances, antiestrogenic effects on the endometrium and cervical mucus. The adverse effect on the endometrium can be identified by routine ultrasound follicular monitoring. If endometrial lining is thin and hyperechoic, supplemental estrogen in the form of transdermal estrogen is given. Since IUI bypasses the cervix, no other intervention is required.

Tamoxifen is chemically and functionally similar to clomiphene and has estrogen agonist action on the vagina and endometrium. It is used orally in dosage of 20 mg to 40 mg daily for 5 days depending on response, starting on day 2–5 of cycle. Despite similar pregnancy rates and favorable endometrial morphology and cervical score, its use is reserved for patients who experience severe visual side effects on CC[12] or resistant to CC.

Aromatase Inhibitors

Aromatase inhibitors (AIs) block the action of the enzyme aromatase, which converts androstenedione to estrogens. The suppressed estrogen biosynthesis decreases negative feedback on the hypothalamus which in-turn increases GnRH release and FSH synthesis. Aromatase inhibitors also increase the intrafollicular androgen concentration with the concomitant FSH receptor up-regulation augmenting follicular sensitivity to FSH. Unlike CC, AIs do not deplete estrogen receptors in central or peripheral target, tissues and hence have no deleterious effect on endometrium and cervical mucus. The intact negative feedback loop limits FSH response and atresia of small follicles, resulting in mono-ovulation.[13,14]

Letrozole and recently Anastrozole have been increasingly used in COH protocols. To achieve COH in IUI cycles these are usually used in combination with exogenous gonadotropins. Mitwally and Casper[13,14] and Badawy et al[15-17] found similar ovulation and pregnancy rates (PRs) for CC, anastrozole and letrozole. Letrozole-FSH co-treatment in IUI cycles caused comparable PRs to FSH-only treatment, with associated lower Estradiol (E2) levels, lower FSH dose and cost, fewer cancelled cycles than FSH treatment alone in poor responders,[14,18-22] and significantly lower multiple pregnancy rates than in CC + FSH cycles.[23,24]

The recommended regimen in ovarian stimulation for IUI includes the use of letrozole 2.5 mg/day (from Day 3–7 of cycle) plus FSH (usually 100 IU/day from day 8, although doses can vary depending on the characteristics of the patients).[22] A recent study by Gregoriou et al. has shown that ovarian stimulation with letrozole was equally effective to stimulation with gonadotrophins for couples who had failed to conceive after treatment with CC

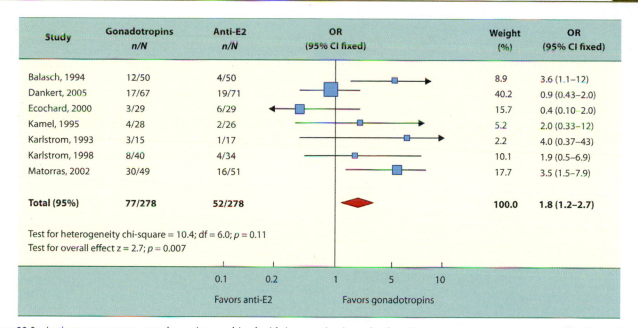

Study	Gonadotropins n/N	Anti-E2 n/N	OR (95% CI fixed)	Weight (%)	OR (95% CI fixed)
Balasch, 1994	12/50	4/50		8.9	3.6 (1.1–12)
Dankert, 2005	17/67	19/71		40.2	0.9 (0.43–2.0)
Ecochard, 2000	3/29	6/29		15.7	0.4 (0.10–2.0)
Kamel, 1995	4/28	2/26		5.2	2.0 (0.33–12)
Karlstrom, 1993	3/15	1/17		2.2	4.0 (0.37–43)
Karlstrom, 1998	8/40	4/34		10.1	1.9 (0.5–6.9)
Matorras, 2002	30/49	16/51		17.7	3.5 (1.5–7.9)
Total (95%)	**77/278**	**52/278**		**100.0**	**1.8 (1.2–2.7)**

Test for heterogeneity chi-square = 10.4; df = 6.0; p = 0.11
Test for overall effect z = 2.7; p = 0.007

0.1   0.2   1   5   10

Favors anti-E2   Favors gonadotropins

Figure 22.2: Antiestrogens versus gonadotropins combined with intrauterine insemination. Outcome: pregnancy rate per couple. *Source*: Modified with permission from Cantineau AE, Cohlen BJ, Heineman MJ. Ovarian stimulation protocols (antioestrogens, gonadotrophins with and without GnRH agonists/antagonists) for intrauterine insemination (IUI) in women with subfertility. Cochrane Database Systematic Reviews 2007;2:CD005356.

Study or subgroup	Aromatase inhibitor n/N	Antiestrogens n/N	Odds ratio M-H, Fixed, 95%	Weight (%)	Odds ratio M-H, Fixed, 95% CI
Al-Fozan, 2004	13/74	15/80		57.8	0.92 (0.41–2.10)
El Helw, 2002	5/27	3/26		12.1	1.74 (0.37–8.18)
Fatemi, 2003	2/7	3/8		9.7	0.67 (0.08–5.88)
Ozmen, 2005	4/22	3/21		12.2	1.33 (0.26–6.83)
Sammour, 2001	4/24	2/24		8.1	2.20 (0.36–3.34)
Total (95% CI)	**154**	**159**		**100.0**	**1.15 (0.64–2.08)**

Total events: 28 (aromatase inhibitor), 26 (anti-estrogens)
Heterogeneity: CHi^2 = 1.32; df = 4 (P = 0.86); I^2 = 0.0%
Test for subgroup differences: Not applicable

0.1 0.2 0.5 1 2 5 10

Favors anti-E2   Favors aromatase inhibitors

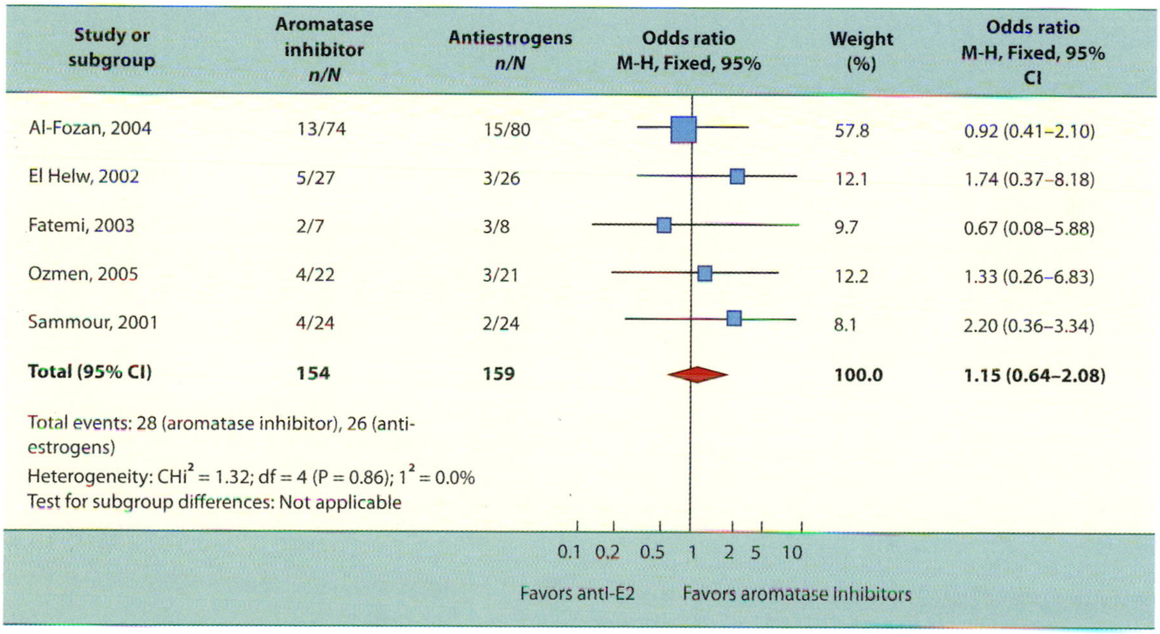

Figure 22.3: Antiestrogens versus aromatase inhibitors. Outcome: pregnancy rate per couple. *Source*: Modified with permission from Cantineau AE, Cohlen BJ, Heineman MJ. Ovarian stimulation protocols (anti-oestrogens, gonadotrophins with and without GnRH agonists/antagonists) for intrauterine insemination (IUI) in women with subfertility. Cochrane Database of Systematic Reviews 2007;2:CD005356.

combined with IUI.[25] The increased risk for OHSS and multiple gestations, cost, inconvenience and discomfort with gonadotrophins therapy favors letrozole as an attractive alternative before proceeding to IVF. A recent Cochrane review concluded from 5 studies (n = 313) that there is no convincing evidence that letrozole is superior to CC (OR 1.2 95% CI 0.64 to 2.1) (**Fig. 22.3**), and therefore the cost should be taken into account when using antiestrogens.[11]

Gonadotropins

Gonadotropins (Gn) have been long used for ovulation induction. They are more potent but expensive and invasive compared with CC. Currently, multiple formulations like human menopausal gonadotropins (hMG- FSH: LHratio of 1:1), urinary FSH, recombinant FSH and LH are widely available. Most of the standard protocols use 75-150IU of FSH/HMG SC/IM from day 3 of cycle. For those who are sensitive, like patients with polycystic ovaries, much lower doses like 25IU or 37.5IU is administered. The response is monitored by ultrasound and estradiol assessment and the dose is adjusted until a lead follicle of 17–18 mm and 2-3 follicles > 15 mm in size are detected.[26] IUI is usually done within 36–40 hrs of hCG administration. A recent cochrane review found no evidence of benefit in using hMG compared to FSH or significant difference in terms of pregnancy, miscarriage or OHSS between hMG, u-FSH or r-FSH[11] (**Fig. 22.4**). Recombinant FSH preparations are purer and have batch to batch consistency and increased bioactivity. However, they are more expensive.

In 1999, multicenter clinical trial by Guzick et al. found 33 percent of couples pregnant over 4 treatment cycles following Gn/IUI (9% per cycle), and reported that 30 percent of all pregnancies with gonadotropins were multiple gestations.[27] Whereas the cochrane review reported multiple pregnancy rate of 10 percent with gonadotropins and 9.8 percent with anti-estrogens[11] (**Fig. 22.5**). The recent 2010 fast track and standard treatment trial (FASTT) found a pregnancy rate similar to that of Guzick et al. when Gn/IUI followed 3 cycles of CC/IUI (9.7 vs 7.6%),[28] which is lower than retrospective reports of 15–20 percent

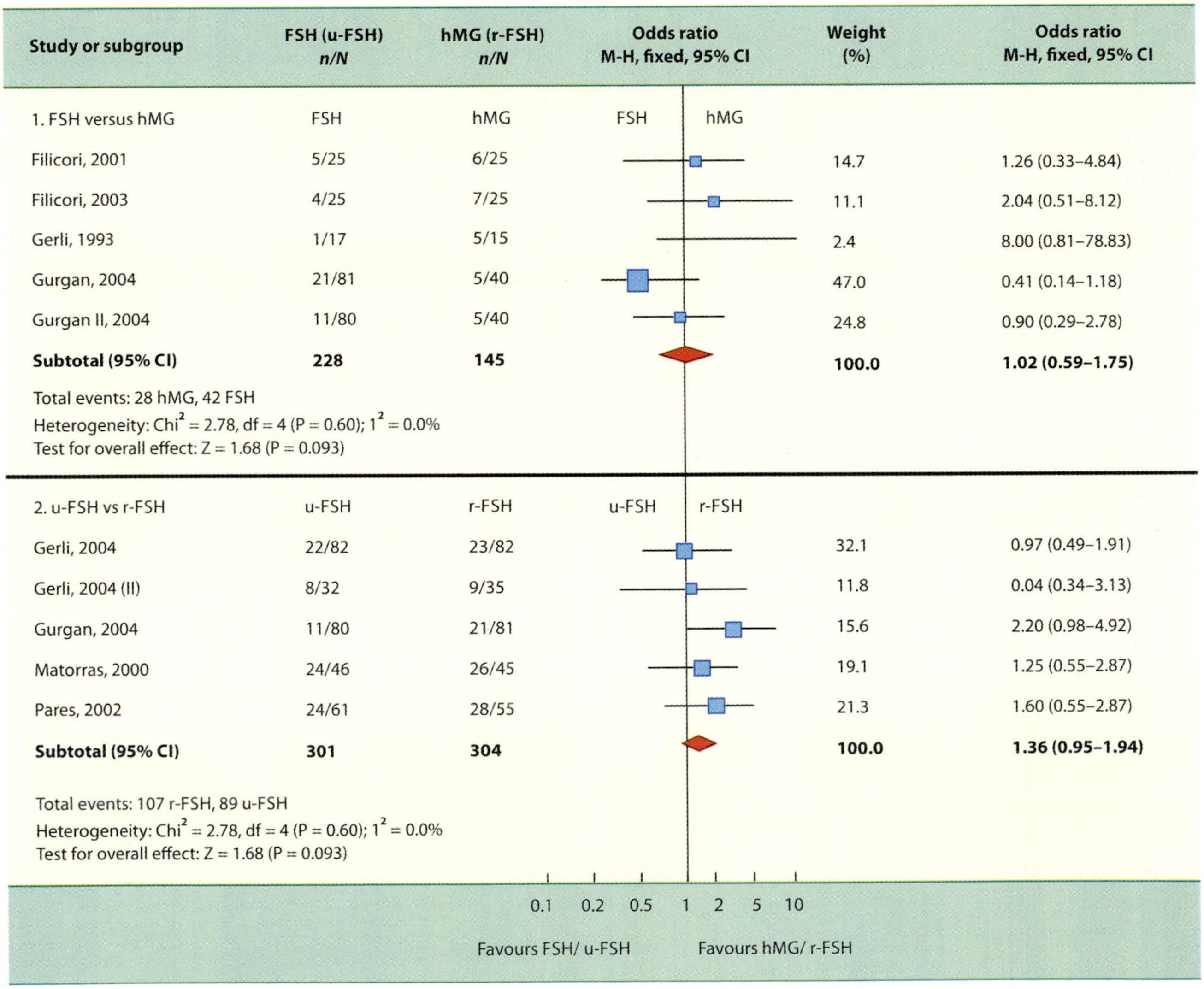
Study or subgroup
FSH (u-FSH) n/N
hMG (r-FSH) n/N
Odds ratio M-H, fixed, 95% CI
Weight (%)
Odds ratio M-H, fixed, 95% CI
1. FSH versus hMG
FSH
hMG
FSH
hMG
Filicori, 2001 5/25 6/25 14.7 1.26 (0.33–4.84)
Filicori, 2003 4/25 7/25 11.1 2.04 (0.51–8.12)
Gerli, 1993 1/17 5/15 2.4 8.00 (0.81–78.83)
Gurgan, 2004 21/81 5/40 47.0 0.41 (0.14–1.18)
Gurgan II, 2004 11/80 5/40 24.8 0.90 (0.29–2.78)
Subtotal (95% CI) 228 145 100.0 1.02 (0.59–1.75)
Total events: 28 hMG, 42 FSH
Heterogeneity: Chi² = 2.78, df = 4 (P = 0.60); 1² = 0.0%
Test for overall effect: Z = 1.68 (P = 0.093)
2. u-FSH vs r-FSH
u-FSH
r-FSH
u-FSH
r-FSH
Gerli, 2004 22/82 23/82 32.1 0.97 (0.49–1.91)
Gerli, 2004 (II) 8/32 9/35 11.8 0.04 (0.34–3.13)
Gurgan, 2004 11/80 21/81 15.6 2.20 (0.98–4.92)
Matorras, 2000 24/46 26/45 19.1 1.25 (0.55–2.87)
Pares, 2002 24/61 28/55 21.3 1.60 (0.55–2.87)
Subtotal (95% CI) 301 304 100.0 1.36 (0.95–1.94)
Total events: 107 r-FSH, 89 u-FSH
Heterogeneity: Chi² = 2.78, df = 4 (P = 0.60); 1² = 0.0%
Test for overall effect: Z = 1.68 (P = 0.093)
0.1 0.2 0.5 1 2 5 10
Favours FSH/ u-FSH
Favours hMG/ r-FSH

Figure 22.4: Comparison of different types of gonadotropins. Outcome: pregnancy rate per couple. *Source*: Modified with permission from Cantineau AE, Cohlen BJ, Heineman MJ. Ovarian stimulation protocols (anti-oestrogens, gonadotrophins with and without GnRH agonists/antagonists) for intrauterine insemination (IUI) in women with subfertility. Cochrane Database of Systematic Reviews 2007;2:CD005356.

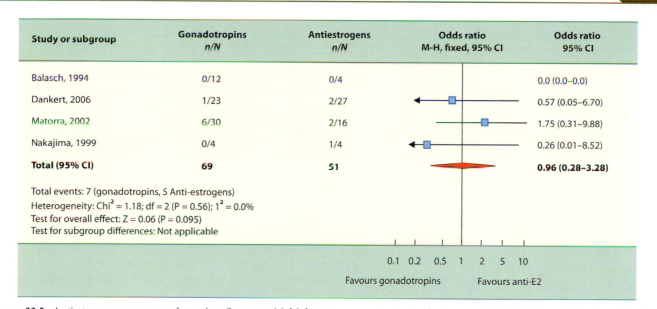

Study or subgroup	Gonadotropins n/N	Antiestrogens n/N	Odds ratio M-H, fixed, 95% CI	Odds ratio 95% CI
Balasch, 1994	0/12	0/4		0.0 (0.0–0.0)
Dankert, 2006	1/23	2/27		0.57 (0.05–6.70)
Matorra, 2002	6/30	2/16		1.75 (0.31–9.88)
Nakajima, 1999	0/4	1/4		0.26 (0.01–8.52)
Total (95% CI)	**69**	**51**		**0.96 (0.28–3.28)**

Total events: 7 (gonadotropins, 5 Anti-estrogens)
Heterogeneity: Chi^2 = 1.18; df = 2 (P = 0.56); I^2 = 0.0%
Test for overall effect: Z = 0.06 (P = 0.095)
Test for subgroup differences: Not applicable

0.1 0.2 0.5 1 2 5 10

Favours gonadotropins   Favours anti-E2

Figure 22.5: Antiestrogens versus gonadotropins. Outcome: Multiple pregnancy rate per couple. *Source*: Modified with permission from Cantineau AE, Cohlen BJ, Heineman MJ. Ovarian stimulation protocols (anti-oestrogens, gonadotrophins with and without GnRH agonists/antagonists) for intrauterine insemination (IUI) in women with subfertility. Cochrane Database of Systematic Reviews 2007;2:CD005356.

per cycle.[29,30] Gn/IUI carries a significant risk of high-order multiple birth (11.6%) more than double the IVF triplet rate.[31] Society for assisted reproductive technology (SART) reports[32] from the year 2009 show that < 2 percent of all IVF births involve 3 or more babies. Dickey et al. (2009) in their updated analysis[33] concluded that risk factors for high-order multiple pregnancy includes ≥ 7 preovulatory follicles (≥ 10–12 mm), E2 >1,000 pg/mL, early cycles of treatment, age < 32, low BMI, and use of donor sperm. Cancellation of cycles in which elevated estradiol levels (> 1200 pg/mL) or an excessive number of follicles (≥ 5) develop would not reduce high order births to acceptable levels.[31] Conversion to rescue IVF and embryo transfer (IVF-ET) or aspiration of supernumerary follicles have been attempted by some investigators.[34-36] Concerns with multiple birth epidemic and the burden of high health care cost together with unavoidable higher order births with Gn/IUI has brought this drug under scrutiny. The FASST trial has concluded eliminating Gn/IUI from the stepwise infertility paradigm will result in pregnancies with the lowest possible risk for multiple births and when the woman is younger than 40 years, an accelerated approach to IVF that starts with CC/IUI, but eliminates Gn/IUI, results in a shorter time to pregnancy, with fewer treatment cycles, and at a suggested cost savings.[29]

Low dose protocols in which 50–75 IU hMG/FSH is given for 5 days from day 3 of cycle found lower risk of OHSS and multiple births without compromising pregnancy rates[37,38] which is supported by meta-analysis.[11] In step-up regimen dose of FSH is increased after 7 days if serum estradiol is < 200 pg/mL or if no lead follicle > 10 mm, weekly increments of 75 IU are given until adequate response is achieved. In step-down regimen dose of FSH is tapered as follows: 150 IU/day till lead follicle of > 10 mm –112.5 IU × 3 days –75 IU/day till hCG trigger.[39]

Role of GnRH Agonists and Antagonists in Combination with Gonadotropins for IUI Protocol

Gonadotropins increase estradiol secretion which activates positive feedback effect on the anterior pituitary. This induces LH surge even before maturation of developing follicles, which is seen in up to one-third of stimulated IUI cycles.[40] GnRH agonists combined with gonadotropins suppress LH before and during ovarian stimulation and are extensively used in long down regulation protocols of IVF. Its use in IUI is limited as it takes longer time, requires higher dose of gonadotropins, and has increased prevalence of multifollicular development, increased cycle cancellation rate, OHSS and multiple pregnancy. A cochrane review found evidence that agonist when added to gonadotropins does not improve pregnancy rates (**Fig. 22.6**), while increasing the probability of achieving a multiple pregnancy (MPR per pregnancy 14 vs 39% for Gn and Gn + agonist respectively) and cost in the setting of IUI where mild ovarian hyperstimulation is applied.[11]

GnRH antagonists by competitive binding modulate degree of hormonal suppression within few hours of treatment. Unlike GnRH agonists, antagonists have no flare up effect or lag in resumption of gonadal function following their discontinuation. Ragni et al.[41] proposed the use of GnRH antagonist in combination with Gn for IUI cycles. GnRH-antagonist given in single or multiple doses when a leading follicle is > 16 mm until the day of hCG trigger reduces premature luteinization and significantly increases clinical pregnancy rate (CPR 22 vs 11% and premature luteinization rate 1.7 vs 17.5% for FSH + GnRH-antagonist vs FSH only respectively).[42] The promising effect of adding antagonists to Gn in IUI protocol is summarized (**Fig. 22.7**). Cochrane review

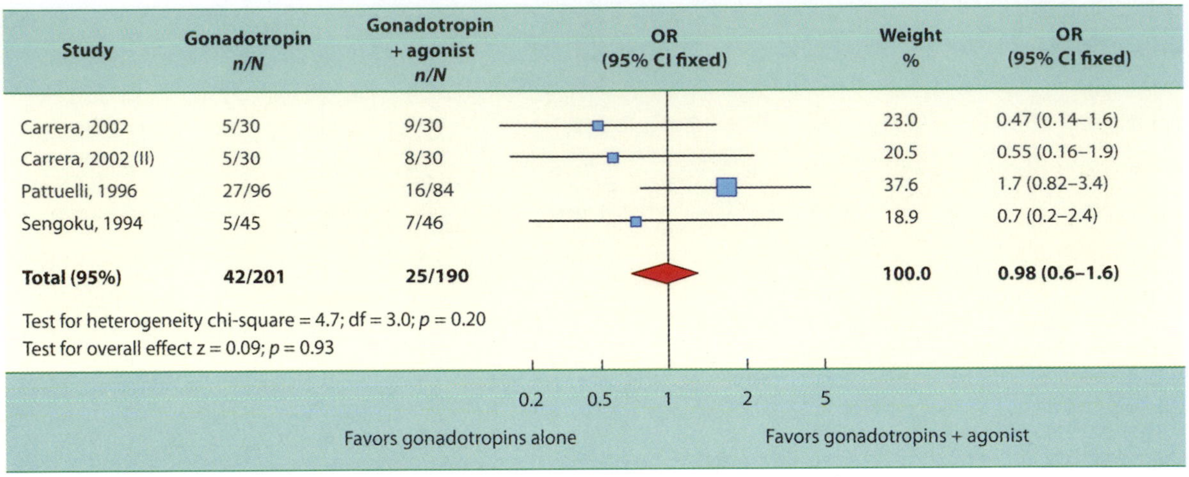

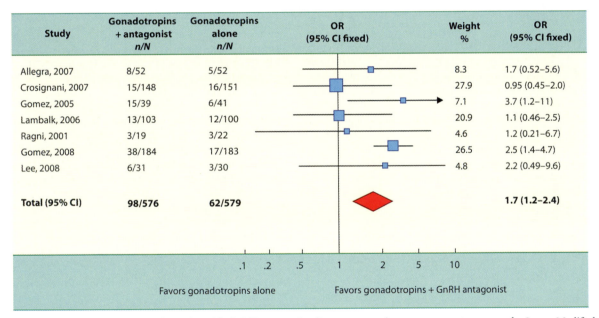

Figure 22.6: Gonadotropins alone vs gonadotropins with GnRH-agonist. Outcome: pregnancy rate per couple. *Source*: Modified with permission from Cantineau AE, Cohlen BJ, Heinerman MJ. Ovarian stimulation protocols (antioestrogens, gonadotrophins with and without GnRH agonists/antagonists) for intrauterine insemination (IUI) in women with subfertility. Cochrane Database Systematic Reviews 2007;2:CD005356.

Figure 22.7: Gonadotropins alone vs gonadotropins with GnRH-antagonist. Outcome: ongoing pregnancy rate per couple. *Source*: Modified with permission from Cohlen B, Cantineau AE. Mild ovarian hyperstimulation in combination with intrauterine insemination. In: Aboulghar M, Rizk B (Eds.). Ovarian Stimulation. Cambridge: Cambridge University Press, 2011. Chapter 3, 30.

analyzing 3 studies also found a significant difference in pregnancy rate favoring treatment with GnRH antagonist in combination with gonadotropins.[11] They concluded that since the studies are not blinded, clinicians would have stimulated more aggressively when antagonists are added leading to higher pregnancy rates and hence the role of antagonists need to be determined in future trials. While Kosmos et al. reported higher pregnancy rates with an odds ratio of 2.3 in a meta-analysis comparing Gn + GnRH-antagonists Gn with Gn alone COH/IUI protocol,[43] Crosignani et al. (2007) found no significant difference in their multicenter randomized trial.[44] It is amazing that even in the era of advanced assisted reproduction, IUI still has an important role to play. History teaches us that old concepts live forever if they are true.

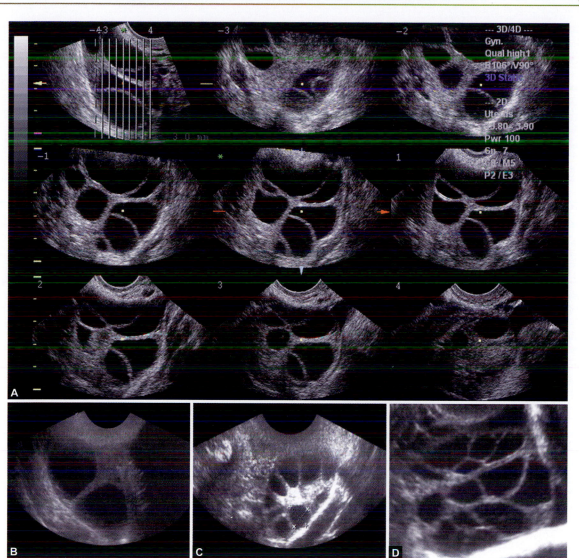

Figures 22.8A to D: (A) Hyperstimulated ovary. TUI mode allows obtaining millimetric images of the selected structure. Modified with permission from Puente M, Garcia JA. 3D Ultrasonography and infertility. In: Rizk B (ed). Ultrasonography in Reproductive Medicine and Infertility. Cambridge: Cambridge University Press, 2010. Chapter 8, 68; (B) Controlled ovarian hyperstimulation on day 9 in a patient with PCOS. Modified with permission from Alexander C. Ultrasonography and the treatment of infertility in polycystic ovary syndrome. In: Rizk B (ed). Ultrasonography in Reproductive Medicine and Infertility. Cambridge: Cambridge University Press, 2010. Chapter 10, 84; (C) : Image of a patient undergoing controlled ovarian hyperstimulation with FSH 150 IU on day 5 stimulation. Modified with permissionfrom Alexander C. Ultrasonography and the treatment of infertility in polycystic ovary syndrome. In: Rizk B (ed). Ultrasonography in Reproductive Medicine and Infertility. Cambridge: Cambridge University Press, 2010. Chapter 10, 85; (D) Image of a 39-year-old with PCOS after ovarian hyperstimulation with FSH 225 IU and human menopausal gonadotropin 150 IU for 6 days. Modified with permission from Alexander C. Ultrasonography and the treatment of infertility in polycystic ovary syndrome. In: Rizk B (ed). Ultrasonography in Reproductive Medicine and Infertility. Cambridge: Cambridge University Press, 2010. Chapter 10, 85

■ KEY POINTS

- Intrauterine insemination in natural cycles could be beneficial for mild male factor infertility and cervical hostility.
- For unexplained infertility and mild endometriosis IUI + COH is recommended for up to 3–4 cycles before proceeding to IVF.

- Antiestrogens although less effective than gonadotropins, appear to be the most cost effective and less invasive for IUI programs.
- Letrazole + FSH co-treatment is associated with lower FSH dose, cost, fewer cancelled cycles and lower multiple pregnancy rates.
- Gonadotropins are more potent, but expensive and invasive compared with anti-estrogens and aromatase inhibitors.

Low dose protocols are recommended as they have advantages of lower risk of OHSS and cost without compromising pregnancy rates.

- The role of GnRH agonists is limited in IUI programs owing to increased time, cost, OHSS and multiple pregnancy rates without improving pregnancy rate.
- GnRH antagonists when combined with Gn in COH + IUI program significantly improves pregnancy rate, and studies are ongoing to determine its definitive role in IUI programs.

■ REFERENCES

1. Angell NF, Moustafa HF, Rizk B, et al. Intra-uterine Insemination in Infertility and Assisted Reproduction. In: Rizk B, Velasco JG Sallam H, Makrigiannakis A, (Eds). Cambridge: Cambridge University Press 2008. Ch 46, 416-27.

2. Cohlen BJ, Te Velde ER, Van Kooij RJ, et al. Controlled ovarian hyperstimulation and intrauterine insemination for treating male subfertility: a controlled study. Hum Reprod 1998;13(6):1553-8.

3. National Institute of Clinical Excellence. Fertility: assessment and treatment of people with fertility problems, Clinical guidelines No11 2004. London, UK.

4. Verhulst SM, Cohlen BJ, Hughes E, et al. Intra-uterine insemination for unexplained subfertility. Cochrane Database Syst Rev 2006;(4):CD0014.

5. Mahani IM, Afnan M. The pregnancy rates with intrauterine insemination (IUI) in superovulated cycles employing different protocols (clomiphene citrate (CC), human menopausal gonadotropin (HMG) and HMG + CC) and in natural ovulatory cycle. J Pak Med Assoc 2004;54:503-5.

6. Arcaini L, Bianchi S, Baglioni A, et al. Superovulation and intrauterine insemination vs. superovulation alone in the treatment of unexplained infertility. A randomized study. J Reprod Med 1996;41:61-4.

7. Chung CC, Fleming R, Jamieson ME, et al. Randomized comparison of ovulation induction with and without intrauterine insemination in the treatment of unexplained infertility. Hum Reprod 1995;10:3139-42.

8. Zeyneloglu HB, Arici A, Olive DL, et al. Comparison of intrauterine insemination with timed intercourse in superovulated cycles with gonadotropins: a meta-analysis. Fertil Steril 1998;69(3):486-91.

9. The practice committee of the American society of reproductive medicine. Effectiveness and treatment of unexplained infertility. Fertil Steril 2006;86(5):111-4.

10. Rizk B. Epidemiology of ovarian hyperstimulation syndrome: iatrogenic and spontaneous. In: Rizk B (Ed). Ovarian Hyperstimulation Syndrome. Cambridge: Cambridge University Press 2006. Ch 2,10-42.

11. Cantineau AEP, Cohlen BJ. Ovarian stimulation protocols (antioestrogens, gonadotrophins with and without GnRH agonists/antagonists) for intrauterine insemination (IUI) in women with subfertility. Cochrane Database of Systematic Reviews 2007, Issue 2. Art. No.: CD005356. DOI: 10.1002/14651858.CD005356.pub2.

12. Patel M. Tamoxifen citrate for ovulation induction in (Gautam Allahbadia, Ed) Manual of ovulation induction 2001;21-26.

13. Mitwally MF, Casper RF. Use of an aromatase inhibitor for induction of ovulation in patients with an inadequate response to clomiphene citrate. Fertil Steril 2001;75: 305-9.

14. Casper RF, Mitwally MF. Review: aromatase inhibitors for ovulation induction. J Clin Endocrinol Metab 2006;91(3):760-71.

15. Badawy A, Abdel Aal I, Abulatta M, et al. Clomiphene citrate or anastrozole for ovulation induction in women with polycystic ovary syndrome? A prospective controlled trial. Fertil Steril 2009;92:860-3.

16. Badawy A, Abdel Aal I, Abulatta M, et al. Clomiphene citrate or letrozole for ovulation induction in women with polycystic ovarian syndrome: a prospective randomized trial. Fertil Steril 2009;92:849-52.

17. Badawy A, Mosbah A, Shady M, et al. Anastrozole or letrozole for ovulation induction in clomiphene-resistant women with polycystic ovarian syndrome: a prospective randomized trial. Fertil Steril 2008;89:1209-12.

18. Mitwally MF, Casper RF. Aromatase inhibition improves ovarian response to follicle-stimulating hormone in poor responders. Fertil Steril 2002;77:776-80.

19. Healey S, Tan SL, Tulandi T, et al. Effects of letrozole on superovulation with gonadotropins in women undergoing intrauterine insemination. Fertil Steril 2003;80:1325-9.

20. Mitwally MF, Casper RF. Aromatase inhibition reduces the dose of gonadotropin required for controlled ovarian hyperstimulation. J Soc Gynecol Investig 2004;11:406-15.

21. Badawy A, Shokry M, et al. Letrozole co-treatment in infertile women 40 years old and older receiving controlled ovarian stimulation and intrauterine insemination. Fertil steril 2009;91: 2501-7.

22. Requena A, Herrero J, Landoras J, et al. Use of letrozole in assisted reproduction: a systematic review and meta-analysis. Human Reproduction Update 2008;14(6):571-82.

23. Mitwally MF, Biljan MM, Casper RF. Pregnancy outcome after the use of an aromatase inhibitor for ovarian stimulation. Am J Obstet Gynecol 2005;192:381-6.

24. Tredway D, Schertz J. Anastrozole versus clomiphene citrate: which is better for ovulation induction? Fertil Steril 2011;95: 1549-51.

25. Gregoriou O, Vlahos NF, Konidaris S, et al. Randomized controlled trial comparing superovulation with letrozole versus recombinant follicle-stimulating hormone combined to intrauterine insemination for couples with unexplained infertility who had failed clomiphene citrate stimulation and intrauterine insemination. Fertil Steril 2008;90:3:678-83.

26. Rizk B, Sallam HN. Intrauterine insemination. In: Rizk B, sallam HN, (Eds). Clinical Infertility and In Vitro Fertilization. Jaypee Brothers Medical Publishers 2010. Ch 28, 233-9.

27. Guzick DS, Carson SA, Coutifaris C, et al. Efficacy of superovulation and intrauterine inseminationin the treatment of infertility. National Cooperative Reproductive Medicine Network. N Engl J Med 1999;340:177-83.

28. Reindollar RH, Regan M, Neumann PJ, et. al. A randomized clinical trial to evaluate optimal treatment for unexplained infertility: the fast track and standard treatment (FASTT) trial. Fertil Steril 2010;94:888-99.

29. Gurgan T, Kisnisci H, Yarali H, et.al. The value of human menopausal gonadotropin treatment in patients with unexplained infertility. Int J Gynaecol Obstet 1991;35:327-30.

30. Assisted reproductive technology in the United States and Canada: 1993 results generated from the American Society for Reproductive Medicine/Society for Assisted Reproductive Technology Registry. Fertil Steril 1995; 64:13-21.

31. Fong S, Palta V, Cheongeun O, et al. Multiple Pregnancy after Gonadotropin-Intrauterine Insemination: An Unavoidable Event? ISRN Obstetrics and Gynecology Volume 2011, Article ID 465483, 5 pages,doi:10.5402/2011/465483.

32. National Summary Data, http://www.sart.org/, 2009.

33. Dickey RP. Strategies to reduce multiple pregnancies due to ovulation stimulation. Fertil Steril 2009;91(1):1-17.

34. Olufowobi O, Sharif K, Papaioannou S, et al. Role of rescue IVF-ET treatment in the management of high response in stimulated IUI cycles. J Obstet Gynaecol 2005;25(2):166-8.

35. De Geyter C, De Geyter M, Castro E, et al. Experience with transvaginal ultrasound-guided aspiration of supernumerary follicles for the prevention of multiple pregnancies after ovulation induction and intrauterine insemination. Fertil Steril 1996;65:1163-8.

36. De Geyter C, De Geyter M, Nieschlag E, et al. Low multiple pregnancy rates and reduced frequency of cancellation after ovulation induction with gonadotropins, if eventual supernumerary follicles are aspirated to prevent polyovulation. J Assist Reprod Genet 1998;15:111-6.

37. Raslan A. Low Dose hMG As a First choice for Ovarian Stimulation in IUI cycles. Evidencebased Women's Health Society Journal 2011;1(1):19-23.

38. Dhaliwal LK, Sialy RK, Gopalan S, et al. Minimal stimulation protocol for use with intrauterine insemination in the treatment of infertility. Int J Fertil Womens Med 2000;45(3):232-5.

39. Weissman A. Ovarian stimulation protocols for IUI. In: Allahbadia G (Ed). Manual of ovulation induction 2001:78-84.

40. Cantineau AE, Cohlen BJ. Dutch IUI Study Group. The prevalence and influence of luteinizing hormone surges in stimulated cycles combined with intrauterine insemination during a prospective cohort study. Fertil Steril 2007;88:107-12.

41. Ragni G, Alagna F, Brigante C, et al. GnRH antagonists and mild ovarian stimulation for intrauterine insemination: a randomized study comparing different gonadotropin dosages. Hum Reprod 2004;19(1):54-8.

42. Bakas P, Konidaris S, Liapis A, et al. Role of gonadotropin-releasing hormone antagonist in the management of subfertile couples with intrauterine insemination and controlled ovarian stimulation. Fertil Steril 2011;95:2024-8.

43. Kosmas I, Tatsioni A, Kolibianakis E, et al. Effects and clinical significance of GnRH antagonist administration for IUI timing in FSH super ovulated cycles: a meta-analysis. Fertil Steril 2008;90:367-72.

44. Crosignani PG, Somigliana E. Effect of GnRH antagonists in FSH mildly stimulated intrauterine insemination cycles: a multi-center randomized trial. Hum Reprod 2007;22:500-5.

23

The Impact of Male Infertility on the Outcome of Intrauterine Insemination

Marwa Badr, Botros RMB Rizk

INTRODUCTION

Couples with male subfertility have repeated semen analyzes below the criteria for normal semen as defined by the World Health Organization (WHO).[1] In many cases, the first treatment for subfertile couples consists of intrauterine insemination (IUI), which can be combined with ovarian stimulation. The probability of conceiving with IUI depends on various factors including semen quality and ovarian stimulation.[2-25]

Interestingly, many studies have shown that men with abnormal semen analysis can still produce spontaneous pregnancies.[3] In this chapter, we will discuss the impact of semen parameters on the IUI outcome.

PREDICTIVE VALUE OF SPERM MORPHOLOGY IN INTRAUTERINE INSEMINATION

Sperm morphology is a good predictor of semen quality, as it has a significant impact on the success of fertilization (**Figs 23.1 and 23.2**).[3-4]

The pregnancy rate or cumulative live birth rate following IUI treatment decreased significantly when the percentage of normal sperm was low.[3-4] Grigoriou et al. (2005) demonstrated that the pregnancies per cycle were significantly decreased in the teratozoospermia group when compared to the normozoospermia group.[5] Burr et al. (1996) reported a normal morphology value of 10 percent to distinguish between the patients with good and poor IUI outcome.[6]

Van Waart et al. (2001) data found eighteen articles that stated a definitive predictive value of normal sperm morphology.[7] Those articles were divided into a Tygerberg 'strict' criteria group[24,25] and a WHO group.[1] Of the nine articles that used the Tygerberg 'strict' criteria[24,25] (**Table 23.1**), six found a positive predictive value for sperm morphology and three found no predictive value at all.[8-15] Of the nine articles that used the WHO criteria[1] for normal sperm morphology (**Table 23.2**), six found a positive predictive value and three found no predictive value at all.[16-23] Van Waart et al. (2001) reviewed the eighteen articles and found eight of them to have sufficient data to be reanalyzed statistically. Six used the Tygerberg 'strict' criteria (**Table 23.3**), and two (Burr et al., 1996; Tomlinson et al., 1996)[6,17] used the WHO criteria.

Menkveld et al. (2010) suggested that the sperm morphology is the best discriminating parameter between the fertile and subfertile populations, with the cut-off value for sperm morphology set at 4 percent, which is less than previously stated values.[26,27] The world wide acceptance of 'strict' criteria for evaluation of sperm morphology is the main reason behind the decreased value for morphologically normal sperm. Menkveld et al. (**Table 23.4**) used an initial sperm count of $< 20 \times 10^6$/ml as a subfertile population and the WHO cut off point of 31 percent normal spermatozoa.[11] The authors concluded that a sperm morphology threshold of 12 percent normal forms would yield a 69 percent sensitivity and 67 percent specificity.[26,27]

There is some controversy regarding the relationship between sperm morphology (**Fig. 23.2**) and IUI success.[29,30] Ombelet et al. (1997), conducted a retrospective study to establish the influence of the inseminating motile count (IMC) and sperm morphology on the success rate in clomiphene citrate intrauterine insemination (CC-IUI) cycles.[29] The authors concluded that sperm morphology was a useful predictive tool in patients with an IMC of $< 1 \times 10^6$. In terms of therapeutic strategy, this finding means that above a cut-off limit of 1×10^6 motile spermatozoa recovered after washing, CC-IUI can be promoted as a first-line therapy with an expected baby take home (BTH) rate of 21–25 percent after three cycles. Furthermore, in cases with $< 1 \times 10^6$ motile spermatozoa, CC-IUI remains important as a first-line option, provided the sperm morphology score is greater than or equal to 4 percent.

Ombelet et al. (1997) calculated their values using the 10th percentile as a cut off value of the fertile population, and the following results were obtained: 14.3×10^6/mL for sperm concentration, 28 percent for progressive motility and 5 percent for sperm morphology.[29,30]

Sperm morphology evaluation is an integral part of male factor evaluation.[2-29] In the IUI setting, morphology by strict criteria is a good predictor of IUI outcome. If morphology is > 4 percent, then IUI should be performed, irrespective of other parameters. However, if morphology is < 4 percent, and other parameters are adequate (IMC $> 13 \times 10^6$, motility > 50 percent, two or more follicles available), then four IUI cycles are recommended.[6] If morphology is < 4 percent and IMC $< 13 \times 10^6$ and motility <50 percent, then other treatment modalities should

Pregnancy rate per cycle					
Study	≤ 4%	> 4%	Risk difference (95% CI)	Weight	Risk difference (95% CI)
Idiopathic					
Montanaro-Gauci et al. (2001)	1/38	35/274		77.9	−0.10 (−0.17 to −0.04)
Matorras et al. (1995)	13/120	3/23		22.1	−0.02 (−0.17 to 0.13)
Subtotal	$\chi^2 = 1.22$ (df = 1)			100	−0.08 (−0.16 to −0.01)
Whole population					
Toner et al. (1995)	6/86	35/309		20.9	−0.04 (−0.11 to 0.02)
Ombelet et al. (1997)	40/335	76/460		24.7	−0.05 (−0.09 to 0.00)
Karabinus & Gelety (1997)	3/53	44/485		20.3	−0.03 (−0.10 to 0.03)
Lindheim et al. (1996)	1/99	15/77		15.5	−0.19 (−0.28 to −0.09)
*Matorras et al. (1995)	18/172	10/99		18.6	−0.00 (−0.07 to 0.08)
Subtotal	$\chi^2 = 10.74$ (df = 4)			100	−0.06 (−0.11 to −0.01)
Total	$\chi^2 = 11.79$ (df = 5)			100	−0.07 (−0.11 to −0.03)

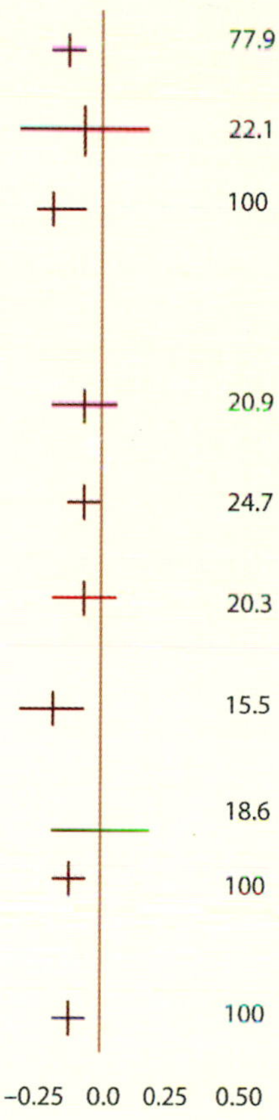

−0.50   −0.25   0.0   0.25   0.50

Figure 23.1: Predictive value of normal sperm morphology in intrauterine insemination (IUI). Risk difference for pregnancy rate (strict criteria, 4% threshold). Value not included (whole population) in final meta-analysis; *Source*: Reproduced with permission from Van Waart et al. Predictive value of normal sperm morphology in intrauterine insemination (IUI): A structured literature review. Hum Reprod Update 2001;7:497

be considered, such as intracytoplasmic sperm injection (ICSI). Ombelet et al. (1997) suggested that a normal sperm morphology group with greater than or equal to 5 percent has a significantly higher pregnancy rate per cycle compared with the group with less than 5 percent normal forms.[29,30] Because of the high cost of assisted reproduction, IUI can be offered as a treatment option with good results. At least four insemination cycles can be an alternative approach for males within semen parameters, where at least 1 million motile spermatozoa per mL can be retrieved after wash and swim-up.[12]

Ombelet et al. (1997) showed that an IMC of < 13 × 10⁶ was highly predictive of IUI failure if the morphology was

<4 percent.[28-30] No pregnancies were achieved when parameters were unfavorable.[29,30] Males with a poor fertility potential with these two features should be therefore referred to assisted reproduction programs.

PREDICTIVE VALUE OF TOTAL SPERM MOTILITY

Total motile sperm (TMS) count is an important prognostic criterion in IUI cycles and reflects both sperm concentration and motility in sperm analysis. Various studies in the literature have given different cut-off values for TMS that are correlated with optimal success rates in IUI cycles.

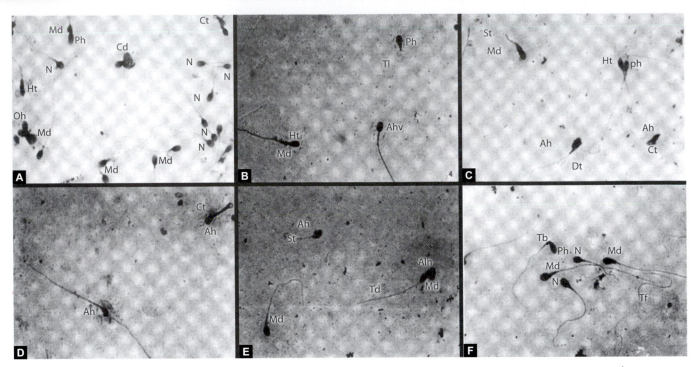

Figures 23.2A to F: Normal and abnormal morphology. Photomicrographs (1000 x) of Diff-Quick stained spermatozoa: N = Normal spermatozoa; Dh = Double head; Ph = pyriform head; Ah = Amorphous head; Alh = Amorphous large head; Ahv = Vacuolated head; Ht = Tapering head; Md = Neck and midpiece defect; Cd = Cytoplasmic droplet; Td = Tail defect; Dt = Double tail; St = Short tail; Ct = Coiled tail; TI = Without tail; Tb = Bent tail. *Source*: Reproduced with permission from MZ Iqbal Khan. Role of sperm morphology in an IUI program. In: Allahbadia GN, (Ed). Intrauterine Insemination. London and New York: Taylor & Francis Group, 2005. Chapter 14, 169-78.

Table 23.1: Predictive value of normal sperm morphology in intrauterine insemination (IUI) using Tygerberg strict criteria

Reference value	Cycles	Predictive	Thresholds
Montanaro-Gauci et al., 2001	495	Positive	<4%; 5–14%; > 14%
Schulman et al.,1998	544	None	No cut-off indicated
Karabinus and Gelety, 1997	538	None	< 4%; 5–9%; 10–19%; 20–29%; > 30%
Ombelet et al.,1997	792	Positive	4%
Lindheim et al., 1996	172	Positive	4%
Ombelet et al.,1996	283	Positive	4%
Toner et al.,1995	395	Positive	< 4%; 5–14%; > 14%
Matorras et al.,1995	271	None	4%; 10%
Irianni et al.,1993	208	Positive	4%

Source: Modified with permission from Van Waart et al. Predictive value of normal sperm morphology in intrauterine insemination (IUI): a structured literature review. Human Reproduction Update 2001;7(5);496

For motility, the cut-off value was at 20 percent motile spermatozoa. Gunalp et al. (2001), showed the best discriminative values between fertile and subfertile males are the threshold value of the progressive motility of 42 percent and the sperm morphology.[31] If we consider the positive and negative predictive value to screen the general population to identify the subfertile group, a 5 percent normal morphology threshold was indicated, with 14 percent progressive motility, 30 percent motility and a concentration of 9×10^6/mL or lower.[13]

Badawy et al. (2009) and Francavilla et al. (1990) reported that the pregnancy rate was significantly lower when TMS was < 5×10^6.[32,33] Van Voorhis et al. (2001) and Miller et al. (2002) suggested that TMS < 10×10^6 was significantly related with a low pregnancy rate.[34,35]

Table 23.2: Predictive value of normal sperm morphology in intrauterine insemination (IUI)
using World Health Organization criteria

Reference value	Cycle	Predictive	Threshold
Chung et al.,1997	56	Positive	No cut-off indicated
Burr et al.,1996	326	Positive	10%; 11–20%; > 30%
Tomlinson et al.,1996	260	None	30%
Milingos et al.,1996	Unknown	None	No cut-off indicated
Comhaire et al.,1995	367	Positive	8%
Johnston et al.,1994	10 797	Positive	No cut-off indicated
Francavilla et al.,1990	441	Positive	50%
Bostofte et al.,1990	1086	Positive	No cut-off indicated
Bolton et al.,1989	Unknown	None	40%

Source: Modified with permission from Van Waart et al. Predictive value of normal sperm morphology in intrauterine insemination (IUI): a structured literature review. Human Reproduction Update 2001;7(5);496

Table 23.3: Predictive value of normal sperm morphology in intrauterine insemination (IUI). Studies with data in which 4% strict criteria threshold could be used to evaluate predictive value of normal sperm morphology (all numbers are given as pregnancy rate per cycle). Predictive value of normal sperm morphology in intrauterine insemination (IUI)

References	<4%	>4%	P	Risk difference (95% CI)
Montanaro-Gauci et al., 2001	2.6%	15.6%	_	–0.10
	(1/38)	(35/274)	_	(–0.17, –0.04)
Toner et al.,1995	7%	11.3%	_	–0.04
	(6/86)	(35/309)	_	(–11,0.02)
Ombelet et al.,1997	12.1%	16.5%	_	–0.05
	(40/335)	(76/460)	_	(–0.09, 0.00)
Karabinus and Gelety, 1997	6.5%	9%	_	–0.03
	(3/53)	(44/485)	_	(–0.10,0.03)
Lindheim et al.,1996	1%	19.5%	_	–0.19
	(1/99)	(15/77)	_	(–0.28, –0.09)
Matorras et al.,1995	10.9%	13%	_	–0.02
	(13/120)	(3/23)	_	(–0.17, 0.13)
Total	_	_	< 0.001	–0.07
				(–0.11, –0.03)

Source: Modified with permission from Van Waart et al. Predictive value of normal sperm morphology in intrauterine insemination (IUI): a structured literature review. Human Reproduction Update 2001;7(5);498

Table 23.4: Possible lower thresholds for the general population to distinguish between subfertile and
fertile men, raised on the assumed incidences of subfertile males in their populations

	Motility (%)	Morphology (%)	Progressive motility (%)	Concentration (10^6/mL)
Menkveld et al.	3	20		14
Gunalp et al.	5	30	14	20
Ombelet et al.	28	5		14.3

Source: Modified with permission from Kruger TF, Oehninger SC. The basic semen analysis: interpretation and clinical application. In Rizk B, Garcia-Velasco J, Sallam HN, Makrigiannakis A (Eds). Infertility and Assisted Reproduction. Cambridge: Cambridge University Press, 2008. Chapter 18, 157-59.

PREDICTIVE VALUE OF THE SPERM COUNT

Sperm count significantly influences the clinical pregnancy rate. The oligozoospermia patients (< 20 million per mL) had the lowest clinical pregnancy rate (5.5%). Male patients with oligozoospermia (low count in sperm) and asthenozoospermia (low progressive motility in sperm) were associated with poor outcome; between 0 and 3 percent pregnancy rate.[36-40] This association suggests that IUI is inappropriate for men with sluggish sperm motility and severely low sperm counts, and that IVF or ICSI should be the first-line treatment in these cases.

There is no consensus on cut-off values for the semen parameters for selection of primary treatment strategy such as IUI. ESHRE Capri Workshop Group (2009) has defined different optimal values in various studies for the rate of teratozoospermia and total motile sperms after preparation.[36-42]

CONCLUSION

Since ancient times, fertility has been a topic of prime importance for all civilizations. Sperm morphology evaluation is an integral part of male factor evaluation. In the IUI setting, morphology (by strict criteria) is a good predictor of IUI outcome. We recommend that if morphology is < 4 percent and other parameters are adequate (IMC > 13×10^6, motility > 50 percent, two or more follicles available, and TMS count per insemination, with > 10×10^6), then four IUI cycles could be performed. If morphology is < 4 percent, IMC < 13×10^6 and motility < 50 percent, then ICSI should be considered, for example ICSI IVF or combined.

REFERENCES

1. World Health Organization. WHO laboratory manual for the examination of human semen and sperm cervical mucus interaction. Cambridge: Cambridge University Press, 1992.
2. Mitwally MF, Abdel-Razeq S, Casper RF. Human chorionic gonadotropin administration is associated with high pregnancy rates during ovarian stimulation and timed intercourse or intrauterine insemination. Reproductive Biology and Endocrinology 2004;2:55-62.
3. Nallella KP, Sharma RK, Aziz N, Agarwal A. Significance of sperm characteristics in the evaluation of male infertility. Fertil Steril 2006;85(3):629-34.
4. Wainer R, Albert M, Dorion A, Bailly M, Berge`re M, Lombroso R, Gombault M, Selva J. Influence of the number of motile spermatozoa inseminated and of their morphology on the success of intrauterine insemination. Hum Reprod 2004;19:2060-65.
5. Grigoriou O, Pantos K, Makrakis E, Hassiakos D, Konidaris S, Creatsas G. Impact of isolated teratozoospermia on the outcome of intrauterine insemination. Fertil Steril 2005;83:773-5.
6. Burr RW, Siegberg R, Flaherty SP, Wang XJ, Matthews CD. The influence of sperm morphology and the number of motile sperm inseminated on the outcome of intrauterine insemination combined with mild ovarian stimulation. Fertil Steril 1996;65:127-32.
7. Van Waart J, Kruger TF, Lombard CJ, et al. Predictive value of normal sperm morphology in intrauterine insemination (IUI): A structured literature review. Hum Reprod Update 2001;7:495-500.
8. Montanaro-Gauci M, Kruger TF, Coetzee K, et al. Stepwise regression analysis on 495 cycles to study male and female factors impacting on pregnancy rate in an IUI program. Andrologia 2001;33:1-9.
9. Schulman A, Hauser R, Lipitz S, et al. Sperm motility is a major determinant of pregnancy outcome following intrauterine insemination. J Assits Reprod Genet 1998;6:381-5.
10. Karabinus DS, Gelety TJ. The impact of sperm morphology evaluated by strict criteria on intrauterine insemination success. Fertil Steril 1997;67:536-41.
11. Lindheim S, Barad D, Zinger M, et al. Abnormal sperm morphology is highly predictive of pregnancy outcome during controlled ovarian hyperstimulation and intrauterine insemination. J Assist Reprod Genet 1996;13:569-72.
12. Ombelet W, Cox A, Janssen M, et al. Artificial insemination 2: using the husband's sperm. In: Acosta AA, Kruger, TF (Eds). Human Spermatozoa in Assisted Reproduction. 2nd edition. Parthenon Publishing Group, New York 1996;pp.399-412.
13. Toner JP, Mossad H, Grow DR, et al. Value of sperm morphology assessed by strict criteria for prediction of the outcome of artificial (intrauterine) insemination. Andrologia 1995;27:143-8.
14. Matorras R, Corcostegui B, Perez C, et al. Sperm morphology analysis (strict criteria) in male infertility is not a prognostic factor in intrauterine insemination with husband's sperm. Fertil Steril 1995;3:608-11.
15. Irianni FM, Ramey J, Vaintraub MT, et al. Therapeutic intrauterine insemination improves with gonadotrophin ovarian stimulation. Arch Androl 1993;31:55-62.
16. Chung PH, Verhauf BS, Mola R, et al. Correlation between semen prarameters of electro ejaculates and achieving pregnancy by intrauterine insemination. Fertil Steril 1997;67:129-32.
17. Tomlinson M, Amissah-Arthur J, Thompson KA, et al. Prognostic indicators for intrauterine insemination (IUI): statistical model for success. Hum Reprod 1996;11:1892-6.
18. Milingos S, Comhaire FH, Liapi A, et al. The value of semen characteristics and tests of sperm function in selecting couples for intrauterine insemination. Eur J Obstet Gynecol 1996;64: 115-8.
19. Comhaire F, Milingos S, Gordts S, et al. The effective cumulative pregnancy rate of different modes of treatment of male infertility. Andrologia 1995;27:217-21.
20. Johnston RC, Gabor TK, Cording DH, et al. Correlation of semen variables and pregnancy rates for donor insemination: a 15 year retrospective. Fertil Steril 1994;61:355-9.
21. Francavilla F, Romano R, Sanctucci R, et al. Effect of sperm morphology and motile sperm count on outcome of intrauterine insemination in oligospermia and/or asthenozoospermia. Fertil Steril 1990;53:892-7.
22. Bostofte F, Bagger P, Michael A, et al. Fertility prognosis for infertile men: results of follow-up study of semen analysis in infertile men from two different populations evaluated by the Cox regression model. Fertil Steril 1990;54:1100-6.
23. Bolton VM, Braude PR, Ockenden K, et al. An evaluation of semen analysis and *in vitro* tests of sperm function in the prediction of the outcome of intrauterine AIH. Hum Reprod 1989;4:674-9.
24. Kruger TF, Menkveld R, Strander FS, Lombard CJ, et al. Sperm morphologic features as a prognostic factor in *in vitro* fertilization. Fertil Steril 1986;46:1118-23.

25. Kruger TF, Acosta AA, Simmons KF, Swanson RJ, et al. Predictive value of abnormal sperm morphology in *in vitro* fertilization. Fertil Steril 1988;49:112-17.

26. Menkveld R. Clinical significance of the low normal sperm morphology value as proposed in the fifth edition of the WHO Laboratory Manual for the Examination and Processing of Human Semen. Asian J Androl 2010;12:47-58.

27. Menkveld R, Wong WY, Lombard CJ, et al. Semen parameters, including WHO and strict criteria morphology, in a fertile and infertile population: an effort towards standardization of *in vivo* thresholds. Hum Reprod 2001;16:1165-71.

28. Kruger TF, Acosta AA, Simmons KF, Swanson RJ, Matta JF, Veeck LL, Morshedi M, Brugo S. New method of evaluating sperm morphology with predictive value for human in vitro fertilization. Urology 1987;30:248-51.

29. Ombelet W, Bosmans E, Janssen M, et al. Semen parameters in a fertile versus sub-fertile population: a need for change in the interpretation of semen testing. Hum Reprod 1997;12:987-93.

30. Ombelet W, Vandeput H, Van de Putte G, et al. Intrauterine insemination after ovarian stimulation with clomiphene citrate: Predictive potential of inseminating motile count and sperm morphology. Hum Reprod 1997;12:1458-65.

31. Gunalp S, Onculoglu C, Gurgan T, et al. A study of semen parameters with emphasis on sperm morphology in a fertile population: An attempt to develop clinical thresholds. Hum Reprod 2001;16:110-14.

32. Francavilla F, Romano R, Santucci R, Poccia G. Effect of sperm morphology and motile sperm count on outcome of intrauterine insemination in oligozoospermia and/or asthenozoospermia. Fertil Steril 1990;53:892-7.

33. Badawy A, Elnashar A, Eltotongy M. Effect of sperm morphology and number on success of intrauterine insemination. Fertility and Sterility 2009;91:777-81.

34. Van Voorhis BJ, Barnett M, Sparks AE, Syrop CH, Rosenthal G, Dawson J. Effect of the total motile sperm count on the efficacy and cost-effectiveness of intrauterine insemination and *in vitro* fertilization. Fertil Steril 2001;75:661-8.

35. Miller DC, Hollenbeck BK, Smith GD, Randolph JF, Christman GM, Smith YR, et al. Processed total motile sperm count correlates with pregnancy outcome after intrauterine insemination. Urology 2002;60:497-50.

36. ESHRE Capri Workshop Group. Intrauterine insemination. Human Reproduction Update 2009;15:265-77.

37. Byrd W, Drobnis EZ, Kutteh WH, Marshburn P, Carr BR. Intrauterine insemination with frozen donor sperm: a prospective randomized trial comparing three different sperm preparation techniques. Fertil Steril 1994;62:850-6.

38. Dodson WC, Moessner J, Miller J, Legro RS, Gnatuk CL. A randomized comparison of the methods of sperm preparation for intrauterine insemination. Fertil Steril 1998;70(3):574–5.

39. Grigoriou O, Makrakis E, Konidaris S, Hassiakos D, Papadias K, Baka S, Creatsas G. Effect of sperm treatment with exogenous platelet-activating factor on the outcome of intrauterine insemination. Fertil Steril 2005;83(3): 618-21.

40. Posada MN, Azuero AM, Arango AM, Raigosa GC, Cano JF, Perez AL. Sperm washing with swim-up versus gradients in intrauterine insemination (IUI): results of a prospective randomized study comparing pregnancy rates and costs. Fertility and Sterility Abstract book 61st ASRM meeting 2005; Vol. 84 Suppl 1:361.

41. Silber J. The relationship of abnormal semen parameters to male infertility. Hum Repord 1989;4:947-53.

42. Van der Steeg J, Sterures P, Eijkemans M, et al. Role of semen analysis in subfertile couples. Fertil Steril 2011;95;1013-19.

Section VI

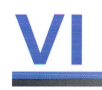

Assisted Reproduction

Assisted Reproduction and Gamete Manipulation Techniques for Male Infertility

Hassan N Sallam, Botros RMB Rizk, Sherman J Silber

INTRODUCTION

The birth of Louise Brown in July 1978, the first baby resulting from *in vitro* fertilization (IVF) of an ovum removed from her mother's ovary with sperm obtained from the father, marked the beginning of a new era in the treatment of infertility (**Figs 24.1A to D**).[1,2] Since then, the technique of *in vitro* fertilization and embryo transfer (IVF-ET) has surpassed the stage of experimentation and has become the most successful procedure for treating infertility in millions of couples who could

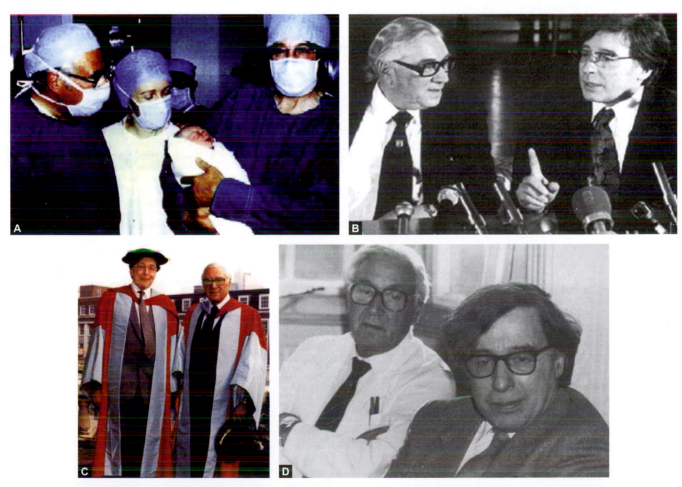

Figures 24.1A to D: (A) Robert Edwards and Patrick Steptoe at the birth of Louise Brown, July 25, 1978 in Oldham, England; (B) Robert Edwards and Patrick Steptoe announcing the scientific developments that led to *in vitro* fertilization at the Royal College in 1978; (C) Robert Edwards and Patrick Steptoe honored by the Royal College in London in 1978; (D) Robert Edwards and Steptoe

not be helped in the past.[3] It has been estimated that by the end of 1998, about 300,000 (IVF) babies had been born worldwide.[4] Amazingly, 4,000,000 babies have been born by 2012.[2] The technique was originally used for the treatment of tubal factor infertility (**Figs 24.2A and B**) but subsequently, couples with endometriosis (**Figs 24.3 to 24.24**) unexplained infertility and male factor infertility have also been treated with IVF.

The success of IVF has been a strong stimulus for the development of other techniques for the treatment of infertility.[3-10] These are collectively known as assisted reproduction technologies (ART). In 1986, Dr Ricardo Asch and his colleagues working in San Antonio, Texas reported the treatment of unexplained infertility using the technique of gamete intrafallopian transfer (GIFT) where the oocyte(s), collected laparoscopically, are replaced during the same setting with the previously prepared

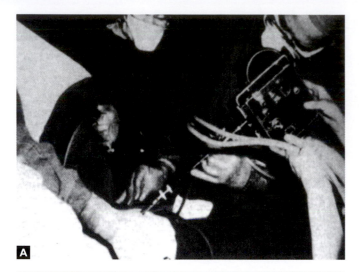

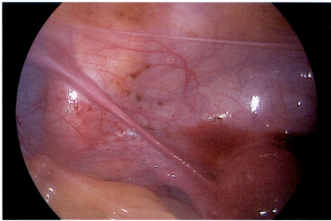

Figure 24.3: Endometriosis seen as burnt powder and copper stains above and below the left round ligament. Small amount of old blood in anterior cul-de-sac, which is frequently observed in women with endometriosis. *Courtesy* of John LaFleur

LAPAROSCOPY IN GYNAECOLOGY

PATRICK C. STEPTOE
F.R.C.S.(Edin.), F.R.C.O.G.

Consultant Gynaecologist to the Oldham Hospital Group, Lancashire

With a foreword by

W. I. C. MORRIS
M.B., Ch.B., F.R.C.S.(Edin.), F.R.C.O.G.
Professor of Obstetrics and Gynaecology. The University of Manchester

DR. H. FRANGENHEIM, M.D.
of the Rheinischen Landesfrauenklinik, Wuppertal,
W. Germany, contributes a section on Sterility

E. & S. LIVINGSTONE LTD.
EDINBURGH & LONDON
1967

Figures 24.2A and B: (A) Patrick Steptoe performing laparoscopic oocyte retrieval recorded by videography; (B) Patrick Steptoe on original monograph on laparoscopy in gynecology

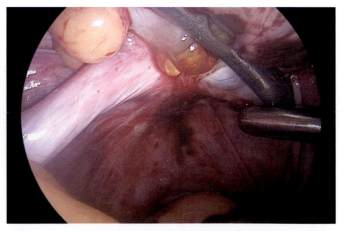

Figure 24.4: Deep endometriosis in left ovarian fossa demonstrating scarring and burnt powder. *Courtesy* of John LaFleur

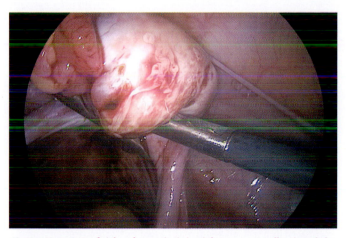

Figure 24.5: Superficial endometriosis in right ovary as well as in cul-de-sac, in between the two uterosacral ligaments. *Courtesy* of John LaFleur

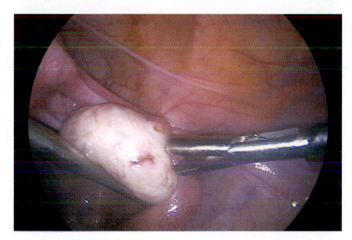

Figure 24.6: Superficial endometriosis in right ovary.
Courtesy of John LaFleur

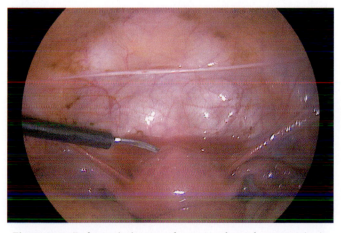

Figure 24.7: Endometriosis seen as burnt powder and copper stains in the anterior cul-de-sac and surface of bladder. *Courtesy* of John LaFleur

husband's spermatozoa in the fallopian tube using the laparoscope (Asch et al., 1985; Asch et al., 1986).[5,6] Subsequently, Jansen and Anderson working in Sydney, Australia, reported the treatment of these patients with transvaginal GIFT, where the oocytes are collected by the transvaginal ultrasound-directed route and replaced inside the fallopian tube after mixing them with the previously prepared husband's spermatozoa, using a special cannula passed through the cervix (Jansen and Anderson, 1993).[9]

Although all the previously mentioned techniques have been used for the treatment of couples with male factor infertility, the success rate was much lower, compared to tubal factor infertility and unexplained infertility (Trounson, 1994).[11] Micromanipulation techniques, have been suggested and different variants have been reported including zona drilling (ZD), partial zona dissection (PZD), subzonal insemination (SUZI) and intracytoplasmic sperm injection (ICSI). The latter technique, first reported by the group of the Dutch-speaking Free University of Belgium, working under the leadership of Andre van Steirteghem, soon showed its superiority over the other variants and is now the technique of choice for the treatment of male factor infertility (Palermo et al., 1992).[10] ICSI and microepididymal sperm aspiration, and testicular sperm extraction pioneered by Sherman J Silber in 1994 are now essential components of most assisted reproduction programs.[2]

These milestones opened the door for further developments that are being reported all the time.[10-18] For example, the development of sperm preparation techniques has led to a revival of the procedure of controlled ovarian hyperstimulation and intrauterine insemination (COh+1UI) in couples with cervical factor infertility (Marinho et al., 1982; Hackeloer and Sallam et al., 1983).[7,12] Similarly, the diminished implantation rates observed after IVF has led to the introduction of assisted hatching either mechanically or by using a YAG-erbium LASER beam (Payne et al., 1991; Strohmer and Feichtinger, 1992).[14,15] As the incidence of multiple pregnancies has been increased with these novel procedures (**Figs 24.25A and B**), the techniques of cryopreservation of embryos, and even gametes, have been introduced in order to maximize the chances of pregnancy resulting from a single attempt of IVF, GIFT or ICSI (Mohr et al., 1985).[13]

In an effort to further diminish the incidence of genetic diseases in the newborn, the technique of preimplantation genetic diagnosis (PGD) has been introduced and the first birth following this technique was reported by the group of the Hammersmith Hospital in London working under the leadership of Robert Winston (Handyside et al., 1990).[8] In PGD, the techniques of molecular biology are used to perform the diagnosis of a possible chromosomal or genetic defect by studying the chromosomes (by fluoro *in situ* hybridization, FISH) or the specific genes (by polymerase chain reaction, PCR, followed by Southern blotting) on a single blastomere removed from the 8-cell embryo.

ASSISTED REPRODUCTION IN MALE INFERTILITY

Male infertility should be properly investigated and the treatment given according to the etiology. The treatment should be followed by repeated semen analyzes. However, if pregnancy

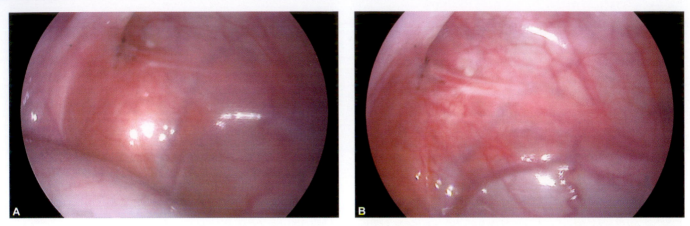

Figures 24.8A and B: Deep pelvic endometriosis around the left uterosacral ligament before surgery. *Courtesy* of Botros Rizk

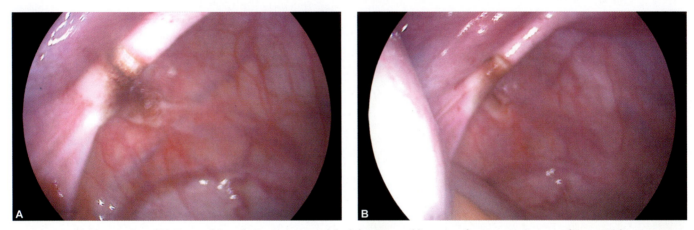

Figures 24.9A and B: Deep pelvic endometriosis around the left uterosacral ligament after surgery. *Courtesy* of Botros Rizk

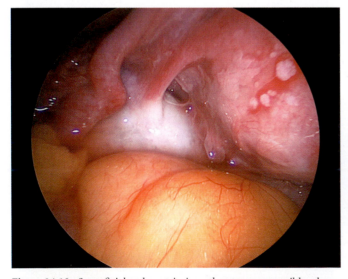

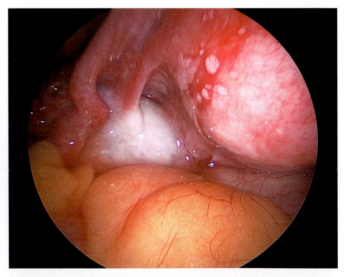

Figure 24.10: Superficial endometriosis on the uterus or possible adenomyosis. Adhesions of left ovary and posterior surface of uterus on the left and left uterosacral ligament. Courtesy of Botros Rizk

Figure 24.11: Endometriosis in the cul-de-sac. Adhesions between right ovary and uterus. Courtesy of Botros Rizk

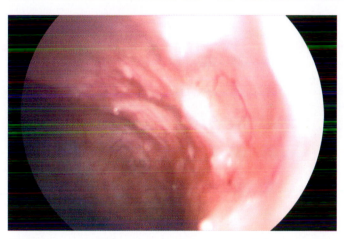

Figure 24.12: Multiple vesicles of endometriosis in cul-de-sac and right uterosacral ligament. Courtesy of Botros Rizk

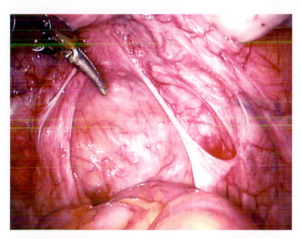

Figure 24.15: Robotic laparoscopy showing deep endometriosis in the cul-de-sac and flimsy adhesions. Courtesy of Botros Rizk

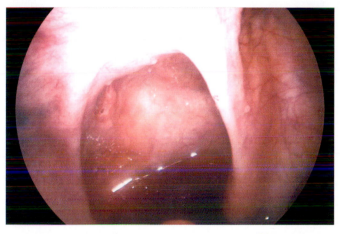

Figure 24.13: Old blood in cul-de-sac, suggesting possible endometriosis. Vesicles are suggestive of possible endometriosis in inside and outside of uterosacral ligament. Courtesy of Botros Rizk

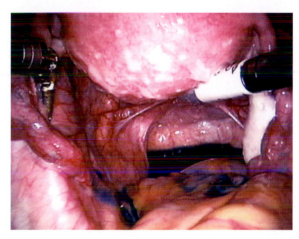

Figure 24.16: Robotic laparoscopy showing patent fallopian tubes despite deep endometriosis. Courtesy of Botros Rizk

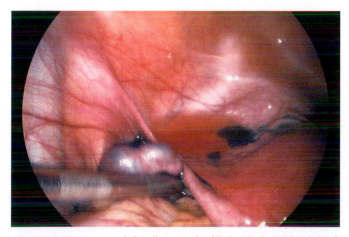

Figure 24.14: Tortuous left Fallopian tube filled with dye with minimal spillage of methylene blue dye. Courtesy of Botros Rizk

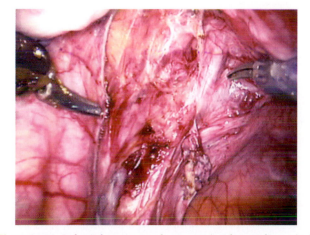

Figure 24.17: Robotic laparoscopy demonstrating deep endometriosis in the left broad ligament. Courtesy of Botros Rizk

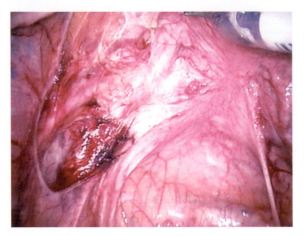

Figure 24.18: Robotic laparoscopy demonstrating deep pelvic endometriosis during resection of left broad ligament. Courtesy of Botros Rizk

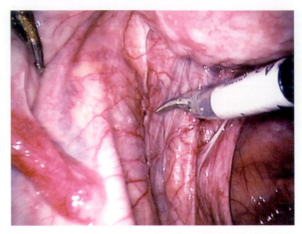

Figure 24.21: Robotic laparoscopy showing adhesions in the left broad ligament. Courtesy of Botros Rizk

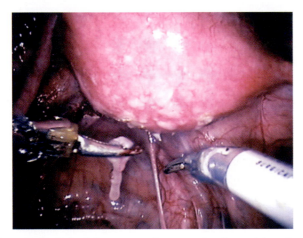

Figure 24.19: Robotic laparoscopy demonstrating deep pelvic endometriosis during resection of left broad ligament. Courtesy of Botros Rizk

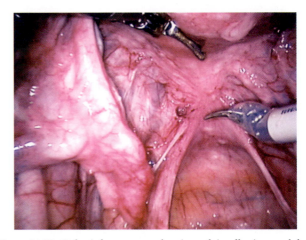

Figure 24.22: Robotic laparoscopy showing pelvic adhesions and deep endometriosis. Courtesy of Botros Rizk

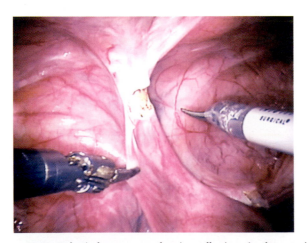

Figure 24.20: Robotic laparoscopy showing adhesions in the anterior cul-de-sac in left side of pelvis, not necessarily related to endometriosis. Courtesy of Botros Rizk

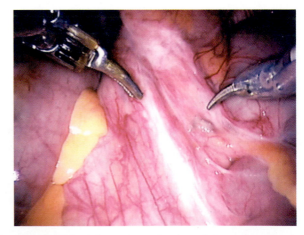

Figure 24.23: Robotic laparoscopy showing pelvic scarring. Courtesy of Botros Rizk

does not result in a reasonable period of time, one can resort to one of the following techniques:

- *Intrauterine insemination (IUI) (chapter 21)*: Although many pregnancies have resulted from IUI in infertile couples with male infertility, most clinicians currently perform it for 3 or 4 cycles before resorting to ICSI.
- *In vitro fertilization*: Although IVF was initially used for the treatment of tubal infertility, it was later used in the treatment of male infertility and unexplained infertility. However, the results are diminished in cases of male infertility due to failure of fertilization in many instances because of the bad quality of the semen. Mahadevan and Trounson reported no

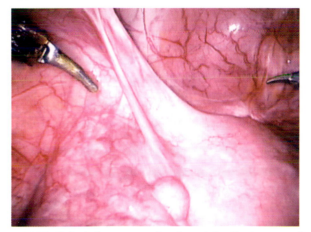

Figure 24.24: Robotic laparoscopy showing pelvic adhesions not related to endometriosis. Courtesy of Botros Rizk

fertilization when motility of the sperm was less than 20% (Mahadevan and Trounson, 1984).[19] Sperm morphology was found to be the most important parameter which correlates with fertilization; and Kruger and Koetzee found that total failure of fertilization occurs if strict morphology of the spermatozoa is less than 4 percent (Kruger and Coetzee, 1999).[20] The following procedures have been suggested to improve the chances of fertilization in cases of male factor infertility treated with IVF:

- *Better sperm preparation techniques (e.g. Percoll, Ficoll and Nicodenz)*: Using these filtration sperm recovery methods, the most fertile fraction of the semen sample can be separated and used for the insemination (Mortimer, 1994).[21]
- *Microdroplet insemination*: The processed semen is condensed and a microdroplet containing a very high concentration of sperm is added to the oocyte, which is placed in a droplet of culture medium kept under paraffin oil (Trounson et al., 1994).[11]
- *Micromanipulation techniques*: The fertilization process is helped by the use of micromanipulators attached to the inverted microscope. The following micromanipulation procedures (**Fig. 24.26A**) have been used for this purpose:
  - *Zona drilling*: In this technique, a hole is made in the zona pellucida using a microjet of acid Tyrode's solution (Payne et al., 1991)[14] or a beam of erbium LASER (Strohmer and Feichtinger, 1992) to facilitate the entry of the spermatozoa into the zona pellucida.[15]
  - *Partial zona dissection*: In this technique, a slit is opened in the zona pellucida to facilitate entrance of one or more

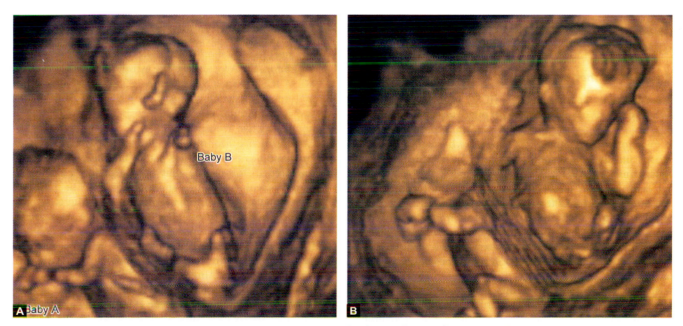

Figures 24.25A and B: 3D ultrasounds of twins. Courtesy by Botros Rizk

28. Tournaye H. Surgical sperm recovery for intracytoplasmic sperm injection: which method is to be preferred? Hum. Reprod 1999;14(Suppl 1):71-81.

29. Tsujimura A. Microdissection testicular sperm extraction: prediction, outcome, and complications. Int J Urol 2007;14: 883-9.

30. Chan PT, Libman J. Feasibility of microsurgical reconstruction of the male reproductive tract after percutaneous epididymal sperm aspiration (PESA). Can J Urol 2003;10: 2070-3.

31. Van Peperstraten A, Proctor ML, Johnson NP, Philipson G. Techniques for surgical retrieval of sperm prior to intra-cyto-plasmic sperm injection (ICSI) for azoospermia. Cochrane Database Syst Rev 2008;(2):CD002807.

32. Yamamoto M, et al. Microsurgical epididymal sperm aspiration versus epididymal micropuncture with perivascular nerve stimulation for intracytoplasmic sperm injection to treat unreconstructable obstructive azoospermia. Arch Androl 1996;36:217-24.

33. Belenky A, et al. Ultrasound-guided testicular sperm aspiration in azoospermic patients: a new sperm retrieval method for intra-cytoplasmic sperm injection. J Clin Ultrasound 2001;29:339-43.

34. AbdelHafez F, Bedaiwy M, El-Nashar SA, Sabanegh E, Desai N. Techniques for cryopreservation of individual or small numbers of human spermatozoa: a systematic review. Hum Reprod Update 2009;15:153-64.

35. Desai NN, Blackmon H, Goldfarb J. Single sperm cryopreservation on cryoloops: an alternative to hamster zona for freezing individual spermatozoa. Reprod Biomed Online 2004;9:47-53.

36. Isachenko E, et al. DNA integrity and motility of human spermatozoa after standard slow freezing versus cryoprotectant-free vitrification. Hum Reprod 2004;19:932-9.

37. Hauser R, et al. Severe hypospermatogenesis in cases of nonobstructive azoospermia: should we use fresh or frozen testicular spermatozoa? J Androl 2005;26:772-8.

38. Ishikawa T, et al. Fertilization and pregnancy using cryopreserved testicular sperm for intracytoplasmic sperm injection with azoospermia. Fertil Steril 2009;92:174-9.

39. Wu B, et al. Optimal use of fresh and frozen-thawed testicular sperm for intracytoplasmic sperm injection in azoospermic patients. J Assist Reprod Genet 2005;22:389-94.

40. Van Rumste MM, Evers JL, Farquhar CM. Intra-cytoplasmic sperm injection versus conventional techniques for oocyte insemination during *in vitro* fertilisation in patients with non-male subfertility. Cochrane Database Syst Rev 2003;(2): CD001301.

41. National Summary Report. (2011).at <http://apps.nccd.cdc. gov/art/Apps/National Summary Report.aspx.

42. Patient fact sheet Intracytoplasmic Sperm Injection (ICSI). (2008). at <http://www.asrm.org/Patients/FactSheets/ICSI-Fact. pdf.

43. Kanto S, et al. Fresh motile testicular sperm retrieved from nonobstructive azoospermic patients has the same potential to achieve fertilization and pregnancy via ICSI as sperm retrieved from obstructive azoospermic patients. Fertil. Steril 2010;90:. e5-2010.e7 (2008).

44. Palermo GD, et al. Fertilization and pregnancy outcome with intracytoplasmic sperm injection for azoospermic men Hum Reprod 1999;14:741-8.

45. De Croo I, Van der Elst J, Everaert K, De Sutter P, Dhont M. Fertilization, pregnancy and embryo implantation rates after ICSI in cases of obstructive and non-obstructive azoospermia. Hum Reprod 2000;15:1383-8.

46. Vernaeve V, et al. Pregnancy outcome and neonatal data of children born after ICSI using testicular sperm in obstructive and non-obstructive azoospermia. Hum Reprod 2003;18:2093-7.

47. Vernaeve V, et al. Intracytoplasmic sperm injection with testicular spermatozoa is less successful in men with nonobstructive azoospermia than in men with obstructive azoospermia. Fertil Steril 2003;79:529-33.

48. Alukal JP, Lamb DJ. Intracytoplasmic sperm injection (ICSI)—what are the risks? Urol Clin North Am 2008;35:277-88, ix-x.

49. Shebl O, Ebner T, Sommergruber M, Sir A, Tews G. Risk in twin pregnancies after the use of assisted reproductive techniques. J Reprod Med 2008;53:798-802.

50. La Sala GB, et al. Lower embryonic loss rates among twin gestations following assisted reproduction. J. Assist Reprod Genet 2005;22:181-4.

51. Lambers MJ, et al. Factors determining early pregnancy loss in singleton and multiple implantations. Hum Reprod 2007;22: 275-9.

52. Al-Fifi S, et al. Congenital anomalies and other perinatal outcomes in ICSI vs. naturally conceived pregnancies: a comparative study. J Assist Reprod Genet 2009;26:377-81.

53. Shebl O, Ebner T, Sommergruber M, Sir A, Tews G. Birth weight is lower for survivors of the vanishing twin syndrome: a case-control study. Fertil Steril 2008;90:310-4.

54. Pinborg A, Lidegaard O, Freiesleben NC, Andersen AN. Vanishing twins: a predictor of small-for-gestational age in IVF singletons. Hum Reprod 2007;22:2707-14.

55. Tarlatzis BC, Bili H. Intracytoplasmic sperm injection. Survey of world results. Ann NYAcad Sci 2000;900:336-44.

56. Allen VM, Wilson RD, Cheung A. Genetics Committee of the Society of Obstetricians and Gynaecologists of Canada (SOGC) and Reproductive Endocrinology Infertility Committee of the Society of Obstetricians and Gynaecologists of Canada (SOGC). Pregnancy outcomes after assisted reproductive technology. J Obstet Gynaecol Can 2006;28:220-50.

57. ESHRE Capri Workshop Group Intracytoplasmic sperm injection (ICSI) in 2006: evidence and evolution. Hum Reprod Update 2007;13:515-26.

58. Jozwiak EA, Ulug U, Mesut A, Erden HF, Bahceci M. Prenatal karyotypes of fetuses conceived by intracytoplasmic sperm injection. Fertil Steril 2004;82:628-33.

59. Reefhuis J, et al. Assisted reproductive technology and major structural birth defects in the United States. Hum Reprod 2009;24:360-6.

60. Belva F, et al. Medical outcome of 8-year-old singleton ICSI children (born >or=32 weeks' gestation) and a spontaneously conceived comparison group. Hum Reprod 2007;22:506-15.

61. Watkins AJ, Papenbrock T, Fleming TP. The preimplantation embryo: handle with care. Semin Reprod Med 2008;26:175-85.

62. Ludwig M, et al. Increased prevalence of imprinting defects in patients with Angelman syndrome born to subfertile couples. J Med Genet 2005;42:289-91.

63. Maher ER, et al. Beckwith-Wiedemann syndrome and assisted reproduction technology (ART). J Med Genet 2003;40:62-4.

64. Leunens L, Celestin-Westreich S, Bonduelle M, Liebaers I, Ponjaert-Kristoffersen I. Follow-up of cognitive and motor development of 10-year-old singleton children born after ICSI compared with spontaneously conceived children. Hum Reprod 2008;23:105-11.

65. Middelburg KJ, Heineman MJ, Bos AF, Hadders-Algra M. Neuromotor, cognitive, language and behavioural outcome in children born following IVF or ICSI-a systematic review. Hum Reprod Update 2008;14:219-31.

66. Friedler S, et al. Testicular sperm retrieval by percutaneous fine needle sperm aspiration compared with testicular sperm extraction by open biopsy in men with nonobstructive azoospermia. Hum Reprod 1997;12:1488-93.

67. Meniru GI, Gorgy A, Podsiadly BT, Craft IL. Results of percutaneous epididymal sperm aspiration and intracytoplasmic sperm injection in two major groups of patients with obstructive azoospermia. Hum Reprod 1997;12:2443-6.

68. Devroey P, et al. Outcome of intracytoplasmic sperm injection with testicular spermatozoa in obstructive and non-obstructive azoospermia. Hum Reprod 1996;11:1015-8.

69. Desai N, AbdelHafez F, Sabanegh E, Goldfarb J. Paternal effect on genomic activation, clinical pregnancy and live birth rate after ICSI with cryopreserved epididymal versus testicular spermatozoa. Reprod Biol Endocrinol 2009;7:142.

70. Ghanem M, et al. Comparison of the outcome of intracytoplasmic sperm injection in obstructive and non-obstructive azoospermia in the first cycle: a report of case series and meta-analysis. Int J Androl 2005;28:16-21.

71. Gil-Salom M, Minguez Y, Rubio C, Remohi J, Pellicer A. Intracytoplasmic testicular sperm injection: an effective treatment for otherwise intractable obstructive azoospermia. J Urol 1995;154:2074-7.

72. Kahraman S, et al. High implantation and pregnancy rates with testicular sperm extraction and intracytoplasmic sperm injection in obstructive and non-obstructive azoospermia. Hum Reprod 1996;11:673-6.

73. Okada H, et al. Assisted reproduction technology for patients with congenital bilateral absence of vas deferens. J Urol 1999;161:1157-62.

74. Araki Y, et al. Intracytoplasmic injection with late spermatids: a successful procedure in achieving childbirth for couples in which the male partner suffers from azoospermia due to deficient spermatogenesis. Fertil Steril 1997;67:559-61.

75. Ben-Yosef D, et al. Testicular sperm retrieval and cryopreservation prior to initiating ovarian stimulation as the first line approach in patients with non-obstructive azoospermia. Hum Reprod 1999;14:1794-1801.

76. Damani MN, et al. Postchemotherapy ejaculatory azoospermia: fatherhood with sperm from testis tissue with intracytoplasmic sperm injection. J Clin Oncol 2002;20:930-6.

77. Friedler S, et al. Factors influencing the outcome of ICSI in patients with obstructive and non-obstructive azoospermia: a comparative study. Hum Reprod 2002;17:3114-21.

78. Gil-Salom M, et al. Testicular sperm extraction and intracytoplasmic sperm injection: a chance of fertility in nonobstructive azoospermia. J Urol 1998;160:2063-7.

79. Haimov-Kochman R, Prus D, Farchat M, Bdolah Y, Hurwitz A. Reproductive outcome of men with azoospermia due to cryptorchidism using assisted techniques. Int J Androl 2010;33:e139-43.

80. Hauser R, et al. Multiple testicular sampling in non-obstructive azoospermia-is it necessary? Hum Reprod 1998;13:3081-5.

81. Haydardedeoglu B, Turunc T, Kilicdag EB, Gul U, Bagis T. The effect of prior varicocelectomy in patients with nonobstructive azoospermia on intracytoplasmic sperm injection outcomes: a retrospective pilot study. Urology 2010;75:83-6.

82. Inci K, et al. Sperm retrieval and intracytoplasmic sperm injection in men with nonobstructive azoospermia, and treated and untreated varicocele. J Urol 2009;182:1500-5.

83. Kahraman S, et al. Fertility with testicular sperm extraction and intracytoplasmic sperm injection in non-obstructive azoospermic men. Hum Reprod 1996;11:756-60.

84. Khadra AA, Abdulhadi I, Ghunain S, Kilani Z. Efficiency of percutaneous testicular sperm aspiration as a mode of sperm collection for intracytoplasmic sperm injection in nonobstructive azoospermia. J Urol 2003;169:603-5.

85. Lewin A, et al. Testicular fine needle aspiration: the alternative method for sperm retrieval in non-obstructive azoospermia. Hum Reprod 1999;14:1785-90.

86. Meseguer M, et al. Testicular sperm extraction (TESE) and ICSI in patients with permanent azoospermia after chemotherapy. Hum Reprod 2003;18:1281-5.

87. Ramasamy R, et al. Successful fertility treatment for Klinefelter's syndrome. J Urol 2009;182:1108-13.

88. Ravizzini P, et al. Microdissection testicular sperm extraction and IVF-ICSI outcome in nonobstructive azoospermia. Andrologia 2008;40:219-26.

89. Schiff JD, et al. Success of testicular sperm extraction [corrected] and intracytoplasmic sperm injection in men with Klinefelter syndrome. J Clin Endocrinol Metab 2005;90:6263-7.

90. Schlegel PN, et al. Testicular sperm extraction with intracytoplasmic sperm injection for nonobstructive azoospermia. Urology 1997;49:435-40.

91. Silber SJ, et al. Normal pregnancies resulting from testicular sperm extraction and intracytoplasmic sperm injection for azoospermia due to maturation arrest. Fertil Steril 1996;66:110-7.

92. Su LM, et al. Testicular sperm extraction with intracytoplasmic sperm injection for nonobstructive azoospermia: testicular histology can predict success of sperm retrieval. J Urol 1999;161:112-6.

93. Tournaye H, et al. Testicular sperm recovery in nine 47,XXY Klinefelter patients. Hum Reprod 1996;11:1644-9.

94. Turunc T, et al. Conventional testicular sperm extraction combined with the microdissection technique in nonobstructive azoospermic patients: a prospective comparative study. Fertil Steril 2010;94:2157-60.

95. Vernaeve V, et al. Outcome of testicular sperm recovery and ICSI in patients with non-obstructive azoospermia with a history of orchidopexy. Hum Reprod 2004;19:2307-12.

96. Yarali H, et al. TESE-ICSI in patients with non-mosaic Klinefelter syndrome: a comparative study. Reprod Biomed Online 2009;18:756-60.

26

Fertility Management in Spinal Cord Injury and Ejaculatory Dysfunction

Viacheslav Iremashvili, Nancy L Brackett, Dana A Ohl, Jens Sønksen, Charles M Lynne

■ INTRODUCTION

The number of people living with spinal cord injury in the United States has been estimated to be approximately 259,000 persons with more than 10,000 new injuries occurring annually.[1] The majority of individuals affected by spinal cord injury are men aged between 18 and 35 years, i.e. men in their prime parenting years. Fertility is severely impaired in the vast majority of these men. This impairment results from the combination of erectile dysfunction, ejaculatory dysfunction and semen abnormalities. Management of infertility in these patients can present challenges due to the unique nature of their condition. In *this review, emphasis* has been placed on the most important clinical problems faced by physicians treating infertility in men with spinal cord injury.

Methods of treating erectile dysfunction in the able-bodied population are highly effective in men with spinal cord injury. Although erectile dysfunction contributes to the development of infertility in men with spinal cord injury and negatively affects their quality of life, restoration of erection usually is not a prerequisite for treating infertility in these men. Ejaculatory dysfunction, on the contrary, represents a major obstacle as about 90 percent of patients with spinal cord injury are unable to ejaculate during sexual intercourse, even if erectile function is restored.[2] As a result, the first clinical problem faced by the physician managing infertility in men with spinal cord injury is:

How to Get the Semen?

Treatment of anejaculation is the most extensively studied area in the management of fertility problems in men with spinal cord injury. Currently, there are two widely used methods of medically assisted ejaculation: *Electroejaculation* and *penile vibratory stimulation*. Both techniques are reasonably effective and safe. However, they are characterized by several important differences which require consideration.

Electroejaculation was popularized in the 1980s by a veterinarian Stephen Seager. This practitioner adapted for humans a sperm retrieval technique which had been used for many years in a variety of animal species. Electroejaculation is performed by placing a probe containing electrodes into the patient's rectum and delivering electrical stimulation until semen is released. It is

assumed that ejaculation results from the stimulation of peripheral pelvic nerve fibers innervating the genital tract.[2,3] Studies have shown that total motile sperm recovery by electroejaculation is optimized when the current is delivered in an interrupted pattern versus a continuous pattern.[4,5] **Figure 26.1** shows the Seager electroejaculation machine.

Penile vibratory stimulation has become increasingly popular during the last 15 years, especially after the research and development of a high amplitude vibrator (**Fig. 26.2**) by Jens Sonksen, MD, PhD.[6,7] This method of semen retrieval is performed by delivering vibratory mechanical stimulation to the glans penis.[8,9] Penile vibratory stimulation causes ejaculation by eliciting the ejaculatory reflex via stimulation of the dorsal penile nerve and is most effective in patients with the level of injury of at or rostral to T10.[10,11] High amplitude vibration (2.5 mm) is optimal for inducing ejaculation in men with spinal cord injury.[12]

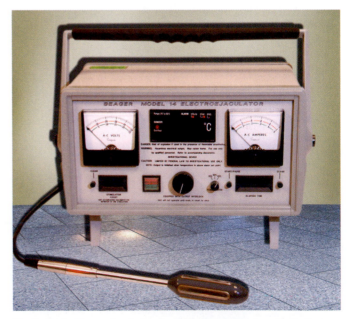

Figure 26.1: Electroejaculation is a safe and effective method of semen retrieval in men with spinal cord injury. The Seager electroejaculator is the only commercially available electroejaculation device

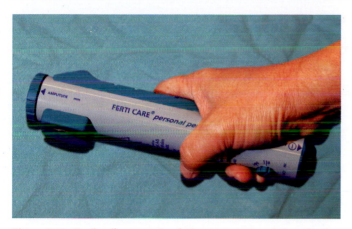

Figure 26.2: Penile vibratory stimulation is recommended as the first line of treatment for semen retrieval in men with spinal cord injury. The FERTI CARE® personal vibrator is a commercially available device developed specifically for inducing ejaculation in men with spinal cord injury

Penile vibratory stimulation is usually preferred over electroejaculation as the first method of sperm retrieval in an ejaculatory men with spinal cord injury. The advantages of penile vibratory stimulation include lower cost, higher patient preference and better semen quality.[13,14] Penile vibratory stimulation can also be combined with abdominal electrical stimulation. This combined procedure has been reported to rescue some failures to penile vibratory stimulation alone.[15] **Figure 26.2** shows an example of the FertiCare vibrator developed by Dr Sonksen.

In a retrospective review of a large single-center experience, we presented our algorithm of sperm retrieval in patients with spinal cord injury,[16] (**Flow chart 26.1**). Patients unable to ejaculate with masturbation should be administered a trial of penile vibratory stimulation with one vibrator. Failures with one vibrator should be administered a trial with two vibrators (also known as the "sandwich" technique)[8] unless:

• Their level of injury is T11 or caudal
• They have complete absence of somatic responses, i.e. an absence of muscle contractions below the level of injury. Such subjects have abnormal nerve conduction in the T11-S4 segments which disrupts the ejaculatory reflex and renders penile vibratory stimulation ineffective. These cases should proceed to electroejaculation. Patients who fail with two vibrators may, prior to electroejaculation, undergo some optional (unproven, non-standard) treatments, such as:
• Prostatic massage
• Penile vibratory stimulation combined with midodrine
• Penile vibratory stimulation combined with oral inhibitors of phosphodiesterase type 5
• Penile vibratory stimulation combined with abdominal electrical stimulation.

Failures of electroejaculation should proceed to surgical sperm retrieval. Patients who experience pain during electroejaculation (a minority, typically those with retained pelvic sensation) may be offered electroejaculation under sedation prior to

being offered surgical sperm retrieval. Performing electroejaculation under general anesthesia is not cost-effective in the United States.[17]

The above mentioned study found that, overall, the methods of penile vibratory stimulation and electroejaculation were highly effective. Of 435 patients who went through the algorithm, sperm were obtained from 422 (97%) without resorting to surgical sperm retrieval. These results are important in the context of a recent tendency of practitioners to not examine the ejaculate as a source of sperm in men with spinal cord injury. In some centers, these patients are offered surgical sperm retrieval as a first treatment option. Our survey of professionals showed that a lack of familiarity with simpler methods was the primary reason.[18] Other reasons mentioned by respondents were a lack of necessary equipment or training. Logistics presented additional problems for some respondents. For example, when the date of semen retrieval must be timed to ovulation, it may be difficult to schedule a urologist to perform a sperm retrieval when the lead time is short, i.e. 1–2 days which is common in these cases.

Surgical sperm retrieval is more expensive, invasive, and risky than penile vibratory stimulation or electroejaculation. Surgical sperm retrieval has been associated with serious adverse effects including testicular hematoma, edema and post-surgical testicular fibrosis.[19] Furthermore, surgical sperm retrieval rarely yields enough motile sperm for use in any assisted conception procedure other than intracytoplasmic sperm injection. (This issue will be discussed later in the chapter).

Thus, penile vibratory stimulation and electroejaculation are the primary methods of semen retrieval in men with spinal cord injury. These techniques are effective in nearly all patients. Invasive methods of sperm retrieval are rarely indicated in this group of patients.

In addition to ejaculatory and erectile dysfunction, most men with spinal cord injury have poor semen quality. Low sperm motility and low sperm viability are the most common abnormalities. Although sperm concentration is normal in most men with spinal cord injury, a minority are azoospermic.[18] This relatively small group of spinal cord injured patients represents a major clinical challenge.

What to do If there is no Sperm in the Ejaculation?

While the management of anejaculation in men with spinal cord injuries has been thoroughly studied, as described above, the consensus management strategy for azoospermia in these patients remains to be established. A recent study found that the probability of finding any sperm in subsequent ejaculates of patients with spinal cord injury who were found to be azoospermic in their first ejaculate was relatively higher if electroejaculation versus penile vibratory stimulation was used as a method of semen retrieval.[20]

Once a sperm-containing ejaculate has been obtained from a man with spinal cord injury, it may be used to attempt pregnancy. Various methodologies are available to induce pregnancy with sperm from men with spinal cord injury. The clinician is thus confronted with the next question:

Flow chart 26.1: Algorithm for sperm retrieval in men with spinal cord injury

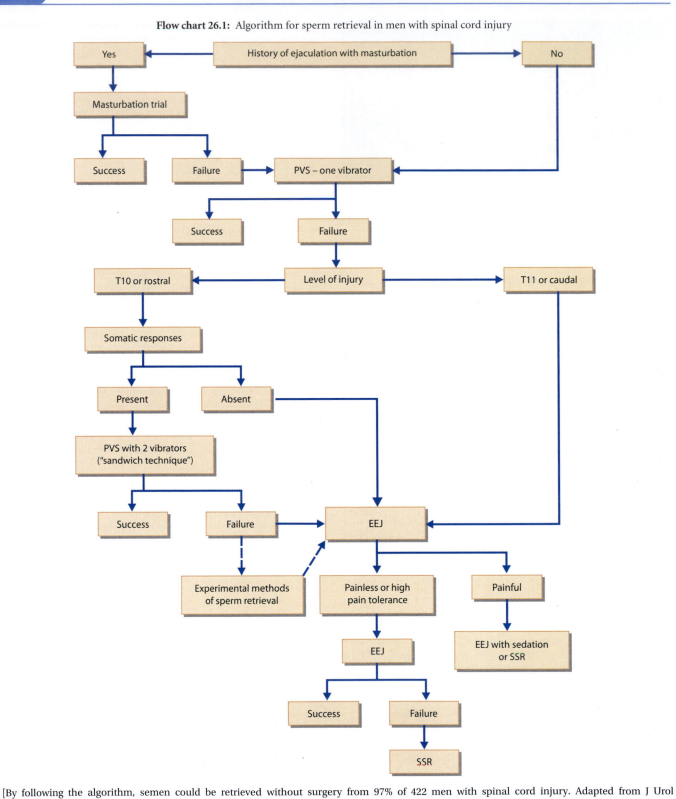

[By following the algorithm, semen could be retrieved without surgery from 97% of 422 men with spinal cord injury. Adapted from J Urol 2010;183:2304-2308]

Which Method of Assisted Conception is Recommended for the Couple with Male Factor Infertility due to Spinal Cord Injury?

The key issue to consider when choosing a specific method of insemination or assisted reproduction is the quality of semen. Among different semen parameters, the total number of motile spermatozoa is the factor which most heavily influences the choice of procedure.

Only a minority of men with spinal cord injury have normal semen quality. For example, in a recent study we found that only 30 out of 400 subjects (7.5%) had at least one normal semen analysis.[21] In these patients, or in those who have relatively minor semen abnormalities, intravaginal insemination is a viable treatment option. This method is usually used in combination with penile vibratory stimulation. In selected couples who can learn to independently perform penile vibratory stimulation, home intravaginal insemination is an option. The female partner should have an evaluation of her fertility potential prior to the treatment.

The pregnancy rate of intravaginal insemination in couples with a male partner with spinal cord injury ranged from 25 percent to more than 50 percent in the few published studies. A recent international study showed that 60 of 140 cases (43%) with spinal cord injured male partners achieved a pregnancy by intravaginal insemination performed at home.[22] Another recent study found that 17 of 45 couples with spinal cord injured male partners (38%) achieved pregnancy with intravaginal insemination at home.[22a] Although the inclusion criteria and number of ovulation cycles differed between these studies, their results show that intravaginal insemination is a successful and cost-effective technique in men with spinal cord injury who have a relatively high quality of semen.

Another relatively simple assisted insemination procedure which could be used in some couples with spinal cord injured male partners is intrauterine insemination. The objective of this procedure is to bypass the vaginal and cervical barriers, and deposit good quality spermatozoa, i.e. spermatozoa with progressive motility, directly into the uterine cavity. Correspondingly, the success of this procedure depends on the number of available motile spermatozoa. The minimal number of motile spermatozoa required for successful intrauterine insemination is not clear. A majority of practitioners accept that intrauterine insemination may be considered when, after semen preparation, at least 5×10^6 motile spermatozoa can be harvested.[23] For example, in a study of 121 couples, 87 of whom had male partners with spinal cord injury, the pregnancy rate with intrauterine insemination was only 1.1 percent per cycle if the total motile sperm count was less than 4×10^6. If the total motile sperm count was more than 40×10^6, the pregnancy rate per cycle was 17.6 percent.[17] According to our experience in men with spinal cord injury, total motile sperm counts exceed 5×10^6 in 62.8 percent of all ejaculates and in 71.4 percent of the antegrade ejaculates collected by penile vibratory stimulation.[16] Thus, in the majority of men with spinal cord injury, sufficient numbers of motile spermatozoa can be obtained to consider intrauterine insemination as a treatment option.

A considerable body of evidence shows that intrauterine insemination is associated with reasonable pregnancy success rates (i.e. about 10% per cycle) when used in couples with spinal cord injured male partners. (see.[18] for review). If pregnancy is not achieved after 3–6 cycles of intrauterine insemination, more advanced techniques such as in vitro fertilization or intracytoplasmic sperm injection should be considered.[2] These techniques are also the treatment of choice when fewer than 5×10^6 progressively motile spermatozoa are available after preparation. For spinal cord injured patients in whom surgical sperm retrieval was used, intracytoplasmic sperm injection is the only feasible technique in order to obtain fertilization in vitro. Overall, the pregnancy success rates of in vitro fertilization techniques in couples with spinal cord injured male partners are comparable to those in couples with general male factor infertility.[18]

Penile vibratory stimulation and electroejaculation typically yield sufficient numbers of motile sperm for consideration in simple assisted conception procedures such as intravaginal insemination or intrauterine insemination. It is unfortunate, then, that these simple procedures are frequently bypassed in favor of more expensive and advanced techniques that may not be necessary in this population. Simple procedures are less risky, less invasive and less expensive options compared to advanced ones. An added benefit of intravaginal insemination is that it may be taught to couples and performed at home. Surgical sperm retrieval rarely yields sufficient total motile sperm for simple insemination procedures, and this outcome resigns couples to higher cost, higher risk, and more invasive options.

Is there Any Way to Improve the Quality of Semen in Men with Spinal Cord Injury?

Although impairments in semen quality are well-documented consequences of spinal cord injury, the underlying mechanism for such defects has not been determined. A number of mechanisms have been postulated, and some of them could be potential targets of treatment aimed at improving semen quality.

It is important to point out that the pathological process leading to abnormal semen quality in men with spinal cord injury does not seem to be progressive. For example, results of cross-sectional[24] and longitudinal studies[25] indicate that there is not a significant decline in semen parameters with ensuing years postinjury. From a practical point of view it means that patients and their spouses do not have to consider the number of years postinjury as a major risk factor in family planning. Although a rare patient may progress from severe oligospermia to azoospermia, measures such as sperm freezing soon after injury are currently not indicated in this patient population.

The negative effect of elevated scrotal temperature on spermatogenesis was initially considered to be a plausible etiologic factor for the development of semen abnormalities in men with spinal cord injury.[26] It was assumed that men with spinal cord injury could have generalized scrotal thermoregulatory dysfunction or elevated scrotal temperature as a result of long periods of sitting in wheelchairs. The presence of elevated scrotal temperature in men with spinal cord injury, however, has never been conclusively established.[27]

It has also been hypothesized that, because most men with spinal cord injury are anejaculatory, long periods between ejaculations may lead to reproductive tract stasis which can negatively affect sperm. If this were the case, semen quality could be improved as a result of repeated medically assisted ejaculations. However, nearly all studies investigating the effect of repeated ejaculation on semen quality in men with spinal cord injury failed to find significant improvement in semen parameters.[2]

Nevertheless, reproductive tract stasis, although not directly related to the frequency of ejaculation, could still be an important factor in the pathogenesis of semen abnormalities in men with spinal cord injury. It is well known that in normal men, mature sperm cells are stored in the epididymis and vas deferens, but not in seminal vesicles. Ohl et al. showed that spinal cord injury could be associated with fundamental changes in mature sperm transport and storage.[28] In this study, bilateral seminal vesicle aspiration was performed immediately before electroejaculation or penile vibratory stimulation. These aspirates contained large numbers of poor quality sperm. It is particularly remarkable that the duration of abstinence was not associated with the number of seminal vesicle sperm. Furthermore, the semen parameters in samples obtained immediately after seminal vesicle aspiration were significantly better compared to historical ejaculated parameters. These data indicate that altered transport with sperm stagnation in the seminal vesicles could contribute to the development of semen abnormalities in men with spinal cord injury. The clinical value of these data remains to be established.

In selected able-bodied infertile men, correction of severe hormonal abnormalities may result in induction of fertility.[29] Different alterations in the serum levels of pituitary and gonadal hormones are present in up to one half of spinal cord injured patients. However, no consistent correlation between these abnormalities and semen quality has been shown.[30]

The role of changes in the composition of the seminal plasma in the pathogenesis of semen abnormalities in men with spinal cord injury has been an active area of study over the last decade. Seminal plasma from men with spinal cord injury was shown to be toxic to sperm and could be a major contributing factor to poor sperm quality. For example, mixing seminal plasma from men with spinal cord injury with normal sperm obtained from healthy, able-bodied men resulted in a rapid decrease in the healthy men's sperm motility.[31] At the same time, sperm aspirated from the vas deferens in men with spinal cord injury had significantly higher motility compared to the sperm in the ejaculate (i.e. mixed with seminal plasma) in the same subjects.[32]

Several constituents of the seminal plasma in subjects with spinal cord injury could be responsible for its toxicity. A significant increase in the seminal concentration of leukocytes is present in most men with spinal cord injury.[33,34] Seminal vesicles are the most likely origin of this leukocytospermia.[2] Cytofluorographic analysis of leukocyte subtypes in the semen of men with spinal cord injury revealed increased numbers of activated T lymphocytes,[35] known to produce cytotoxic cytokines.[36] Seminal plasma from men with spinal cord injury contains elevated levels of different cytokines including proinflammatory interleukin 1 beta, interleukin 6, and tumor necrosis factor

alpha.[37] Inactivation of these cytokines, by adding monoclonal antibodies or receptor blockers improves sperm motility.[38,39]

There is also an increasing awareness of the importance of reactive oxygen species in the development of semen abnormalities in men with spinal cord injury. Several studies have shown that reactive oxygen species levels are much higher in semen from men with spinal cord injury compared to normal and infertile able-bodied men.[40,41] Semen abnormalities characteristic in men with spinal cord injury, such as decreased sperm motility, decreased sperm viability, sperm DNA damage, impaired sperm function, and hyperviscosity of the semen, could be a direct result of sperm oxidative stress.

The potential sources of elevated levels of reactive oxygen species in semen of men with spinal cord injury are activated leukocytes and increased numbers of immature sperm. Of different leukocyte subtypes, cells which are peroxidase-positive (namely neutrophils and macrophages), are predominant sources of reactive oxygen species production. These white blood cell subpopulations are principal contributors to leukocytospermia in men with spinal cord injury.[34] Furthermore, in an activated state, these white blood cells can produce up to a 100-fold increase in reactive oxygen species compared with non-activated cells.[42]

Functionally immature sperm and morphologically abnormal sperm with retained cytoplasm are other sources of reactive oxygen species both in able-bodied men and men with spinal cord injury. In the latter group, increased numbers of immature sperm were found.[43] Although leukocytes produce more reactive oxygen species compared to immature sperm, this "intrinsic" production could result in greater damage of the spermatozoa especially to the integrity of sperm DNA.

Increased oxidative stress could be a potential target for treatment aimed at improving semen quality in men with spinal cord injury. In one study, it was shown that feeding vitamin E to spinal cord injured rats was associated with improved sperm motility, viability, and morphology, as well as partial restoration of prostate and seminal vesicle weight.[44] These effects could result from the antioxidant effects of vitamin E. Further studies are needed to establish the place of vitamin E and other antioxidants in the treatment of infertility in men with spinal cord injury.

■ CONCLUSION

Treatment of infertility in men with spinal cord injury is a dynamic and continuously evolving field. While some problems are studied relatively well, others are far from being settled. Current methods of assisted ejaculation not only are effective and safe, but also in many cases allow clinicians to use less invasive assisted reproductive technologies. Unfortunately, some clinics tend to bypass more simple techniques in favor of more expensive and advanced procedures. Physicians must critically appraise the benefits of techniques which are more widely used in general andrological practice (including surgical sperm retrieval and intracytoplasmic sperm injection) from the standpoint of their invasiveness, cost, and potential complications in couples with spinal cord injured male partners.

Improvement of semen quality is an important but still poorly understood area of research. Although several factors were shown to be associated with semen abnormalities, the practical significance of these findings remains to be established. It is hoped that future studies will provide insights into and possible ways of correcting factors that are responsible for decreased semen quality in men with spinal cord injury.

■ REFERENCES

1. National Spinal Cord Injury Statistical Center. Spinal Cord Injury - Facts and Figures at a Glance 2009 (Accessed September 10, 2009, at http://www.spinalcord.uab.edu/).

2. Brackett NL, Lynne CM, Ibrahim E, Ohl DA, Sonksen J. Treatment of infertility in men with spinal cord injury. Nat Rev Urol 2010;7:162-72.

3. Brindley GS. Electroejaculation: its technique, neurological implications and uses. J Neurol Neurosurg Psychiatry 1981;44:9-18.

4. Brackett NL, Ead DN, Aballa TC, Ferrell SM, Lynne CM. Semen retrieval in men with spinal cord injury is improved by interrupting current delivery during electroejaculation. J Urol 2002;167:201-3.

5. Sonksen J, Ohl DA, Wedemeyer G. Sphincteric events during penile vibratory ejaculation and electroejaculation in men with spinal cord injuries. J Urol 2001;165:426-9.

6. Sonksen J, Biering-Sorensen F, Kristensen JK. Ejaculation induced by penile vibratory stimulation in men with spinal cord injuries. The importance of the vibratory amplitude. Paraplegia 1994;32:651-60.

7. FERTI CARE® personal. In. Albertslund, Denmark: Multicept A/S.

8. Brackett NL, Kafetsoulis A, Ibrahim E, Aballa TC, Lynne CM. Application of 2 vibrators salvages ejaculatory failures to 1 vibrator during penile vibratory stimulation in men with spinal cord injuries. J Urol 2007;177:660-3.

9. Brackett NL. Semen retrieval by penile vibratory stimulation in men with spinal cord injury. Hum Reprod Update 1999;5:216-22.

10. Brackett NL, Ferrell SM, Aballa TC, et al. An analysis of 653 trials of penile vibratory stimulation in men with spinal cord injury. J Urol 1998;159:1931-4.

11. Wieder JA, Brackett NL, Lynne CM, Green JT, Aballa TC. Anesthetic block of the dorsal penile nerve inhibits vibratory-induced ejaculation in men with spinal cord injuries. Urology 2000;55:915-7.

12. Ohl DA, Quallich SA, Sonksen J, Brackett NL, Lynne CM. Anejaculation: an electrifying approach. Semin Reprod Med 2009;27:179-85.

13. Brackett NL, Padron OF, Lynne CM. Semen quality of spinal cord injured men is better when obtained by vibratory stimulation versus electroejaculation. J Urol 1997;157:151-7.

14. Ohl DA, Sonksen J, Menge AC, McCabe M, Keller LM. Electroejaculation versus vibratory stimulation in spinal cord injured men: sperm quality and patient preference. J Urol 1997;157:2147-9.

15. Kafetsoulis A, Ibrahim E, Aballa TC, Goetz LL, Lynne CM, Brackett NL. Abdominal electrical stimulation rescues failures to penile vibratory stimulation in men with spinal cord injury: a report of two cases. Urology 2006;68:9-11.

16. Brackett NL, Ibrahim E, Iremashvili V, Aballa TC, Lynne CM. Treatment for ejaculatory dysfunction in men with spinal cord injury: an 18-year single center experience. J Urol 2010;183:2304-8.

17. Ohl DA, Wolf LJ, Menge AC, et al. Electroejaculation and assisted reproductive technologies in the treatment of anejaculatory infertility. Fertil Steril 2001;76:1249-55.

18. Kafetsoulis A, Brackett NL, Ibrahim E, Attia GR, Lynne CM. Current trends in the treatment of infertility in men with spinal cord injury. Fertil Steril 2006;86:781-9.

19. Van Peperstraten A, Proctor ML, Johnson NP, Philipson G. Techniques for surgical retrieval of sperm prior to intra-cytoplasmic sperm injection (ICSI) for azoospermia. Cochrane Database Syst Rev 2008:CD002807.

20. Iremashvili V, Brackett NL, Ibrahim E, Aballa TC, Lynne CM. The choice of assisted ejaculation method is relevant for the diagnosis of azoospermia in men with spinal cord injuries. Spinal Cord 2011;49:55-9.

21. Iremashvili VV, Brackett NL, Ibrahim E, Aballa TC, Lynne CM. A minority of men with spinal cord injury have normal semen quality-can we learn from them? A case-control study. Urology 2010;76:347-51.

22. Sonksen J, Fode M, Lochner-Ernst D, Ohl DA. Vibratory ejaculation in 140 spinal cord injured men and home insemination of their partners. Spinal Cord 2012;50:63-66.

22a. Kathiresan ASQ, Ibrahim E, Aballa TC, Attia GR, Lynne CM, Brackett NL. Pregnancy outcomes by intravaginal and intra-uterine insemination in 82 couples with male factor infertility due to spinal cord injuries. Fertil Steril 2011;96:328-31.

23. Merviel P, Heraud MH, Grenier N, Lourdel E, Sanguinet P, Copin H. Predictive factors for pregnancy after intrauterine insemination (IUI): an analysis of 1038 cycles and a review of the literature. Fertil Steril 2010;93:79-88.

24. Brackett NL, Ferrell SM, Aballa TC, Amador MJ, Lynne CM. Semen quality in spinal cord injured men: does it progressively decline postinjury? Arch Phys Med Rehabil 1998;79:625-8.

25. Iremashvili V, Brackett NL, Ibrahim E, Aballa TC, Lynne CM. Semen quality remains stable during the chronic phase of spinal cord injury. J Urol 2010;184:2073-7.

26. Brindley GS. Deep scrotal temperature and the effect on it of clothing, air temperature, activity, posture and paraplegia. Br J Urol 1982;54:49-55.

27. Brackett NL, Lynne CM, Weizman MS, Bloch WE, Padron OF. Scrotal and oral temperatures are not related to semen quality of serum gonadotropin levels in spinal cord-injured men. J Androl 1994;15:614-9.

28. Ohl DA, Menge AC, Jarow JP. Seminal vesicle aspiration in spinal cord injured men: insight into poor sperm quality. J Urol 1999;162:2048-51.

29. Madhukar D, Rajender S. Hormonal treatment of male infertility: promises and pitfalls. J Androl 2009;30:95-112.

30. Brackett NL, Lynne CM, Weizman MS, Bloch WE, Abae M. Endocrine profiles and semen quality of spinal cord injured men. J Urol 1994;151:114-9.

31. Brackett NL, Davi RC, Padron OF, Lynne CM. Seminal plasma of spinal cord injured men inhibits sperm motility of normal men. J Urol 1996;155:1632-5.

32. Brackett NL, Lynne CM, Aballa TC, Ferrell SM. Sperm motility from the vas deferens of spinal cord injured men is higher than from the ejaculate. J Urol 2000;164:712-5.

33. Aird IA, Vince GS, Bates MD, Johnson PM, Lewis-Jones ID. Leukocytes in semen from men with spinal cord injuries. Fertil Steril 1999;72:97-103.

34. Trabulsi EJ, Shupp-Byrne D, Sedor J, Hirsch IH. Leukocyte subtypes in electroejaculates of spinal cord injured men. Arch Phys Med Rehabil 2002;83:31-4.

35. Basu S, Lynne CM, Ruiz P, Aballa TC, Ferrell SM, Brackett NL. Cytofluorographic identification of activated T-cell subpopulations in the semen of men with spinal cord injuries. J Androl 2002;23:551-6.

36. Charo IF, Ransohoff RM. The many roles of chemokines and chemokine receptors in inflammation. N Engl J Med 2006;354:610-21.

37. Basu S, Aballa TC, Ferrell SM, Lynne CM, Brackett NL. Inflammatory cytokine concentrations are elevated in seminal plasma of men with spinal cord injuries. J Androl 2004;25:250-4.

38. Brackett NL, Cohen DR, Ibrahim E, Aballa TC, Lynne CM. Neutralization of cytokine activity at the receptor level improves sperm motility in men with spinal cord injuries. J Androl 2007;28:717-21.

39. Cohen Dr, Basu S, Randall JM, Aballa TC, Lynne CM, Brackett NL. Sperm motility in men with spinal cord injuries is enhanced by inactivating cytokines in the seminal plasma. J Androl 2004;25:922-5.

40. Padron OF, Brackett NL, Sharma RK, Lynne CM, Thomas AJ Jr, Agarwal A. Seminal reactive oxygen species and sperm motility and morphology in men with spinal cord injury. Fertil Steril 1997;67:1115-20.

41. de Lamirande E, Leduc BE, Iwasaki A, Hassouna M, Gagnon C. Increased reactive oxygen species formation in semen of patients with spinal cord injury. Fertil Steril 1995;63:637-42.

42. Plante M, de Lamirande E, Gagnon C. Reactive oxygen species released by activated neutrophils, but not by deficient spermatozoa, are sufficient to affect normal sperm motility. Fertil Steril 1994;62:387-93.

43. Iremashvili V, Brackett NL, Ibrahim E, Aballa TC, Bruck D, Lynne CM. Hyaluronic acid binding and acrosin activity are decreased in sperm from men with spinal cord injury. Fertil Steril 2010;94:1925-7.

44. Wang S, Wang G, Barton BE, Murphy TF, Huang HF. Beneficial effects of vitamin E in sperm functions in the rat after spinal cord injury. J Androl 2007;28:334-41.

27

Challenges Facing the Embryologist at the Bench

Karen Schnauffer, Stephen Troup

INTRODUCTION

Assisted conception is now commonly accepted by the vast majority of society as a way-of-life, and it is estimated that over 4 million babies have been born as a result of interventional assisted conception techniques. It is often said that everyone will know at least someone who has had some form of assisted conception treatment or indeed, a child born as a result of treatment! The treatments involved are largely laboratory based and range from the relatively straightforward intrauterine insemination (IUI) of prepared sperm through to the more 'high-tech' approaches of in vitro fertilization (IVF) and intracytoplasmic sperm injection (ICSI), perhaps using sperm derived surgically directly from the testes. In the UK, approximately 50,000 cycles of IVF and ICSI are performed annually (Human Fertilization and Embryology Authority, 2009) and in common to every single one of those cycles was the need to assess and appropriately prepare human sperm (of highly variable quality) in order to optimize the chance of the patients achieving a pregnancy. Techniques used to prepare human sperm for therapeutic purposes vary according to the way in which the sperm is to be used, although all techniques generally seek to firstly remove the sperm from the surrounding seminal plasma, and secondly, to obtain a preparation which contains a large number of highly motile, morphologically normal sperm (Zavos PM, 1992; Boomsma CM et al. 1997; Erel et al., 2000; Moohan and Lindsay, 1995). Whilst these endpoints of the preparation process remain desirable for ICSI, it is important to remember that the numbers and quality of sperm may be hugely reduced (Liu et al, 1994; Al-Hasani et al, 1995; Bourne et al, 1995).

Over the last 20 years or so, a new 'breed' of scientist has emerged who has the necessary expertise and experience to critically analyze and prepare human sperm for therapeutic purposes. Recognized training programs have emerged worldwide with one of the first being set up in the UK in the early 1990s.

The assisted conception sector is an almost unique area of medicine in that it is often subject to regulatory control, although the degree of regulation varies widely around the world with some of the most prescriptive legislation being in place in Europe. Whilst rarely perfect, such legislation provides a sound framework in around which assisted conception services can be provided, more often than not placing the patient at the top of the list of considerations. This is perhaps particularly evident within the UK where the Human Fertilization and Embryology Act (1990) has been in force since 1991 and although it has been subject to several bouts of fine-tuning, retains its fundamental principles.

This chapter seeks to explore in more detail some of the challenges that face the laboratory scientists involved in assisted conception as they go about their day-to-day duties. These challenges have different causes, with some arising from the nature of the biological material being handled and the desired outcome and others from the relevant regulation or indeed the fundamentally important nature of the work being undertaken.

TRAINING

If we look back 25 years or so, to the emergence of laboratory based assisted conception techniques we find an ill-defined, disparate group of scientists becoming involved. Many had gained experience of handling gametes and embryos by virtue of using animal models (e.g. mice, hamsters, etc.) for research purposes and often had Masters degrees or even PhDs. Others had a more 'diagnostic' background, gaining experience within a pathology environment. Nevertheless, as assisted conception began to find its feet, a new breed of laboratory scientist began to emerge. These individuals almost invariably had biological sciences first degrees and had chosen to work within the assisted conception field rather than 'falling' into it from a research background. And so, the profession of 'clinical embryology' was born leading to the formation within the UK, of the Association of Clinical Embryologists (ACE) with other similar professional bodies emerging worldwide. One of the fundamental roles of ACE, was to provide a structured training scheme that would be recognized by the powers that be and provide a route by which state registration could be gained. The first Diploma in Clinical Embryology was awarded in 1997, with a significant section of the training being directed towards the diagnosis and treatment of male infertility and all the associated necessary laboratory methodologies. The Diploma in Clinical Embryology has been superseded by the Certificate in Clinical Embryology (now in its second version) and over 200 clinical embryologists now hold this qualification.

Nowadays, the vast majority of sperm preparation for assisted conception purposes is undertaken by clinical embryologists within specialized, dedicated assisted conception units, many of which are within the private sector. A relatively small proportion of sperm preparation for intrauterine insemination purposes is undertaken in less specialized centers, although such services are now subject to identical regulatory requirements.

Although the UK has over 60 specialist assisted conception units, the vast majority of diagnostic andrology (i.e. routine semen analyses) is performed within the more conventional hospital laboratory, often taking place within a pathology environment. In recognition of this specialism the Association of Biomedical Andrologists (ABA) was founded in 2004. ABA now boasts a membership of over 300 with one of its fundamental roles being to provide education. Three log-book driven, experiential courses are now available covering subjects such as diagnostic semen analysis, sperm preparation for diagnosis or therapeutic intervention and sperm cryopreservation in assisted reproduction. Importantly, these courses lead to the award of professionally recognized qualifications (see *www.aba.uk.net*).

REGULATION

In 2007, the European Union Cells and Tissues Directive came into force in the UK. The purpose of this EU-wide legislation is summarized by the following extract from the Directive itself:

'Directive 2004/23/EC lays down standards of quality and safety for the donation, procurement, testing processing, preservation, storage and distribution of human tissues and cells intended for human applications, and of manufactured products derived from human tissues and cells intended for human applications, so as to ensure a high level of human health protection'

Within the complexity of these regulations was the requirement for each EU member state to appoint a 'competent authority' to administer the requirements of the Directive. As such, the speed at which the legislation has been introduced varies widely across Europe. In countries such as the UK, with regulation and a regulatory authority (the HFEA) already in place, implementation of the EU Directive was relatively straightforward. Other EU member states (e.g. Greece), have not been in a position to implement the EU Directive quite so readily. Ironically, although the EU Directive sets out to fundamentally unify the way in which cells and tissues are dealt with across the EU, the way in which it has been implemented has in itself generated some frustrating challenges. More specifically, there are perhaps three elements of UK and European regulation that particularly challenge those working in the field on a day-to-day basis. These are, firstly, to do with the standard of laboratory facilities that are now required for the safe handling of cells and tissues and in particular the air quality in which gametes and embryos are handled. Secondly, the requirement to witness either 'manually' or 'electronically' all points during a process at which an error may occur and thirdly, the need to be able to trace, in a standardized way, all gametes from 'procurement' through to use or disposal. Each of these three challenges is discussed in more detail below.

Laboratory Minimum Standards

The EU Directive specifies that, in simple terms, cells and tissues should be handled in a 'clean air' environment. Such an approach has been widely accepted by those dealing with gametes and embryos although any beneficial effect in terms of improved clinical outcome is yet to be proven. The EU legislators have, however, allowed each competent authority to interpret this particular aspect individually, leading to perhaps inevitable variations in air quality requirements between member states. For example, the Irish Medicine's Board (IMB), the competent authority in the Republic of Ireland, requires gametes and embryos to be handled in air of 'Grade D' quality as specified by the Medicines and Healthcare products Regulatory Agency (MHRA) (MHRA, 2002). The HFEA in the UK, however, require gametes and embryos to be handled in air if 'Grade C' quality with background air being of 'Grade D' quality (although exceptions are permitted in the HFEA's Code of Practice (HFEA, 2009) where the techniques being employed (e.g. ICSI) make the use of Class II safety cabinets problematic). Nevertheless, the standard of laboratories in which gametes and embryos are now routinely handled has risen (dramatically in some instances) with assisted conception laboratories being constructed to extremely stringent clean-room standards and appropriate cleaning and monitoring regimens. High efficiency particulate air (HEPA) filtration systems are now common place in such laboratories together with specialist clean-room design features and strict uniform and access control.

Although the subject of considerable debate during the development and implementation of the EU Directive, the preparation of sperm for intrauterine insemination (IUI) falls under this legislation. Previously many nonspecialist laboratories felt comfortable with the relatively straightforward laboratory techniques required to process sperm for IUI facilitating the provision of IUI in many hospital laboratories. The effect of the EU Directive has been threefold. Some laboratories which perform sperm preparation for IUI have raised the standard of their facilities to meet the EU Directive requirements whereas others have diverted patients to nearby specialist assisted conception laboratories. Unfortunately, however, some IUI services have been withdrawn as the resource commitment required to maintain a service under EU Directive legislation has not been found to be cost-effective.

WITNESSING

In 2002, one of the most highly publicized errors in laboratory medicine in the UK took place in which a white couple gave birth to black twins following assisted conception treatment (Dyer, 2002). It became apparent that human error had lead to eggs being inseminated with incorrect sperm within an assisted conception lab setting. An independent investigation, headed by Prof Brian Toft, highlighted that, although additional contributory factors were relevant, it seemed quite clear that a process of procedure witnessing was likely to significantly lessen the chance of such an unthinkable event occurring again (Toft, 2004). The

Toft report also raised concerns about a phenomenon known as 'involuntary automaticity' in which individuals fail to perform tasks competently (although they remain unaware of their failure) by virtue of the fact that they repeat the same task over and over again. Nevertheless, the HFEA in the UK responded rapidly, requiring that all key procedures in which gametes or embryos are handled be witnessed with such practice now being routine in most assisted conception laboratories worldwide.

Considerable time and effort now has to be devoted to the witnessing of procedures. It has been estimated that approximately 17 minutes will be spent on just manually witnessing procedures throughout an IVF or ICSI treatment cycle (Schnauffer et al, 2005). In addition, manual witnessing, by its very nature, requires the presence of a second individual who needs to have been appropriately trained and be familiar with both the process and methods of witnessing. It is inappropriate to simply ask a colleague to briefly glance at a label as they are passing, and as such manual witnessing is considerably more onerous than might be apparent. It also goes without saying that being involved in manual witnessing is necessarily distracting to the witness, particularly if they are already occupied dealing with gametes belonging to another patient. Indeed, many have questioned whether the distraction caused by manual witnessing may outweigh its benefit! In order to mitigate the distraction caused by manual witnessing several laboratories have chosen to employ individuals whose prime role is simply to act as witness.

In rapid response to the requirement to witness procedures within assisted conception laboratories, the commercial sector, with considerable input from experts within the field began to look for more high-tech solutions to the witnessing requirements. Two technologies emerged as being suitable: bar-coding and the use of radio frequency identification (RFID). Bar-coding had already proved its worth within the medical environment particularly in the labeling of blood for transfusion and although RFID tagging was still a relatively new technology its potential was self-evident.

As the use of these technologies developed into systems designed specifically for the therapeutic assisted conception environment, in 2004 the HFEA formed an expert 'Safety and New Technologies' (SANT) group to objectively examine their use. Not only did the SANT group examine the efficacy of these new systems but they dedicated considerable effort to ensure, so far as possible, that the use of these systems would not cause any adverse effect upon the gametes or embryos in their vicinity. In relation to the bar-code system, concerns were voiced regarding the exposure of gametes and embryos to additional light and even laser-light necessary to read the bar-codes. The major concern regarding the RFID systems was exposure of gametes and embryos to radio-waves, particularly as this coincided with adverse publicity around the use of mobile telephones. Fortunately, the HFEA's SANT group were provided with evidence suggesting that the risk of damage to gametes and embryos using these technologies was exceptionally small and as such permitted their use in the UK. The requirement to witness procedures, either manually or electronically now remains enshrined in the HFEA's Code of Practice (HFEA, 2009) in the UK

with many other countries following suit. Electronic witnessing systems are now commonplace in many laboratories in which human gametes are handled although it remains to be seen if their use will genuinely reduce the incident of serious adverse clinical events.

TRACEABILITY

Once again, the HFEA's Code of Practice sets standards in relation to a laboratories ability to trace not only a semen sample from its production to its use therapeutically but also to be able to identify anything which, or anyone who may have come into contact with the sample during this journey. These requirements are evident in the following extract of the mandatory requirements from the HFEA's Code of Practice:

"Traceability" means the ability:

- *To identify and locate gametes and embryos during any step from procurement to use for human application or disposal*
- *Identify the donor [i.e. the provider] and recipient of particular gametes or embryos*
- *To identify any person who has carried out any activity in relation to particular gametes or embryos*
- *To identify and locate all relevant data relating to products and materials coming into contact with particular gametes or embryos and which can affect their quality or safety.*

Therefore, highly accurate and robust labelling and data recording systems are now commonplace. In addition, the EU legislators are keen to regularise the way in which samples are labelled leading to the HFEA, for example, currently requiring the following, once again, extracted from the HFEA's Code of Practice:

All samples of gametes and embryos should be labelled with at least the patient's or donor's full name and a unique identifier. If at some stages (e.g. labeling donor sperm) it is not possible to label the dishes or tubes with the donor name:

- The donor code should uniquely identify that donor
- The dishes or tubes should be labelled with the female patient's name and unique identifier as soon as possible.

In relation to the above extract, the term unique identifier, in practical terms, refers more often than not to a unique hospital or clinic number and not simply a date of birth—although exceptionally rare, it is not unheard of to have two patients with the same name and the same date of birth attending an assisted conception unit for treatment on the same day!

The days of the marker-pen or china-graph pencil are clearly numbered with several commercial PC-driven labeling systems now being available and being commonly utilised within the embryology and therapeutic andrology setting.

PRACTICAL DIFFICULTIES

The advent of micromanipulation techniques and in particular intracytoplasmic sperm injection (ICSI) has revolutionized the treatment of male subfertility (Van Steirteghem et al, 1993). However, the ability to alleviate subfertility by injecting a single sperm directly into an egg faces those embryologists tasked with performing the micro-injection procedure with two practical difficulties. Firstly, the embryologist must assume the responsibility for selecting the sperm that will penetrate the egg, and secondly, ICSI facilitates conception in cases where there may be fewer sperm available than there are eggs!

The dogmatic approach to selecting sperm for injection with ICSI persists, and relies on an embryologist being able to recognize a sperm which is moving (and therefore demonstrably viable) but one which is also morphologically normal. At first consideration this may not appear (with appropriate training) particularly onerous. However, consider the situation where there may be numerous sperm available for selection, but none are motile or all are morphologically abnormal, or sometimes both—should one consider injecting immotile or morphologically abnormal sperm? Should one ask the patient to produce a second sample? Will the second sample be more 'useable'? Such practical challenges are faced by clinical embryologists on a day-to-day basis.

A correlation exists between the number of sperm present in a semen sample and the chances of natural conception. The WHO has taken cognisance of this when deriving 'normal ranges' in relation to achieving conception (WHO, 2010). However, when considering ICSI, such a correlation is largely irrelevant as in reality 'we only really need one-sperm-per-egg'. This too poses a significant challenge to the embryologist. In recent years a condition known as 'crypotozoopsermia' has emerged. This is where a conventional semen analysis will fail to identify any sperm in an ejaculate. However, the use of centrifugation techniques to 'concentrate' the ejaculate, combined with systematic microscopic examination may lead to the identification of extremely small numbers of sperm being present—sufficient numbers to undertake ICSI.

Similarly, several surgical procedures are now commonplace whereby sperm can be retrieved directly from the epididymis or testis. Several variations of 'surgical sperm retrieval' now exist including microepididymal sperm aspiration (MESA), percutaneous epididymal sperm aspiration (PESA) and testicular sperm aspiration or extraction (TESA or TESE) although, once again, the numbers of sperm recovered can be extremely small (Troup et al, 1998). As such is it not uncommon for embryologists to spend many, many hours simply looking for sperm and treatment cycles do occur occasionally where more eggs are available than there are sperm!

With the advent of ICSI, every time an embryologist sits down to carry out an ICSI procedure, they are faced with having to choose which sperm are suitable to be injected into the egg(s). Clearly, during natural conception or indeed IVF, this selection process is performed by virtue of the female reproductive tract (including cervical mucus), the egg vestments, and the inherent characteristics of the sperm. In the laboratory, however, the selection process rests with the embryologist and there are relatively few 'tools' to assist in this process. Routinely, sperm motility and morphology remain the principal desirable characteristics, with the former indicating viability and the latter desirable as it is known that sperm which have 'normal' morphology pass preferentially through cervical mucus. Embryologists, therefore,

routinely choose motile sperm with normal morphology for injection with ICSI. However, two scenarios are common. Firstly, embryologists can be faced with samples in which all sperm are immotile (although sperm may be viable). The reasons why a man's sperm are viable yet immotile are more often than not unexplained although can be due to ultrastructural deficiencies as is the case with Immotile Cilia Syndrome or Kartagener's Syndrome. In these conditions microtubular ultrastructural abnormalities (often a lack of dynein arms) renders sperm immotile. In such conditions, the rest of the sperm remains functionally competent and as such can be treated using ICSI. In addition, some have suggested the use of a hypo-osmotic swelling test to facilitate identification of viable (immotile) sperm although the benefits of such an approach remain questionable (Peeraer et al, 2004). More latterly, the use of high powered microscopy together with ICSI (known as intracytoplasmic morphologically selected sperm injection or IMSI) has been suggested to more reliably select morphologically normal and functionally competent sperm (Nadali et al, 2009).

CONCLUSION

Clearly, it is unlikely that the desire to have children will diminish, this perhaps being the most fundamental of human functions. As such, for so long as fertility deficiencies persist there will remain a need to provide treatment to sub-fertile couples. Therefore, the role of the clinical embryologist seems guaranteed for some considerable time to come. This chapter has given a snapshot of the challenges facing embryologists at the start of the 21st century, with particular emphasis on the 'andrological' aspects of their role. The need for assisted conception treatments will continue to increase, but alongside this understanding of the fundamental biological processes will also improve. It seems inevitable, therefore, that embryologists will continue to face a barrage of fascinating and rapidly ever-changing challenges.

BIBLIOGRAPHY

1. Al Hasani S, Küpker W, Baschat AA, Sturm R, Bauer O, Diedrich C, Diedrich K. J Mini-swim-up: a new technique of sperm preparation for intracytoplasmic sperm injection. Assist Reprod Genet 1995;12(7):428-33.
2. Black twins are born to white twins after infertility treatment. BMJ 2002; 325: 64 doi: 10.1136/bmj.325.7355.64 (Published 6 July 2002).
3. Boomsma CM, Heineman MJ, Cohlen BJ, Farquhar C. Semen preparation techniques for intrauterine insemination. Cochrane Database Syst Rev. 2007 Oct 17;(4):CD004507. Review. PMID: 17943816.
4. Bourne H, Richings N, Liu DY, Clarke GN, Harari O, Baker HW. Sperm preparation for intracytoplasmic injection: methods and relationship to fertilization results. Reprod Fertil Dev 1995;7(2):177-83.
5. Erel CT, Senturk LM, Irez T, Ercan L, Elter K, Colgar U, Ertungealp E. Sperm-preparation techniques for men with normal and abnormal semen analysis. A comparison. J Reprod Med 2000;45(11):917-22.

6. European Society for Human Reproduction (ESHRE) Annual Meeting, Copenhagen, June, 2005.

7. Human Fertilisation and Embryology Authority, Code of Practice, Edition 8 first published 2009.

8. Human Fertilisation and Embryology Authority, F-2010-00197 – Number of IVF cycles in 2009.

9. Liu J, Nagy Z, Joris H, Tournaye H, Devroey P, Van Steirteghem AC. Intracytoplasmic sperm injection does not require special treatment of the spermatozoa. Hum Reprod 1994;9(6):1127-30.

10. MHRA–Rules and Guidance for Pharmaceutical Manufacturers and Distributors 2002.

11. Moohan JM, Lindsay KS. Spermatozoa selected by a discontinuous Percoll density gradient exhibit better motion characteristics, more hyperactivation, and longer survival than direct swim-up. Fertil Steril 1995;64(1):160-5.

12. Nadalini M, Tarozzi N, Distratis V, Scaravelli G, Borini A. Impact of intracytoplasmic morphologically selected sperm injection on assisted reproduction outcome: a review. Reprod Biomed Online 2009;(19 Suppl)3:45-55.

13. Peeraer K, Nijs M, Raick D, Ombelet W. Pregnancy after ICSI with ejaculated immotile spermatozoa from a patient with immotile cilia syndrome: a case report and review of the literature. Reprod Biomed Online 2004;9(6):659-63.

14. Schnauffer K, Kingsland C, Troup S. (presented by Hannah Marsden). Prospective and systematic evaluation of a barcode witnessing system. Fertility 2009;7-9 January 2009, Edinburgh International Conference Centre.

15. Schnauffer K, Kingsland C, Troup S. Barcode labeling in the IVF laboratory.

16. Toft B. Independent review of the circumstances surrounding four adverse events that occurred in the Reproductive Medicine Units at The Leeds Teaching Hospitals NHS Trust, West Yorkshire, 2004, Department of Health.

17. Troup SA, Falconer DA, Payne SR, Lieberman BA. Testicular sperm extraction (TESE): quantification, and the effect of culture and cryopreservation on sperm motility. International Symposium on Male Sterility for Motility Disorders: Etiological Factor and Treatment. Serono Symposia Series, Springer Verlag, New York, 1998.

18. Van Steirteghem AC, Nagy Z, Joris H, Liu J, Staessen C, Smitz J, Wisanto A, Devroey P. High fertilization and implantation rates after intracytoplasmic sperm injection. Hum Reprod 1993;8:1061-6.

19. World Health Organization (2010). WHO laboratory manual for the examination and processing of human semen. 5th edition. ISBN 9789241547789.

20. Zavos PM. Preparation of human frozen-thawed seminal specimens using the SpermPrep filtration method: improvements over the conventional swim-up method. Fertil Steril 1992;57(6):1326-30.

28

Sperm Banking via Cryopreservation

Sajal Gupta, Ashok Agarwal, Reecha Sharma, Ali Ahmady

Sperm banking with cryopreservation is an important procedure that can be used to preserve the future fertility of men who are facing the prospect of permanent loss of fertility for several reasons. For example, some patients who choose sperm banking have been diagnosed with cancer and are about to undergo gonadal surgery or gonadotoxic treatment such as chemotherapy and/or radiation therapy. In other cases, men are already infertile due to azoospermia or sexual dysfunction but have some viable sperm that can be successfully harvested and frozen. In any case, when pregnancy is desired, the sperm sample can be thawed and used in a number of assisted reproductive techniques (ARTs): intracytoplasmic sperm injection (ICSI), intrauterine insemination (IUI) and *in vitro* fertilization (IVF). This chapter will discuss the current role of sperm banking with cryopreservation, including the main indications, procedures used to extract, process and freeze sperm, and ART outcomes. We will also discuss the need to educate patients about sperm banking before treatment.

INDICATIONS FOR SPERM BANKING

Absent Partner

When either the male or female partner is often absent (due to travelling, for example) it can be difficult to time intercourse with ovulation.

Male Factor Infertility

About 12 percent of couples are unable to conceive after one year of unprotected intercourse and are therefore considered infertile.[1] About 30–40 percent of these couples are unable to conceive due to male factor infertility. Approximately 10 percent of male factor infertility is caused by azoospermia. In the most severe cases of male infertility, couples may decide to use cryopreserved sperm from a healthy third-party donor.[2]

Cancer

Hodgkin's disease, testicular cancer, leukemia, and non-Hodgkin's lymphoma are the most common malignancies seen in men of reproductive age.[3] Sperm quality in men diagnosed with testicular tumors is suboptimal, even prior to the initiation of chemo/radiotherapy, due to in part the local negative effects exerted by the tumors. In one study, sperm concentration was significantly lower in patients with a testicular malignancy than in those with systemic malignancy and healthy donors with proven fertility. Motility was found to be significantly lower in patients with testicular and systemic malignancy than in healthy proven fertile donors.[4]

Anti-neoplastic therapy is associated with significant morbidity, and testicular dysfunction is among the most common long-term side effects of cytotoxic chemotherapy in men. Cancer patients receiving radiotherapy are at high-risk for developing infertility, and cancer surgery can reduce sperm concentration, causing erectile dysfunction or dry ejaculation.[27] Between 15 and 30 percent of male patients undergoing gonadotoxic treatments do not regain fertility.[5] Most patients undergoing chemotherapy develop azoospermia by 12 weeks.

The degree to which testicular function is affected depends on the dose and agent.[6] Alkylating agents (e.g. cyclophosphamide and busulfan) and ionizing radiation frequently induce azoospermia, rendering the patient infertile. Another major reason to freeze sperm before treatment is the concern for potential chromosomal aberrations in sperm that are exposed to chemotherapy.[7] Although no increase in malformation rates have been reported in children born to patients who have had chemotherapy or radiotherapy, the available data and follow-up are still limited.

Chemotherapy targets cells outside the G0 phase, destroying proliferating spermatogonias.[8] The majority of chemotherapy patients develop azoospermia during treatment, and it is difficult to predict if and when spermatogenesis will recover. Recovery tends to be dose dependent. Patients receiving low doses of these agents may recover spermatogenesis within 12 weeks after completing chemotherapy. However more than 50 percent of patients will receive high dose chemotherapy and may contribute to the 15–30 percent of all patients who remain sterile in the long term. It is estimated that up to 15 percent of male patients will already be azoospermic before undergoing any type of treatment. Semen should be cryopreserved before cancer treatment begins. It is optimal to have multiple samples cryopreserved.[9] Patients who are most at risk are those who undergo a treatment that includes successive and multiple toxicities, such as bone marrow transplantation.[10]

Prostate/Testicular Surgery/Biopsy

One study found that non-germ cell urological cancer was independently associated with the desire for sperm cryopreservation.[11]

Severe Oligozoospermia/Poor Sperm Quality

Azoospermia may occur in some healthy men, and natural fertilization may be impossible for them, however, cryopreservation and IVF may allow these men to father children. The recovery of viable sperms is comparatively low with less than 60 percent of cells retaining motility on thawing. This loss of viability becomes a major issue in case of oligozoospermic samples. For these cases there is a growing need to store low numbers of sperm by developing improved freezing techniques. The use of frozen-thawed testicular biopsies in ICSI is very helpful in patients with obstructive azoospermia with normal spermatogenesis.[12]

Erectile/Ejaculatory Dysfunction

Erectile dysfunction and anxiety issues may prevent a couple from successfully conceiving, so cryopreservation and IUI can allow these couples to conceive in a clinical setting.

Vasectomy

Although there is a high success rate with vasectomy reversall it is an expensive procedure and requires hospitalization. It is therefore far more cost-effective to cryopreserve semen before vasectomy, which then can be stored indefinitely at lesser cost.[13] The availability of ICSI technology has made cryopreservation of sperm during vasectomy reversals possible.[14]

High-risk Occupations

Exposure to environmental factors such as air pollution, pesticides, phthalates, PCBs (polychlorinated biphenyls) and the use of mobile phones affects semen quality.[15] Men who work with chemicals, pesticides, etc. are considered at high-risk for developing infertility, and those engaged in these high-risk occupations should be offered and counseled about sperm banking as an option.

Failure to Ejaculate

A man may have difficulty ejaculating for a number of reasons: psychogenic ejaculation, spinal cord injury, and premature ejaculation (the latter of which varies from 8 to 30 percent for all age groups).[16] Sperm can be extracted from patients with failure of ejaculation by vibrator therapy, electro-ejaculation, medical and surgical treatment. If surgery fails, or is not possible, then pregnancy can be achieved by aspirating sperm from the epididymis and using these sperm for ICSI.

■ SURGICAL SPERM RETRIEVAL

Surgical sperm retrieval techniques can be used for patients with azoospermia. Percutaneous epididymal sperm aspiration (PESA) and microsurgical epididymal sperm aspiration (MESA) are used in cases of obstructive azoospermia whereas testicular sperm aspiration (TESA) and testicular sperm extraction (TESE) are used in cases of non-obstructive azoospermia.

Obstructive Azoospermia

Percutaneous Epididymal Sperm Aspiration

Percutaneous epididymal sperm aspiration (PESA) is performed without surgical scrotal exploration. It does not require an operating microscope or expertise in microsurgery. To perform this procedure, a butterfly needle (attached to a 10–20 mL syringe) is inserted into the caput epididymis. The tip of the needle is gradually moved within the epididymis until clear or opalescent fluid seen in the needle tubing as shown in **Figure 28.1**. The procedure is repeated until adequate amounts of epididymal fluid are retrieved.[17] The aspirate is then flushed into a sterile tube before it is sent to a lab for evaluation and processing.

Microsurgical Epididymal Sperm Aspiration

For this procedure, the patient is placed under local anesthesia. After opening the tunica vaginalis and exposing the epididymis, single epididymal tubules are identified under an operating microscope. The tubules are then punctured, and the effluent

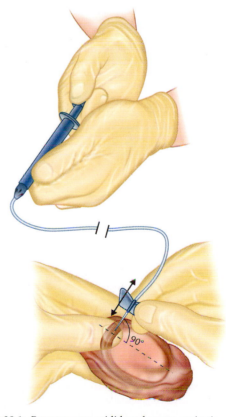

Figure 28.1: Percutaneous epididymal sperm aspiration (PESA)

is aspirated into an aspiration device (syringe). Sequential aspirations are performed until an optimal number of sperm are obtained.[18,19] Sperm with the best quality are found in the proximal epididymis close to the testes. The aspirates are then sent to a lab for evaluation and processing.

Testicular Sperm Retrieval Techniques for Non-obstructive Azoospermia

Mature spermatozoa can be recovered in some testicular areas in men with non-obstructive azoospermia (percentage recovery). When examining the testes of infertile men, Levin found a mixed histological pattern of germinal cell aplasia and minute foci (focal) spermatogenesis.[20] A similar histology (different patterns of focal spermatogenesis and Sertoli-cell syndrome) was observed in men with non-obstructive azoospermia.[21,22] Therefore, multiple focal testicular sperm retrievals are needed to ensure the presence of sperm in any testicular sample.[23]

The most common methods for retrieving the testicular sperm are needle biopsies (testicular sperm aspiration, TESA) and open testicular biopsy (testicular sperm extraction TESE). Recently, however, optical loupe magnification TESE was used to retrieve sperm from men with non-obstructive azoospermia.[24] The TESA and TESE procedures are performed with the patient under anesthesia (general, or local). Generally, the scrotum is opened via a median raphe incision, and all layers are cut until the testis is fully exposed.

Testicular Sperm Aspiration

Multifocal testicular sperm aspiration (TESA) is usually performed in 3 different locations—in the center of the testis and in the upper and lower poles—with the aim of aspirating testicular tissue from the depth of the testis. After the testis is exposed, the needle is inserted into the center of the testis as demonstrated (**Fig. 28.2**) and negative suction pressure is applied. While maintaining negative pressure, the needle is partially withdrawn and inserted again at different angles. The sampling is performed using a needle biopsy gun that allows for controlled and accurate sampling as well as the creation and maintenance of a substantial negative pressure. A separate 20-mL syringe containing 0.5 mL of culture medium and an 18-gauge needle are used for each sample. The aspirated samples are transferred immediately to the laboratory for sperm identification and isolation.[25]

Testicular Sperm Extraction

For testicular sperm extraction (TESE), the tunica albuginea is incised transversely in three locations (the center, upper, and lower poles) in each testis. The testis is then gently squeezed and the protruding tissues are excised, each of which weighs approximately 50 mg. The biopsy material is placed in culture and transferred immediately to the laboratory for sperm cell isolation.[25]

Laboratory Preparation of TESE and TESA Sample

Upon receipt of the biopsy tissues, they are shredded into small pieces with a sterile 25-gauge needle or fine seizers. The presence of spermatozoa is assessed using an inverted microscope. The effluents and the shredded biopsy tissue can be centrifuged. The pellet is re-suspended in culture medium and incubated in a few droplets under mineral oil for ~1 h prior to the selection of spermatozoa. Motile spermatozoa usually 'swim out' to the edge of the drop.[26,27] Alternatively, the original shredded specimen can

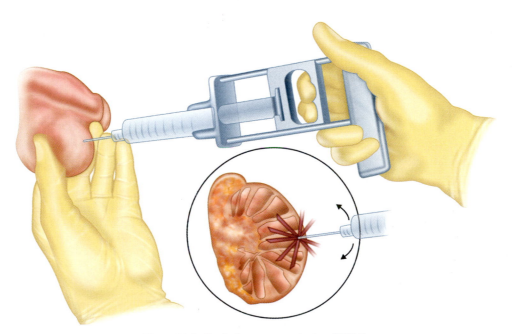

Figure 28.2: Testicular sperm aspiration (TESA)

be incubated in droplets under oil without centrifugation prior to selection of sperm. The selected spermatozoa can be washed in PVP droplets before proceeding to injection into oocyte.

BARRIERS TO SPERM BANKING

Even though sperm banking is a safe and effective procedure for storing sperm, only few patients who could benefit from it actually choose to do so.[28] Authors of a qualitative study of 20 cancer survivors and 18 health care professionals conducted in-depth interviews to examine their perspectives on factors that facilitate or hinder sperm banking. The study found six factors that have an impact on sperm banking:

Priority

Sperm banking is usually not a priority for patients who have already completed their family and those who do not want to have children. Patients who are too young fail to understand the impact of infertility and do not consider sperm banking as a priority.[28]

Cost

The cost of sperm banking is not covered by most insurance companies and may be a very important factor for patients with low incomes. Healthcare professionals are likely to presume that the costs are too high for their patients,[27] and therefore may fail to mention it as an option.

Time Interval

Many patients with cancer or other serious diseases understandably want to start therapy as soon as they receive a diagnosis. As a result, they may not want to postpone their treatment to bank their sperm.

Lack of Information

Surveys show that the lack of timely information is the most common reason for not banking sperm.[10] According to a study that surveyed oncologists to determine their knowledge, attitudes, and practices regarding sperm banking, 91 percent of respondents agreed that it should be offered to all men at risk of infertility as a result of cancer treatment. However, almost half reported that they did not mention the option to all eligible male patients due to a lack of time for the discussion, perceived high cost, and lack of convenient facilities. HIV-positive men, patients with a poor prognosis, or those with aggressive tumors are even less likely to be offered the option of sperm banking.[29]

Religious or Ethical Concerns about Sperm Banking

The practice of sperm donation is opposed by many religions and hence, the option of sperm banking may not be acceptable to couples or physicians due to religious reasons. Many ethical issues are raised regarding the rights and obligations of the mother, the husband, and the child.[30]

Psychosocial Issues with Sperm Banking— Anxiety and Emotional Stress

A cancer diagnosis and the threat of infertility can cause tremendous stress on a patient.[31] Schover formulated certain hypotheses for psychological stress in cancer patients such as:

- Cancer survivors might have higher infertility distress compared to infertility patients without a major medical disorder.
- Adolescents survivors being more distressed about parenthood compared to adults.
- Women are more often distressed than men about infertility and their children's health than men.
- Those with inheritable cancers more frequently distressed about childbearing issues than those with non-inheritable cancers.
- Patients who rate their overall quality of life more negatively are less concerned about infertility and more quick to give up having children.
- Cancer survivors who do have children after treatment will perceive them more positively than non cancer patients.[31,32] These factors need to be acknowledged by health care professionals and utilized in proper care and treatment of these patients.

SCREENING OF PATIENTS PRIOR TO BANKING

All sperm donors are required to complete a physical examination, including a genital exam, no more than twelve months prior to the first storage appointment. Most sperm banks also require every potential donor to schedule a physical semen analysis prior to sperm retrieval and storage. Donors are screened for infectious diseases with blood tests for HIV-1/2, HTLV-1/2, hepatitis B, hepatitis C, syphilis, and sometimes CMV. Genetic testing of the sperm donor is required by certain states like New York.[33] Some banks also request that donors complete an HIV risk assessment form and a personal and family health history form as well as undergo blood testing to identify blood type and Rh factor.

PREPARATION AND SELECTION MECHANISMS PRIOR TO BANKING

Before sperm samples can be frozen, they must be processed first to increase their chances of successfully surviving the freeze and thaw cycle. The swim-up and density gradient techniques are the two most widely used methods for sperm washing and processing. Sperm washing techniques separate ejaculated spermatozoa from the seminal environment and eliminate dead spermatozoa along with exfoliated epithelial cells, cellular debris, leukocytes, and amorphous material.[34]

The swim-up method involves centrifuging a semen sample into pellets, which are then covered with culture medium. The sperm with better motion characteristics and motility swim up into the culture medium where they can be selected for cryopreservation.[35] In comparison to untreated specimens, swim-up cryopreserved sperm have been shown to exhibit faster velocity and progression, higher percentages of intact acrosomes, increased ability to undergo acrosome reaction and better performance in the sperm penetration assay after thawing.[35,36]

There are two types of density gradient centrifugation: continuous[37] and discontinuous.[38] In continuous density gradient centrifugation, the density gradually increases from the top of the gradient to the bottom. In the discontinuous method, there is a clear boundary between each layer. The ejaculate is placed on top of the density gradient and centrifuged for 15–30 minutes. During this procedure, highly motile spermatozoa move in the direction of the sedimentation gradient and penetrate the boundary more quickly than poorly motile or immotile sperm, enriching the soft pellet at the bottom with highly motile sperm.

A number of substances can be used for density gradient centrifugation, including Nycodenz (Nyegaard and Co, Oslo, Norway), IxaPrep® (MediCult, Copenhagen, Denmark), SilSelect® (FertiPro NV, Beernem, Belgium), PureSperm® (NidaCon Laboratories AB, Gothenburg, Sweden) and ISolate® (Irvine Scientific, Santa Ana, CA, USA). These are replacements to a substance that was once widely used called Percoll, which is now recommended for research purposes only. Studies have shown that use of these newer substances produce populations of highly motile spermatozoa with better yields and survival than those seen with either the swim-up technique or gradient centrifugation with Percoll® in oligozoospermic and asthenozoospermic semen samples.[11,39,40,59] Percoll® replacement procedure shows superior results in zona-free hamster egg penetration test as compared to the swim-up procedure.[41] Thus, this technique clearly has great potential in the preparation of motile spermatozoa from poor quality semen.

Techniques of Cryopreservation

Cryoprotectant

Since Polge and Rowson[42] first successful report of glycerol as a cryoprotectant for bull spermatozoa cryopreservation, there have been many reports on its use in the cryopreservation of spermatozoa of other species including horse,[43] pig,[44] sheep,[45] dog,[46] rabbit,[47] and man.[48] It is the most widely used and successful cryoprotectant for human sperm. A final concentration of 7.5 percent has been shown to be an optimal concentration of glycerol for a freezing solution. Egg yolk, on the other hand, which is not a cryoprotectant itself and is often used in combination with glycerol, seems to confer improved sperm plasma membrane fluidity, resulting in improved cryo-survival.[49]

Prins et al. compared eight different cryopreservatives and concluded that sperm frozen with egg yolk buffer demonstrated the highest post-thaw survival.[50] Mahadevan and Trounson have developed a modified Tyrod's medium containing 7.5 percent glycerol, referred to as Human Sperm Preservation Medium (HSPM). When HSPM was used, higher pregnancy rates were achieved as compared to use of egg yolk-citrate-glycerol medium. However, it did not show any difference in post-thaw motility and motility.[51]

When comparing three cryopreservatives (TEST yolk, glycerol, and HSPM), Centola et al. demonstrated that HSPM led to the best recovery rates in regards to concentration and motility. Glycerol showed better recovery rates in progressive velocity as compared to the TEST yolk.[52] These data suggest that HSPM is a superior cryopreservative based on post-thaw recovery of motile sperm, which confirms the earlier report by Mahadevan and Trounson.[51]

Slow Freezing

Slow freezing is based on the principal of dehydration, where equilibration is achieved by combining low levels of cryoprotectant and slow rate of cooling. This allows dehydration to occur during cooling. It is the method of choice for cryopreservation of human spermatozoa. In this method, semen samples (raw and washed) are diluted by drop-wise addition of the freezing medium until a final ratio of 1:1 (volume-in-volume) is achieved. The samples are then loaded into straws or transferred into cryovials before being exposing to a temperature of –20°C for 15–30 minutes and to –79°C for another 15–30 minutes. They are placed in liquid nitrogen for storage (WHO 5th edn). This slow rate can be achieved by using the freeze programmer or manual vapour liquid nitrogen.

Various techniques have been proposed to freeze sperm that have been surgically retrieved (where few sperm are present). In one approach, isolated sperm cells were injected into an empty zona pellucida of a hamster oocyte and placed between 2 air bubbles inside a straw so that it could be easily located after thawing.[53,54] Others have suggested freezing under a layer of paraffin oil with glycerol.[26] Romero et al have described a frozen "testicular pill" that is composed of a mixture of sperm and testicular tissue.[55]

Vitrification

Vitrification is preservation at extremely low temperatures without freezing. Freezing involves ice crystal formation, which damages delicate organelles. Vitrification involves the formation of a glassy or amorphous solid state which, unlike freezing, it does not intrinsically damage the most complicated living systems. In this process, the ice formation during cooling is inhibited by high concentration of viscous solutions that produce a glass-like state at low temperatures.

Recently, a new technique of ice- and cryoprotectant-free cryopreservation (vitrification) was developed in which a sperm suspension is plunged directly into liquid nitrogen.[56,57] After storage, warming is achieved using direct melting. This is a simple, straightforward approach that preserves the motility and fertilizing ability of the spermatozoa. This newer method leads to better results (better pregnancy rates) compared with the conventional slow freezing (ice-equilibrium) method, partially because it omits the need for permeable cryoprotectants, thereby preventing the lethal effects of osmotic shock.[58] Vitrification of sperm is a relatively new technique and has not been standardized for clinical use.

Effect of Cryopreservation on Sperm Functions

DNA Stability

Semen cryopreservation has been reported to induce DNA damage, but the exact mechanism by which this damage occurs is not known. One theory is that it increases levels of oxidative stress in the semen. Some reports have proposed that it stimulates caspases, but the addition of caspase inhibitors to the medium has been shown to have no significant effect on post-thaw motility. Other reports have suggested that cryopreservation induces apoptosis.

Cryopreservation can cause and exacerbate DNA fragmentation in spermatozoa.[59] Some studies indicate that cryopreservation can increase inappropriate chromatin condensation in human sperm.[60] DNA integrity can be determined by several methods, including the TUNEL assay, (direct measure of DNA damage), and the Comet assay, (electrophoresis assay evaluating packaging of DNA within the nucleus).[60,61] The sperm chromatic structure assay (SCSA) measures the extent of DNA denaturation.[62] This method can determine whether the DNA within a sperm cell is normal, native chromatin that is structurally intact or if it is abnormal chromatin.

Oxidative damage caused by increased levels of reactive oxygen species may play a role in cryo-injury of sperm DNA. Antioxidants such as genistein (a plant-derived phyto-estrogen) and those found in native semen protect sperm from oxidative stress and lipid peroxidation and thereby reduce DNA fragmentation.[59] An increase in the activation of the intrinsic apoptotic cascade might result from insults to structural integrity of sperm that occurs during cryopreservation, but this is most likely not responsible for DNA damage in sperm.

Acrosomal Integrity

The zona-free hamster oocyte penetration test evaluates the ability of a sperm population to capacitate, acrosome react, bind and penetrate the membrane of an oocyte lacking a zona pellucida.[63] Especially when conducted with acrosomal stimulants such as TEST-yolk buffer, the penetration test correlates well with IVF success. Poor test results of male patients with deficient acrosomal integrity require the use of intracytoplasmic sperm injection (ICSI) to achieve pregnancy.

The acrosome is an organelle that facilitates the passage of the spermatozoa through the zona pellucida of the oocyte just prior to fertilization. Studies have shown that acrosomes are affected by cryopreservation more severely than any other organelle.[64] Acrosomes are characterized by fragile membranes that are susceptible to changes in osmolarity and physical or chemical conditions, which are extreme in the case of cryopreservation of gametes. Cryopreservation of sperm can lead to acrosomal abnormalities such as cracks or peelings due to low temperatures, which can increase cytoplasmic Ca^{2+} levels, capacitation-like reactions, ionic leakage, and exocytosis of the acrosomal content.

Motility and Viability

Post-thaw motility depends on the pre-freeze motility of the sperm sample. Generally speaking, it is reduced in cryopreserved semen samples.[64] Most studies indicate that viability and motility—the most important sperm parameters determining independent fertilization capacity—are reduced by 50 percent between the pre-freeze and post-thaw semen samples. It is likely that much (but not all) of the reduced motility is a direct result of reduced viability caused by damage to sperm cell membranes when they are frozen. In addition, reactive oxygen species can be formed during the freezing and thawing processes, leading to decreased motility through peroxidation of the plasma lipid membrane. However, seminal plasma contains innate antioxidants, which is one benefit of using unaltered semen during freezing

Fertilization Capacity

Sperm morphology can change with cryopreservation, leading to lower motility and less potential for fertilization. Fertilization capacity is impacted negatively because capacitation and the acrosome reaction can be inhibited when cryopreservation damages the membrane around the sperm head. Pentoxifyline treatment significantly increases sperm motility and the frequency of spontaneous acrosome reactions prior to freezing.[65,66]

Cryopreserved spermatozoa may have decreased function due to reactive oxidative species and acrosomal dysfunction as well as cellular changes that mark the spermatozoa for apoptosis. Pentoxifylline was found to have antioxidant properties that stabilize the acrosomal membrane and maintain the spontaneous acrosomal reaction. Pentoxifylline has beneficial effects of spermatozoa prior to cryopreservation and is proposed to improve the fertilization ability of cryopreserved spermatozoa.

Outcomes of ART Using Cryopreserved Sperm

Cryopreservation is a technique that provides a source of sperm that can be used for ART. ICSI has a higher success rate than IUI and IVF. Kelleher et al reported 29 pregnancies with frozen sperm from 64 men who underwent 85 ART cycles (35 IUI, 28 IVF cycles and 22 IVF-ICSI cycles).[67] Success rates of IVF and ICSI using cryopreserved semen was comparable to that of fresh semen-the average pregnancy rate was 54 percent (range, 33–73%).[68] Limited data is available regarding the ART treatment outcomes of cryopreserved sperm from male cancer survivors.[69] Audrins et al reported in their series of 258 patients who cryopreserved their semen prior to chemotherapy, 18 used their frozen sperm for treatment, and this resulted in six pregnancies.[13]

Hourvitz et al. described the ART outcome in 118 male cancer survivors undergoing 169 IVF-ICSI cycles—the largest series of couples treated with IVF-ICSI using cryopreserved sperm stored before cancer therapy.[70] They reported a clinical pregnancy rate of 56.8 percent, which is comparable to the average pregnancy rate achieved with other male-factor patients in their center. In another study 6 of 231 patients with cryopreserved sperm for malignant diseases returned for infertility treatment after chemotherapy. 2 of the 6 couples achieved pregnancy after IUI, 1 couple after IVF, and 2 couples after ICSI.[71] Schmidt et al reported a total of 151 ART cycles with cryopreserved sperm resulted in a clinical pregnancy rate of 14.8 percent after IUI and 38.6 percent following ICSI.[72]

A recent review on comparing successful retrievals from microsurgical TESE from standard TESE reported a mean success rate of 52 percent.[73] In cases associated with cryptorchidism, success rates were significantly higher than those associated with unexplained non obstructive azoospermia (NOA).[74,75] Earlier studies that compared ICSI outcomes in fresh vs. frozen-thawed cycles in patients with NOA of all degrees of severity demonstrated that pregnancy rates were similar.[76] Hauser et al evaluated the outcomes of fresh and frozen TESE in the most difficult subgroup of NOA patients-those with very few, and sometimes exclusively immotile sperm (severe hypospermatogenesis).[77] Their results indicated that pregnancies can be achieved at rates similar to those when fresh testicular sperm are used, even when motility is lost during the cryopreservation process. The initial lack of motility correlated with a significant reduction in fertilization rates and with a similar magnitude for both the fresh and frozen-thawed cycles. Thus, suggesting that post-thaw loss of motility should be considered in a different way than a primary lack of motility of fresh sperm. Motile sperm cells that lost motility during the freezing-thawing process might still be viable and their fertilizing capacity might be preserved. This capacity may be better than the fertilizing capacity of primarily immotile sperm cells retrieved from the testes.[77]

█ UTILIZATION OF BANKED SAMPLES

Interestingly, few patients (less than 10%) who bank sperm before cancer treatment return for infertility treatments. In a study with 256 men who cryopreserved their semen before undergoing vasectomy, only 4 men later returned to use their cryostored sperm with the aim of achieving a pregnancy.[78] The interval between storage and use ranged from 11 months to 10 years. Audrins et al found that out of 256 men who cryopreserved their semen before chemotherapy and/or radiation therapy, only 18 men returned to use their stored semen.[78] The duration of storage since the diagnosis of their disease in the men who continued the storage ranged from 1 month to 16 years, and the interval between storage and use ranged from 1 month to 7 years.[13]

There are a number of reasons why male patients do not return for fertility treatment: lack of a desire for children, anxiety regarding ART, financial considerations, and uncertainty about long-term prognosis.[70] However, the most common reason is patient demise.

█ ETHICAL ISSUES

The ethical challenges arise after the death of the patient regarding ownership and use of the cryopreserved material of the patient. Clear and precise instructions regarding the posthumous use of stored gametes or gonadal tissue taken from the patient along with informed consent is recognize by law.[79]

Patient Education

It is of crucial importance that all newly diagnosed male cancer patients be advised to cryopreserve their sperm at the earliest stage of their disease and, most importantly, before starting treatment. Although many cancer patients have poor pre-treatment semen quality, most have suitable sperm for freezing with good expectations for sperm survival. All young males 12 years of age or older should be offered the opportunity to bank their sperm before administration of any treatment that may have an adverse affect on the spermatogenesis process.[8] Semen cryopreservation should be performed before cancer treatment begins, and it is preferable that multiple samples are preserved. All males of reproductive age should consider banking semen samples before undergoing any type of chemotherapy or radiation therapy, and physicians should always provide them with the education they need to decide for or against cryopreservation.

Sperm banking can be a difficult subject to discuss with young patients and their parents. Topics such as developing sexuality, the grief associated with facing infertility as a side effect, and masturbation as a means of collecting a sample are sensitive. But it is still very important to preserve the right to trust of a reproductive future of the patient if possible.[5] One study suggested that the majority of physicians and about half of the patients preferred to have initial discussions on sperm banking without the patient's parents present.[10] Semen cryopreservation is the standard of care for these individuals. Failure to offer this option ignores the patient's only reproductive option.[3]

The staff at the oncologist's office can educate the patient thus reducing the amount of physician time invested in explaining sperm banking. Self help books can be provided to patients that discuss cancer, male infertility, and sperm banking. The availability of home kit for sperm collection and express shipping to the sperm bank makes it even easier for patients to collected a sample.[29] Patients who are clearly educated about the high-risk of infertility associated with chemotherapy treatment and the potential benefits of sperm banking are most likely to pursue this option.[28,29]

█ CONCLUSION

The gonadotoxic effects of cancer chemotherapy and radiation therapy or combination of both lead to impairment of sperm quality that leads to infertility. Fertility preservation options should be discussed at an early stage during treatment planning for cancer. Effective promotion of sperm banking involves adequate communication regarding the severity and estimated risk for infertility, assessment of the patient needs regarding having children in future, emphasis on the benefits of banking and addressing possible obstacles such as cost, misperceptions and cultural/other factors.[28]

Although usage rates of stored sperm are low, at least half of the couples can benefit from getting pregnant with ART techniques utilising cryopreserved sperm. Continuing research needs to focus on further improving cryopreservation protocols. There is a need for national guidance, training and support, for a strong collaborative effort between the different health and social care sectors that are involved. These sectors along with appropriate information systems need to be organized to face all the challenges of sperm banking services from diagnosis of the patient to eventual discharge from the health system.[80] Fertility preservation of younger cancer patients also requires coordinated efforts and attention by oncologists and fertility specialists to legal and ethical issues and to use of posthumous stored material after patient's death.[79]

■ REFERENCES

1. Eisenberg ML, Smith JF, Millstein SG, Walsh TJ, Breyer BN, Katz PP. Perceived negative consequences of donor gametes from male and female members of infertile couples. Fertil Steril 2009.p.10.

2. Abdel Hafez F, Bedaiwy M, El-Nashar SA, Sabanegh E, Desai N. Techniques for cryopreservation of individual or small numbers of human spermatozoa: a systematic review. Hum Reprod Update 2009;15(2):153-64.

3. Hourvitz A, Goldschlag DE, Davis OK, Gosden LV, Palermo GD, Rosenwaks Z. Intracytoplasmic sperm injection (ICSI) using cryopreserved sperm from men with malignant neoplasm yields high pregnancy rates. Fertil Steril 2008;90(3):557-63.

4. Williams DH, Karpman E, Sander JC, Spiess PE, Pisters LL, Lipshultz LI. Pretreatment semen parameters in men with cancer. J Urol 2009;181(2):736-40.

5. Menon S, Rives N, Mousset-Simeon N, Sibert L, Vannier JP, Mazurier S, et al. Fertility preservation in adolescent males: experience over 22 years at Rouen University Hospital. Hum Reprod 2009;24(1):37-44.

6. Palermo G, Joris H, Devroey P, Van Steirteghem AC. Pregnancies after intracytoplasmic injection of single spermatozoon into an oocyte. Lancet 1992;340(8810):17-8.

7. Lass A, Akagbosu F, Brinsden P. Sperm banking and assisted reproduction treatment for couples following cancer treatment of the male partner. Hum Reprod Update 2001;7(4):370-7.

8. Bonetti TCS, Pasqualotto FF, Queiroz P, Iaconelli A, Borges E. Sperm banking for male cancer patients: social and semen profiles. Int Braz J Urol 2009;35(2):190-7.

9. Bonetti TC, Pasqualotto FF, Queiroz P, Iaconelli A Jr, Borges E Jr. Sperm banking for male cancer patients: social and semen profiles. Int Braz J Urol 2009;35(2):190-7; discussion 7-8.

10. de Vries MC, Bresters D, Engberts DP, Wit JM, van Leeuwen E. Attitudes of physicians and parents towards discussing infertility risks and semen cryopreservation with male adolescents diagnosed with cancer. Pediatr Blood Cancer 2009;53(3):386-91.

11. Salonia A, Gallina A, Matloob R, Rocchini L, Sacca A, Abdollah F, et al. Is sperm banking of interest to patients with nongerm cell urological cancer before potentially fertility damaging treatments? J Urol 2009;182(3):1101-7.

12. Bagchi A, Woods EJ, Critser JK. Cryopreservation and vitrification: recent advances in fertility preservation technologies. Expert Rev Med Devices 2008;5(3):359-70.

13. Audrins P, Holden CA, McLachlan RI, Kovacs GT. Semen storage for special purposes at Monash IVF from 1977 to 1997. Fertil Steril 1999;72(1):179-81.

14. Vasectomy reversal. Fertil Steril 2006;86 (5 Suppl 1):S268-71.

15. Jurewicz J, Hanke W, Radwan M, Bonde JP. Environmental factors and semen quality. Int J Occup Med Environ Health 2009;22(4):305-29.

16. Corona G, Jannini EA, Lotti F, Boddi V, De Vita G, Forti G, et al. Premature and delayed ejaculation: two ends of a single continuum influenced by hormonal milieu. Int J Androl Mar 19.

17. Craft IL, Khalifa Y, Boulos A, Pelekanos M, Foster C, Tsirigotis M. Factors influencing the outcome of in vitro fertilization with percutaneous aspirated epididymal spermatozoa and intracytoplasmic sperm injection in azoospermic men. Hum Reprod 1995;10(7):1791-4.

18. Schlegel PN, Berkeley AS, Goldstein M, Cohen J, Alikani M, Adler A, et al. Epididymal micropuncture with in vitro fertilization and oocyte micromanipulation for the treatment of unreconstructable obstructive azoospermia. Fertil Steril 1994;61(5):895-901.

19. Tournaye H, Devroey P, Liu J, Nagy Z, Lissens W, Van Steirteghem A. Microsurgical epididymal sperm aspiration and intracytoplasmic sperm injection: a new effective approach to infertility as a result of congenital bilateral absence of the vas deferens. Fertil Steril 1994;61(6):1045-51.

20. Levin HS. Testicular biopsy in the study of male infertility: its current usefulness, histologic techniques, and prospects for the future. Hum Pathol 1979;10(5):569-84.

21. Gil-Salom M, Minguez Y, Rubio C, De los Santos MJ, Remohi J, Pellicer A. Efficacy of intracytoplasmic sperm injection using testicular spermatozoa. Hum Reprod 1995;10(12):3166-70.

22. Devroey P, Liu J, Nagy Z, Goossens A, Tournaye H, Camus M, et al. Pregnancies after testicular sperm extraction and intracytoplasmic sperm injection in non-obstructive azoospermia. Hum Reprod 1995;10(6):1457-60.

23. Hauser R, Botchan A, Amit A, Ben Yosef D, Gamzu R, Paz G, et al. Multiple testicular sampling in non-obstructive azoospermia— is it necessary? Hum Reprod 1998;13(11):3081-5.

24. Mulhall JP, Ghaly SW, Aviv N, Ahmed A. The utility of optical loupe magnification for testis sperm extraction in men with nonobstructive azoospermia. J Androl 2005;26(2):178-81.

25. Hauser R, Yogev L, Paz G, Yavetz H, Azem F, Lessing JB, et al. Comparison of efficacy of two techniques for testicular sperm retrieval in nonobstructive azoospermia: multifocal testicular sperm extraction versus multifocal testicular sperm aspiration. J Androl 2006;27(1):28-33.

26. Craft I, Tsirigotis M. Simplified recovery, preparation and cryopreservation of testicular spermatozoa. Hum Reprod 1995;10(7):1623-6.

27. Nijs M, Vanderzwalmen P, Vandamme B, Segal-Bertin G, Lejeune B, Segal L, et al. Fertilizing ability of immotile spermatozoa after intracytoplasmic sperm injection. Hum Reprod 1996;11(10):2180-5.

28. Achille MA, Rosberger Z, Robitaille R, Lebel S, Gouin JP, Bultz BD, et al. Facilitators and obstacles to sperm banking in young men receiving gonadotoxic chemotherapy for cancer: the perspective of survivors and health care professionals. Hum Reprod 2006;21(12):3206-16.

29. Schover LR, Brey K, Lichtin A, Lipshultz LI, Jeha S. Oncologists' attitudes and practices regarding banking sperm before cancer treatment. J Clin Oncol 2002;20(7):1890-7.

30. Meirow D, Schenker JG. The current status of sperm donation in assisted reproduction technology: ethical and legal considerations. J Assist Reprod Genet 1997;14(3):133-8.

31. Tschudin S, Bitzer J. Psychological aspects of fertility preservation in men and women affected by cancer and other life-threatening diseases. Hum Reprod Update 2009;15(5):587-97.

32. Schover LR. Psychosocial aspects of infertility and decisions about reproduction in young cancer survivors: a review. Med Pediatr Oncol 1999;33(1):53-9.

33. The Screening Process. California: The sperm bank of california; [cited 2010]; Available from: http://thespermbankofca.org/content/comprehensive-donor-screening.

34. Berger T, Marrs RP, Moyer DL. Comparison of techniques for selection of motile spermatozoa. Fertil Steril 1985;43(2):268-73.

35. Esteves SC, Sharma RK, Thomas AJ Jr, Agarwal A. Improvement in motion characteristics and acrosome status in cryopreserved human spermatozoa by swim-up processing before freezing. Hum Reprod 2000;15(10):2173-9.

36. Russell LD, Rogers BJ. Improvement in the quality and fertilization potential of a human sperm population using the rise technique. J Androl 1987;8(1):25-33.

37. Bolton VN, Braude PR. Preparation of human spermatozoa for in vitro fertilization by isopycnic centrifugation on self-generating density gradients. Arch Androl 1984;13(2-3):167-76.

38. Pousette A, Akerlof E, Rosenborg L, Fredricsson B. Increase in progressive motility and improved morphology of human spermatozoa following their migration through Percoll gradients. Int J Androl 1986;9(1):1-13.

39. Mortimer D. Sperm recovery techniques to maximize fertilizing capacity. Reprod Fertil Dev 1994;6(1):25-31.

40. Gellert-Mortimer ST, Clarke GN, Baker HW, Hyne RV, Johnston WI. Evaluation of Nycodenz and Percoll density gradients for the selection of motile human spermatozoa. Fertil Steril 1988;49(2):335-41.

41. Serafini P, Blank W, Tran C, Mansourian M, Tan T, Batzofin J. Enhanced penetration of zona-free hamster ova by sperm prepared by Nycodenz and Percoll gradient centrifugation. Fertil Steril 1990;53(3):551-5.

42. Polge C. Fertilizing capacity of bull spermatozoa after freezing at 79 degrees C. Nature 1952;169(4302):626-7.

43. Nishikawa Y. Studies on the preservation of raw and frozen horse semen. J Reprod Fertil Suppl 1975;(23):99-104.

44. Pursel VG, Johnson LA. Freezing of boar spermatozoa: fertilizing capacity with concentrated semen and a new thawing procedure. J Anim Sci 1975;40(1):99-102.

45. Colas G. Effect of initial freezing temperature, addition of glycerol and dilution on the survival and fertilizing ability of deep-frozen ram semen. J Reprod Fertil 1975;42(2):277-85.

46. Seager SW, Fletcher WS. Progress on the use of frozen semen in the dog. Vet Rec 1973;92(1):6-10.

47. Fox RR. Preservation of rabbit spermatozoa: fertility results from frozen semen. Proc Soc Exp Biol Med 1961;108:663-5.

48. Bunge RG, Sherman JK. Fertilizing capacity of frozen human spermatozoa. Nature 1953;172(4382):767-8.

49. Hallak J, Sharma RK, Wellstead C, Agarwal A. Cryopreservation of human spermatozoa: comparison of TEST-yolk buffer and glycerol. Int J Fertil Womens Med 2000;45(1):38-42.

50. Prins GS, Weidel L. A comparative study of buffer systems as cryoprotectants for human spermatozoa. Fertil Steril 1986;46(1):147-9.

51. Mahadevan M, Trounson AO. Effect of cryoprotective media and dilution methods on the preservation of human spermatozoa. Andrologia 1983;15(4):355-66.

52. Centola GM, Raubertas RF, Mattox JH. Cryopreservation of human semen. Comparison of cryopreservatives, sources of variability, and prediction of post-thaw survival. J Androl 1992;13(3):283-8.

53. Cohen J, Garrisi GJ, Congedo-Ferrara TA, Kieck KA, Schimmel TW, Scott RT. Cryopreservation of single human spermatozoa. Hum Reprod 1997;12(5):994-1001.

54. Hsieh Y, Tsai H, Chang C, Lo H. Cryopreservation of human spermatozoa within human or mouse empty zona pellucidae. Fertil Steril 2000;73(4):694-8.

55. Romero J, Remohi J, Minguez Y, Rubio C, Pellicer A, Gil-Salom M. Fertilization after intracytoplasmic sperm injection with cryopreserved testicular spermatozoa. Fertil Steril 1996;65(4):877-9.

56. Nawroth F, Isachenko V, Dessole S, Rahimi G, Farina M, Vargiu N, et al. Vitrification of human spermatozoa without cryoprotectants. Cryo Letters 2002;23(2):93-102.

57. Isachenko E, Isachenko V, Katkov II, Dessole S, Nawroth F. Vitrification of mammalian spermatozoa in the absence of cryoprotectants: from past practical difficulties to present success. Reprod Biomed Online 2003;6(2):191-200.

58. Isachenko V, Isachenko E, Katkov II, Montag M, Dessole S, Nawroth F, et al. Cryoprotectant-free cryopreservation of human spermatozoa by vitrification and freezing in vapor: effect on motility, DNA integrity, and fertilization ability. Biol Reprod 2004;71(4):1167-73.

59. Thomson LK, Fleming SD, Aitken RJ, De Iuliis GN, Zieschang JA, Clark AM. Cryopreservation-induced human sperm DNA damage is predominantly mediated by oxidative stress rather than apoptosis. Hum Reprod 2009;24(9):2061-70.

60. Yildiz C, Ottaviani P, Law N, Ayearst R, Liu L, McKerlie C. Effects of cryopreservation on sperm quality, nuclear DNA integrity, in vitro fertilization, and in vitro embryo development in the mouse. Reproduction 2007;133(3):585-95.

61. Bakos HW, Thompson JG, Feil D, Lane M. Sperm DNA damage is associated with assisted reproductive technology pregnancy. Int J Androl 2008;31(5):518-26.

62. Kobayashi H, Larson K, Sharma RK, Nelson DR, Evenson DP, Toma H, et al. DNA damage in patients with untreated cancer as measured by the sperm chromatin structure assay. Fertil Steril 2001;75(3):469-75.

63. Wallach E. Infertility: Overview and Initial Evaluation, General Strategy of Management, 1998.

64. Ozkavukcu S, Erdemli E, Isik A, Oztuna D, Karahuseyinoglu S. Effects of cryopreservation on sperm parameters and ultrastructural morphology of human spermatozoa. J Assist Reprod Genet 2008;25(8):403-11.

65. Schmidt KLT, Larsen E, Bangsboll S, Meinertz H, Carlsen E, Andersen AN. Assisted reproduction in male cancer survivors: fertility treatment and outcome in 67 couples. Hum Reprod 2004;19(12):2806-10.

66. Esteves SC, Sharma RK, Thomas AJ, Agarwal A. Effect of in vitro incubation on spontaneous acrosome reaction in fresh and cryopreserved human spermatozoa. Int J Fertil Womens Med 1998;43(5):235-42.

67. Kelleher S, Wishart SM, Liu PY, Turner L, Di Pierro I, Conway AJ, et al. Long-term outcomes of elective human sperm cryostorage. Hum Reprod 2001;16(12):2632-9.

68. VanCasteren NJ. Use rate and assisted reproduction technologies outcome of cryopreserved semen from 629 cancer patients. Fertility and Sterility 2008;90(6):2245-50.

69. Tournaye H, Goossens E, Verheyen G, Frederickx V, De Block G, Devroey P, et al. Preserving the reproductive potential of men and boys with cancer: current concepts and future prospects. Hum Reprod Update 2004;10(6):525-32.

70. Hourvitz A, Goldschlag DE, Davis OK, Gosden LV, Palermo GD, Rosenwaks Z. Intracytoplasmic sperm injection (ICSI) using cryopreserved sperm from men with malignant neoplasm yields high pregnancy rates. Fertil Steril 2008;90(3):557-63.

71. Lass A, Akagbosu F, Abusheikha N, Hassouneh M, Blayney M, Avery S, et al. A programme of semen cryopreservation for patients with malignant disease in a tertiary infertility centre: lessons from 8 years' experience. Hum Reprod 1998;13(11): 3256-61.

72. Schmidt KL, Larsen E, Bangsboll S, Meinertz H, Carlsen E, Andersen AN. Assisted reproduction in male cancer survivors: fertility treatment and outcome in 67 couples. Hum Reprod 2004;19(12):2806-10.

73. Colpi GM, Piediferro G, Nerva F, Giacchetta D, Colpi EM, Piatti E. Sperm retrieval for intracytoplasmic sperm injection in nonobstructive azoospermia. Minerva Urol Nefrol 2005;57(2): 99-107.

74. Raman JD, Schlegel PN. Testicular sperm extraction with intra-cytoplasmic sperm injection is successful for the treatment of nonobstructive azoospermia associated with cryptorchidism. J Urol 2003;170(4 Pt 1):1287-90.

75. Vernaeve V, Krikilion A, Verheyen G, Van Steirteghem A, Devroey P, Tournaye H. Outcome of testicular sperm recovery and ICSI in patients with non-obstructive azoospermia with a history of orchidopexy. Hum Reprod 2004;19(10):2307-12.

76. Ben-Yosef D, Yogev L, Hauser R, Yavetz H, Azem F, Yovel I, et al. Testicular sperm retrieval and cryopreservation prior to initiating ovarian stimulation as the first line approach in patients with nonobstructive azoospermia. Hum Reprod 1999;14(7):1794-801.

77. Hauser R, Yogev L, Amit A, Yavetz H, Botchan A, Azem F, et al. Severe hypospermatogenesis in cases of nonobstructive azoospermia: should we use fresh or frozen testicular spermatozoa? J Androl 2005;26(6):772-8.

78. Audrins P, Holden CA, McLachlan RI, Kovacs GT. Semen storage for special purposes at Monash IVF from 1977 to 1997. Fertil Steril 1999;72(1):179-81.

79. Robertson JA. Cancer and fertility: ethical and legal challenges. J Natl Cancer Inst Monogr 2005;(34):104-6.

80. Crawshaw M, Glaser A, Hale J, Sloper P. Professionals' views on the issues and challenges arising from providing a fertility preservation service through sperm banking to teenage males with cancer. Hum Fertil (Camb) 2004;7(1):23-30.

29

Sperm Preparation and Selection Techniques

Tahir Beydola, Rakesh K Sharma, Ashok Agarwal

ABSTRACT

This chapter will discuss the various sperm preparation and selection techniques used to process sperm for use with assisted reproductive techniques: swim-down, swim-up, migration-sedimentation, density gradient centrifugation, magnetic activated cell sorting, and glass wool filtration. It will also explain the procedures used to prepare viscous semen samples as well as when to obtain and prepare semen samples using epididymal and testicular spermatozoa, assisted ejaculation, and retrograde ejaculation.

INTRODUCTION

Approximately 2–4 percent of births in developed countries involve the use of assisted reproductive techniques (ART).[1] With ART, semen samples must first be processed before they can be used for insemination. Specifically, sperm preparation methods seek to replicate *in vitro* the natural process in which viable sperm are separated from other constituents of the ejaculate as they actively migrate through the cervical mucus.[2]

During processing, viable sperm cells are first separated from other constituents of the ejaculate as early as possible. If spermatozoa are not separated from seminal plasma within 30 minutes of ejaculation, the *in vitro* fertilization (IVF) capacity permanently diminishes.[3] The World Health Organization (WHO)[4] recommends separating sperm cells from the seminal plasma within one hour after ejaculation to limit damage from leukocytes and other cells present in the semen.

Various sperm separation or isolation methods exist to select sperm cells. These include swim-up methods, two-layer discontinuous gradient centrifugation, pentoxifylline wash, test-yolk buffer, sedimentation methods, polyvinylpyrrolidone (PVP) droplet swim-out, electrophoresis and fluorescence cell sorting methods.[5] A number of these have been developed to separate viable sperm from the seminal ejaculate for use in ART such as swim-down, swim-up, migration-sedimentation, density gradient centrifugation, magnetic activated cell sorting, and glass wool filtration. This chapter will discuss these techniques—the more commonly used procedures are explained in detail. It will also explain the procedures used to prepare viscous semen samples as well as when to obtain and prepare semen samples using epididymal and testicular spermatozoa, assisted ejaculation, and retrograde ejaculation.

SIMPLE WASH METHOD

In the simple wash method, following complete liquefaction, culture medium is added to the ejaculate and centrifuged twice to remove the seminal plasma. It is essential to use lower centrifugal forces (less than 500 g) and fewer centrifugation steps to minimize the damage caused by formation of reactive oxygen species (ROS) by non-viable spermatozoa and leukocytes.[3] Increased levels of ROS result in DNA damage in spermatozoa, decreased sperm motility, increased numbers of apoptotic spermatozoa, and decreased sperm plasma membrane integrity.[6] Additionally, the presence of large numbers of non-viable spermatozoa in the prepared sample can inhibit capacitation—a physiological process that confers spermatozoa with the ability to fertilize an oocyte.[6]

The simple wash technique is usually used when the semen sample has optimal parameters. This technique is often used to prepare sperm cells for intrauterine insemination because it produces very high yields of spermatozoa.

MIGRATION-BASED TECHNIQUES

Swim-Up

Swim-up is one of the most commonly used techniques for sperm preparation. Swim-up can be performed using a cell pellet or a liquefied semen sample. In conventional swim-up, a pre-washed sperm pellet obtained by a soft spin is placed in an overlaying culture medium in a conical tube (**Fig. 29.1**). The common steps of this method (using a cell pellet) are as follows:

- Allow specimen to liquefy completely for 15–30 minutes in a 37°C incubator before processing.
- Measure volume using a sterile 2 mL pipet.
- Transfer specimen from a plastic cup to a sterile 15 mL—conical centrifuge tube. If specimen is >3 mL, split the specimen into two aliquots.
- Gently mix the specimen with Quinn's Sperm Wash Media (HTF) in a ratio of 1:4 using a sterile pasteur pipet.
- Centrifuge the tubes at 1600 rpm for 10 minutes.

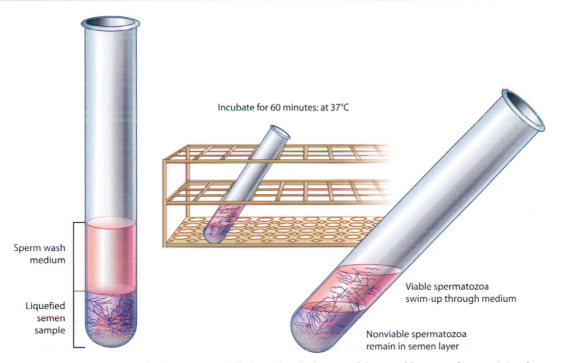

Incubate for 60 minutes: at 37°C

Sperm wash medium

Liquefied semen sample

Viable spermatozoa swim-up through medium

Nonviable spermatozoa remain in semen layer

Figure 29.1: The swim-up technique. Liquefied semen is carefully layered at the bottom of the round bottom tube containing the sperm wash medium. The tube is placed at an angle of 45° and incubated for 60 minutes. Active, motile sperm move out of the sample into the clear medium which is then aspirated

- Examine for sperm count and motility.
- Carefully aspirate the supernatant without disturbing the pellet and resuspend the pellet in 3 mL of fresh HTF. Transfer the resuspended sample into two 15 mL sterile round bottom tubes using a sterile serological pipette (1.5 mL in each).
- Centrifuge the tubes at 500 rpm for 5 minutes.
- Incubate the tubes at a 45° angle for 1 hour for swim-up in vertical rack in a 37°C incubator.
- After the incubation period, aspirate the entire supernatant from the round bottom tube. Use a pasteur pipet, with the tip placed just about the pellet surface.
- Pool supernatant from the two round bottom tubes into a single 15 mL conical centrifuge tube. Centrifuge the tube at 1600 rpm for 7 minutes.
- Aspirate the supernatant from the top of the meniscus using a pasteur pipet.
- Resuspend the pellet in a volume of 0.5 mL HTF using a 1 mL sterile pipet. Record the final volume.

Note: Sterile techniques should be used throughout specimen processing. When examining the specimen, it is important to pay particular attention to extraneous round cells, debris, and bacteria that may be present.

The medium used in this technique provides the sperm with a nourishing environment and attracts the sperm cells. The spermatozoa leave the pellet and swim into the medium. The sperm cells furthest away from the pellet are retrieved since they have the greatest probability of being motile and morphologically normal.

The swim-up method has been modified for oligozoospermic men.[7] This modified method is called direct swim-up and involves swim-up from semen rather than swim-up from the cell pellet. Direct swim-up is the simplest and fastest method for separating sperm by migration. Round-bottom tubes are used for direct swim-up to maximize the surface area between the semen and medium.[3] Multiple tubes with small volumes can be used to further increase this interface area and increase the number of motile sperm retrieved.[7] With this particular procedure, incubation is performed at 34.5°C, which has been reported to result in higher motility than incubation at 37°C.[8]

The swim-up method is simple and relatively inexpensive.[9] Yet, it has some disadvantages:

- Centrifugation, which is performed to create a cell pellet before conventional swim-up, has been shown to generate ROS[10]
- The amount of motile spermatozoa retrieved is relatively low
- Only 5–10 percent of the sperm cells subjected to swim-up are retrieved
- When a concentrated cell pellet is used, some motile spermatozoa may be trapped in the middle of the pellet and thus may not travel as far as the sperm cells at the edges of the pellet.

Migration-Sedimentation

Direct swim-up from semen is used for sperm samples with average or good motility. On the other hand, migration-sedimentation is usually used for samples with low motility.[11]

Migration-sedimentation uses the swim-up technique but also relies on the natural settling of spermatozoa due to gravity. Sperm cells migrate from a ring-shaped well into a culture medium above and then settle through the central hole of the ring. Special tubes called Tea-Jondet tubes are used for migration-sedimentation.[11]

The advantage of this technique is that it is a gentle method, and thus the amount of ROS produced is not very significant. On the other hand, the special tubes that are needed are relatively expensive.[9]

Swim-Down

This technique relies on the natural movement of spermatozoa. A discontinuous bovine serum albumin medium is prepared. This medium becomes progressively less concentrated moving from top to bottom. The semen sample is placed onto the top of the medium, and the tube is incubated at 37°C for one hour.[11] During migration, the most motile sperm move downward into the gradient.

Density Gradient Centrifugation

Density gradient centrifugation separates sperm cells based on their density. Thus, at the end of centrifugation, each spermatozoon is located at the gradient level that matches its density.[3] Morphologically normal and abnormal spermatozoa have different densities. A mature morphologically normal spermatozoon has a density of at least 1.10 g/mL whereas an immature and morphologically abnormal spermatozoon has a density between 1.06 and 1.09 g/mL.[12] As a result, the resulting interphases between seminal plasma and 45 percent, 45 percent and

90 percent containing the leukocytes, cell debris and morphologically abnormal sperm with poor motility, are discarded. The highly motile, morphologically normal, viable spermatozoa form a pellet at the bottom of the tube. Centrifugal force and time should be kept at the lowest possible values (<300 g) in order to minimize the production of ROS by leukocytes and non-viable sperm cells.[13] Also, non-viable sperm cells and debris should be separated from viable sperm cells as soon as possible to minimize oxidative damage.[13]

Density gradients can either be continuous or discontinuous. Density gradually increases from the top of a continuous gradient to its bottom. There are clear boundaries between layers of discontinuous gradients.[9] The latter gradient is formed when a number of layers of decreasing density are placed on top of each other.[3] Double density gradients comprise the commonly used sperm preparation protocol for ART.[3]

Components of the density gradient sperm separation procedure include a colloidal suspension of silica particles stabilized with covalently bonded hydrophilic silane supplied in HEPES. There are two gradients: a lower phase (90%) and an upper phase (45%). Sperm washing medium (Modified HTF with 5.0 mg/mL human albumin) is used to wash and resuspend the final pellet (**Fig. 29.2**).

Below are some of the main steps of the process:
- Place all components of the upper and lower phase and semen samples in an incubator at 37°C for 20 minutes.
- Transfer 2 mL of the lower phase into a sterile conical–bottom, disposable centrifuge tube.
- Layer 2 mL of the upper phase on top of the lower phase using a transfer pipet. Slowly dispense the upper phase lifting the pipet up the side of the tube as the level of the

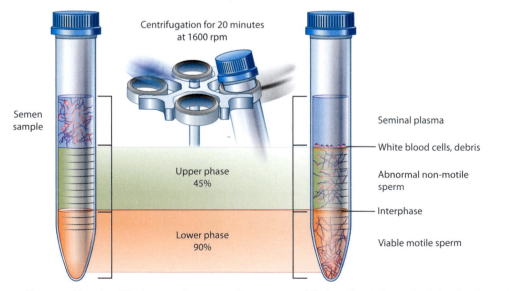

Figure 29.2: Density gradient centrifugation. The lower and upper gradients are carefully layerd and the seminal ejaculate layered on the top. The sample is centrifuged at 1600 rpm for 20 minutes. Clear seminal plasma is retained on the uppermost part of the gradient followed by a clear separation of white blood cells, debris and other cells. The immature, abnormal sperm are seen along the gradient based on their density and motility. Highly motile normal sperm move actively to the bottom of the gradient and collected as a pellet

upper phase rises. A distinct line separating the two layers will be observed. This two-layer gradient is stable for up to two hours.

- Measure semen volume to be loaded using a sterile 2 mL pipet. Remove a drop of semen using sterile technique for count, percent motility and presence of round cells.
- Gently place up to 3 mL of liquefied semen onto the upper phase (leaving approximately 0.1 mL in original container for a prewash analysis). If volume is greater than 3 mL, it may be necessary to split the specimen into two tubes before processing.
- Centrifuge for 20 minutes at 1600 rpm.

Note: Occasionally, samples that do not liquefy properly and remain too viscous to pass through the gradient will be encountered. Increasing the centrifugal force up to but no more than 600Xg will aid in separating the sperm in these cases.

- Using a transfer pipet, add 2 mL of HTF and resuspend pellet. Mix gently with pipet until sperm pellet is in suspension.
- Centrifuge for 7 minutes at 1600 rpm.
- Again, remove supernatant from the centrifuge tube using a transfer pipet down to the pellet.
- Resuspend the final pellet in a volume of 0.5 mL using a 1 mL sterile pipet with HTF. Record the final volume.

The advantages and disadvantages of density gradient centrifugation are listed in **Table 29.1**.

Tips to Maximize the Sperm Yield

- It is important to make sure that all components of the gradient and sperm wash medium are at room to body temperature before use. This will protect spermatozoa from "cold shock." In addition, any condensation on the media bottles will disappear, which aids in the visual detection of contamination. Any bottle whose contents appear in any way cloudy or hazy should not be used.
- Do not use the same pipet in more than one bottle of media.
- Prolonged exposure to a 5 percent CO_2 environment will alter the pH of these products, which may in turn affect their nature and performance.

- Highly viscous semen usually should be treated with 5 mg of trypsin, dissolved in 1.0 mL of sperm washing media and added to the ejaculate 5 minutes before loading on the upper gradient. This will increase the motile sperm yield without causing any measurable damage to the motile sperm.
- Avoid overloading the gradient as it causes a phenomenon called 'rafting'. Rafting is the aggregation of desirable as well as undesirable components of the semen that will be present in the postcentrifugation pellet.
- Use the gradient within one hour after creating it—eventually the two phases over time blend into each other and a sharp interface will not exist.
- Percoll™, a colloidal suspension of silica particles coated with polyvinylpyrrolidone, was widely used by ART laboratories until it was withdrawn from the market for clinical use. Nowadays, media containing silane-coated silica particles are commonly used. Isolate™ (Irvine Scientific, Santa Ana, CA), IxaPrep™, Sperm preparation medium™ and Suprasperm™ (Origio, MediCult, Copenhagen, Denmark), SpermGrad™ (Vitrolife, San Diego, CA), SilSelect™ (Ferti Pro NV, Beernem, Belgium) and PureSperm™ (NidaCon Laboratories AB, Gothenburg, Sweden) are commonly used.[9]

■ MAGNETIC ACTIVATED CELL SORTING

Magnetic activated cell sorting (MACS) separates apoptotic spermatozoa from non-apoptotic spermatozoa. During apoptosis (programmed cell death), phosphatidyl serine residues are translocated from the inner membrane of the spermatozoa to the outside. Annexin V has a strong affinity for phosphatidyl serine but cannot pass through the intact sperm membrane. Colloidal superparamagnetic beads (~50 nm in diameter) are conjugated to highly specific antibodies to annexin V and used to separate dead and apoptotic spermatozoa by MACS. Annexin V binding to spermatozoa indicates compromised sperm membrane integrity.

A 100 µL sperm sample is mixed with 100 µL of MACS microbeads and incubated at room temperature for 15 minutes. The

Table 29.1: Advantages and disadvantages of density gradient centrifugation

Advantages of density gradient centrifugation	Disadvantages of density gradient centrifugation
Density gradient centrifugation requires maximally a thirty-minute centrifugation. It takes less time than the swim-up technique which requires one-hour incubation.	Production of good interphases between layers can take some time.
Density gradient centrifugation is relatively easy to perform under sterile conditions.	There is a risk of contamination with endotoxins.
Spermatozoa from oligozoospermic semen can be effectively separated with density gradient centrifugation.[9]	Some scientists have claimed that density gradient centrifugation negatively affects sperm DNA integrity. For instance, Zini et al.[20] found that spermatozoa recovered after density gradient centrifugation possess lower DNA integrity than spermatozoa recovered after swim-up.
Density gradient centrifugation eliminates the majority of leukocytes in the ejaculate.	

mixture is loaded on top of the separation column which is placed in the magnetic field [0.5 Tesla (T) between the poles of the magnet and 1.5 T within the iron globes of the column]; 1 Tesla = 10,000 gauss (**Figs 29.3A and B**). The column is rinsed with buffer. All the unlabeled (annexin V-negative) non-apoptotic spermatozoa pass through the column (**Fig. 29.3C**). The annexin V-positive (apoptotic) fraction is retained in the column. The column is removed from the magnetic field, and annexin V-positive fraction is eluted using the annexin V-binding buffer.[5]

Spermatozoa prepared by density gradient centrifugation followed by MACS have a higher percentage of motility, a higher percentage viability, and a lower expression of apoptotic markers than spermatozoa prepared by density gradient centrifugation alone.[14] Annexin V-negative spermatozoa have a higher motility, lower caspase activation, lower membrane mitochondrial potential disruption, lower amounts of DNA damage, and higher oocyte penetration capacity than annexin V-positive spermatozoa.[15] Magnetic activated cell sorting improves the acrosome reaction in couples with unexplained fertility.[16] Annexin V-negative sperm cells show significantly higher motility and survival rates following cryopreservation than annexin V-positive

sperm cells.[17] Dirican et al.[18] reported that spematozoa selected by MACS were associated with higher cleavage and pregnancy rates than spermatozoa selected by density gradient centrifugation in oligoasthenozoospermic cases.

The advantages and disadvantages of magnetic activated cell sorting are outlined in **Table 29.2**.

GLASS WOOL FILTRATION

Glass wool filtration separates motile sperm cells from other contents of semen by filtration through densely packed glass wool fibers.[9] The filtration separates out immotile sperm cells, leukocytes and debris. Henkel et al.[19] reported that glass wool filtration eliminates 87.5 percent of leukocytes in semen. This is important since leukocytes are the main source of ROS in semen. After filtration, the semen is centrifuged to remove seminal plasma from viable sperm cells. The fact that centrifugation is carried out without leukocytes and non-viable spermatozoa are important since the absence of these populations limits the production of ROS. The advantages and disadvantages of this method are shown in **Table 29.3**.

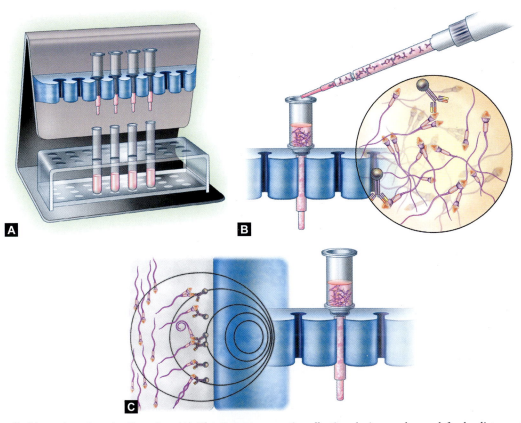

Figures 29.3A to C: Magnetic activated cell sorting: (A) The Octatet magnetic collection device can be used for loading up to a maximum of 8 samples. The tubes are placed between each open slot surrounded by the magnetic field, (B) The apoptotic and the nonapoptotic cells are labeled with the annexin V antibody beads (magnetic). These attach to the outer surface of the sperm that are apoptotic. Annexin V beads (magnetic) do not bind to the sperm that are non apoptotic and have intact membranes, (C) Apoptotic sperm with annexin V beads (magnetic) are retained in the column while the nonapoptotic sperm are eluted out and collected in a tube below the collection device

Table 29.2: Advantages and disadvantages of magnetic activated cell sorting (MACS)

Advantages of MACS	Disadvantages of MACS
MACS acts at the molecular level as opposed to routine sperm preparation techniques that rely on sperm density and motility.	Viable spermatozoa ought to be separated from all substances in the ejaculate such as apoptotic sperma- tozoa, leukocytes, and seminal plasma. MACS, which removes apoptotic spermatozoa, needs to be used in conjunction with other techniques such as density gradient centrifugation to remove the other substances.
MACS is the only known technique which separates apoptotic spermatozoa from non-apoptotic spermatozoa.	
MACS is rapid, convenient and non-invasive.	
Bead detachment after MACS is not necessary.	
MACS provides optimal purity and recovery with reliable and consistent results.	
MACS can used to optimize the cryopreservation-thawing outcome and enhance cryosurvival rates following cryopreservation.	

Table 29.3: Advantages and disadvantages of glass wool filtration

Advantages of glass wool filtration	Disadvantages of glass wool filtration
Glass wool filtration has been shown to select for sperm cells with normal chromatin condensation.	Glass wool filtration is relatively expensive.
Glass wool filtration has been reported to lead to a higher percentage of spermatozoa with intact acrosome than both density gradient centrifugation and a simple two-step centrifugation procedure.	Some debris is usually still present in the sample after glass wool filtration.

REDUCTION OF SEMEN VISCOSITY

Human semen normally liquefies within 5–20 minutes after ejaculation.[9] However, some ejaculates fail to liquefy and some are viscous by nature. Semen viscosity is a problem since it can reduce sperm motility. To reduce viscosity, the semen can be mixed with a medium. Liquefaction achieved by this method might not be adequate for highly viscous samples. Forcing the viscous semen through a needle with a narrow gauge is another option. However, this technique damages the sperm cells.[9] A commonly used viscosity treatment system involves enzymatic liquefaction using trypsin (5 mg). These can also be obtained prepackaged in 5 mg vials (VTS; Vitrolife, San Diego, CA). If the sample fails to completely liquefy following 20 minutes of incu- bation at 37°C, trypsin is added directly to the semen specimen. The specimen is then swirled and incubated for an additional 10 minutes. This results in complete liquefaction of the sample.

WHEN TO USE A PARTICULAR SPERM PREPARATION TECHNIQUE

The choice of sperm preparation method depends on the char- acteristics of the semen sample. When sperm parameters such as concentration and motility are within the normal ranges, the direct swim-up technique is preferred.[4] For significantly oligo- zoospermic, teratozoospermic and asthenozoospermic samples, density gradient centrifugation is preferred since density gradient centrifugation leads to a higher recovery of motile sperm cells than the swim-up technique. Also, density gradient centrifuga- tion can be modified to address the issues of each individual specimen, and it is the method of choice for sperm preparation in the majority of ART and andrology laboratories.[4] Glass wool filtration is also effective for the separation of sperm cells from semen with suboptimal parameters.[4]

SPERM SELECTION BASED ON MEMBRANE CHARGE

Mature sperm possess an electric charge of –16 to –20 mV called zeta potential (electrokinetic potential).[5] In this method, washed sperm (0.1 mL) is pipetted into the tube and diluted with 5 mL of serum-free HEPES–HTF medium. The positive charged (+2 up to +4 kV at 1 inch) on the tube is maintained by placing the tube inside a latex glove up to the cap and by grasping the cap, the tube is rotated two or three turns and rapidly pulled out. The electrostatic charge is verified using electrostatic voltmeters.

To allow adherence of the charged sperm to the wall of the centrifuge tube, each tube is kept at room temperature (22°C) for 1 minute. The tube is held by the cap to avoid grounding the tube. After 1 minute, the tube(s) are centrifuged at 300 g for 5 minutes and each tube is simply inverted to remove the nonadhering sperm and other cell types and excess liquid is blotted off at the mouth of each tube. To detach the charged adhering sperm, serum supplemented HEPES–HTF medium (0.2 mL) is pipetted into each tube allowing the medium to trickle down the side of the tube. The collected medium at the bottom of each tube is repipetted and used to rinse the wall of the same tube several times to increase the number of recovered sperm.

- The zeta method can be carried out immediately as sperm cells loose the charge with the onset of capacitation.
- To maximize the charge, a new centrifuge tube must be used.
- The use of culture medium with a higher percentage of serum or discharging the tube may improve recovery of detached sperm in low sperm concentration situations.

The zeta method of sperm processing is simple to perform, inexpensive, and permits rapid recovery of sperm with improved sperm parameters, particularly strict normal morphology, DNA normal integrity, and aniline blue maturity. These parameters are associated with improved fertilization and pregnancy after intracytoplasmic sperm injection (ICSI). Sperm progressive motility and hyperactivation (predictive of successful pregnancies after ART procedures) is improved in this method, suggesting that the brief exposure to the serum-free condition or the manipulation from the attaching—detaching process triggers sperm metabolic activity without causing premature acrosome reactions. To maximize the isolation of motile sperm, it is recommended that the sperm are preprocessed on density gradient.

The zeta method does not require the use of expensive electrophoresis equipment, Tris buffers, extreme pH environments, and UV irradiation. A limitation of the zeta method is the low recovery of processed sperm, and thereby limiting its usefulness especially in oligozoospermic patients. This method is not be useful for testicular or epididymal sperm aspirates as they lack sufficient net electrical charge on the sperm membrane surface.

◼ SPERM PREPARATION FOR ART

Density gradient centrifugation is usually used to prepare sperm cells for standard *in vitro* fertilization (IVF). If the semen sample is poor in terms of motility and concentration, intracytoplasmic sperm injection (ICSI) should be considered.[13]

The sperm sample can be prepared for ICSI with density gradient centrifugation or swim-up. Oligozoospermic samples can be prepared using the swim-up technique if there are some viable spermatozoa with forward motility.[13] If needed, sperm cells in oligozoospermic samples can be concentrated with a wash and re-suspension. These concentrated samples can be used directly or be subjected to density gradient centrifugation or swim-up before being used. Density gradient centrifugation is a better option than swim-up for significantly oligozoospermic and significantly asthenozoospermic samples as well as

for samples with high quantities of debris.[13] The hypo-osmotic swelling test is also an efficient method for selecting sperm for ICSI.[20]

Preparation of Epididymal and Testicular Spermatozoa

In case of epididymal obstruction or complete azoospermia, spermatozoa can be obtained from the epididymis or the testicular tissue, both require special preparation. Usually, large numbers of sperm cells can be collected from the epididymis.[4] Sperm samples obtained from the epididymis do not contain a significant amount of non-germ cells such as red blood cells. If sufficient numbers of epididymal sperm cells are collected, density gradient centrifugation can be used to prepare the spermatozoa for ART. On the other hand, the simple wash technique will be used if the number of spermatozoa aspirated is low.[4]

Spermatozoa can be retrieved from the testes by open biopsy or by percutaneous needle biopsy.[4] Testicular samples contain large numbers of non-germ cells such as red blood cells. Spermatozoa need to be separated from these non-germ cells. Also, the elongated spermatids, which are bound to the seminiferous tubules, must be freed. Sperm cells collected from the testes are used in ICSI because low numbers of spermatozoa with poor motility are generally aspirated. Pentoxifylline is occasionally used to increase the motility of epididymal and testicular spermatozoa before ICSI.[9]

Preparation of Assisted Ejaculation Samples

Direct penile vibratory stimulation or indirect rectal stimulation is used to retrieve semen from men who have disturbed ejaculation or who cannot ejaculate due to health issues such as spinal cord injury.[4] Patients with spinal cord injury often have ejaculates with a high sperm concentration and low sperm motility.[4] These ejaculates are also contaminated with red blood cells and white blood cells.[4] Ejaculates obtained by electroejaculation are most effectively prepared with density gradient centrifugation.[4] It has been reported that semen obtained by vibratory stimulation is of better quality than semen obtained by electroejaculation for men with spinal cord injuries.[21]

Preparation of Retrograde Ejaculation Samples

Retrograde ejaculation occurs when semen is directed into the urinary bladder during ejaculation. If there is an inadequate number of spermatozoa in the ejaculate, sperm cells in the urine need to be retrieved. At the laboratory, the patient is first asked to urinate without entirely emptying his bladder.[4] Then, he is asked to ejaculate and urinate again into another specimen cup containing 5–6 mL of culture medium, which alkalinizes the urine.[4] The urine sample volume is noted and analyzed after centrifugation.[4] The concentrated retrograde specimen and the antegrade specimen are usually prepared with density gradient centrifugation.[4]

The Liverpool solution given orally to alkalinize urine have been recently described and was demonstrated to be associated with improved sperm motility.[22]

CONCLUSION

In summary, a number of sperm preparation methods are available to process sperm for use in ART. Each infertile couple must be carefully examined to determine the best sperm preparation method. Future research should seek to improve the efficacy and the safety of the sperm preparation techniques.

REFERENCES

1. Poenicke K, Grunewald S, Glander H, Paasch U. Sperm Selection in Assisted Reproductive Techniques. In: Rao KA, Agarwal A, Srinivas MS (Eds). Andrology Laboratory Manual. 1st edn. India: Jaypee Brothers Pvt Ltd 2010.pp.173-87.
2. Franken DR, Claasens OE, Henkel RR. Sperm Preparation Techniques, X/Y Chromosome Separation. In: Acosta AA, Kruger TF (Eds). Human Spermatozoa in Assisted Reproduction. 2nd edn. USA: Informa Healthcare 1996.p.277-94.
3. Bjorndahl L, Mortimer D, Barratt CLR, Castilla JA, Menkveld R, Kvist U, et al. Sperm Preparation. A Practical Guide to Basic Laboratory Andrology. 1st edn. USA: Cambridge University Press 2010.pp.167-87.
4. Sperm Preparation Techniques. In: Cooper TG, Aitken J, Auger J, Baker GHW, Barratt CLR, Behre HM, et al, (Eds). World Health Organization Laboratory Manual for the Examination and Processing of Human Semen. 5th edn. Switzerland: WHO Press 2010.pp.161-8.
5. Chan PJ, Jacobson JD, Corselli JU, Patton WC. A simple zeta method for sperm selection based on membrane charge. Fertil Steril 2006;85(2):481-6.
6. Makker K, Agarwal A, Sharma R. Oxidative stress and male infertility. Indian J Med Res 2009;129(4):357-67.
7. Jameel T. Sperm swim-up: a simple and effective technique of semen processing for intrauterine insemination. J Pak Med Assoc 2008;58(2):71-4.
8. Otsuki J, Chuko M, Momma Y, Takahashi K, Nagai Y. A comparison of the swim-up procedure at body and testis temperatures. J Assist Reprod Genet 2008;25(8):413-5.
9. Henkel RR, Schill WB. Sperm preparation for ART. Reprod Biol Endocrinol 2003;1:108.
10. Ren SS, Sun GH, Ku CH, Chen DC, Wu GJ. Comparison of four methods for sperm preparation for IUI. Arch Androl 2004;50(3):139-43.
11. Mortimer D. Sperm Washing In: Mortimer D (Ed). Practical Laboratory Andrology. 1st edn. USA: Oxford University Press 1994.pp.267-86.
12. Oshio S, Kaneko S, Iizuka R, Mohri H. Effects of gradient centrifugation on human sperm. Arch Androl 1987;19(1):85-93.
13. Bourne H, Edgar DH, Baker HWG. Sperm Preparation Techniques. In: Gardner DK, Weissman A, Howles CM, Shoham Z (Eds). Textbook of Assisted Reproductive Techniques: Laboratory and Clinical Perspectives. 2nd edn. USA: Informa Healthcare 2004.pp.79-91.
14. Said TM, Agarwal A, Grunewald S, Rasch M, Glander HJ, Paasch U. Evaluation of sperm recovery following annexin V magnetic-activated cell sorting separation. Reprod Biomed Online 2006;13(3):336-9.
15. Said T, Agarwal A, Grunewald S, Rasch M, Baumann T, Kriegel C, et al. Selection of nonapoptotic spermatozoa as a new tool for enhancing assisted reproduction outcomes: an *in vitro* model. Biol Reprod 2006;74(3):530-7.
16. Lee TH, Liu CH, Shih YT, Tsao HM, Huang CC, Chen HH, et al. Magnetic-activated cell sorting for sperm preparation reduces spermatozoa with apoptotic markers and improves the acrosome reaction in couples with unexplained infertility. Hum Reprod 2010;25(4):839-46.
17. Said TM, Grunewald S, Paasch U, Rasch M, Agarwal A, Glander HJ. Effects of magnetic-activated cell sorting on sperm motility and cryosurvival rates. Fertil Steril 2005;83(5):1442-6.
18. Dirican EK, Ozgun OD, Akarsu S, Akin KO, Ercan O, Ugurlu M, et al. Clinical outcome of magnetic activated cell sorting of non-apoptotic spermatozoa before density gradient centrifugation for assisted reproduction. J Assist Reprod Genet 2008;25(8): 375-81.
19. Henkel R, Ichikawa T, Sanchez R, Miska W, Ohmori H, Schill WB. Differentiation of ejaculates showing reactive oxygen species production by spermatozoa or leukocytes. Andrologia 1997;29(6):295-301.
20. Liu J, Tsai YL, Katz E, Compton G, Garcia JE, Baramki TA. High fertilization rate obtained after intracytoplasmic sperm injection with 100% nonmotile spermatozoa selected by using a simple modified hypo-osmotic swelling test. Fertil Steril 1997;68(2):373-5.
21. Brackett NL, Padron OF, Lynne CM. Semen quality of spinal cord injured men is better when obtained by vibratory stimulation versus electroejaculation. J Urol 1997;157(1):151-7.
22. Aust TR, Brookes S, Troup SA, Fraser WD, Lewis-Jones DI. Development and *in vitro* testing of a new method of urine preparation for retrograde ejaculation; the Liverpool solution. Fertil Steril 2008;89:885-91.

INDUCTION AND INHIBITION OF SPERM APOPTOSIS SIGNALING

Oxidative Stress

Although the direct negative impact of oxidative stress on the sperm DNA integrity is proven by several studies, its impact on sperm apoptosis signaling activation is not fully clarified. One study measuring the level of oxidative stress and caspase-9 and -3 activation in sperm from males with idiopathic infertility documented a positive correlation of oxidative stress and caspase activation (Wang et al, 2003b), this relationship could not be verified in induction studies. Oxidative stress-induced apoptosis appears to be caspase-independent. In detail, incubation with low and high concentrations of HOCl and H_2O_2 respectively did not result in caspase activation in human sperm (Grunewald et al, 2005a; Taylor et al, 2004). Nevertheless, a recent study showed caspase-activation in boar spermatozoa after incubation with extremely high levels of NO (Moran et al, 2008).

Cryopreservation

Cryopreservation of human semen is the most commonly accepted method of preserving male reproductive capacity. Cryopreserved spermatozoa may be used in assisted reproductive techniques, especially in cases when a patient is diagnosed with cancer and the treatment may render him infertile. The indications for sperm cryobanking have been greatly expanded by recent breakthroughs in ART, in which immotile but viable sperm can be used successfully for oocyte fertilization through intracytoplasmic sperm injection (ICSI).

Cryopreservation leads to a significantly increased percentage of sperm showing activation of all types of caspases and is associated with externalization of phosphatidylserine at the outer side of the sperm membrane (Grunewald et al, 2001). The highest cryopreservation-induced increase in caspase activation was found in sperm positive for active CP-3 (+32.6%) underlining the central role of the effector caspase-3 (Paasch et al, 2004a). Hence caspase-3 marks a "point of no return" in the apoptosis signalling cascade, the pronounced activation of the protease by cryopreservation and thawing displays the deleterious influence of this process on sperm. Moreover, cryopreservation and thawing related caspase activation is significantly increased in semen samples from subfertile males (Grunewald et al, 2005b). The increase in caspase activation is dependant on the applied sperm preparation and cryopreservation protocol (Grunewald et al, 2005b). Comparative studies showed clearly a strong caspase activation when sperm were shock frozen (>90% of sperm contained active caspases), while stepwise cryopreservation protocols induce caspase activation to a significantly lower extent (Said et al, 2005b). On the other hand, density gradient centrifugation (DGC) enables selection of sperm with improved cryotolerance.

Caspase activation following the cryopreservation and thawing process was also seen in animal germ cells, e.g. in bovine (Martin et al, 2007; Martin et al, 2004) and equine spermatozoa (Brum et al, 2008; Ortega-Ferrusola et al, 2008). However, supplementation of cryopreservation media with caspase inhibitors does not improve the cryosurvival rates of sperm (Peter et al, 2005). The study was performed on canine sperm, but it is likely that the results can be transferred to human sperm.

Sperm Immaturity

Incomplete maturation of human ejaculated spermatozoa is associated with an increase of initiator and effector caspase activity (Paasch et al, 2004c). This caspase activation is also associated with the disruption of mitochondrial membrane potential in the immature sperm subpopulation. However, the activated apoptotic process does not immediately affect the levels of DNA fragmentation (Paasch et al, 2004c). Particularly cytoplasmic droplets of immature sperm contain activated caspases (Paasch et al, 2003) supporting the theory of abortive apoptosis following incomplete spermatogenesis (Sakkas et al, 1999). In addition, the presence of the anti-apoptotic regulator protein Bcl-xL in mature sperm reduces caspase-3 activation (Cayli et al, 2004). Recent studies proved the decreased activity of caspase-3 in mature sperm by double probing using aniline blue and caspase-3 immunostaining on the same slide (Sati et al, 2008). Reaching maturity may implicate a deactivation of the apoptosis-signaling cascade in human sperm.

Capacitation-related Inhibition of Apoptosis

The impact of capacitation on apoptosis-related signal transduction in human sperm was only subject to very few investigations. While some studies observed the externalization of phosphatidylserine (in somatic cells marker of terminal apoptosis) under capacitating conditions (De Vries et al, 2003; Gadella et al, 2002), it could not be verified in later studies (Grunewald et al, 2006a; Muratori et al, 2004). Capacitation of the mature sperm fraction obtained by density gradient centrifugation leads to a significant reduction of sperm with active apoptosis signalling. Remarkably, the inactivation is more pronounced at the level of initiator caspases (CP-9) than effector caspases (CP-3) (Grunewald et al, 2009a). This underlines, that in sperm the activation of the effector caspase-3 marks a "point of no return" in the apoptosis signaling cascade as known from somatic cells (Green et al, 1998), while activation of initiator caspases is a reversible process. The capacitation-induced inhibition of apoptosis signaling is most prominent in the mitochondria; the mitochondria membrane potential integrity was preserved during the capacitation process (Grunewald et al, 2009a). Intact mitochondria are essential for energy supply and the basis of sperm motility (Marchetti et al, 2004). Possibly, the improved mitochondrial function allows the hyperactivated motility during capacitation.

Impact of Activated Apoptosis Signaling on Sperm Fertilization Capacity

Male infertility is only a symptom for a variety of spermatozoal defects originating from different andrological diseases. Possibly, the increased susceptibility on proapoptotic stimuli and activation of apoptosis signaling is a common mechanism for various sperm pathologies.

Several studies indicate that semen samples from infertility patients contain higher levels of activated caspases and disrupted mitochondrial membrane potential compared to healthy donors (Gandini et al, 2000; Grunewald et al, 2005b; Grunewald et al, 2010; Grunewald et al, 2009b; Shen et al, 2002).

Subgrouping analysis of the infertility patients revealed that the percentage of caspase-positive sperm was elevated in patients with pathological spermiogram compared to fertile donors, but almost equally elevated in those patients showing normal spermiogram parameter (Grunewald et al, 2005b).

Semen samples with oligoasthenozoospermia show higher incidences of sperm with apoptotic features compared to samples with normozoospermia (Marchiani et al, 2007). This might be explained by alterations of the mitochondrial membrane potential, which severely affect sperm motility.

Another example are semen samples from patients with varicocele, which contain significantly more sperm with active apoptosis cascade than samples from donors without varicocele. The effect may be explained by the higher testicular temperatures in the varicocele patients (Chen et al, 2004).

A negative impact of activated apoptosis signaling on sperm fertilizing capacity was assumed and recent studies using hamster oocytes proved this relationship. All studies used animal models to simulate either *in vitro* fertilization (IVF) by the zona-free hamster oocyte sperm penetration assay (SPA) or the intracytoplasmic sperm injection (ICSI) by hamster oocyte-ICSI (H-ICSI).

Using the SPA, increased oocyte penetration potential was directly correlated with the absence of apoptosis markers in human donor sperm (Said et al, 2006; Sion et al, 2004). Analyzes of semen samples of infertility patients revealed an even stronger negative correlation between the apoptosis-related parameters: disruption of the mitochondria membrane potential, activation of caspase-3 as well as externalized phosphatidylserine and the performance of the spermatozoa in the hamster oocyte penetration assay. Semen samples showing subnormal SPA values (<20% penetrated oocytes) were characterized by significantly increased levels of disruption of the mitochondrial membrane potential, activation of caspase-3 and externalized phosphatidylserine (Grunewald et al, 2008), indicating an impact of apoptosis-related processes not only at the plasma membrane but also at the mitochondrial and cytoplasmic level on the spermatozoal capacity to penetrate oocytes.

Analysis of sperm performance in hamster oocyte-ICSI revealed a negative correlation of fertilization rates with the percentage of apoptotic sperm in samples from infertility patients (Grunewald et al, 2009b).

Due to the limitation of the animal model, the assessment of embryonic development was not possible, but many other studies proved the correlation of DNA fragmentation with later stages of the fertilization process such as embryonic development, the blastocyst development rate and clinical pregnancy rates (Zini et al, 2008).

SELECTION OF NON-APOPTOTIC SPERMATOZOA

Potential of Standard Sperm Separation Methods

Over the last decades a variety of standard procedures have been developed with certain modifications (conventional selection strategies). These sperm selection techniques can be classified by their basis on centrifugation, filtration or sperm migration. Among the centrifugation techniques, density gradient centrifugation (DGC) has been proposed as the gold standard for sperm preparation.

As mentioned above, semen samples of subfertile patients contain higher levels of spermatozoa with activated apoptosis signaling which is likely to impair their fertiliy.

Own investigations of semen samples from healthy donors showed a significant reduction of sperm with activated apoptosis signaling by DGC (Said et al, 2005a). Moreover, ejaculates of 20 subfertile men were investigated before and after DGC followed by a swim up procedure. While the amount of apoptotic sperm was reduced in the majority of the samples, profound inter individual differences in the separation effect ranging from <1 percent up to >65 percent were observed (Grunewald et al, 2010). Therefore, further development of specific, molecular-based separation methods to deplete apoptotic spermatozoa is needed.

Annexin-V Based Depletion of Sperm with Active Apoptosis Signaling

Currently available molecular-based methods to deplete sperm with activated apoptosis signaling are based on the specific binding of Annexin-V to externalized phosphatidylserine.

As mentioned before, externalization of phosphatidylserine (EPS) is the main apoptotic event detectable at the sperm surface, although it usually is present only on the inner leaflet of the sperm plasma membrane (Oosterhuis et al, 2004). Annexin V is a phospholipid-binding protein that has high affinity for phosphatidylserine and lacks the ability to pass through an intact membrane (van Heerde et al, 1995). Therefore, annexin V binding to spermatozoa may be used to label sperm that have compromised membrane integrity and that are less capable to fertilize eggs (Glander et al, 1999).

Annexin V conjugated superparamagnetic microbeads can effectively separate non-apoptotic spermatozoa from those with deteriorated plasma membranes based on the externalization of phosphatidylserine using magnetic-activated cell sorting (MACS, Miltenyi Biotec, Bergisch Gladbach, Germany). Annexin-V MACS separation of sperm yields two fractions: EPS-negative (intact membranes, nonapoptotic) and EPS-positive (apoptotic) which is retained in the magnetic field (Grunewald et al, 2001; Paasch et al, 2003).

Many own studies proved the ability of annexin-V MACS to enrich vital, motile sperm with inactivated apoptosis signaling and lower DNA fragmentation rate (Grunewald et al, 2001; Grunewald et al, 2006b; Paasch et al, 2004a; Paasch et al, 2003). Moreover, selected non-apoptotic sperm are characterized by a superior ability to undergo capacitation and acrosome reaction

Table 30.1: Overview of own studies on the separation effect of annexin-V MACS on sperm from healthy donors and subfertile patients (n.d. not detected, reduced, elevated compared to native donor sperm)

Sperm parameter	Healthy donors	Infertility patients	After cryopreservation and thawing	Annexin-V MACS	
				EPS-negative	EPS-positive
Progressive motility [%]	59.6 ± 14.3	↓	↓	Enrichment	Depletion
Pan-Caspase+ [%]	21.8 ± 8.3	↑	↑	Depletion	Enrichment
Caspase 8+ [%]	16.0 ± 3.8	n.d.	↑	Depletion	Enrichment
Caspase 9+ [%]	14.9 ± 6.5	n.d.	↑	Depletion	Enrichment
Caspase 3+ [%]	18.1 ± 7.5	↑	↑	Depletion	Enrichment
Disrupted MMP [%]	19.9 ± 7.2	↑	↑	Depletion	Enrichment
DNA-fragmentation [%]	9.7 ± 10.6	↑	↑	Depletion	Enrichment
Aneuploidies [%]	6.0 ± 6.7	↑	n.d.	Depletion	Enrichment
Induction of capacitation	yes	n.d.	n.d.	Improved	Reduced
Induction of acrosome reaction	yes	n.d.	n.d.	Improved	Reduced
Sperm penetration assay [% penetrated oocytes]	33.8 ± 6.9	↓	↓	Improved	Reduced
Sperm chromatin decondensation after hamster-ICSI [% oocytes]	34.0 ± 13.1	↓	–	Improved	Reduced

(not spontaneous acrosome reaction!) (Grunewald et al, 2006a; Lee et al, 2010). The depletion of sperm with activated apoptosis signaling is able to increase cryosurvival rates by integration of MACS before or after cryopreservation and thawing of sperm said (Grunewald et al, 2006b; Paasch et al, 2004a; Said et al, 2005b). An overview is given in the **Table 30.1**.

Sperm preparation that combines MACS with double-density centrifugation provides spermatozoa of higher quality in terms of motility, viability and apoptosis indices (caspase activation, mitochondrial membrane disruption and DNA fragmentation) compared with other conventional sperm preparation methods (Said et al, 2005a). Furthermore, sperm prepared according to this protocol showed improved ability to fertilize eggs using the hamster oocyte penetration assay and hamster oocyte ICSI (Grunewald et al, 2009b; Said et al, 2006).

An alternative approach to select EPS-negative sperm is annexin-V glass wool, which has similar separation potential compared to annexin-V MACS (Grunewald et al, 2007). However, it is currently not commercially available.

In recent years, several clinical studies and reports proved the advantage of integrating annexin-V MACS in conventional sperm preparation protocols. The combination leads to superior pregnancy rates and so far, healthy babies (Dirican et al, 2008; Rawe et al, 2010).

CONCLUSION

Many studies prove the presence and activation of apoptosis signaling in human sperm. High levels of sperm with activated apoptosis signaling are seen frequently following cryopreservation and thawing of the germ cells and in semen samples from subfertile males.

The initial theory of a sole abortive form of apoptosis cannot be further supported, although it might play a role in immature sperm. Due to the compartmentation of the mitochondria in the midpiece region, sperm are highly susceptible to mitochondria-associated apoptosis signaling. Although activated apoptosis signaling does not always lead directly to DNA fragmentation, caspase activation, disrupted transmembrane mitochondrial potential and externalized phosphatidylserine are correlated negatively with the oocyte penetration capacity and sperm chromatin decondensation rate.

Subsequently, the depletion of sperm with activated apoptosis signaling by implementation of annexin V-based methods in sperm preparation protocols may enhance the outcome of assisted reproduction techniques.

BIBLIOGRAPHY

1. Aitken RJ, Koppers AJ. Apoptosis and DNA damage in human spermatozoa. Asian J Androl 2011;13:36-42.
2. Blanc-Layrac G, Bringuier AF, Guillot R, Feldmann G. Morphological and biochemical analysis of cell death in human ejaculated spermatozoa. Cell Mol Biol (Noisy.-le-grand) 2000;46:187-97.
3. Bohring C, Krause E, Habermann B, Krause W. Isolation and identification of sperm membrane antigens recognized by anti-sperm antibodies, and their possible role in immunological infertility disease. Mol Hum Reprod 2001;7:113-8.
4. Brum AM, Sabeur K, Ball BA. Apoptotic-like changes in equine spermatozoa separated by density-gradient centrifugation or after cryopreservation. Theriogenology 2008;69:1041-55.
5. Cayli S, Sakkas D, Vigue L, Demir R, Huszar G. Cellular maturity and apoptosis in human sperm: creatine kinase, caspase-3 and

Bcl-XL levels in mature and diminished maturity sperm. Mol Hum Reprod 2004;10:365-72.

6. Chen CH, Lee SS, Chen DC, Chien HH, Chen IC, Chu YN, Liu JY, Chen WH, Wu GJ. Apoptosis and kinematics of ejaculated spermatozoa in patients with varicocele. J Androl 2004;25:348-53.

7. De Vries KJ, Wiedmer T, Sims PJ, Gadella BM. Caspase-independent exposure of aminophospholipids and tyrosine phosphorylation in bicarbonate responsive human sperm cells. Biol Reprod 2003;68:2122-34.

8. Dirican EK, Ozgun OD, Akarsu S, Akin KO, Ercan O, Ugurlu M, Camsari C, Kanyilmaz O, Kaya A, Unsal A. Clinical outcome of magnetic activated cell sorting of non-apoptotic spermatozoa before density gradient centrifugation for assisted reproduction. J Assist Reprod Genet 2008;25:375-81.

9. Espinoza JA, Paasch U, Villegas JV. Mitochondrial membrane potential disruption pattern in human sperm. Hum Reprod 2009;24:2079-85.

10. Gadella BM, Harrison RA. Capacitation induces cyclic adenosine 3',5'-monophosphate-dependent, but apoptosis-unrelated, exposure of aminophospholipids at the apical head plasma membrane of boar sperm cells. Biol Reprod 2002;67:340-50.

11. Gandini L, Lombardo F, Paoli D, Caponecchia L, Familiari G, Verlengia C, Dondero F, Lenzi A. Study of apoptotic DNA fragmentation in human spermatozoa. Hum Reprod 2000;15:830-9.

12. Glander HJ, Schaller J. Binding of annexin V to plasma membranes of human spermatozoa: a rapid assay for detection of membrane changes after cryostorage. Mol Hum Reprod 1999;5:109-15.

13. Green DR, Amarante-Mendes GP. The point of no return: mitochondria, caspases, and the commitment to cell death. Results Probl. Cell Differ 1998;24:45-61.

14. Green DR. Apoptotic pathways: the roads to ruin. Cell 1998;94:695-8.

15. Grunewald S, Baumann T, Paasch U, Glander HJ. Capacitation and acrosome reaction in non-apoptotic human spermatozoa. Ann NY Acad Sci 2006a;1090:138-46.

16. Grunewald S, Kriegel C, Baumann T, Glander HJ, Paasch U. Interactions between apoptotic signal transduction and capacitation in human spermatozoa. Hum Reprod 2009a;24:2071-8.

17. Grunewald S, Miska W, Miska G, Rasch M, Reinhardt M, Glander HJ, Paasch U. Molecular glass wool filtration as a new tool for sperm preparation. Hum Reprod 2007;22:1405-12.

18. Grunewald S, Paasch U, Glander HJ. Enrichment of non-apoptotic human spermatozoa after cryopreservation by immuno-magnetic cell sorting. Cell Tissue Bank 2001;2:127-33.

19. Grunewald S, Paasch U, Said TM, Rasch M, Agarwal A, Glander HJ. Magnetic-activated Cell Sorting before Cryopreservation Preserves Mitochondrial Integrity in Human Spermatozoa. Cell Tissue Bank 2006b;7:99-104.

20. Grunewald S, Paasch U, Said TM, Sharma RK, Glander HJ, Agarwal A. Caspase activation in human spermatozoa in response to physiological and pathological stimuli. Fertil Steril 2005a;(83 Suppl)1:1106-12.

21. Grunewald S, Paasch U, Wuendrich K, Glander HJ. Sperm caspases become more activated in infertility patients than in healthy donors during cryopreservation. Arch Androl 2005b;51:449-60.

22. Grunewald S, Reinhardt M, Blumenauer V, Hmeidan AF, Glander HJ, Paasch U. Effects of post-density gradient swim-up

on apoptosis signaling in human spermatozoa. Andrologia 2010;42:127-31.

23. Grunewald S, Reinhardt M, Blumenauer V, Said TM, Agarwal A, Abu HF, Glander HJ, Paasch U. Increased sperm chromatin decondensation in selected non-apoptotic spermatozoa of patients with male infertility. Fertil Steril 2009b;92:572-7.

24. Grunewald S, Said TM, Paasch U, Glander HJ, Agarwal A. Relationship between sperm apoptosis signaling and oocyte penetration capacity. Int J Androl 2008;31:325-30.

25. Kerr JF, Wyllie AH, Currie AR. Apoptosis: a basic biological phenomenon with wide-ranging implications in tissue kinetics. Br J Cancer 1972;26:239-57.

26. Kotwicka M, Filipiak K, Jedrzejczak P, Warchol JB. Caspase-3 activation and phosphatidylserine membrane translocation in human spermatozoa: is there a relationship? Reprod Biomed Online 2008;16:657-63.

27. Lee TH, Liu CH, Shih YT, Tsao HM, Huang CC, Chen HH, Lee MS. Magnetic-activated cell sorting for sperm preparation reduces spermatozoa with apoptotic markers and improves the acrosome reaction in couples with unexplained infertility dagger. Hum Reprod 2010;25:839-46.

28. Marchetti C, Gallego MA, Defossez A, Formstecher P, Marchetti P. Staining of human sperm with fluorochrome-labeled inhibitor of caspases to detect activated caspases: correlation with apoptosis and sperm parameters. Hum Reprod 2004;19:1127-34.

29. Marchiani S, Tamburrino L, Maoggi A, Vannelli GB, Forti G, Baldi E, Muratori M. Characterization of M540 bodies in human semen: evidence that they are apoptotic bodies. Mol Hum Reprod 2007;13:621-31.

30. Martin G, Cagnon N, Sabido O, Sion B, Grizard G, Durand P, Levy R. Kinetics of occurrence of some features of apoptosis during the cryopreservation process of bovine spermatozoa. Hum Reprod 2007;22:380-8.

31. Martin G, Sabido O, Durand P, Levy R. Cryopreservation induces an apoptosis-like mechanism in bull sperm. Biol Reprod 2004;71:28-37.

32. Moran JM, Madejon L, Ortega FC, Pena FJ. Nitric oxide induces caspase activity in boar spermatozoa. Theriogenology 2008;70:91-6.

33. Muratori M, Porazzi I, Luconi M, Marchiani S, Forti G, Baldi E. AnnexinV binding and merocyanine staining fail to detect human sperm capacitation. J Androl 2004;25:797-810.

34. Oehninger S, Morshedi M, Weng SL, Taylor S, Duran H, Beebe S. Presence and significance of somatic cell apoptosis markers in human ejaculated spermatozoa. Reproductive Biomedicine Online 2003;7:469-76.

35. Oosterhuis GJ, Vermes I. Apoptosis in human ejaculated spermatozoa. J Biol Regul Homeost Agents 2004;18:115-9.

36. Ortega-Ferrusola C, Sotillo-Galan Y, Varela-Fernandez E, Gallardo-Bolanos JM, Muriel A, Gonzalez-Fernandez L, Tapia JA, Pena FJ. Detection of "apoptosis-like" changes during the cryopreservation process in equine sperm. J Androl 2008;29:213-21.

37. Paasch U, Grunewald S, Agarwal A, Glandera HJ. Activation pattern of caspases in human spermatozoa. Fertil Steril 2004a;(81 Suppl)1:802-9.

38. Paasch U, Grunewald S, Dathe S, Glander HJ. Mitochondria of human spermatozoa are preferentially susceptible to apoptosis. Ann NY Acad Sci 2004b;1030:403-9.

39. Paasch U, Grunewald S, Fitzl G, Glander HJ. Deterioration of plasma membrane is associated with activated caspases in human spermatozoa. J Androl 2003;24:246-52.

40. Paasch U, Grunewald S, Wuendrich K, Jope T, Glander HJ. Immunomagnetic removal of cryo-damaged human spermatozoa. Asian J Androl 2005;7:61-9.

41. Paasch U, Sharma RK, Gupta AK, Grunewald S, Mascha EJ, Thomas AJ Jr, Glander HJ, Agarwal A. Cryopreservation and thawing is associated with varying extend of activation of apoptotic machinery in subsets of ejaculated human spermatozoa. Biol Reprod 2004c;71:1828-37.

42. Paasch U. Der programmierte Zelltod humaner Spermatogenesezellen und ejakulierter Spermatozoen— Mechanismend der Signaltrasnduktion und assoziierte Membranveränderungen im physiologischen und pathologischen Kontext im Hinblick auf eine potentielle diagnostische und therapeutische Konsequenz. The programmed cell death of human spermatogenesis and ejaculated spermatozoa - mechanisms of signal transduction under physiological and pathological conditions and the consequences for diagnostic and treatment. Shaker Verlag, Aachen, Germany, 2002.

43. Perticarari S, Ricci G, Boscolo R, De SM, Pagnini G, Martinelli M, Presani G. Fas receptor is not present on ejaculated human sperm. Hum Reprod 2008;23:1271-9.

44. Peter AT, Colenbrander B, Gadella B. Effect of caspase inhibitors on the post-thaw motility, and integrity of acrosome and plasma membrane of cryopreserved equine spermatozoa. Indian J Exp Biol 2005;43:483-7.

45. Rawe VY, Boudri HU, Sedo CA, Carro M, Papier S, Nodar F. Healthy baby born after reduction of sperm DNA fragmentation using cell sorting before ICSI. Reprod Biomed Online 2010;20: 320-3.

46. Said TM, Agarwal A, Grunewald S, Rasch M, Baumann T, Kriegel C, Li L, Glander HJ, Thomas AJ Jr, Paasch U. Selection of nonapoptotic spermatozoa as a new tool for enhancing assisted reproduction outcomes: an *in vitro* model. Biol Reprod 2006;74:530-7.

47. Said TM, Grunewald S, Paasch U, Glander HJ, Baumann T, Kriegel C, Li L, Agarwal A. Advantage of combining magnetic cell separation with sperm preparation techniques. Reprod Biomed Online 2005a;10:740-6.

48. Said TM, Grunewald S, Paasch U, Rasch M, Agarwal A, Glander HJ. Effects of magnetic-activated cell sorting on sperm motility and cryosurvival rates. Fertil Steril 2005b;83:1442-6.

49. Sakkas D, Mariethoz E, St John JC. Abnormal sperm parameters in humans are indicative of an abortive apoptotic mechanism linked to the Fas-mediated pathway. Exp Cell Res 1999;251:350-5.

50. Sakkas D, Moffatt O, Manicardi GC, Mariethoz E, Tarozzi N, Bizzaro D. Nature of DNA damage in ejaculated human spermatozoa and the possible involvement of apoptosis. Biol Reprod 2002;66:1061-7.

51. Salvesen GS, Dixit VM. Caspases: intracellular signaling by proteolysis. Cell 1997;91:443-6.

52. Sati L, Ovari L, Bennett D, Simon SD, Demir R, Huszar G. Double probing of human spermatozoa for persistent histones, surplus cytoplasm, apoptosis and DNA fragmentation. Reprod Biomed Online 2008;16:570-9.

53. Schuffner A, Morshedi M, Oehninger S. Cryopreservation of fractionated, highly motile human spermatozoa: effect on membrane phosphatidylserine externalization and lipid peroxidation. Hum Reprod 2001;16:2148-53.

54. Sharlip ID, Jarow JP, Belker AM, Lipshultz LI, Sigman M, Thomas AJ, Schlegel PN, Howards SS, Nehra A, Damewood MD, Overstreet JW, Sadovsky R. Best practice policies for male infertility. Fertil Steril 2002;77:873-82.

55. Shen HM, Dai J, Chia SE, Lim A, Ong CN. Detection of apoptotic alterations in sperm in subfertile patients and their correlations with sperm quality. Hum Reprod 2002;17:1266-73.

56. Sion B, Janny L, Boucher D, Grizard G. Annexin V binding to plasma membrane predicts the quality of human cryopreserved spermatozoa. International Journal of Andrology 2004;27:108-14.

57. Taylor SL, Weng SL, Fox P, Duran EH, Morshedi MS, Oehninger S, Beebe SJ. Somatic cell apoptosis markers and pathways in human ejaculated sperm: potential utility as indicators of sperm quality. Mol Hum Reprod 2004;10:825-34.

58. Van Heerde WL, de Groot PG, Reutelingsperger CP. The complexity of the phospholipid binding protein Annexin V. Thromb Haemost 1995;73:172-9.

59. Vermes I, Haanen C, Steffens-Nakken H, Reutelingsperger CP. A novel assay for apoptosis: Flow cytometric detection of phosphatidylserine expression of early apoptotic cells using fluorescein labeled Annexin VJ Immunol Methods 1995;184:39-51.

60. Von Schonfeldt V, Krishnamurthy H, Foppiani L, Schlatt S. Magnetic cell sorting is a fast and effective method of enriching viable spermatogonia from Djungarian hamster, mouse, and marmoset monkey testes. Biol Reprod 1999;61:582-9.

61. Wang X, Sharma RK, Gupta A, George V, Thomas AJ, Falcone T, Agarwal A. Alterations in mitochondria membrane potential and oxidative stress in infertile men: a prospective observational study. Fertil Steril 2003a;(80 Suppl)2:844-50.

62. Wang X, Sharma RK, Sikka SC, Thomas AJ Jr, Falcone T, Agarwal A. Oxidative stress is associated with increased apoptosis leading to spermatozoa DNA damage in patients with male factor infertility. Fertil Steril 2003b;80:531-5.

63. Weil M, Jacobson MD, Raff MC. Are caspases involved in the death of cells with a transcriptionally inactive nucleus? Sperm and chicken erythrocytes. J Cell Sci 111 1998; (Pt 18):2707-15.

64. Weng SL, Taylor SL, Morshedi M, Schuffner A, Duran EH, Beebe S, Oehninger S. Caspase activity and apoptotic markers in ejaculated human sperm. Mol Hum Reprod 2002;8:984-91.

65. World Health Organization. WHO laboratory manual for the examination and processing of human semen 2010;5th edition.

66. Zini A, Boman JM, Belzile E, Ciampi A. Sperm DNA damage is associated with an increased risk of pregnancy loss after IVF and ICSI: systematic review and meta-analysis. Hum Reprod 2008;23:2663-8.

Antisperm Antibodies Detection and Management

Tamer M Said, Iryna Kuznyetsova

ABSTRACT

Antioocyte and antizona pellucida antibodies are not found frequently in females; however, it has been proven that antisperm antibodies (ASA) play important roles in male and female immunological infertility. Several methods have been described for the detection of ASA. Despite the multiplicity of testing methods, the World Health Organization (WHO) Special Programme of Research Development and Research Training in Human Reproduction has consistently recommended the inclusion of only the mixed antiglobulin reaction test and the immunobead test for the assessment of human semen.

There is no established consensus regarding the extent of clinical significance of ASA testing. Nevertheless, the identification of ASA bound to the sperm is more relevant for fertility assessment than their presence in seminal plasma or serum. The hemizona assay is a reasonable method for selection of a treatment strategy for males with antisperm antibodies. Treatment of severe male immunological infertility by intracytoplasmic sperm injection (ICSI) is the best option known to date for these patients.

INTRODUCTION

Antisperm antibodies (ASA) have been documented as a potential cause for male infertility via several mechanisms that include interference with sperm motility, impedance of cervical mucus penetration, decreasing capacitation and sperm-ovum interaction as well as cytotoxicity.[1] There are several classes of ASA that have been discovered. ASA appear to exert detrimental effects on male fertility only if found on spermatozoa and in the male reproductive tract. Their presence in serum does not have clinical significance related to human reproduction.[2] One of the ASA, IgM, has not been detected in the male reproductive system and was only found in the circulation. On the other hand, IgG and IgA are locally produced in the genital tract and are found in semen.[3,4] Therefore in the context of male fertility management, investigations should focus only on IgG and IgA and not IgM.[5]

The chapter of this book aims at describing the management of ASA as a cause for male infertility including different methods used for detection, testing and treatment. Testing for ASA has been a subject of controversies due to several factors.

The different methodologies described in the literature vary in terms of indications, standardization and clinical interpretation of their results. Recent reports argue the absence of sufficient evidence to substantiate the inclusion of ASA testing in routine clinical andrology practice.[6] However, testing for ASA may allow the identification of the exact cause of infertility. If ASA are found to be a contributing factor, this could influence the decision of which assisted reproductive technique to be used for treatment.[7] Therefore, inefficient expensive treatments may be avoided and success rates may be boosted to alleviate patients' burden.[8]

DETECTION OF ANTISPERM ANTIBODIES

The several methods described for the detection and quantitation of ASA can be categorized into three groups:
1. Live sperm assays such as macroagglutination, microagglutination, immobilization, or sperm-cervical mucus interaction tests.
2. Sperm extract assays such as enzyme linked immunoassays and immunofluorescence.
3. Fixed sperm assays such as mixed antiglobulin tests and immunobead test.[9] At present, the mixed antiglobulin reaction test and the immunobead test are the most commonly used and recommended techniques in clinical andrology laboratories to investigate ASA.[10]

Macro/Microagglutination and Immobilization

Macro and microagglutination tests were initially developed to detect the presence of ASA in serum. The tube slide agglutination test (TSAT) is conducted by mixing donor semen with complement-inactivated patient serum. The presence of sperm agglutination is evaluated microscopically.[11] The gelatin agglutination test (GAT) is also conducted using the same approach but the mixture in placed in gelatin mix and sperm agglutination is observed without a microscope.[12] Both TSAT and GAT were used mainly for the assessment of sera from suspected subfertile men. Therefore, their clinical significance is extremely limited.

Similarly, the sperm immobilization test (SIT) procedure is based on the same concept with the addition of complement in the form of rabbit or guinea pig. The results are evaluated microscopically for the number of motile sperm (normal = >50%).[13]

The steps of complement fixation renders the SIT not capable to identifying IgA, only IgG and IgM can be detected.[14]

Cervical Mucus Penetration Tests

Antisperm antibodies (ASA) presence in the cervical mucus is one of the leading causes of immunological infertility. Assessment for the presence of IgG and IgA can be done via an *in vitro* or *in vivo* approach. An *in vitro* test, sperm-cervical mucus contact (SCMC) test, has been developed based on mixing drops of semen and cervical mucus. The test is evaluated by examining the mixture for the presence of a special sperm motility pattern that appears as shaking movement. On the other hand, the *in vivo* post-coital test (PCT) is conducted by evaluating spermatozoa present in the cervical mucus several hours after intercourse as regards their number and pattern of motility. The presence of less than 10 sperm/HPF or more than 25 percent of spermatozoa showing shaking pattern is interpreted as positive for ASA.[15] Both SCMC and PCT correlate very well as evidenced by a study that showed that 15/17 couples who repeatedly demonstrated unexpected poor post coital tests, had a positive SCMC test.[16]

Enzyme-linked Immunosorbent Assay and Immunofluorescence

Enzyme-linked immunosorbent assay (ELISA) utilizes specific antigen-antibody reaction and the degradation of chromogenic substrate by an enzyme to detect the presence of ASA. ELISA assessment of ASA has been described with various materials and methods such as solid phase materials (silicon rubber, glass); carriers (tubes, beads, disks); enzymes (alkaline phosphatase, horseradish peroxidase) and substrates (*p*-nitrophenyl phosphate).[17] The disadvantages of ELISA include being a complex assay that requires expensive instrumentation and experienced labor. These disadvantages have obstructed the implementation of the assay in the workup of male immunological infertility. Similarly, flow cytometry is not currently widely used for the detection of ASA due to its complexity, expense and instrumentation requirement. Despite its specificity, flow cytometry is not available in standard andrology laboratories. It is important to note that flow cytometry not only can detect sperm-bound antibodies but also can quantitate the sperm antibody load (antibody molecules/spermatozoa). Quantization of the sperm antibody load can be used to compare different patients or to follow-up with the same patient.[18]

Mixed Antiglobulin Reaction Test

The mixed antiglobulin reaction (MAR) test was developed based on modification of the Coombs test to detect surface ASA.[19] The assay initially included mixing semen sample with a suspension of group O, Rh-positive, human red cells of $R_1 R_2$ type, sensitized with human IgG in addition to rabbit or goat, undiluted, monospecific anti-IgG antiserum. Agglutination can be seen under light microscope after 10 minutes as mixed clumps of spermatozoa and red blood cells with a slow "shaky" movement. MAR test results can be expressed as percentages of motile

spermatozoa incorporated into the mixed agglutinates. The site of attachment can be also assessed. A MAR test can be reported as positive when >50 percent agglutination is seen.[10]

The MAR test has many advantages as it is quick, simple, consistent, inexpensive and can be applied directly to fresh, untreated semen samples. Therefore, the MAR test is one of the most commonly used methods for screening of ASA. Nevertheless, the assay has several limitations that should be considered. The MAR test cannot be used in patients with low sperm counts or motility. Also, variables such as debris, semen viscosity, mucus and microbial factors can affect the accuracy of the results.[20]

There are sperm MAR kits that are commercially available and are a better alternative to erythrocyte MAR. The commercially available kits are time and cost effective, and allow for assessments of both IgA and IgG classes. They include latex beads conjugated with human IgG or IgA and an antiserum against human IgG to induce mixed agglutination between antibody-coated.[21] The assay has been used routinely for the evaluation of male partners of infertile couples as a component of the semen analysis.[22] An indirect MAR test has been described to test for the presence of ASA in cases of azoospemia using donor sperm. However, the assay is difficult to interpret.

Immunobead Test

The immunobead test (IBT) has been described to be similar to the MAR test since it is a relatively simple procedure that does not require expensive instrumentation and employs commercially available beads (latex beads coated with antihuman IgG, IgA and IgM).[23] The test detects specifically ASA bound to sperm. Advantages of IBT also include allowing the localization of antibodies on the sperm and the identification of the antibody class attached to spermatozoa, as well as the proportions of spermatozoa bound to antibodies.[23]

Initially, spermatozoa are washed to discard any free immunoglobulins which may be in the seminal plasma and have the possibility of interfering with the assay results. Thereafter, sperm concentrations are adjusted to $10-25 \times 10^6$ motile sperm/mL to optimize the microscopic assessment of sperm. Unlike MAR test, the IBT can produce reliable results when conducted indirectly on reproductive fluids, seminal plasma, follicular fluid, cervical mucus and serum.[21] Both intra- and inter-assay reproducibility were evaluated using antisperm antibody-positive sera from two different patients against the same donor sperm sample and a positive serum sample with different sperm samples from the same donor and different donors. Based on these results, the assay has been confirmed to have a very low intra-assay variation and a high inter-assay variability.[24]

■ OPTIONS FOR ANTISPERM ANTIBODIES TESTING

Based on the presence of various methodologies as described above, it is critical to define to the documented relationships between these methods in order to identify which ASA is most suitable for each indication. The selection of ASA test to be used should be also based on its clinical significance. Understanding the correlation between the MAR test and the IBT is of extreme importance as both assays are the most commonly used and recommended ASA tests in routine clinical practice.[10] In principle, the two testing protocols similarly aim at identifying immunoglobulins attached to the sperm surfaces.

Mixed antiglobulin reaction (MAR) test correlates well with most other ASA tests including IBT.[19] Results from both assays were confirmed to be in correspondence with each other. However, there is a reported tendency for the MAR test to be slightly more sensitive than the IBT.[21] A contradicting report has shown that the IBT is more accurate than MAR.[25] IBT requires washing of spermatozoa free of seminal plasma, which makes it more cumbersome and time consuming than the MAR test. It also requires larger semen volume and higher sperm concentration in comparison to the MAR test.[26,27] It has been suggested that the MAR test can be easily implemented into routine semen analysis as a screening test, however, positive results should be confirmed by IBT.[28] Nevertheless, caution should be exercised during the interpretation of the results since sperm agglutination may occur due to non-immunological factors.[23]

CLINICAL SIGNIFICANCE OF ANTISPERM ANTIBODIES

It is not yet clear how extensive is the role of ASA in male infertility. However, data supports the negative impact of ASA in cases previously diagnosed with unexplained infertility. In clinical practice, the MAR test and the IBT are currently being used for the detection of ASA. The current threshold for considering a semen sample as immunocompromised is more than 50 percent of spermatozoa show binding in the MAR test or the IBT.[10] The presence of ASA was not correlated with other abnormalities in the sperm parameters. The sperm concentration, motility, morphology and leukocytes were shown to be normal in some cases with positive MAR test and spontaneous sperm autoagglutination.[29] These findings do not hold true in all cases as reported in a contradicting study conducted on 1176 infertile males.[30] In the aforementioned study, positive results obtained from the MAR test significantly correlated sperm concentration and motility. In support of the role of ASA as an etiological factor in unexplained infertility, IgG antisperm antibodies were found to be present in about 10 percent of men who had normal sperm parameters. Moreover, significantly elevated ASA levels were found in 18 percent of males diagnosed with unexplained infertility compared to fertile individuals.[31]

TREATMENT STRATEGIES FOR MALES WITH ANTISPERM ANTIBODIES

Several approaches were attempted to combat the potentially deleterious effects of ASA-mediated infertility and obtain antibody-free sperm. These approaches include sperm washing, swim up, immunoadsorption and immunocompetition. Using strict laboratory criteria to evaluate the immunological value of such reductions in the percentage of bound sperm after

in vitro manipulation, none of the protocols tested was capable of decreasing detectable sperm surface ASA positivity.[32] The most common empiric medical treatments are based on corticosteroid treatment with various dosages and administration methods. Suppressing the immune system with high doses of corticosteroids may decrease the production of antibodies but can result in serious side effects. Therefore, the use of low dose of steroids for treating male immunological infertility remains controversial and is no longer advised. Omu et al. showed that low dose prednisolone is useful in antisperm antibody associated infertility, by improving the sperm quality and giving rise to natural pregnancies without any side effects.[33] However in another study, corticosteroid treatment did not improve the results of intrauterine insemination in male subfertility caused by antisperm antibodies.[34] Similarly, Lombardo et al. found that corticosteroid therapy does not significantly reduce the titer and binding percentage.[35]

Hemizona Assay

For infertile males with ASA, diagnosis using the hemizona assay (HZA) may be carried out as the basis for decision making (**Figs 31.1 and 31.2**). Hemizona index (HZI) of <30 was

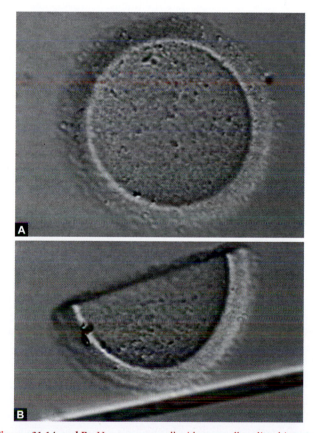

Figures 31.1A and B: Human zona pellucida manually splitted into two hemizonae. Upper hemizona—top view, lower hemizona—side view. Hoffman modulation contrast, magnification 200X

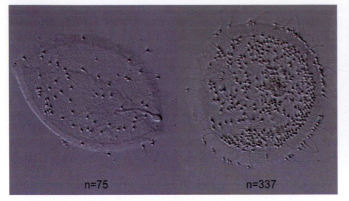

Figure 31.2: Hemizona assay with low hemizona index (HZI = 22), number of sperm bound is shown on the left compared to control sample on the right. Wet mount slide, phase contrast, magnification 400X

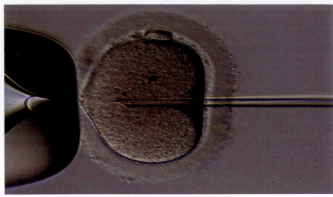

Figure 31.3: Intracytoplasmic sperm injection. Hoffman modulation contrast, magnification 400X

associated with lower pregnancy rate compared to patients with and HZI of ≥30 undergoing controlled ovarian hyperstimulation and intrauterine insemination (IUI).[36] If the patient with ASA has an abnormal hemizona index, it seems reasonable to advise selecting intracytoplasmic sperm injection-embryo transfer (ICSI-ET) as a primary treatment. However, it has been shown that some immunologically infertile males with normal fertilizing ability established pregnancy by timed intercourse (TI) or IUI. In such patients with ASA having normal hemizona index, TI or IUI can be selected based on the postcoital test result. Therefore, the treatment strategy for males with ASA is similar to that for infertile males with oligozoospermia or asthenozoospermia.[37]

Intracytoplasmic Sperm Injection

There are several pathways by which ASA can decrease the sperm fertilizing potential by affecting sperm progression through the female genital tract and by interfering with the fertilization process. It has been shown that ASA impair sperm motility and penetration into the cervical mucus.[38] ASA can also inhibit fertilization by binding to specific membrane antigenic structures involved in acrosome reaction and sperm-oocyte interaction.[39] Lower fertilization and cleavage rates are expected when ASA bound sperm are used in conventional *in vitro* fertilization (IVF).[40] Fertilization rates tended to decrease as the amount of antibody increased in the IBT,[41] and very low fertilization rates have been observed when >70 percent of inseminated spermatozoa were coated with ASA. Once fertilization had occurred, the pregnancy rate was not affected by the severity of immunological factors.[42]

Microinjection of the immunocompromised spermatozoa into the oocyte cytoplasm (ICSI) bypasses sperm-oocyte membrane interaction (**Fig. 31.3**). It has been also shown that the use of ICSI increases fertilization rates when compared to conventional IVF in cases of male immunologic infertility. Many findings demonstrated that fertilization rates, embryo

development, embryos' quality, pregnancy success and miscarriage rates after ICSI were not influenced by the ASA levels on sperm. This could be due to ASA becoming inactive within the ooplasm after microinjection, or that a segregation process may take place during the first cleavage divisions.[42] These hypotheses seem reasonable to explain why no differences on ICSI outcome are seen in ASA patients, since inactivation and segregation also occur with the acrosome and sperm tail after microinjection.[7]

■ CONCLUSION

The integration of ASA testing in the routine male infertility investigation panel has been controversial. There are several testing options that have been described with variable sensitivity and specificity levels. The MAR and IBT tests are the only candidates for implementation in clinical andrology laboratories. Whether the detection of ASA is associated with other deficiencies in the semen analysis or should not infringe on the importance of the assay, which may be of significance in identifying the etiology of infertility. One of the valid indications for ASA testing is cases diagnosed with unexplained infertility. The HZA is useful technique for selection of treatment strategy for males with ASA. The presence of antisperm antibodies in the semen does not affect the ICSI outcomes. Therefore, ICSI is the best treatment option for infertile men in the presence of high level of antisperm antibodies.

■ REFERENCES

1. Naz RK, Menge AC. Antisperm antibodies: origin, regulation, and sperm reactivity in human infertility. Fertil Steril 1994;61(6):1001-13.
2. Dondero F, Gandini L, Lombardo F, Salacone P, Caponecchia L, Lenzi A. Antisperm antibody detection: 1. Methods and standard protocol. Am J Reprod Immunol 1997;38(3):218-23.
3. Haas GG Jr, Cunningham ME. Identification of anti body-laden sperm by cytofluorometry. Fertil Steril 1984;42(4):606-13.

4. Witkin SS, Zelikovsky G, Good RA, Day NK. Demonstration of 11S IgA antibody to spermatozoa in human seminal fluid. Clin Exp Immunol 1981;44(2):368-74.

5. Rumke P. The origin of immunoglobulins in semen. Clin Exp Immunol 1974;17(2):287-97.

6. Kallen CB, Arici A. Immune testing in fertility practice: truth or deception? Curr Opin Obstet Gynecol 2003;15(3):225-31.

7. Clarke GN, Bourne H, Baker HW. Intracytoplasmic sperm injection for treating infertility associated with sperm autoimmunity. Fertil Steril 1997;68(1):112-7.

8. Bronson R. Detection of antisperm antibodies: an argument against therapeutic nihilism. Hum Reprod 1999;14(7):1671-3.

9. Alexander N, Ackerman S, Windt M-L. Immunology. In: Acosta A, Swanson R, Ackerman S, Kruger T, van Zyl J, Menkveld R (Eds). Human Spermatozoa in Assisted Reproduction. Baltimore: Williams and Wilkins 1990.pp.208-22.

10. World Health Organization: WHO laboratory manual for the examination of human semen and sperm-cervical mucus interaction. Cambridge University Press, 1999;4.

11. Franklin RR, Dukes CD. Antispermatozoal Antibody and Unexplained Infertility. Am J Obstet Gynecol 1964;89:6-9.

12. Kibrick S, Belding DL, Merrill B. Methods for the detection of antibodies against mammalian spermatozoa. II. A gelatin agglutination test. Fertil Steril 1952;3(5):430-8.

13. Isojima S, Tsuchiya K, Koyama K, Tanaka C, Naka O, Adachi H. Further studies on sperm-immobilizing antibody found in sera of unexplained cases of sterility in women. Am J Obstet Gynecol 1972;112(2):199-207.

14. Bronson RA, Cooper GW, Rosenfeld DL. Correlation between regional specificity of antisperm antibodies to the spermatozoan surface and complement-mediated sperm immobilization. Am J Reprod Immunol 1982;2(4):222-4.

15. Mortimer D. Clinical relevance of diagnostic procedures. In: Mortimer D (Ed). Practical Laboratory Andrology. New York: Oxford University Press; 1994.pp.241-67.

16. Franken DR, Slabber CF, Grobler S. The SCMC test: a screening test for spermatozoal antibodies. Andrologia 1983;15(3):270-3.

17. Ackerman SB, Wortham JW, Swanson RJ. An indirect enzyme-linked immunosorbent assay (ELISA) for the detection and quantitation of antisperm antibodies. Am J Reprod Immunol 1981;1(4):199-205.

18. Ke RW, Dockter ME, Majumdar G, Buster JE, Carson SA. Flow cytometry provides rapid and highly accurate detection of antisperm antibodies. Fertil Steril 1995;63(4):902-6.

19. Jager S, Kremer J, van Slochteren-Draaisma T. A simple method of screening for antisperm antibodies in the human male. Detection of spermatozoal surface IgG with the direct mixed antiglobulin reaction carried out on untreated fresh human semen. Int J Fertil 1978;23(1):12-21.

20. Mathur S, Williamson HO, Landgrebe SC, Smith CL, Fudenberg HH. Application of passive hemagglutination for evaluation of antisperm antibodies and a modified Coomb's test for detecting male autoimmunity to sperm antigens. J Immunol Methods 1979;30(4):381-93.

21. Kay DJ, Boettcher B. Comparison of the Sperm MAR test with currently accepted procedures for detecting human sperm antibodies. Reprod Fertil Dev 1992;4(2):175-81.

22. Sinisi AA, Di Finizio B, Pasquali D, Scurini C, D'Apuzzo A, Bellastella A. Prevalence of antisperm antibodies by Sperm MAR test in subjects undergoing a routine sperm analysis for infertility. Int J Androl 1993;16(5):311-4.

23. Franco JG Jr, Schimberni M, Stone SC. An immunobead assay for antibodies to spermatozoa in serum. Comparison with traditional agglutination and immobilization tests. J Reprod Med 1987;32(3):188-90.

24. Franco JG Jr, Schimberni M, Rojas FJ, Moretti-Rojas I, Stone SC. Reproducibility of the indirect immunobead assay for detecting sperm antibodies in serum. J Reprod Med 1989;34(4):259-63.

25. Mahmoud A, Comhaire F. Antisperm antibodies: use of the mixed agglutination reaction (MAR) test using latex beads. Hum Reprod 2000;15(2):231-3.

26. Ackerman S, McGuire G, Fulgham DL, Alexander NJ. An evaluation of a commercially available assay for the detection of antisperm antibodies. Fertil Steril 1988;49(4):732-4.

27. Rasanen M, Lahteenmaki A, Saarikoski S, Agrawal YP. Comparison of flow cytometric measurement of seminal antisperm antibodies with the mixed antiglobulin reaction and the serum tray agglutination test. Fertil Steril 1994;61(1):143-50.

28. Hellstrom WJ, Samuels SJ, Waits AB, Overstreet JW. A comparison of the usefulness of Sperm MAR and immunobead tests for the detection of antisperm antibodies. Fertil Steril 1989;52(6):1027-31.

29. Cerasaro M, Valenti M, Massacesi A, Lenzi A, Dondero F. Correlation between the direct IgG MAR test (mixed antiglobulin reaction test) and seminal analysis in men from infertile couples. Fertil Steril 1985;44(3):390-5.

30. La Sala GB, Torelli MG, Salvatore V, Dessanti L, Dall'Asta D, Cantarelli M, et al. The direct IgG-MAR test (mixed antiglobulin reaction test): results and correlations with seminal analysis in 1176 men from infertile couples. Acta Eur Fertil 1987;18(6):385-90.

31. Fichorova RN, Boulanov ID. Anti-seminal plasma antibodies associated with infertility: I. Serum antibodies against normozoospermic seminal plasma in patients with unexplained infertility. Am J Reprod Immunol 1996;36(4):198-203.

32. Haas GG Jr, Lambert H, Stern JE, Manganiello P. Comparison of the direct radiolabeled antiglobulin assay and the direct immunobead binding test for detection of sperm-associated antibodies. Am J Reprod Immunol 1990;22(3-4):130-2.

33. Omu AE, al-Qattan F, Abdul Hamada B. Effect of low dose continuous corticosteroid therapy in men with antisperm antibodies on spermatozoal quality and conception rate. Eur J Obstet Gynecol Reprod Biol 1996;69(2):129-34.

34. Grigoriou O, Konidaris S, Antonaki V, Papadias C, Antoniou G, Gargaropoulos A. Corticosteroid treatment does not improve the results of intrauterine insemination in male subfertility caused by antisperm antibodies. Eur J Obstet Gynecol Reprod Biol 1996;65(2):227-30.

35. Lombardo F, Gandini L, Dondero F, Lenzi A. Antisperm immunity in natural and assisted reproduction. Hum Reprod Update 2001;7(5):450-6.

36. Arslan M, Morshedi M, Arslan EO, Taylor S, Kanik A, Duran HE, et al. Predictive value of the hemizona assay for pregnancy outcome in patients undergoing controlled ovarian

hyperstimulation with intrauterine insemination. Fertil Steril 2006;85(6):1697-707.

37. Shibahara H, Shiraishi Y, Suzuki M. Diagnosis and treatment of immunologically infertile males with antisperm antibodies. Reprod Med Biol 2005;4(2):133-41.

38. Barratt CL, Dunphy BC, McLeod I, Cooke ID. The poor prognostic value of low to moderate levels of sperm surface-bound antibodies. Hum Reprod 1992;7(1):95-8.

39. Shibahara H, Burkman LJ, Isojima S, Alexander NJ. Effects of sperm-immobilizing antibodies on sperm-zona pellucida tight binding. Fertil Steril 1993;60:533-9.

40. Chang TH, Jih MH, Wu TC. Relationship of sperm antibodies in women and men to human *in vitro* fertilization, cleavage, and pregnancy rate. Am J Reprod Immunol 1993;30(2-3):108-12.

41. Ford WC, Williams KM, McLaughlin EA, Harrison S, Ray B, Hull MG. The indirect immunobead test for seminal antisperm antibodies and fertilization rates at *in vitro* fertilization. Hum Reprod 1996;11(7):1418-22.

42. Esteves SC, Schneider DT, Verza S. influence of antisperm antibodies in the semen on intracytoplasmic injection outcome. Intl Braz J Urol 2007;33(6):797-802.

Management of Nonobstructive Azoospermia

Ibrahim Fahmy, Ahmed El-Guindi

■ INTRODUCTION

Azoospermia, the absence of spermatozoa in the ejaculate, is observed in 1 percent of the general population and in 10–15 percent of infertile men. Azoospermia may result from pretesticular or testicular causes having adverse effects on spermatogenesis or posttesticular causes leading to obstruction of the genital tract. Pretesticular causes are infrequent in infertility clinics and include lesions in the hypothalamus or pituitary gland leading to defective production of follicle stimulating hormone (FSH) and/or LH resulting in secondary spermatogenic (testicular) failure. Testicular causes include all conditions leading to spermatogenic alteration other than hypothalamic and pituitary diseases. The severe forms of primary spermatogenic failure lead to azoospermia or severe oligozoospermia. Testicular causes of azoospermia are collectively referred to as non-obstructive azoospermia (NOA). The estimated prevalence of NOA in patients with severe male factor ranges between 40 and 60 percent.[1] In the past patients with proven NOA were considered hopeless. Since, testicular pathology is usually heterogeneous, foci of complete spermatogenesis might be present in a testis with severe impaired spermatogenesis. The introduction of ICSI opened the possibility to achieve pregnancy when only few spermatozoa could be retrieved from testicular biopsies in men having NOA with a reasonable probability of success.

■ ETIOLOGY

Non-obstructive azoospermia (NOA) may be caused by a variety of congenital and acquired conditions (**Table 32.1**). In a significant proportion of men with NOA the underlying etiology remains unknown.

Congenital Causes

Klinefelter's syndrome is the most common chromosomal abnormality affecting about 1 in 500 newly born babies. Up to 11 percent of azoospermic and 0.7 percent of oligozoospermic men have 47,XXY karyotype. The majority of patients have a uniform 47,XXY karyotype. The others are either 47,XXY/46,XY mosaics or have higher-grade sex chromosomal aneuploidy. The classic Klinefelter's syndrome is characterized by gynecomastia,

Table 32.1: Causes of nonobstructive azoospermia

- Congenital Causes
  - Genetic disorders
    - i. Klinefelter's syndrome
    - ii. Y-chromosome microdeletions
    - iii. Myotonic dystrophy
    - iv. Kennedy's syndrome
    - v. Androgen insensitivity syndromes
    - vi. Noonan's syndrome
    - vii. Sex reversal syndrome (XX male)
  - Other disorders
    - i. Maldescended testes
    - ii. Anorchia
    - iii. Testicular dysgenesis
- Acquired Causes
  - Trauma
  - Testicular torsion
  - Testicular tumors
  - Medications
    - i. Cytotoxic drugs
    - ii. Hormones (androgens, antiandrogens, estrogens, progestagens, anabolics)
    - iii. Hormonally active drugs (cimetidine, spironolactone, digoxin, ketoconazole)
    - iv. Psychotropic drugs, certain antiepileptics, antiemetics
    - v. Anthelmintics (niridazole)
    - vi. Salazosulphapyridine
  - Radiotherapy
  - Surgeries that can cause devascularization of the testes
  - Infections
    - i. Viral infections (mumps orchitis, influenza)
    - ii. Bacterial (brucellosis, typhoid fever)
    - iii. Specific granulomas (syphilis, leprosy)
  - Environmental factors (toxins, irradiation, heat)
  - Systemic diseases (liver cirrhosis, renal failure)
- Idiopathic

small, firm testes with hyalinization of the seminiferous tubules, hypergonadotrophic hypogonadism and azoospermia, though these features are reported to be variable.[2]

Deletions of the Y-chromosome represents other common causes of NOA. Molecular techniques have allowed identification of four non-overlapping regions, designated as azoospermia factor (AZF) a, b, c and d, in interval 6 of the long arm of the Y-chromosome. Contrary to AZFd, deletions of AZFa, AZFb, or AZFc result in spermatogenic impairment. These microdeletions are typically *de novo* mutations with a prevalence ranging from 3–15 percent, although in rare cases it can be transmitted through natural pregnancy. It is postulated that these three regions on the Y-chromosome correspond to different phenotypes. In this hypothesis AZFa is associated with complete absence of germ cells and AZFb is associated with spermatogenic arrest. AZFc does not appear to be associated with interruption of a specific phase of spermatogenesis, and can result in either azoospermia or severe oligozoospermia.[3]

Other rare autosomal or X-linked disorders with generalized phenotypic abnormalities may cause spermatogenic failure. Myotonia atrophica and Kennedy's syndrome are neurodegenerative disorders associated with NOA. Incomplete form of androgen resistance (Refenstein syndrome) is characterized by variable degrees of androgen deficiency and impaired spermatogenesis. Noonan's syndrome is characterized by male phenotype similar to female Turner's syndrome and is associated with azoospermia, and very small or undescended testes. XX-Male is a very rare syndrome (1: 20,000 males) caused by translocation of SRY sex determining gene from Y-chromosome to X-chromosome or autosomes.[4]

Other congenital defects may have a profound effect on spermatogenesis. Cryptorchidism is the most frequent congenital abnormality of the male genitalia affecting 2–5 percent of the newly born. The etiology is multifactorial and both disrupted endocrine regulation and several gene defects might be involved. The degeneration of germ cells starts after the first year and continues during childhood. If left untreated, complete loss of germ cells occurs after puberty. Orchiopexy performed before the age of 3 years may save spermatogenesis later. However, azoospermia still can be found in 42 percent of patients who underwent successful orchiopexy. Bilateral anorchia is an extremely rare disorder (1: 20,000 males). The etiology is not fully understood but intrauterine torsion is currently favored.[5]

Acquired Causes

There are wide varieties of acquired disorders that may lead to NOA. Radiation and cancer chemotherapy has a devastating effect on the testicular germinal epithelium. Alkylating agents exert an antimitotic effect on spermatogonia. Other antitumor agents block the cell division during the metaphase. Other drugs that have adverse effects of spermatogenesis include androgens, antiandrogens, estrogens, and thalazopyrine. Testicular tumors whether primary or secondary, may cause azoospermia by direct effect of the neoplasm or through effects of treatment. Post-pubertal mumps orchitis may lead to loss of germ cells and tubular hyalinization. Neglected non-specific epididymorchitis and testicular abscess may lead to total loss of testicular tissue. Other rare infections that may cause testicular fibrosis include brucellosis and leprosy. Testicular torsion if not diagnosed and treated properly will result in testicular atrophy due to interruption of the testicular blood supply. Secondary testicular failure may also results from other environmental factors (toxins, irradiation, heat) and systemic diseases (liver cirrhosis, renal failure).[6]

■ DIAGNOSIS OF NONOBSTRUCTIVE AZOOSPERMIA

Clinical Evaluation

The diagnosis of a man with azoospermia should include careful inspection of the semen sediment obtained by centrifugation. Absence of sperm should be confirmed in at least two specimens. Patients with very few sperm occasionally seen in some of their ejaculates may be termed cryptozoospermia, intermittent or occult azoospermia. These cases should be managed as true azoospermia except that during ICSI, motile normal sperm may be found in the ejaculate thus eliminating the need for surgical sperm retrieval. All patients having azoospermia should undergo a complete andrological workup. The reasons are; to exclude cases amenable to medical treatment, confirm the diagnosis, and counsel the patients for possibilities and success rate of different treatment options as well as for the possibility of transmitting genetic disorders to the offspring.

A thorough medical history and a detailed physical examination should be performed to assess all factors that can affect spermatogenesis. It is important to report size, consistency and symmetry of the testes. Estimation of testicular size by an orchidometer can improve accuracy. The presence or absence of the vas deferens and epididymal distension or nodularity should be established. Exclusion of other abnormalities especially varicocele should be done. The identification and management of co-existent illness is essential as androgen deficiency, testicular neoplasia and psychosexual/erectile problems are more frequent among infertile men.[1]

Laboratory Investigations

Measuring FSH, LH, PRL and testosterone is an important step to diagnose the cause of azoospermia. Hypogonadotrophic hypogonadism is diagnosed if FSH, LH and testosterone are low. Patients usually have a history of delayed puberty and are already undergone hormonal replacement therapy. However, sporadic cases may escape recognition and first present with infertility. Hyperprolactinemia may be caused by medications, concurrent medical illnesses, stress (both physiological and psychological), and pituitary tumors or may be idiopathic. Brain MRI with gadolinium enhancement is diagnostic of pituitary micro and macroadenoma or other anatomic pathology. It is important to identify this group of patients because effective medical treatment is available and can restore fertility.[3]

Generally, FSH reflects the state of spermatogenesis. The levels of FSH are mainly correlated with the number of spermatogonia. When the number of spermatogonia is normal but there is complete spermatocyte or spermatid arrest, FSH values are within normal. However, on an individual basis, FSH levels do not provide an accurate prediction of the status of spermatogenesis.[7]

When the FSH is normal, the differentiation between obstructive azoospermia and NOA, is almost unachievable without testicular biopsy. On the other hand, patients with small testes and elevated FSH should not go any diagnostic biopsy as it may hinder their future chances for sperm retrieval. **Flow chart 32.1** summarizes how to proceed with a patient presenting with azoospermia. Genetic testing, including Y-chromosome microdeletion analysis and karyotype, should be performed. These tests can reinforce the presumptive diagnosis of NOA and can provide useful prognostic information. Other hormones such as Inhibin-B and estrogens are not routinely done, but may add useful information in sporadic cases.[8]

Diagnostic Testicular Biopsy

When NOA is suspected from initial investigations, a diagnostic biopsy should not be performed except in centers experienced in testicular exploration and sperm extraction and cryopreservation is available. However, if the testicular size is normal a unilateral diagnostic biopsy, will confirm the diagnosis and specify testicular pathology. It may also help to council the patient since histopathology remains the best predictor of successful sperm retrieval.[9]

The histopathologic changes found on testicular biopsy can be subdivided into several well-recognized patterns regardless of the etiological factors. Testis biopsy must be assessed not only in regard to spermatogenesis but also for the possibility of co-existent carcinoma-in-situ (CIS). The histological evaluation requires familiarity with the morphological appearance of CIS cells and the use of immunohistochemical staining for suspected cases.

Classification of the Testicular Histopathologic Patterns

Several studies appeared that described the common histopathologic patterns seen in male infertility settings.[10-12] A minority of studies dealing with testicular pathology adheres to a referenced histopathological classification (**Figs 32.1A to F**). More often, the pathologists use general descriptive terms that lack precision and clarity. Most of the classifications describe the following main patterns; normal spermatogenesis, hypospermatogenesis, spermatogenic arrest, Sertoli cell only syndrome (SCOS) and tubular hyalinization. Some classifications included other patterns such as prepubertal, and Klinefelter's-like pattern. **Table 32.2** summarizes the main criteria of each pattern.

The controversies in testicular biopsy evaluation and classification arise from the fact that large proportion of cases has mixed patterns. Different authors may classify these mixed patterns in different ways. Another source of error is the identification of different spermatogenic cells. For example, some apoptotic cells having a fragmented deeply stained nuclei may be wrongly interpreted as late spermatids and a diagnosis of hypospermatogenesis is given instead of complete spermatogenic arrest.[12]

In order to avoid such conflicts, McLachlan et al, 2007[13] described a new classification that included all the mixed patterns

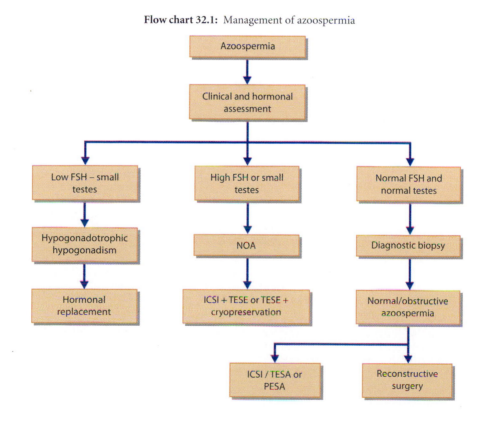

Flow chart 32.1: Management of azoospermia

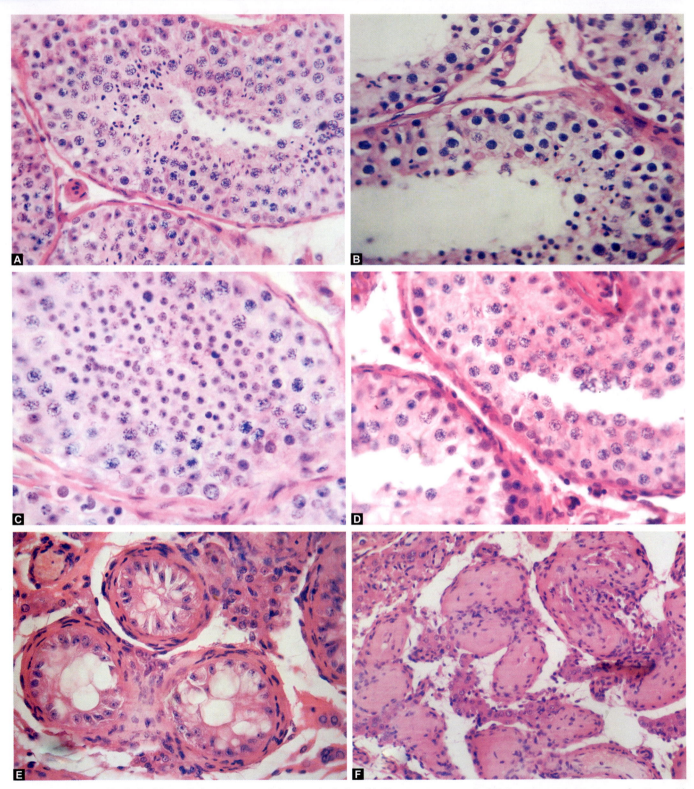

Figures 32.1A to F: Testicular histopathologic patterns: (A) Normal tubules; (B) Hypospermatogenesis; (C) Spermatogenic arrest at early spermatid stage; (D) Spermatogenic arrest at primary spermatocyte stage; (E) Sertoli cell only; (F) Hyalinized tubules

Table 32.2: Main histopathologic patterns encountered during testicular biopsy in infertile males

Histopathologic pattern	Description
Normal spermatogenesis	Most of the tubules show full spermatogenesis and contain >10 late spermatids (sperm heads).
Hypospermatogenesis (germ cell hypoplasia)	Most of the tubules show full spermatogenesis but the population of spermatogenic cells is markedly reduced-the average number of late spermatids is <5-10.

Spermatogenic arrest (maturation arrest)
a. Incomplete (partial)
b. - Complete
  - Early spermatid arrest
  - Primary spermatocyte arrest
  - Spermatogonial arrest
	Most of the tubules show arrested spermatogenesis but some tubules show few late spermatids (<5-10).
	All the tubules show arrested spermatogenesis, early spermatids are present in most tubules.
	All the tubules show arrested spermatogenesis mainly at primary spermatocyte stage.
	All the tubules show arrested spermatogenesis at spermatgonial stage. Exclusion of CIS is important.

Sertoli cell only (germinal aplasia) a. Incomplete (mixed) b. Complete (classical)	Most tubules are devoid of germ cells but foci or areas of normal or arrested spermatogenesis are present. All tubules are devoid of germ cells.
Tubular hyalinization (fibrosis) a. Incomplete b. Complete	Most tubules are devoid of cells and replaced by hyaline material. Some tubules may retain foci of normal or arrested spermatogenesis. All tubules are replaced by hyaline material.
Other specific patterns - Klinefelter's-like pattern - Prepubertal testis - Carcinoma *in situ* (CIS)	Most of the tubules are hyalinized, some tubules may retain Sertoli cells or rarely few spermatogenic cells. There is marked Leydig cell hyperplasia with accumulation of cells into large clumps. All tubules are small, devoid of basement membrane and lined by one type of cells called gonocytes. No Leydig cells are seen. Preinvasive malignant cells, present in the place normally occupied by spermatogonia. In a typical adult pattern, only Sertoli cells are present in tubules with CIS, but sometimes, CIS cells may be seen in tubules with ongoing spermatogenesis.

that show late spermatids, even in very small numbers, under the term "hypospermatogenesis". Thus cases with divergent patterns such as partial arrest, incomplete SCOS, hyalinization with focal spermatogenesis, all are included under one category. Under this classification, only patients with hypospermatogenesis will have the best chance of retrieving spermatozoa in an ICSI program. This facilitates counseling the patients and may put an end to the conflicts arising from the adoption of various classifications.

Quantitative Evaluation of Testicular Biopsy

The use of quantitative techniques like histometry and cell counting offers objectivity and increases precision.[13] However, these methods are rather laborious and are not suitable for clinical practice.

The Johnson score is a widely used simple scoring system for quantitatively describing spermatogenesis. In this score 50–100 tubules are examined and given scores according to the most advanced germ cell present in each tubule starting from 10 (normal) to 1 (fibrotic tubule). During evaluation, the whole profile of scores should be considered, as the 'mean score' might be misleading. To illustrate the problem, consider two settings: a biopsy with 90 percent of the tubules showing SCOS (given

score 2) and 10 percent showing many mature sperm heads (given score 9), the mean Johnson score for this biopsy will be 2.8. Another biopsy having 100 percent tubules showing only spermatocytes (given score 5) will have a mean score 5. Obviously the chances of the patient to have sperm during TESE is much higher in the first biopsy with the lower Johnson score.[13]

The late spermatid score is another simple quantitative method for evaluation of testicular biopsy. In this method, only the elongated dark spermatids are identified and counted in at least 20 rounded seminiferous tubules. Patients with normal spermatogenesis have a late spermatid score 17–35.[14]

TREATMENT OF NONOBSTRUCTIVE AZOOSPERMIA

Sperm extracted from testicular tissue obtained by testis biopsy, called testis exploration and sperm extraction (TESE), was first described in 1994 in obstructive azoospermia.[15] Retrieval of sperm from testes of patient with NOA for use in ICSI was described one year later[16] and is now a well-established standard treatment for men with NOA.

In patients with NOA, multiple biopsies from different sites may show focal areas with full spermatogenic activity.

Obstruction either intra- or post-testicular and too small numbers of spermatozoa that may be missed during routine examination of semen may explain why spermatozoa fail to appear in the ejaculate. Quantitative analysis of diagnostic biopsies performed prior to TESE/ICSI showed that a threshold of four late spermatids per tubule should be present for spermatozoa to appear in the ejaculate.[14]

The efficacy of testicular sperm extraction was reviewed in several studies.

For non-selected cases with NOA, the reported sperm retrieval rates (SRR) varies between 24 and 70 percent. The majority of these studies reported SRR between 40 and 60 percent.[17] A review on TESE including observational studies described a mean sperm retrieval rate (SRR) of 52 percent.[18] The variation of the reported results may be explained by differences in the population studied and differences in patient inclusion to ICSI programs. The difference in surgical techniques and the methods of processing testicular tissue and search for sperm might offer other explanations. Performing TESE prior to ICSI and cryopreservation of retrieved sperm may help to reduce the financial and psychological burden following unsuccessful surgery.[17] Patients with NOA should be clearly counseled as rereads the possibility of sperm retrieval rate prior to participation in ICSI program. For patients undergoing ICS/TESE simultaneously, donor sperm back up may be offered if the cultural and legal issues permit.

Techniques of Testicular Sperm Retrieval

Multiple Open Biopsy

The procedure can be done under local anesthesia and spermatic cord block using a mixture of 1:1 bupovacaine and xylocaine (**Fig. 32.2A**). For anxious patients, sedation, general or spinal anesthesia may be required. The testis is hold keeping the epididymis at a posterior position to avoid its injury. A 2–3 cm skin transverse or a mid line longitudinal incision is made (**Fig. 32.2B**). The advantageous of the longitudinal incision is that both testes can be accessed through a single scrotal incision. The skin incision is deepened to expose the tunica albuginea. The biopsy can be performed through this scrotal incision (window technique) without delivering the testis for full inspection (**Fig. 32.2C**). If the testis is small it can be delivered out the wound (**Fig. 32.2D**). A 5–10 mm incision is made sufficient to induce protrusion of testicular tissue about the size of a pea, which is snipped with sharp scissors (**Fig. 32.2E**). The testicular tissue should be immediately immersed in the appropriate media (modified Earle's salt solution). The biopsy is processed in the operating theater or a near-by embryo lab and examined for the presence of sperm. If no spermatozoa are seen, larger testicular biopsy specimen is taken from the same site or multiple biopsies are taken from different locations. The search should be continued until sperm were found or sufficient tissue is removed. Following adequate hemostasis, the wound is closed in layers (**Fig. 32.2F**).

Microdissection TESE

Schlegel 1999[19] introduced the use of optical magnification during TESE to help the identification of areas with intact spermatogenesis. Seminiferous tubules with active spermatogenesis are usually dilated, whitish and opaque in contrast to tubules where no sperm production occurs. Optical magnification also helps to visualize the blood vessels under the surface of tunica albuginea allowing biopsy incision in the least vascular region. This technique, in addition to improving sperm retrieval, facilitates the removal of smaller amounts of testicular tissue and avoids vascular injury and intratesticular hematomas. This result in less postoperative pain and minimize the possibility of postoperative fibrosis which is crucial for patients with small testes.[14]

The technique is similar to open biopsy except that a long incision is made exposing a wide area of testicular tissue. Inspection is carried out under magnification 15X–40X. The most dilated tubules are excised carefully. Usually, the size of each excised biopsy is 10 µgm. If sperm are found the wound is closed, or another biopsies are performed until the entire exposed testicular tissue is sampled. Micrometer attached to the eyepiece of the surgical microscope may be help to select the most dilated tubule. When the diameter is 300 micron or more, a single tubule biopsy is usually sufficient to harvest enough testicular spermatozoa for ICSI and freezing.[20]

To avoid the need for an operative microscope and surgical team experienced in microsurgical techniques, the use of surgical loupes was suggested.[21] Although surgical loupes (X3.5) did not offer superior sperm retrieval when compared with conventional TESE in non-selected patients with NOA, better rates (42% compared with 27%) of sperm retrieval in men who have testicular volumes of 10 mL or less were reported.[22]

Percutaneous Needle Biopsy

Fine needle aspiration (FNA) was initially used for diagnostic purposes. Different techniques have been described with variations in the needle diameter (18–21 gauge) and the number of testicular punctures (range 1–6). Under local anesthesia, the testis is hold firmly with the epididymis in a posterior position. Butterfly needles, attached to a 20 mL syringes is introduced inside the testis. A negative pressure is applied as the needle is moved in and out in various directions. A wide variety of needles, including Tru-cut needle, Biopty gun needle, wide-bore needles and intravenous catheters were introduced to increase the amount of tissue aspirated.[23]

All the techniques of needle aspiration look simpler, cheaper, and can be carried out as an office procedure. However, the amount of testicular tissue obtained is inadequate. Being a blind procedure, it is more likely to cause unrecognized vascular or epididymal injuries. Therefore, in men with NOA, its effectiveness has been questioned. Colored Doppler US may be used to guide FNA to improve the sperm retrieval rates and limit testicular damage.[24]

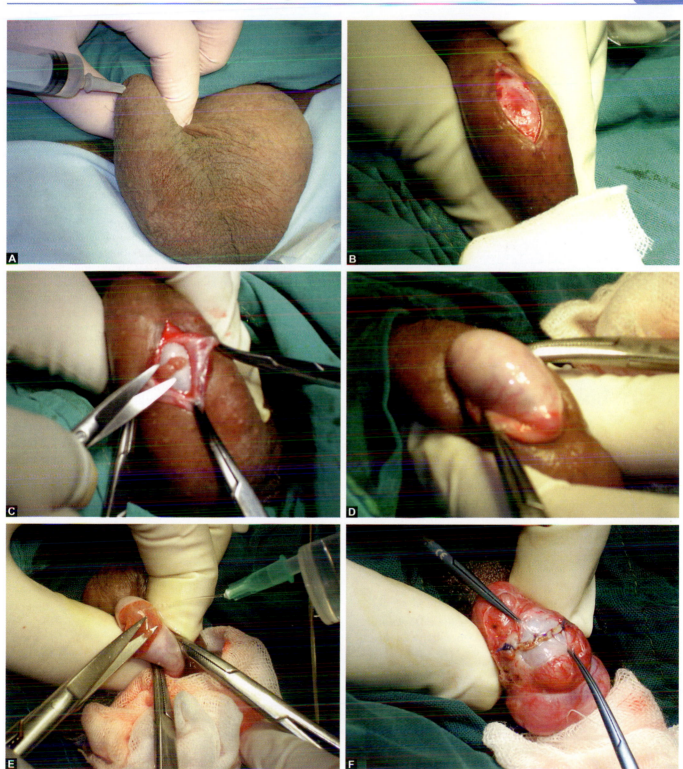

Figures 32.2A to F: Steps of conventional testis biopsy: (A) Local anesthesia - cord block; (B) Skin incision; (C) Window biopsy; (D) Delivering the testis out of wound; (E) Tunical incision and biopsy; (F) Closure of tunica

Prediction of Successful Sperm Retrieval

Multiple factors have been assessed to predict the success of sperm retrieval. Clinical and laboratory findings, such as testicular volume, testosterone and FSH levels, have not demonstrated reliability in predicting success.[8,9] There has been some interest in inhibin B and anti-Mullerian hormone but results using these markers have been inconsistent.[25] Instead of using each value alone, some investigators have combined clinical parameters of FSH, total testosterone, and inhibin B levels in a prognostic equation with a sensitivity of 71 percent and a specificity of 71.4 percent for successful retrieval.[26] Other laboratory parameters including May-Grünwald-Giemsa stain and immunofluorescent to identify spermatids in the ejaculate were used to predict sperm retrieval.[27]

In cases associated with cryptorchidism, a significantly higher SRR than unexplained NOA has been reported. However, this might be a consequence of the inclusion of patients with retractile testes. The reported SRR in patients with Klinefelter's syndrome varied between 30 and 50 percent. Hormonal treatment prior to ICSI especially with aromatase inhibitors and the use of micro-dissection TESE may improve the results.[28]

More reliable predictors of successful sperm retrieval include testicular histology and azoospermia factor (AZF) deletions. There is a strong evidence of negative predictive value in the presence of deletions on the Y-chromosome involving the AZFa and AZFb compared to men with deletions restricted to the AZFc region.[29]

There is wide variation in sperm retrieval rates among commonly recognized histopathologic patterns. For example, in cases of SOCS, SRR varies from 15 to 60 percent of cases. Although this variation may reflect real differences in surgical and laboratory techniques, it may also result from inconsistent interpretation of testicular histopathology.[12] To date, histopathology using the classification outlined by Levin (1979)[11] gives the best prediction of retrieving sperm, especially in SOCS (accuracy 0.83), but not in the cases showing maturation arrest (accuracy 0.55).[9] **Table 32.3** shows the success rates for sperm retrieval based on testicular histology. It seems that the more advanced the level of spermatogenesis, the more likely is the successful retrieval of mature sperm.[30]

Mapping the testes by Doppler ultrasound or FNA prior to conventional TESE has been introduced to improve the SRR and reduce the testicular damage. More studies are required to establish the added value of these techniques.[29]

Comparisons of Different Techniques

While most of the studies showed that TESE is more effective than FNA, few studies showed comparable results. Controversy resulted from the fact that some of these studies did not include histological characterization of the patients. Subgroup analysis showed that FNA might be successful on patients with hypospermatogenesis.[24] Recently updated Cochrane database review concluded that there is insufficient evidence to recommend any particular surgical technique.[31]

The most appropriate number of biopsies to be taken remains controversial. Single large testicular biopsy was proposed based on the finding that spermatogenesis in NOA is multifocal and diffuse rather than regional.[14] One randomized study showed that SRR were similar if the biopsies were performed through a single large incision or multiple incisions.[32] Nevertheless, this approach was refuted by other studies that found a patchy distribution of regions with minimal spermatogenesis throughout the testis.[24] The evidence provided by observational studies favors multiple biopsies. One study revealed that sperm recovery would have been missed in 32 percent of cases if only one biopsy had been performed.[30] Another larger study showed that multiple biopsies enabled a significantly higher SRR compared with single biopsy.[33]

When compared to conventional TESE, several studies showed higher sperm retrieval with microdissection TESE. Subgroup analysis revealed that SCOS had a significantly higher SRR compared to maturation arrest. A possible explanation is that in cases of arrest all tubules are uniform as opposed to SCOS where the difference in tubular diameter enables the identification of sites of active spermatogenesis. Nonetheless, a larger study found a significantly higher SRR only in cases of hypospermatogenesis.[24,29]

Complications of Treatment

The main drawbacks of TESE are the loss of a significant amount of testicular tissue and a disruption in the blood supply leading to fibrosis and atrophy.[34] An autoimmune response, and impaired testosterone synthesis are other possible complications. Although the development of gross hematoma and hematocele are rare, intratesticular hematoma observed by ultrasounds are common. Microdissection TESE has a lower incidence in developing intratesticular hematoma and fibrosis.[35]

As confirmed in several recent series, male offspring will almost certainly inherit the Y-chromosomal deletions if

Table 32.3: SRR according to the main histopathology in patients with NOA*

Histopathologic pattern	SRR range	Remarks
Hypospermatogenesis	79-100%	The definition of hypospermatogenesis is not constant in most studies
Spermatogenic arrest	25-85%	Early and complete forms have lower SRR
Sertoli cell only	16-86%	Complete forms have lower SRR
Hyalinization	10-42%	Includes patients with KF

*Figures are collected from references.[15,20,21,26,28]

present.[3] There were concerns regarding the use of ICSI in passing the genetic abnormalities to the offspring of men with NOA. However, major and minor malformation rates were not affected by the application of ICSI, and neither was the rate of early pregnancy loss. The increased rate of chromosomal abnormalities appeared probably related to pre-existing conditions in the fathers who provided the sperm for ICSI, rather than to the ICSI procedure itself. Genetic counseling, however, should be mandatory for all couples undergoing assisted reproductive techniques.[36]

Timing of Surgical Sperm Retrieval and Repeated TESE

Whether to time the sperm retrieval in-cycle or to perform TESE first and cryopreserve sperm for future use, remains an important issue in patients with NOA. Coordinating in-cycle retrieval can be complex as well as stressful for the couple should a cycle be canceled due to failure of sperm retrieval. On the other hand, if the numbers of retrieved sperm are very low, loss of viability secondary to the freeze-thaw process may occur making a repeat TESE necessary. The possibility of finding sperm during repeated TESE is high (70–85%).[29,33,34,37,38] Studies using frozen sperm have noted fertilization and clinical pregnancy rates comparable to fresh sperm.[29] However, other studies demonstrated a trend toward favoring fresh spermatozoa.[39] Before making the decision to perform in-cycle retrieval or to use frozen sperm, the couple's preferences should be understood especially in societies where donor sperm is not accepted. The best time to perform a repeated biopsy remains controversial. Similar SRR were reported when the second TESE was performed before or after three or six months.[33,38] On the contrary, a higher retrieval rate was reported when the second biopsy was performed after six months.[34]

Processing of Testicular Tissue for Intracytoplasmic Sperm Injection

During TESE, most protocols use mechanical disruption to release sperm from biopsy samples.[24] Enzymatic tissue dispersion with collagenase and the use of erythrocyte lysis in order to remove excess red blood cells that may hamper the field were prescribed to facilitate the search for sperm in testicular tissue.[21,33] The use of stereoscope at a magnification of X40 to isolate the most distended tubules from the rest of the biopsy was described to improve the sperm retrieval.[21]

Another recent innovation aimed at increasing the yield of spermatozoa for ICSI is the use of special culture media, like human tubal fluid FSH-enriched medium for 24 h before ICSI. Besides increasing the motility and fertilization rate, the possibility of *in vitro* differentiation of round spermatids into elongated spermatids, and even spermatozoa by incubation over a period of 3±5 day was reported. However, most of these studies were not properly controlled.[3,29]

Methods Used to Enhance Fertilization Rates and ICSI Outcome

The fertilizing ability of sperm in ICSI was highest with normal semen and lowest with sperm extracted from a testicular biopsy in NOA.[40] Meta-analysis of these studies showed a significantly reduced fertilization and clinical pregnancy rates in men with NOA as compared to obstructive azoospermia.[18] This may be explained by the quality of sperm injected. In NOA, embryologist may find only few sperm after a prolonged search. Therefore, they do not have the option to select the best sperm.

In case impaired or failed fertilization of oocytes during ICSI, artificial oocyte activation either by calcium ionophore[41] or electrical activation[42] can improve the fertilization rate and ICSI outcomes. The injection of morphologically selected sperm under a magnification up to 6000X was recently suggested to improve the fertilization rate.[43] This technique was called IMSSI (intracytoplasmic morphologically selected sperm injection). The use of such magnification allows the observer to see nuclear vacuoles not apparent under the usual magnification X400 used during routine ICSI. A recent meta-analysis demonstrated that the pooled data of IMSI cycles showed a statistically significant improvement in implantation and pregnancy rates and a statistically significant reduction in miscarriage rates.[44] However, more randomized controlled trials are needed to confirm these results.

Microinjection of Immature Spermatogenic Precursor Cells

Several groups have investigated the use of immature spermatogenic precursor cells for oocyte injection in animal models and humans. The ability of elongated spermatids to act as male gametes after injection into human oocytes was confirmed by different groups. However, the exact phase of the elongated spermatids that were used was not clear in most of the studies. Accordingly, there was an overlap between what some authors reported as ELSI and others as ICSI with testicular spermatozoa. The original enthusiasm inspired by reports of births after fertilization with round spermatids was subsequently tempered by the low success rates obtained in a larger series of round spermatid injection.[45] Immature gamete injection may work only in a selected group of men with late spermatids of the subclass "Sc" and "Sd".[46] Because of many concerns about the safety of injecting spermatids and the problem of their identification during ICSI settings, many centers are conservative about spermatid injection. Genomic imprinting, DNA stability, cell cycle asynchronization, the cytosolic sperm factor for oocyte activation and the role of paternal centriols are among such concerns.

Future Therapy for NOA

The successful *in vitro* culture of spermatogenic cells and the progress in studying spermatogonial stem cells (SSC) origins, regulation and activity over the past years, has opened the way for the possibility of treating patients in whom TESE fails to retrieve sperm or spermatids for ICSI. The successful *in vitro* culture of spermatogenic cells may give hope to patients with maturation arrest. Successful fertilization with spermatids obtained by culturing germ cells arrested at the primary spermatocyte stage resulting in the birth of a normal child, was reported.[47] Additionally a co-culture system that led to the *in vitro* release of human male germ cells from patients with maturation arrest was achieved.[48] However, these reports have not been further confirmed. The development of the SSC transplantation technique had a positive impact on the fundamental investigations and the possible clinical application of SSC to restore fertility in selected patients with NOA.[49] The isolation and successful culturing of male germ stem cell-like cells (GSC-LC) from the testicular tissue of patients with NOA, may give hope for this group of patients.[50]

Concluding Remarks

Non-obstructive azoospermia (NOA) results from a wide variety of congenital and acquired causes. Genetic factors play a crucial role. A complete andrological work up including hormonal profile is essential to establish the diagnosis of NOA and exclude frequently associated disorders. Sperm extraction from the testis combined with ICSI is an established standard treatment. Testicular histopathology remains the best predictive indicator for sperm retrieval. Current guidelines on surgical sperm retrieval techniques for NOA are mostly based on observational studies. However, the best available evidence suggests that open biopsy is better than needle aspiration. Multiple biopsies yield better results than a single random biopsy. Microdissection TESE may improve the yield and sacrifice less testicular tissue especially in patients with SCOS. In non-selected cases the overall SRR is about 50 percent. There is no difference in the outcome with the use of fresh or frozen testicular sperm. However, in some cases, the cryopreservation process may not allow adequate recovery of viable sperm. Electro-activation or the injection of morphologically selected sperm may be needed in case of previous failed or poor fertilization. The injection of sperm precursors is still experimental. Finally, further research should focus on new techniques that can help improving the sperm retrieval rates. *In vitro* culture of spermatogenic cells or spermatogonial stem cell transplantation might be the future treatment of NOA.

◼ REFERENCES

1. Jarow JP, Espeland MA, Lipshultz LI. Evaluation of the azoospermic patient. J Urol 1989;142:62-5.
2. Smyth CM, Bremner WJ. Klinefelter syndrome. Arch Intern Med 1998;158:1309-14.
3. Chan P, Schlegel P. Nonobstructive azoospermia. Curr Opin Urol 2000;10:617-24.
4. Meschede D, Behre HM, Nieschlag E. Disorders of androgen targets organs'. In Andrology male reproductive health and function. Nieschlag and Behre (Eds), Springer, Berlin, London, New York 1997.pp.209-23.
5. Nieschlag E, Behre HM, Meschede D, et al. Disorders at the testicular level. In Andrology male reproductive health and function. Nieschlag and Behre (Eds), Springer, Berlin, London, New York 1997.pp.133-59.
6. Mahmoud A, Comhaire F. Systemic causes of male infertility. In andrology for the clinician. Schill, Hragreave, Comhaire (Eds). Springer-Verlag Berlin Heidelberg 2006.pp.57-66.
7. Martin-du-Pan RC, Bischof P. Increased follicle stimulating hormone in infertile men. Is increased plasma FSH always due to damaged germinal epithelium? Hum Reprod 1995;10:1940-5.
8. Anniballo R, Ubaldi F, Cobellis L, et al. Criteria predicting the absence of spermatozoa in the Sertoli cell-only syndrome can be used to improve success rates of sperm retrieval. Hum Reprod 2000;15(11):2269-77.
9. Tournaye H, Verheyen G, Nagy P, et al. Are there any predictive factors for successful testicular sperm recovery in azoospermic patients? Hum Reprod 1997;12:80-6.
10. Girgis SM, Hafez ESE. Evaluation of testicular biopsy. In Hafez ESE (Ed): Techniques of human andrology. Elsevier/North-Holland Biomedical press 1976.pp.83-103.
11. Levin H. Testicular biopsy in the study of male infertility. Hum Path 1979;10:569-84.
12. Cooperberg MR, Chi T, Jad A, et al. Variability in testis biopsy interpretation: implications for male infertility care in the era of intracytoplasmic sperm injection. Fertil Steril 2005;84:672-7.
13. McLachlan RI, Rajpert-De Meyts E, et al. Histological evaluation of the human testis-approaches to optimizing the clinical value of the assessment: mini review. Hum Reprod 2007;22:2-16.
14. Silber SJ. Microsurgical TESE and the distribution of spermatogenesis in non-obstructive azoospermia. Hum Reprod 2000;15:2278-84.
15. Devroey P, Liu J, Nagy Z, et al. Normal fertilization of human oocytes after testicular sperm extraction and intracytoplasmic sperm injection. Fertil Steril 1994;62:639-41.
16. Devroey P, Liu J, Nagy Z, et al. Pregnancies after testicular sperm extraction and intracytoplasmic sperm injection in non-obstructive azoospermia. Hum Reprod 1995;10:1457-60.
17. Colpi GM, Piediferro G, Scroppo FI, et al. Surgery for male infertility: Surgical sperm retrievals. In: Clinical Andrology, EAU/ESAU Course Guidelines. Bjorndahl L, Giwercman A, Tournaye H, Weidner (Eds). Informa UK 2010.pp.95-104.
18. Nicopoullos J, Gilling-Smith C, Almeida P, et al. Use of surgical sperm retrieval in azoospermic men: a meta-analysis. Fertil Steril 2004;82:691-700.
19. Schlegel PN. Testicular sperm extraction: microdissection improves sperm yield with minimal tissue excision. Hum Reprod 1999;14:131-5.
20. Amer M, Zohdy W, Abdel-Naser T, et al. Single tubule biopsy: a new objective microsurgical advancement for testicular sperm retrieval in patients with nonobstructive azoospermia. Fertil Steril 2008;89:592-6.
21. Kamal A, Fahmy I, Mansour RT, et al. Selection of individual testicular tubules from biopsied testicular tissue with a stereomicroscope improves sperm retrieval rate. J Androl 2004;25:123-7.
22. Mulhall JP, Ghaly SW, Aviv N, et al. The utility of optical loupe magnification for testis sperm extraction in men with nonobstructive azoospermia. J Androl 2005;26:178-81.
23. Fahmy I, Kamal A, Aboulghar M, et al. Percutaneous aspiration biopsy using intravenous catheter for testicular sperm retrieval

in patients with obstructive azoospermia. Reprod Biomed Online 2004;9(1):102-5.

24. Donoso P, Tournaye H, Devroey P. Which is the best sperm retrieval technique for non-obstructive azoospermia? A systematic review. Human Reproduction Update 2007;13(6):539-49.

25. Mostafa T, Amer MK, Abdel-Malak G, et al. Seminal plasma anti-Müllerian hormone level correlates with semen parameters but does not predict success of testicular sperm extraction (TESE). Asian J Androl 2007;9:265-70.

26. Tsujimura A, Matsumiya K, Miyagawa, et al. Prediction of successful outcome of microdissection testicular sperm extraction in men with idiopathic nonobstructive azoospermia. J Urol 2004;172(5 Pt 1):1944-7.

27. Amer M, Abd Elnasser T, El Haggar S, et al. May-Grünwald-Giemsa stain for detection of spermatogenic cells in the ejaculate: a simple predictive parameter for successful testicular sperm retrieval. Hum Reprod 2001;16:1427-32.

28. Ramasamy R, Ricci JA, Palermo GD, et al. Successful fertility treatment for Klinefelter's syndrome. J Urol 2009;182(3):1108-13.

29. Harris SE, Sandlow JI. Sperm acquisition in nonobstructive azoospermia: what are the options? Urol Clin N Am 2008;35:235-42.

30. Fahmy I, Kamal A, Mansour R, et al. Relationship between testicular histopathology and the outcome of testicular sperm extraction combined with intracytoplasmic sperm injection in patients with non-obstructive azoospermia MEFSJ 1999;4:45-51.

31. Van Perperstraten AM, Proctor ML, Phillipson G, et al. Techniques for surgical retrieval of sperm prior to ICSI for azoospermia. Cochrane Database Syst Rev 2006;3:CD002807.

32. Hauser R, Botchan A, Amit A, et al. Multiple testicular sampling in non-obstructive azoospermia—is it necessary? Hum Reprod 1998;13:3081-5.

33. Amer M, El Haggar S, Moustafa T, et al. Testicular sperm extraction: impact of testicular histology on outcome, number of biopsies to be performed and optimal time for repetition. Hum Reprod 1999;14:3030-4.

34. Schlegel PN, Su LM. Physiological consequences of testicular sperm extraction. Hum Reprod 1997;12:1688-92.

35. Ramasamy R, Yagan N, Schlegel PN. Structural and functional changes to the testis after conventional versus microdissection testicular sperm extraction. Urol 2005;65:1190-4.

36. Schlegel PN. Debate: is ICSI a genetic time bomb? No: ICSI is safe and effective. J Androl 1999;20:18-21.

37. Kamal A, Fahmy I, Mansour R, et al. Outcome of repeated testicular sperm extraction and ICSI in patients with non-obstructive azoospermia. MEFSJ 2004;9:42-6.

38. Vernaeve V, Verheyen G, Goosens A, et al. How successful is repeat testicular sperm extraction in patients with azoospermia? Hum Reprod 2006;21:1551-4.

39. Friedler S, Raziel A, Soffer Y, et al. Intracytoplasmic injection of fresh and cryopreserved testicular spermatozoa in patients with nonobstructive azoospermiad a comparative study. Fertil Steril 1997;68(5):892-7.

40. Aboulghar MA, Mansour RT, Serour GI, et al. Fertilization and pregnancy rates after intracytoplasmic sperm injection using ejaculate semen and surgically retrieved sperm. Fertil Steril 1997;68(1):108-11.

41. Borges E Jr, de Almeida Ferreira Braga DP, de Sousa Bonetti TC, et al. Artificial oocyte activation with calcium ionophore A23187 in intracytoplasmic sperm injection cycles using surgically retrieved spermatozoa. Fertil Steril 2009;92(1):131-6.

42. Mansour R, Fahmy I, Tawab NA, et al. Electrical activation of oocytes after intracytoplasmic sperm injection: a controlled randomized study. Fertil Steril 2009;91(1):133-9.

43. Bartoov B, Berkovitz A, Eltes F, et al. Pregnancy rates are higher with intracytoplasmic morphologically selected sperm injection than with conventional intracytoplasmic injection. Fertil Steril 2003;80:1413-9.

44. Souza Setti A, Ferreira RC, Paes de Almeida Ferreira Braga D, et al. Intracytoplasmic sperm injection outcome versus intracytoplasmic morphologically selected sperm injection outcome: a meta-analysis. Reprod Biomed Online 2010;21(4):450-5.

45. Tesarik J, Mendoza C. Using the male gamete for assisted reproduction: past, present, and future. J Androl 2003;24(3):317-28.

46. Mansour RT, Fahmy I, Kamal A, et al. Intracytoplasmic spermatid injection can result in the delivery of normal offspring. J Androl 2003;24:757-64.

47. Tesarik J, Bahceci M, Ozcan C, et al. Restoration of fertility by in vitro spermatogenesis. Lancet 1999;353(9152):555-6.

48. Tanaka A, Nagayoshi M, Awata S, et al. Completion of meiosis in human primary spermatocytes through in vitro coculture with Vero cells. Fertil Steril 2003;79 (Suppl 1):795-801.

49. Phillips BT, Gassei K, Orwig KE. Spermatogonial stem cell regulation and spermatogenesis. Philos Trans R Soc Lond B Biol Sci 2010;365(1546):1663-78.

50. Lee DR, Kim KS, Yang YH, et al. Isolation of male germ stem cell-like cells from testicular tissue of non-obstructive azoospermic patients and differentiation into haploid male germ cells in vitro. Hum Reprod 2006;21(2):471-6.

33

Klinefelter Syndrome

Ibrahim Fahmy

INTRODUCTION

In 1942, Dr Harry Klinefelter published a report on nine men with a constellation of features: testicular dysgenesis, elevated urinary gonadotropins, microorchidism, eunuchoidism, azoospermia, and gynecomastia.[1] It was believed to be an endocrine disorder of unknown etiology. In 1949, Barr and Bertram discovered dense chromatin bodies "Barr bodies" detected in smears of stained buccal mucosal cells of phenotypic females and not males. In 1956, Barr bodies were detected in seven patients with Klinefelter syndrome thus suggesting a genetic origin of the disorder.[2] In 1959, Jacobs et al.[3] recognized that Klinefelter syndrome was a chromosomal disorder, with an extra X-chromosome resulting in the karyotype of 47, XXY. During the early 1970s, a number of centers began screening newborns for sex chromosomal abnormalities, because there was a need to obtain accurate information about childhood development in this condition.[4]

Most, but not all XXY males, are infertile with small testicles, a relative increase in the numbers of Leydig cells, tubular sclerosis, and interstitial fibrosis of varying degrees.[5] Their ejaculate is usually azoospermic, and levels of testosterone are typically low to low-normal. At first it was believed that hypogonadism was due to failure of Sertoli cells of the testes, along with deficiency of second testicular hormone—X hormone, which regulates levels of pituitary gonadotropins (later known as inhibin).[1]

The presence of an extra X chromosome is considered the fundamental etiologic factor of KS. The constant components of the disorder remain as Klinefelter et al described, but in contrast to their hypothesis, Leydig cells are hypofunctional. However, testosterone levels may be well within normal range leading to varying degrees of virilization. The hypothesis concerning a second testicular hormone was correct, as shown by studies that inhibin B originating from testicular Sertoli cells correlate well with Sertoli cell function and are found in extremely low levels in KS patients.[6]

GENETICS

The term Klinefelter syndrome (KS) describes a group of chromosomal disorder with at least one extra X chromosome added to a normal male karyotype. The classic form is the most common numerical chromosomal disorder, in which there is one extra X-chromosome resulting in the karyotype of 47, XXY. This classic form is observed in about 80 percent of cases. The other 20 percent are represented either by 46, XY/47, XXY mosaics, one or more additional Y chromosomes (e.g. 48, XXYY), higher-grade X-chromosomal aneuploidies (48, XXXY; 49, XXXXY) or structurally abnormal additional X chromosomes. XXY aneuploidy is the most common disorder of sex chromosomes in humans, with a prevalence of one in 500–1000 male births.[7] Other sex chromosomal aneuploidies are much less frequent with 48, XXYY and 48, XXXY being present in 1 per 17,000 to 1 per 50,000 male births. The incidence of 49, XXXXY is 1 per 85,000–100,000 male births.[8] Men with KS are thought to represent 11 percent of the azoospermic patient and 3 percent of the infertile men.[9]

The numerical chromosomal aberration that characterizes KS arises from non-disjunction of sex chromosomes. Non-disjunction is defined as the failure of homologous chromosomes to segregate symmetrically at cell division. In a person with normal chromosomal constitution, if the pair of homologs comprising a bivalent at meiosis-I fail to separate, one of the daughter cells will have two of the chromosomes, while the other will have none. Non-disjunction may occur during meiosis-II after successful meiosis-I, during which the chromatids fail to separate. During oogenesis, it is more common for non-disjunction to happen during meiosis I, and about one-third occurs in meiosis-II.[10] In contrast to autosomal non-disjunction, as much as half of 47, XXY KS is due to non-disjunction during spermatogenesis, resulting in a 24, XY sperm. X-Y nondisjunction is predisposed following an absence of recombination in the primary pseudoautosomal regions (PAR1) of the X and Y chromosomes at meiosis I.

In 3 percent of apparently nonmosaic KS the error was post-zygotic (mitotic non-disjunction), presumably prior to the formation of the inner cell mass.[11] Most mosaic KS occur due to mitotic non-disjunction in a 47, XXY conceptus, resulting in a cell line with 46, XY, giving rise to a mosaic KS conceptus. The same result may also be due to the mechanism of anaphase lag.[12] Mitotic non-disjunction of sex chromosome can also occur in a normal 46, XY conceptus, resulting in 47, XXY, 46, XY and 45, Y lines, after which the 45, Y dies out resulting in a 46, XY/47, XXY embryo. Sex chromosome polysomies such as XXYY, XXXY and XXXXY are very rare and are due to successive non-disjunction in one parent while the other contributes a single sex chromosome.[13,14]

ETIOLOGY

The most important factor imputed in the etiology of KS is advanced maternal age although this association is less marked than in trisomy 21. The paternal age has no impact on the degree of recombination.[15-17] The maternal age effects in chromosome abnormalities may be a consequence of the long diplotene stage of human oocytes. Ova remain suspended in the prophase of the first meiotic division from birth to ovulation that may take up to 40 years or more. Fathers of paternally originating KS may have marginally elevated levels of disomic XY sperm in comparison with fathers of maternally originating cases, possibly reflecting an inherent tendency among a small minority of these men to produce aneuploid sperm.[18] Woods et al[19] reported two 47, XXY brothers, probably the only reported case, in which both were of paternal origin. A role of radiation, viruses or other environmental toxins as a predisposing factor for KS is not established.

CLINICAL PICTURE

The salient clinical features of the classical Klinefelters syndrome are azoospermia, very small firm testes, gynecomastia and variable grades of eunochoidal features (**Figs 33.1A and B**). However apart from azoospermia, and the small testis other features might be lacking. The hormonal profile show high FSH and LH while testosterone may be low or low normal.

Klinefelter syndrome remains largely undiagnosed in the general population. The newborns and children with 47, XXY have no distinguishing features. As a result, many geneticists reserve the term Klinefelter syndrome for the adult.[20] Between two thirds and 75 percent of the expected number of 47, XXY males are never diagnosed.[21] Ten percent of 47, XXY are diagnosed prenatally during chorionic villus sampling or amniocentesis for late maternal age, due to the absence of prenatal

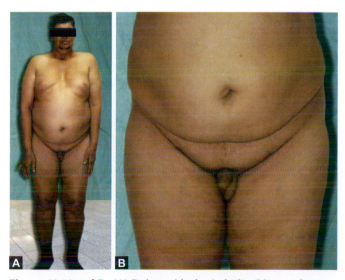

Figures 33.1A and B: (A) Patient with classical Klinefelter syndrome—Note the eunochoidal features; (B) The very small testicles with a relatively small sized penis

ultrasound findings to prompt invasive procedures. The few diagnosed during early childhood are usually due to language delay, learning and behavioral problems, abnormally small testes, and long legs.[22] Another 25 percent are diagnosed during adolescence mostly presenting with gynecomastia, small, firm testes and hypogonadism, with varying degrees of androgen deficiency. In later life, many men present at infertility centers with azoospermia. The majority of the undiagnosed cases are attributed to failure to seek medical advice combined with the failure of health professionals to recognize or consider KS.

Klinefelter patients have a wide variety of associated medical conditions. The height, weight and head circumference of 47, XXY newborns lie within normal range. Fifth finger clinodactyly has been reported more frequently in newborn 47, XXY.[20] Cryptorchidism, hypospadius or smaller than average penile length rarely leads to a diagnosis during infancy. An accelerated linear growth begins around age of 5 years, although weight and head circumference remain around the 50 percent percentile. Heights vary in 47, XXY males, presumably according to parental factors. The increase in length occurs well before puberty suggesting its relation to the KS phenotype rather than due to androgen deficiency, also the increase in length is mainly due to increase in leg length, leading to longer lower body segment (symphysis pubis to soles) compared to upper segment (symphysis pubis to head). Arm span is seldom more than total body height in contrast to typical eunuchoid stature. KS males usually have narrower shoulders and broader hips, in accordance with eunuchoid features. There is also an increase in minor skeletal deformities such as scoliosis and kyphosis due to laxness of the ligaments. Bone age becomes normal around the age of 8 years after an initial delay. There is a delay in closure of ulnar and radial epiphyses of 3–4 years.[20]

Taurodontism, an uncommon condition characterized by enlargement of the pulp along with thin tooth surface, is present in more than 40 percent of KS patients, compared to 3 percent in the general population.[23] Other dental anomalies associated with KS include; congenital absence of permanent teeth, shovel incisors and increased length of teeth.[24]

Sexual development of 47, XXY males during infancy and childhood is no different than normal. Testicular size, penile length, testosterone and gonadotropin levels are within normal range.[25] Testosterone level increases at the onset of puberty, which is of normal onset and timing. Penile size is mostly within normal range due to the initial androgen rise. Increase of testicular size does not occur during puberty, the testicular volume in nonmosaic KS being between 1 mL and 3 mL. Small and firm testes is the most consistent physical finding in postpubertal KS males, differentiating them from men with normal karyotype.[22] Postpubertal Leydig cells undergo a decline in number and function, leading to decreased testosterone levels compared to normal controls, while seminiferous tubules undergo progressive hyalinization and fibrosis, leading to azoospermia.

The testicular histopathology of patients with KS is rather unique and was referred to as "Klinefelter-like" pattern[26] (**Fig. 33.2**). It is characterized by complete atrophy of the seminiferous tubules. The fibrotic tissue around the atrophic tubules

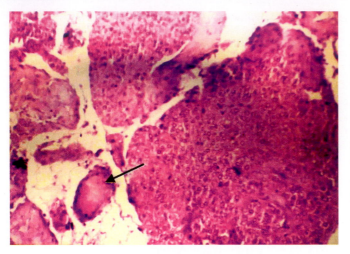

Figure 33.2: Testicular histopathology of Klinefelter syndrome—Note Leydig cell pseudoadenomatous hyperplasia and tubular fibrosis (arrow)

Table 33.1: Incidence of different signs associated with Klinefelter syndrome

Pathological feature	Incidence
Infertility	99-100%
Small testes	99-100%
Gynecomastia	50-75%
Decreased pubic hair	30-60%
Decreased facial hair	60-80%
Decreased testosterone levels	65-85%
Elevated gonadotropin levels	90-100%
Decreased penile size	10-25%

Smyth and Bremner[5]

is arranged in a concentric pattern forming "ghost tubules". Occasionally some tubules may retain few Sertoli cells, and few other tubules may contain residual spermatogenic cells at different grades of maturation. Although the total number of Leydig cells per testis is reduced their number in the cross section is apparently increased due to atrophy of the tubules. Characteristically they clump together to form adenoid like structures. The term pseudoadenomatous hyperplasia is given to describe this histopathologic picture.

Testicular biopsy of 47, XXY infants show only a slight decrease in number of germ cells.[27] Early in puberty, semen may show presence of sperm in KS males, which later disappear from the ejaculate due to the progressive nature of the testicular pathology. The absence of negative feedback of testosterone and inhibin B leads to increase in gonadotropins (FSH and LH) that occurs around the age of 12 years leading eventually to the hypergonadotrophic hypogonadal state of most 47, XXY males. The significant decrease in Sertoli cell population leads to a marked drop of inhibin B levels. This explains the very high levels of FSH that characterize most of the patients with KS. Testosterone levels could be normal or low, and the levels of estradiol (E2) and sex hormone binding globulin (SHBG) are predominantly elevated.

A small proportion of KS males exhibit all the characteristics phenotypic features. **Table 33.1** show the percentages of common abnormalities associated with KS. Faulty inactivation of the extra X chromosome and androgen receptor CAG repeat polymorphism has been implicated in the phenotypic outcome.[22,28] Development of secondary sexual characters including facial, axillary and body hair is extremely variable, ranging from absent to complete virilization. The presence of eunuchoid body habitus and gynecomastia is also variable. The elevated estradiol levels most likely contribute to the pathogenesis of gynecomastia. However, the unique histological changes namely interductal tissue hyperplasia is unlike the ductal hyperplasia present in gynecomastia caused by other high estrogen

states.[29] A slightly higher percentage of 47, XXY adolescents and adults develop gynecomastia compared to the normal population, but it is less likely to recede in KS men. Muscle mass is mostly compromised due to androgen deficiency, although to highly variable degrees. Decrease in sexual activity is more in KS, concerning libido and potency, usually observed after the age of 25 years.[22] Decreased testosterone levels may also lead to osteoporosis due to decreased calcium absorption and bone mineralization and increase bone resorption. Low-grade anemia may also occur.

Previous studies of XXY individuals were extremely biased toward more severely affected individuals, since these patients were drawn largely from mental or penal settings where large numbers of men could be screened. These earlier studies implied a risk for mental deficiency and behavioral problems. As prospective, unbiased studied have reported their results afterwards, it has become clear that most XXY boys demonstrate reductions in speech and language abilities which are correlated with decreased reading and spelling achievement.[30] There has been shown to be mild impairment in coordination, speed, dexterity and strength, leading to poor athletic abilities and avoidance of participation in team sports.[20] The IQ of 47, XXY individuals is within normal range, though slightly below their siblings, especially verbal IQ—including verbal expression, verbal comprehension, verbal reasoning and auditory short-term memory-scores. They show delayed speech and language acquisition, diminished short memory and decreased data retrieval skills, all which may lead to poor academic performance. They may also show a higher incidence of dyslexia and attention deficit disorder.[31-33] Avoidance of athletic activities and delayed language and verbal skills can lead to poor academic achievements and social withdrawal. Some intellectual difficulties seem to arise from the extra X-chromosome, as variants with more X-chromosomes show a higher incidence of mental retardation.[31] Interestingly, 45,X girls show a mirrored pattern of cognitive deficits, suggesting that an altered dose of X-linked pseudoautosomal genes underlies the cognitive changes. Few studies have been conducted concerning the brain morphology of KS males. The studies lean toward a smaller brain, especially temporal lobe gray matter volume. This difference was not apparent in KS males receiving testosterone supplementation.[7,34,35] The estimated incidence of epileptic manifestations occurring in association with Klinefelter syndrome is 5–17 percent.[36]

Common characteristic temperamental differences have been described in 47, XXY boys. Toddlers may be reserved, less active and more adaptable.[37] Adolescents with KS consider themselves more sensitive, introspective, apprehensive and insecure, this may be due to the verbal delay and decreased athletic abilities. They are also later to express an interest in dating and attaining sexual experience.[20] Psychiatric disorders are rare, but clinical depression has been described.

KS men have a higher incidence of various vascular diseases. Varicose veins, leg ulcers, pulmonary embolism, vascular insufficiency and deep venous thrombosis occur more frequently compared to the general population.[38] Varicose veins are more severe and occur at an earlier age.[29] Increased mortality due to subarachnoid hemorrhage, mitral and aortic valves diseases has been observed in KS men.[39,40] The etiology may be due to androgen insufficiency, increased cholesterol levels and/or hypercoagulable states.

Estrogen has always been thought to play a role in autoimmune diseases, so it comes as no surprise that KS men have slightly higher risk of autoimmune disorders. These disorders include systemic lupus, rheumatoid arthritis, Sjogren syndrome and thyroid disease. Frequently obesity, reduced glucose tolerance, diabetes mellitus and metabolic syndrome are observed.[41,42]

Increased incidence of breast cancer and extragonadal germ cell tumors is associated with KS. The typical patient is younger than 30 years and is probably due to incomplete migration of primordial germ cells along with increased level of gonadotropins.[43,44] KS males are relatively protected from cancer prostate due to the decreased testosterone level, but cases of cancer prostate have been reported in KS males receiving androgen supplementation.

In general, men with mosaic 46, XY/47, XXY karyotype have a milder phenotype than those with non-mosaic 47, XXY. Pentasomy 49, XXXXY presents a great variety of morphological abnormalities. The facial dysmorphism is characterized by; a full round face, hypertelorism, telecanthus, upslanted palpebral fissures, and widely spaced nipples.[45] Skeletal defects include delayed bone age, radioulnar synostosis, clinodactyly of fifth fingers, and congenital hip dysplasia. Genital anomalies include micropenis, scrotal hypoplasia, and cryptorchidism.[46] Tetrasomy 48, XXXY shows a phenotype midway between 47, XXY and 49, XXXXY.

■ MANAGEMENT

If the diagnosis is not made prenatally, 47, XXY males may present with a variety of subtle clinical signs according to the age of presentation. In infancy, males with 47,XXY may rarely undergo chromosomal evaluations for having hypospadias, small phallus or cryptorchidism. During the toddler and school years, boys may present with developmental delay, especially with expressive language skills, learning disabilities, or behavioral/social problems. The older child or adolescent may be discovered during an endocrine evaluation for delayed or incomplete

pubertal development with eunuchoid body habitus, gynecomastia, and small testes. Adults are often diagnosed during evaluation for infertility, sexual problems, and less commonly with breast malignancy.

The most consistent symptoms are very low testicular volume (1–3 mL) and firm consistency of the testes. Symptoms described above provide additional indications. The ultimate diagnosis of a Klinefelter syndrome is confirmed cytogenetically by establishing the karyotype. FISH analysis of lymphocytes in the interphase or metaphase offers an additional diagnostic option because it allows analysis of a greater number of cells and better correlation with clinical findings.[47]

Androgen Replacement

Adult KS subjects are characterized by hypergonadotropic hypogonadism of variable degrees. Concentrations of LH and FSH are high; FSH is usually higher. In 65–85 percent of adult KS patients, serum testosterone concentrations are below normal, but some may show normal levels.[5,22] On average, serum concentrations of E2 and SHBG are higher than normal. Serum inhibin B levels in most adult KS subjects are undetectable, and recently it has been shown that serum INSL3 concentration is significantly below normal.[48,49]

All KS men should be offered testosterone replacement therapy. The age at which the patient should start testosterone supplementation is a matter of debate.[37] Some propose the initiation of treatment at puberty, age of 12 years, and others 2–3 years later, with the beginning of the testosterone plateau. The before mentioned lines of treatment can only take place if the diagnosis is made before or around puberty, in order to improve physical development, muscle mass, facial and body hair, fat distribution and mitigate behavioral and learning difficulties. The role of testosterone in improving or preventing gynecomastia is not proven, as the reports are conflicting. The aim of androgen supplementation is to maintain a serum testosterone, FSH, LH and estradiol levels similar to that of men of same age. KS men should receive androgen supplementation on diagnosis, as it improves all androgen dependant processes. It improves the development of facial and body hair, increases muscle mass, drive, energy and libido. Many KS patients under androgen treatment also observe diminished irritability, improved mood and better concentration levels. All this promotes the self-image of a normal male, increasing self-confidence and better functioning as a member of society. Supplementation using androgen increases bone mineralization, thus reducing the incidence of osteoporosis. It also decreases the risk of autoimmune diseases and breast cancer.[20] It leads to stimulation of erythropoiesis. Intramuscular injection of testosterone enanthate or cypionate was the most widely used form of supplementation. It is given every 10–14 days in doses of 200 mg. Intramuscular injection leads to fluctuating levels of serum testosterone which do not simulate normal male physiology, leading to fluctuation of mood and physical functioning. Transdermal patches and gel produce more appropriate bioavailability. Other testosterone preparations include oral preparations, implantable pellets and long-lasting injections. Speech and language therapy should be provided in cases that suffer from difficulties.

Treatment of Infertility

Practically all ejaculates from patients with 47, XXY karyotype show azoospermia. In the adult XXY testes virtually all germ cells disappear.[26,50] Occasionally, isolated foci of spermatogenesis may persist in the testes of patients with Klinefelter syndrome,[51] explaining the presence of sperm in the ejaculate of few cases.[52] KS males who may have sperm in their ejaculate, mostly, but not all, have a mosaic karyotype, with a normal, 46, XY, cell line. A small number of patients with classic KS have been reported to succeed in fathering a child before the era of assisted reproductive technology.[53] Since then more cases have been reported and sperm have been found in 7.7 and 8.4 percent of ejaculated semen samples of non-mosaic Klinefelter patients.[22,54] With the advent of assisted reproductive techniques, namely ICSI-TESE, 47, XXY males now have a chance to attain biological fatherhood. Hinney et al.[55] were the first to report pregnancy after intracytoplasmic sperm injection (ICSI) with ejaculated sperm from a non-mosaic 47, XXY patient. Moreover, in cases of azoospermia, these men can father their own genetic children by performing ICSI with sperm extracted from their testes[51] (**Fig. 33.3**). Successful sperm retrieval from testes of KS men using testicular sperm extraction (TESE) ranges from 28–72 percent (**Table 33.2**).[51,56-69] Micro TESE may yield better results than conventional TESE. As expected, men with mosaic KS have a higher rate of sperm retrieval. The retrieved sperm are used for intracytoplasmic sperm injection with pregnancy and delivery rates similar to men diagnosed with non-obstructive azoospermia.

The success of ICSI in cases of KS, either with ejaculated or testicular sperm, made it essential to evaluate the safety of such procedure as regards chromosomal abnormalities in the offspring. Some studies showed increased percentages of hyper-haploid sex chromosome sperm cells (24, XY and 24, XX) in mosaic as well as in non-mosaic Klinefelter syndrome (0.9–7.5%) compared to 0.4 percent in normal men without chromosomal abnormalities.[56] However, this elevation of sex chromatin abnormalities in sperm of KS patients is comparable to the rate of sperm sex chromosome aneuploidy among other male infertility patients with normal karyotype.[70,71] Other investigators suggested

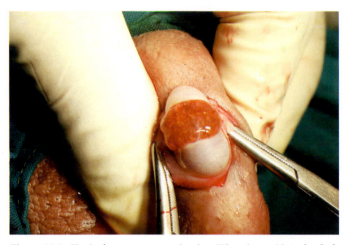

Figure 33.3: Testicular sperm extraction in a KS patient—Note the dark color of testicular tissue and the very small size of testis

Table 33.2: Successful sperm retrieval (SSR) among different studies

Study	Number of patients	Number of attempts	SSR(%)	Procedure
Tournaye (1997)[51]	15	17	47	TESE
Levron (2000)[56]	20	20	40	TESE
Friedler (2001)[57]	12	10	42	TESE
Madgar (2002)[58]	20	20	45	TESE
Westlander (2003)[59]	18	18	28	TESE
Ulug (2003)[60]	11	11	55	-
Vernaeve (2004)[61]	50	-	48	TESE
Seo (2004)[62]	25 KS, 11 mos	36	16 KS, 54 mos	TESE
Okada (2005)[63]	51	51	51	TESE
Schiff (2005)[64]	54	54	72	microT
Okada (2005)[65]	10	10	60	microT
Emre bakiricioglu (2006)[66]	74	74	57	microT
Kyono (2007)[67]	17	17	35	TESE
Koga (2007)[68]	26	26	50	microT
Yarali (2009)[69]	33	39	52	microT

KS = Non-mosaic KS, mos = Mosaic KS, microT = Micro-TESE, - = Unidentified

that spermatogonia bearing XXY are capable of producing normal gamete.[9] Conversely, other authors demonstrated that the testis of non-mosaic KS patients with positive sperm retrieval carry both XY and XXY germ cell lines. Only spermatogonial cells carrying XY are capable of undergoing meiosis.[72] The lack of significant gonosomal aneuploidy in the presence of somatic aneuploidy suggests that abnormal germ cell lines may arrest at a meiotic checkpoint within the testis or that somatic-germ line mosaicism is more common than previously thought.[73]

Denschlag et al.[74] reviewed all the reports that included pregnancies after ICSI procedures with spermatozoa from non-mosaic KS patients. These reports included the births of 39 healthy children. In a triplet pregnancy, chromosome analysis after chorionic villous sampling revealed a 47, XXY karyotype in one fetus. Therefore, the incidence of chromosomal abnormalities in the offspring of KS patients is about 2.5 percent (1 out of 40). Fullerton et al[75] reviewed studies of non-mosaic Klinefelter patients that underwent ICSI-TESE. These studies reported the birth of 101 children. The studies reported two fetuses diagnosed prenatally as 47, XXY genotype. Each fetus was part of a triplet pregnancy, which was later reduced to twin pregnancy.

Since, the incidence of sex chromosome disomy is found to be higher in sperm extracted from 47, XXY men—both mosaic and non-mosaic.[22,74] KS patients undergoing ICSI-TESE should be informed that there is a higher risk of sex chromosome aneuploidy. Also, there is an increased incidence of autosomal disomy, especially chromosomes 13,18 and 21, suggesting an increase in incidence of offspring with trisomy 13, 18 and 21. The parents have to be clearly counseled and the offer of preimplantation and/or prenatal diagnosis is reasonable.[22,74,76]

In non-mosaic KS patients, there is no consensus about the presence of parameters that can accurately predict the success of sperm extraction. Therefore, an objective counseling based on the available predictive parameters may be useful. Different studies showed contradictory conclusions, the majority being conducted on a small number of cases. In the largest series including 50 non-mosaic 47,XXY patients, Vernaeve et al. (2004)[61] found that none of the clinical and biological parameters including age of the patients, testicular volume of the largest testis, FSH value, FSH:LH ratio, testosterone value and androgen sensitivity index, had an acceptable predictive power for sperm retrieval. Westlander et al. (2003)[59] also described 19 non-mosaic Klinefelter patients in whom there were no significant differences in testicular volume, serum T levels, and serum concentrations of FSH between those with and those without successful sperm recovery. On the other hand, Madgar et al. (2002)[58] studied 20 patients and found that the mean testicular volume was significantly higher in patients with testicular sperm after TESE than in those without sperm. He also found that testosterone level was significantly higher following TESE in patients with successful sperm retrieval. Okada et al.[63] and Kyono et al[67] have reported better sperm retrieval results in younger men.

In our experience, of 190 KS patients that underwent ICSI-TESE, testicular size, FSH and testosterone had no predictive value concerning successful sperm retrieval rates. However, the age of the patient was the only parameter of predictive value.

Successful sperm retrieval was higher in patients under the age of 35 years.

Some andrologists have recently started to recommend the cryopreservation of seminal sperm of KS men directly after puberty or even performing micro-TESE to obtain sperm for future fertility.[77] The role of androgen supplementation given to KS males has been disputed. It is postulated that androgen therapy may adversely affect their chances of future fertility. Androgen supplementation should be stopped 3–6 months before undergoing testicular sperm extraction. Premedication with hCG, antiestrogens or aromatase inhibitors have been attempted to increase results of successful sperm retrieval.[64,78]

CONCLUSION

Klinefelter syndrome is the most frequent sex chromosome abnormality affecting newborn males. Many cases may skip recognition during childhood and adolescence and present at infertility centers with azoospermia. Therefore, physicians working in infertility centers should be familiar with the diagnosis and management of KS. The most consistent signs include bilateral small firm testes, azoospermia, and elevated FSH. Gynecomastia, and other signs occur in varying degrees. The phenotype can vary from a normally virilized man to one with all stigmata of androgen deficiency. During recent years, KS males have attained a chance for biologic parenthood. ICSI/TESE can be offered to all KS males with a reasonable chance for success. Since spermatogenic cells start to decline at puberty, early sperm retrieval and cryopreservation may be offered for young adolescents. More research is needed to optimize the timing and conditions, to further increase the chances of successful ICSI-TESE procedures. Androgen supplementation should be given to all KS males to avoid and restore the effects of decreased testosterone levels.

REFERENCES

1. Klinefelter HF, Reifenstein EC, Albright F. Syndrome characterized by gynecomastia aspermatogenes without aleydigism and increased excretion of follicle stimulating hormone. J Clin Endocrinol Metab 1942;2:615-27.
2. Bradbury JT, Bunge RG, Boccabella RA. Chromatin test in Klinefelter's syndrome. J Clin Endocrinal Metab 1956;16:689-90.
3. Jacobs PA, Strong JA. A case of human intersexuality having possible XXY sex-determining mechanism. Nature 1959;2:164-7.
4. Nielsen J, Wohlert M. Sex chromosome abnormalities found among 34,910 newborn children: results from a 13-year incidence study in Arthus, Denmark. In: Evans JA, Hamerton JL (Eds). Children and Young Adults with Sex Chromosome Aneuploidy Birth Defects: Original Article Series. Vol. 26. New York: Wiley-Liss, for the March of Dimes Birth Defects Foundation 1991.pp.209-23.
5. Smyth CM, Bremner WJ. Klinefelter syndrome. Arch Intern Med 1998;158:1309-14.
6. Anawalt BD, Bebb RA, Matsumoto AM, Groome NP, Illingworth PJ, McNeilly AS, Bremner WJ. Serum inhibin B levels reflect Sertoli cell function in normal men and men with testicular dysfunction. J Clin Endocrinol Metab 1996;81:3341-5.

7. Simpson JL, de la Cruz F, Swerdloff RS, Samango-Sprouse C, Skakkebaek NE, Graham JM Jr, Hassold T, Aylstock M, Meyer-Bahlburg HF, Willard HF, Hall JG, Salameh W, Boone K, Staessen C, Geschwind D, Giedd J, Dobs AS, Rogol A, Brinton B, Paulsen CA. Klinefelter syndrome: expanding the phenotype and identifying new research directions. Genet Med 2003;5:460-8.

8. Linden MG, Bender BG, Robinson A. Sex chromosome tetrasomy and pentasomy. Pediatrics 1995;96:672-82.

9. Foresta C, Galeazzi C, Bettella A, Bettella A, Marin P, Rossato M, Garolla A, Ferlin A. Analysis of meiosis in intratesticular germ cells from subjects affected by classic Klinefelter's syndrome. J Clin Endocrinol Metab 1999;84:3807-10.

10. Thomas NS, Ennis S, Sharp AJ, Durkie M, Hassold TJ, Collins AR, Jacobs PA. Maternal sex chromosome nondisjunction: evidence for X chromosome-specific risk factors. Hum Mol Genet 2001;10:243-50.

11. MacDonald M, Hassold T, Harvey J, Wang LH, Morton NE, Jacobs P. The origin of 47,XXY and 47XXX aneuploidy: heterogeneous mechanisms and role of aberrant recombination. Hum Mol Genet 1994;3:1365-71.

12. Robinson WP, Binkert F, Bernasconi F, Lorda-sanchez I, Werder EA, Schinzel AA. Molecular studies of chromosomal mosaicism: relative frequency of chromosome gain or loss and possible role of cell selection. Am J Hum Genet 1995;56:444-51.

13. Hassold T, Pettay D, May K, Robinson A. Analysis of nondisjunction in sex chromosome tetrasomy and pentasomy. Hum Genet 1990;85:648-50.

14. Deng HX, Abe K, Kondo I, Tsukahara M, Inagaki H, Hamada I, Fukushima Y, Niikawa N. Parental origin and mechanism of formation of polysomy X: an XXXXX case and four XXXXY cases determined with RFLPs. Hum Genet 1991;86:541-4.

15. Thomas NS, Collins AR, Hassold TJ, Jacobs PA. A re-investigation of nondisjunction resulting in 47,XXY males of paternal origin. Eur j Hum Genet 2000;8:805-8.

16. Shi Q, Spriggs E, Field LL, Rademaker A, Ko E, Barclay L, Martin RH. Absence of age effect on meiotic recombination between human X and Y chromosomes. Am J Hum Genet 2002;71:254-61.

17. Shi Q, Spriggs E, Field LL, Ko E, Barclay L, Martin RH. Single sperm typing demonstrates that reduced recombination is associated with the production of aneuploid 24,XY human sperm. Am J Hum Genet 2001b;99:34-8.

18. Eskenazi B, Wyrobek AJ, Kidd SA, Lowe X, Moore D, Weisiger K, Aylstock M. Sperm aneuploidy in fathers of children with paternally and maternally inherited Klinefelter syndrome. Hum Reprod 2002;17:576-83.

19. Woods CG, Noble J, Falconer AR. A study of brothers with Klinefelter syndrome. J Med Genet 1997;34:702.

20. Visootsak J, Aylstock M, Graham JM. Klinefelter syndrome and its variants: an update and review for the primary pediatrician. Clin Pediatr 2001;40:639-51.

21. Bojesen A, Juul S, Gravholt CH. Prenatal and postnatal prevalence of Klinefelter syndrome: A national registry study. J Clin Endocrinl Metab 2003;88:622-6.

22. Lanfranco M, Kamischke A, Zitzmann M, Nieschlag E. Klinefelter's syndrome. Lancet 2004;364:273-83.

23. Jorgenson RJ. The conditions manifesting taurodontism. Am J Med Genet 1982;11:435-42.

24. Hunter ML, Collard MM, Razavi T, Hunter B. Increased primary tooth size in a 47, XXY male: a first case report. International journal of pediatric dentistry 2003;13:271-3.

25. Robinson A, Bender BG, Linden MG. Summary of clinical findings in children and adults with sex chromosome anomalies. Birth Defects Orig Artic Sec 1990;26:225-8.

26. Girgis SM, Etriby AN, Ibrahim A, Khalil SA. Testicular biopsy in azoospermia. A review of the last ten years' experiences of over 800 cases. Fertil Steril 1969;20:467-77.

27. Mikamo K, Aguereif M, Hazeglin P, Martin-Du Pan R. Chromatin positive Klinefelter's syndrome: a quantitative analysis of spermatogonadal deficiency at 3,4 and 12 months of age. Fertil Steril 1968;19:731-9.

28. Litsuka Y, Bock A, Nguyen DD, Samango-Sprouse CA, Simpson JL, Bischoff FZ. Evidence of skewed X-chromosome inactivation in 47,XXY and 48,XXYY Klinefelter patients. Am J Med Genet. 2001;98(1):25-31.

29. Becker KL. Clinical and therapeutic experiences with Klinefelter's syndrome. Fertil Steril 1972;23:568-78.

30. Graham JM Jr, Bashir AS, Stark RE, Silbert A, Walzer S. Oral and written language abilities of XXY boys: implications for anticipatory guidance. Pediatrics 1988;81:795-806.

31. Ratcliffe SG, Barcroft J, Axworthy D, McLaren W. Klinefelter's syndrome in adolescence. Arch Dis Child 1982;57:6-12.

32. Bender BA, Puck MH, Salbenblatt JA, Robinson A. Dyslexia in 47XXY boys identified at birth. Behav Genet 1986;16:343-54.

33. Mandoki MW, Sumner GS, Hoffman RP, Riconda DL. A review of Klinefelter's syndrome in children and adolescents. J Am Acad Child Adolesc Psychiatry 1991;30:167-72.

34. Patwardhan AJ, Eliez S, Bender B, Linden MG, Reiss AL. Brain morphology in Klinefelter syndrome: Extra X chromosome and testosterone supplementation. Neurology 2000;54:2218-23.

35. Warwick MM, Doody GA, Lawrie SM, Kestelman JN, Best JJ, Johnstone EC. Volumetric magnetic resonance imaging study of the brain with subjects with sex chromosome aneuploidies. J Neurol Neurosurg Psych 1999;66:628-32.

36. Tatum WO IV, Passaro EA, Elia M, Guerrini R, Gieron M, Genton P. Seizures in Klinefelter's syndrome. Pediatr Neurol 1998;19:275-8.

37. Manning MA, Hoyme HE. Diagnosis and management of the adolescent boy with Klinefelter syndrome. Adolesc Med 2002;13:367-74.

38. Veraart JC, Hamulyak K, Neumann HA. Leg ulcers and Klinefelter's syndrome. Arch Dermatol 1995;131:958-9.

39. Price WH, Clayton JF, Wilson J, Collyer S, De Mey R. Causes of death in X chromatin positive males (Klinefelter's syndrome). J Epidem Commun Health 1985;39:330-6.

40. Fricke GR, Mattern HJ, Schweikert HU, Schwanitz G. Klinefelter's syndrome and mitral valve prolapsed, an echocardiographic study in 22 patients. Biomed Pharmacother 1984;38:88-97.

41. Bojesen A, Juul S, Birkebaek NH, Gravholt CH. Morbidity in Klinefelter syndrome: a Danish register study based on hospital discharge diagnoses. J Clin Endocrinol Metab 2006;91:1254-60.

42. Bojesen A, Kristensen K, Birkebaek NH, Fedder J, Mosekilde L, Bennett P, Laurberg P, Frystyk J, Flyvbjerg A, Christiansen JS, Gravholt CH. The metabolic syndrome is frequent in Klinefelter's syndrome and is associated with abdominal obesity and hypogonadism. Diab Care 2006;29:1591-8.

43. Hasle H, Mellemgaard A, Neilsen J, Hansen J. Cancer incidence in men with Klinefelter syndrome. Br J Cancer 1995;71:416-20.

44. Hultborn R, Hanson C, Kopf I, Verbiené I, Warnhammar E, Weimarck A. Prevalence of Klinefelter syndrome in male breast cancer patients. Anticancer Res 1997;17:4293-7.

45. Kleczkowska A, Fryns JP, Van den Berghe H. X-chromosome polysomy in the male. Hum Genet 1988;80:16-22.

46. Peet J, Weaver DD, Vance GH. 49,XXXXY: a distinct phenotype. Three new cases and review. J Med Genet 1998;35: 420-4.

47. Lenz P, Luetjens CM, Kamischke A, Kühnert B, Kennerknecht I, Nieschlag E. Mosaic status in lymphocytes of infertile men with or without Klinefelter syndrome. Hum Reprod 2005;20:1248-55.

48. Foresta C, Bettella A, Vinanzi C, Dabrilli P, Meriggiola MC, Garolla A, Ferlin A. Insulin-like factor 3: a novel circulating hormone of testis origin in humans. J Clin Endocrinol Metab 2004;89:5952-8.

49. Bay K, Hartung S, Ivell R, Schumacher M, Jurgensen D, Jorgensen N, Holm M, Skakkebaek NE, Andersson AM. Insulin-like factor 3 serum levels in 135 normal men and 85 men with testicular disorders: relationship to the luteinizing hormone-testosterone axis. J Clin Endocrinol Metab 2005;90:3410-8.

50. Gordon DL, Krmpotic E, Thomas W, Gandy HM, Paulsen CA. Pathologic testicular findings in Klinefelter's syndrome 47,XXY vs 46,XY-47,XXY. Arch Intern Med 1972;130:726-9.

51. Tournaye H, Staessen C, Liebaers I, Van Assche E, Devroey P, Bonduelle M, Van Steirteghem A. Testicular sperm recovery in nine 47, XXY Klinefelter patients. Hum Reprod 1996;11:1644-9.

52. Foss GL, Lewis FI. A study of four cases with Klinefelter's syndrome showing motile spermatozoa in their ejaculates. J Reprod Fertil 1971;25:401-8.

53. Kaplan H, Asillaga M, Shelley T, Gardner LI. Possible fertility in Klinefelter's syndrome. Lancet 1963;2:506.

54. Kitamura M, Matsumiya K, Koga M, Nishimura K, Miura H, Tsuji T, Matsumoto M, Okamoto Y, Okuyama A. Ejaculated spermatozoa in patients with non-mosaic Klinefelter's syndrome. Int J Urol 2000;7:88-92.

55. Hinney B, Guttenbach M, Schmid M, Engel W, Michelmann HW. Pregnancy after intracytoplasmic sperm injection with sperm from a man with a 47,XXY Klinefelter's karyotype. Fertil Steril 1997;68:718-20.

56. Levron J, Aviram-Goldring A, Madgar I, Raviv G, Barkai G, Dor J. Sperm chromosome analysis and outcome of IVF in patients with non-mosaic Klinefelter's syndrome. Fertil Steril 2000;74:925-9.

57. Friedler S, Raziel A, Strassburger D, Schachter M, Bern O, Ron-El R. Outcome of ICSI using fresh and cryopreserved-thawed testicular spermatozoa in patients with non-mosaic Klinefelter's syndrome. Hum Reprod 2001;16:2616-20.

58. Madgar I, Jehoshua D, Weissenberg R, Raviv G, Menashe Y, Levron J. Prognostic value of the clinical and laboratory evaluation in patients with non-mosaic Klinefelter syndrome who are receiving assisted reproductive therapy. Fertil Steril 2002;77:1167-9.

59. Westlander G, Ekerhovd E, Bergh C. Low levels of serum inhibin B do not exclude successful sperm recovery in men with nonmosaic Klinefelter syndrome. Fertil Steril 2003; (79 Suppl 3):1680-2.

60. Ulug U, Bener, F, Akman MA, Bahceci M. Partners of men with Klinefelter syndrome can benefit from assisted reproductive technologies. Fertil Steril 2003;80:903-6.

61. Vernaeve V, Staessen C, Verheyen G, Van Steirteghem A, Devroey P, Tournaye, H. Can biological or clinical parameters predict testicular sperm recovery in 47,XXY Klinefelter's syndrome patients? Hum Reprod 2004;19:1135-9.

62. Seo JT, Park YS, Lee JS. Successful testicular sperm extraction in Korean Klinefelter syndrome. Urology 2004;64(6):1208-11.

63. Okada H, Goda K, Yamamoto Y, Sofikitis N, Miyagawa I, Mio Y, Koshida M, Horie S. Age as a limiting factor for successful sperm retrieval in patients with nonmosaic Klinefelter's syndrome. Fertil Steril 2005;84(6):1662-4.

64. Schiff JD, Palermo GD, Veeck LL, Goldstein M, Rosenwaks Z, Schlegel PN. Success of testicular sperm extraction [corrected] and intracytoplasmic sperm injection in men with Klinefelter syndrome. J Clin Endocrinol Metab 2005;90:6263-7.

65. Okada H, Goda K, Muto S, Maruyama O, Koshida M, Horie S. Four pregnancies in nonmosaic Klinefelter's syndrome using cryopreserved-thawed testicular spermatozoa. Fertil Steril 2005;84(5):1508.

66. Emre Bakircioglu M, Erden HF, Kaplancan T, Ciray N, Bener F, Bahceci M. Aging may adversely affect testicular sperm recovery in patients with Klinefelter syndrome. Urology 2006;68(5):1082-6.

67. Kyono K, Uto H, Nakajo Y, Kumagai S, Araki Y, Kanto S. Seven pregnancies and deliveries from non-mosaic Klinefelter syndrome patients using fresh and frozen testicular sperm. J Assist Reprod Genet 2007;24:47-51.

68. Koga M, Tsujimura A, Takeyama M, Kiuchi H, Takao T, Miyagawa Y, Takada S, Matsumiya K, Fujioka H, Okamoto Y, Nonomura N, Okuyama A. Clinical comparison of successful and failed microdissection testicular sperm extraction in patients with nonmosaic Klinefelter syndrome. Urology 2007;70(2):341-5.

69. Yarali H, Polat M, Bozdag G, Gunel M, Alpas I, Esinler I, Dogan U, Tiras B. TESE-ICSI in patients with non-mosaic Klinefelter syndrome: a comparative study. Reprod Biomed Online 2009;18(6):756-60.

70. Pang MG, Hoegerman SF, Cuticchia AJ, Moon, Doncel GF, Acosta AA, Kearns WA. Detection of aneuploidy for chromosomes 4,6,7,8,9,10,11,12,13,17,18,21,X and Y by fluorescence in situ hybridization in spermatozoa from nine patients with oligoasthenoteratozoospermia undergoing intracytoplasmic sperm injection. Hum Reprod 1999;14:1266-73.

71. Giltay JC, Van Golde RJT, Kastrop PMM. Analysis of Spermatozoa from Seven ICSI Males with Constitutional Sex Chromosomal Abnormalities by Fluorescent in situ Hybridization. J Assist Reprod Genet 2000;17:151-5.

72. Bergere M, Wainer R, Nataf V, Bailly M, Gombault M, Ville Y, Selva J. Biopsied testis cells of four 47,XXY patients: fluorescence in situ hybridization and ICSI results. Hum Reprod 2002;17:32-7.

73. Brugh V, Maduro M, Lamb D. Genetic disorders and infertility. Urol Clin North Am 2003;30:143-52.

74. Denschlag D, Tempfar C, Kunze M, Wolff G, Keck C. Assisted reproductive techniques in patients with Klinefelter syndrome: A critical review. Fertil Steril 2004;82:775-9.

75. Fullerton G, Hamilton M, Maheshwari A. Should non-mosaic Klinefelter syndrome men be labeled as infertile in 2009? Hum Reprod. 2010;25(3):588-97.

76. Staessen C, Tournaye H, Van Assche E, Michiels A, Van Landuyt L, Devroey P, Liebaers I, Van Steirteghem A. PGD in 47,XXY Klinefelter's syndrome patients. Hum Reprod Update 2003;9:319-30.

77. Plotton I, Brosse A, Lejeune H. Is it useful to modify the care of Klinefelter's syndrome to improve the chances of paternity? Ann Endocrinol (Paris) 2010;71(6):494-504.

78. Ramasamy R, Ricci JA, Palermo GD, Gosden LV, Rosenwaks Z, Schlegel PN. Successful fertility treatment for Klinefelter's syndrome. J Urol 2009;182(3):1108-13.

34

Y-Chromosome Genetics and Fertility

Nissankararao Mary Praveena, Rachel A Jesudasan

Transmission of genetic material to posterity is the ultimate aim of any organism. This genetic transmission is achieved through sexual reproduction in higher organisms. The role of Y-chromosome in male sex determination is well established.[1] The male determining genes present on the Y-chromosome direct development of the bipotential gonad towards maleness and initiates testis development during early embryonic stages. Y-chromosome is one of the smallest (~60 Mb) chromosomes in the human complement.[2] Y-chromosomes carry very few genes and are constituted mainly by repeats.[3] The known genes on human Y, map to the short arm (Yp) and the X-Y homologous pseudoautosomal regions (PARs) present on the two ends of the chromosome (http://www.ncbi.nlm.nih.gov). The long arm (Yq) is highly repetitive and can be differentiated into two distinct regions, euchromatic and the heterochromatic. High number of repetitive elements homologous to the X-chromosome[4,5] and the few functional genes are restricted to the euchromatic region on Yq. Factors responsible for spermatogenesis localize to the euchromatic portion of the long arm.[6-9] A heterochromatic block poises enigmatically at the distal end of the long arm, recalcitrant to sequencing and functional analysis. Y is subject to a great inter-individual variation in the heterochromatic region[10] which in most cases constitutes > 50 percent of the chromosome.[11]

■ GENES ON THE Y-CHROMOSOME

Short Arm (Yp)

Male sex is determined at fertilization by sperm bearing the Y-chromosome in Homosapiens.[12-14] The minimal region necessary for determining maleness was identified on the short arm of mouse Y-chromosome and called the sex-determining region on the Y (SRY,[15-17]). Initially, this region was identified from the study of XX male mice in a laboratory colony. In the sex reversed (Sxr) mice a small segment from the short arm of the Y-chromosome that is necessary and sufficient to induce testis determination is translocated to the X. Translocations resulting in XX males have now been identified in man also. The XX males have a translocation of the sex-determining region of the Y-chromosome on to one of the X-chromosomes. In XY females, on the other hand the sex-determining region on the Y-chromosome is deleted resulting in the female phenotype regardless of the presence of the Y. The XX

males are however infertile, as the translocated sex-determining region does not contain factors essential for spermatogenesis. Thus the sex-determining region localizes to the short arm of the human Y and the factors responsible for spermatogenesis localize outside the sex-determining region. The male specific region of the human Y-chromosome has been divided into 43 intervals defined using sequence tagged sites (STS) markers in individuals with naturally occurring deletions on the Y (**Fig. 34.1**). These intervals help define deletions in infertile patients.[18]

Euchromatic Long Arm (Yq11)

At least one in 1000 males lacks part of the long arm of the Y-chromosome.[19] The involvement of Y-chromosome in spermatogenesis in man was demonstrated through the study of naturally occurring deletions of the long arm of the Y in men presenting with azoospermia. The region deleted in azoospermia (DAZ) houses the azoospermia factor (AZF). Semen samples from individuals with microdeletions in this region contain few or no sperms. Three distinct non-overlapping sets of deletions are present within the AZF region viz., AZFa, AZFb and AZFc (**Fig. 34.2**). Deletions in the Yq11 proximal region give rise to a Sertoli cell only phenotype, wherein germ cells are absent in all (SCO type I) or most (SCO type II) of the testis tubules. SCO type 1 patients generally have small testes, with volume ranging from 5–10 mL. In, SCO type II, germ cells that have progressed to different stages are present in very few testis tubules. This could be owing to an event that affects spermatogenesis premeiotically, before or during the proliferation phase of spermatogonia. The variation in testis phenotypes of SCO I and II could also be due to secondary degenerative effects.

Deletions in middle region of Yq11 revealed spermatogenic arrest at the primary spermatocyte stage. Spermatogonia and primary spermatocytes were normal in all the tubules, although postmeiotic germ cells are not present in any tubule. Disruption in spermatogenesis in middle Yq11 deletions most likely occurs before or during meiosis at the spermatocyte stage.

In distal Yq11 deletions, only Sertoli cells were present with no germ cells. However, in some tubules germ cells of different developmental stages were recognized, wherein a subgroup also produced a small number of motile sperms, mostly with high degree of sperm morphological abnormalities. The distal Yq11 deletions perhaps affect postmeiotic events. The testis volume in

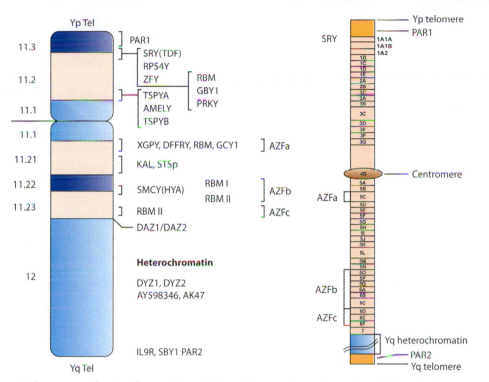

Figure 34.1: The human Y-chromosome showing the sex-determination and spermatogenesis genes localizing to the short arm and the euchromatic long arm respectively. The Yq12 heterochromatic block transcribes two noncoding RNAs from the DYZ1 repeats. The ideogram on the right represents the deletion intervals defined on the Y chromosome

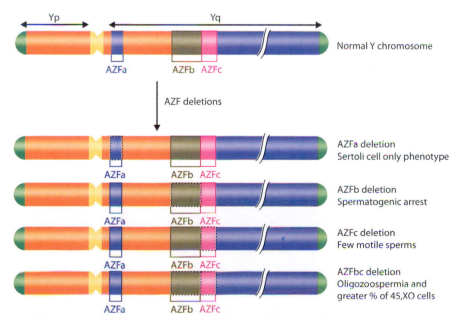

Figure 34.2: Deletion of the AZFa region results in the presence of only Sertoli cells in most of the tubules. In the AZFb deletions most of the tubules are arrested at the spermatocyte stage. In individuals with deletion of the AZFc region few motile sperms are often found. Deletion of the AZFbc regions can also result in a varying ratio of 45,XO/46,XY cells manifesting ambiguous genitalia

these cases ranged between 11 and 23 ml. In contrast to distal Yq11 deletions, proximal and middle Yq11 deletions showed less variation in testicular histology. Also, proximal and middle Yq11 showed a lower frequency of deletions compared to the distal region.[7,20] Microdeletions of the Y-chromosome cause a significantly higher proportion of azoospermia and oligozoospermia in men than do major chromosome abnormalities.[21]

Further studies have shown that the AZFa, AZFb and AZFc deletions are caused by intrachromosomal recombination events between homologous blocks of repetitive sequences located in Yq11.[22,23] Complete AZF microdeletions can now be distinguished from suspected partial deletions or polymorphisms by assessing recombination junctions in the patient sequences. The deletions lie within specific repeat blocks—the AZFa in HERV15 yq1/yq2,[21] AZFb in P5 proximal P1 repeat blocks[23] and AZFc in b2/b4 blocks (**Fig. 34.3**).[24]

For the clinical diagnosis of "complete AZF deletions" a set of STS (sequence tagged sites) loci has been suggested (25 and references therein). The molecular basis behind the plasticity of the AZF locus is still not clear. They might be based on inversions, insertions, or deletions of specific amplicons forming a specific Y lineage.

Y-chromosome Haplogroups

Human Y-chromosome has been classified into different haplogroups based on the substructure of the Y-chromosome.

Organization of the repeats, in terms of sequence and copy number variations define the haplogroups. The Y-chromosome is made of large blocks of repetitive sequences that vary between individuals and within populations, with the result that there is no unique Y-chromosome sequence in human populations. The plasticity of the Y-chromosome has been characterized using sets of markers and 18 Y-chromosomal haplogroups 'A-R' have been defined.[26] The GenBank Y-chromosome sequence is from a man from R haplogroup. Partial AZFc deletions have been reported from 14 different lineages.[27] The frequency of these deletions is higher in men with spermatogenic failure, although it is not clear whether this association is true in all the Y lineages.[25]

The Danish population in Europe that belongs to the haplotype Hg26 has a low sperm count compared to the rest of the Europeans. This haplotype has also been found in severely oligozoospermic and azoospermic men. This effect observed in Denmark could perhaps be due to a negative selection pressure by unknown factors in spermatogenesis, on the haplotype or this specific class of Y-chromosome. Further studies are required to determine the molecular mechanism of this susceptibility and to check if this has any correlation with other populations that have differences in semen quality and different Y-chromosome ancestry.

Epidemiological data clearly suggests a genetic component associated with male infertility, although majority of men with idiopathic azoospermia or oligozoospermia appear to have largely intact Y-chromosome. Therefore cause of infertility

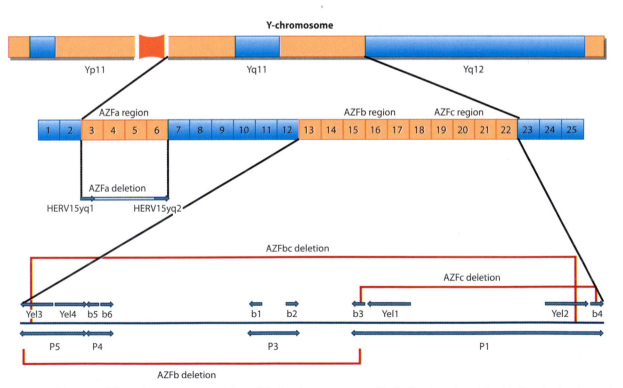

Figure 34.3: The long arm of the Y-chromosome comprises of blocks of repeats arranged in both orientations. The deletions in the AZF region are caused by recombination between different palindromes. The repeats involved in the deletion of the AZFa, b and c regions are shown above

remains uncertain in these individuals. An effect of the Y chromosomal background has been envisaged in men with idiopathic infertility. Partial AZFc deletions in men with Y-haplogroup N do not cause infertility. They probably arise by an intrachromosomal recombination between amplicons g1 and g3, after an inversion of b2/b3 amplicons such that the AZFc sequence of N haplogroup should be reduced by more than 50 percent.[25] Copy number of the Y-specific DAZ gene family associated with fertility varies in different human populations.[7] This would suggest that the multicopy genes in AZFc and probably in AZFb are functionally redundant.

The availability of the AZF genomic sequence and extensive testis cDNA screening programs[28,29,24] show that AZFb contains eight protein coding genes, *CDY2, EIFIAY, HSFY, PRY, RBMY1, RPS4Y2, SMCY* and *XKRY. AZFc* contains five protein-coding genes, *BPY2, CDY1, CSPG4LY, DAZ* and *GOLGA2LY.* All these genes are transcribed in testis[3] and are candidate functional genes in spermatogenesis. The precise biological role of genes or gene families in spermatogenesis is yet to be determined. Gene-specific mutations associated with specific testicular dysfunction in spermatogenesis have not been reported in the above genes, suggesting the necessity of complete deletions for causing male infertility. Smaller deletions are probably compensated for owing to copy number redundancy in AZFc. On the contrary, partial AZFb deletion is associated with variable testicular pathologies, different from that of complete AZFb deletion.

Between 10 and 20 percent of phenotypically normal men with idiopathic infertility and a cytogenetically normal Y-chromosome, carry microdeletions in the euchromatic region of the Y long arm. Infertility associated with microdeletions of various regions of the Y-chromosomes, indicates that factors encoded by the Y-chromosome are necessary for spermatogenesis. Three regions necessary for fertility in the long arm of the Y-chromosome are AZFa, AZFb and AZFc respectively.[30] Large submicroscopic Yq deletions are associated with significantly increased percentages of 45,XO cells in lymphocytes and sperms.[31] Large Yq deletions are also associated with sperms either nullisomic for gonosomes, or containing isodicentric Y-chromosomes.[32] The risk of genetically abnormal offspring being born to fathers carrying Y microdeletions is far greater, compared to males with normal Y-chromosomes. Such offspring could have increased phenotypic abnormalities like sex chromosome mosaicism and ambiguous genitalia. This should caution the infertile individuals against the use of artificial reproductive techniques for siring children. Study of 600 cases of Y aneuploidy by Hsu[33] also shows presence of 45,XO cell lines in more than half of the cases of postnatally diagnosed carriers of aberrant chromosomes. The frequency of microdeletions in Yq11 in infertile men ranges from 5-20 percent.[30,34,35] The high frequency of deletion on Y suggests that this chromosome is susceptible to the spontaneous loss of genetic material and is hence of great clinical significance. It is interesting to note that there is no concordance in lesions reported from different studies;[29] noncontiguous lesions are also found in this region.[36,37] Microdeletions in the Yq11 region has been shown to cause oligospermy and/or azoospermy and pairing anomalies of chromosomes at meiosis.

A region of pairing between the X and the Y-chromosomes, besides those at the pseudoautosomal regions has been conjectured at Yq11. Numerical aberrations such as 47,XXY, 48,XXYY 45,XO, etc. result from chromosomal non-disjunctions.

Infertile men with microscopically visible aberrations in Yq11 usually have a mosaic karyotype (46,XYq-/45,XO or 46,X idicY/45,XO with a variable number of XO cells.[7,38,39] A wide spectrum of phenotypes like Turner syndrome, mixed gonadal dysgenesis, male pseudohermaphroditism, mild mental retardation and autism was reported by an international survey of prenatally-diagnosed embryos with 45,X/46,XY mosaicism. A 100 percent transmission of AZFc deletions to the offspring has been reported on using sperm from such fathers for ICSI.[40-42] An increased risk of Turner's syndrome and mosaicism has been reported in babies born by ICSI.[43,44] Nevertheless, there is no clinical data describing genital abnormalities or other somatic defects in the ICSI-AZFc offspring. Turner syndrome patients usually lack the paternal X-chromosome and an increased frequency of X-Y nondisjunction in meiosis I as has been shown in some fathers of affected girls.[45] The presence of 45,XO/46,XY mosaicism in the father's gonads could also lead either to the formation of a monosomic X embryo or to the transmission of a potentially unstable Y-chromosome to a male fetus. In the latter case, a 45,XO/46,XY mosaicism could develop in the early steps of embryo development, resulting in ambiguous genitalia or mixed gonadal dysgenesis.[33,46] The general instability and heterogeneity of human Y-chromosome suggests that AZFc microdeletions can become premutations for subsequent complete loss of Y-chromosome. This inherent instability and heterogeneity of AZF region should be weighed seriously when counseling men with deletions of the region regarding ICSI. The frequency of nullisomic spermatozoa is greater, when compared to 45,XO lymphocytes in an individual;[32] therefore, spermatozoa rather than lymphocytes should be analyzed in infertile individuals, especially for those whom assisted reproductive procedures are suggested.

Heterochromatic Long Arm (Yq12)

There is very little information on the heterochromatic block at the distal end of the long arm of human Y. Classical male specific repeats used for identification of the Y were described from this region.[47] As late as 2007, Jesudasan's group described two testis-specific non-coding transcripts from this block of heterochromatin.[48] One of these noncoding RNAs forms a chimeric transcript with *CDC2L2* mRNA in testis. In this chimeric transcript, a 67-nucleotide stretch from the noncoding Yq12 RNA becomes the 5'UTR of *CDC2L2* mRNA only in testis. *CDC2L2* localizes to the map position 1p36.3 and is transcribed from all the tissues with 25–30 isoforms in all. In this example, a chimeric RNA is made in testis, between the noncoding RNA from Yq12 and *CDC2L2* mRNA from chromosome number 1, for putative translational regulation of *CDC2L2* mRNA in testis. This is the first example of regulation of an autosomal RNA by Y chromosomal noncoding RNA. Here the Y-chromosome apparently controls the translation of a testicular isoform of *CDC2L2.*

CHROMOSOMAL REARRANGEMENTS INVOLVING THE Y-CHROMOSOME

A greater proportion of chromosomal abnormalities are found in infertile males when compared to the general population. These include both numerical anomalies and structural chromosome reorganizations. The structural reorganizations may be microdeletions mainly of the euchromatic long arm of Y, deletions or duplications in the PARs or gross rearrangements involving two or more chromosomes.

Y-to-X Translocations

Y-to-X translocation is a rare type of chromosomal rearrangement in man, for which a few more sporadic cases have been reported[49-56] than familial cases.[49,57-60]

Translocation of Yp on to X resulting in male phenotype (**Fig. 34.4**) has been reported more often than translocation of Yq. Translocation of Yq material to the X chromosome results in excess of Yq material in the male with the translocated X and a normal Y that may result in sterility, although sterility status has been studied only in a few cases. Such translocations are mostly due to t(X,Y)(p22;q11) and often are associated with mental disturbances and dysmorphic features. Excess of Yq material may not be responsible for the phenotype as XYY males are fertile and do not show such phenotypic abnormalities.[60] Morel et al.[56] show that spermatogenesis can proceed to completion in at least some cells in such cases, resulting in severe oligozoospermy.

Translocations Between Acrocentric Chromosomes and Yq12

Y-autosome translocations have been reported in male infertility. The incidence of Y-autosome translocations in the general population is approximately 1:2000.[61,62] Translocations involving the Y and non-acrocentric chromosomes are rare when compared to those involving acrocentric chromosomes and may involve any segment of the Y.[63] Only 1.5 percent of the translocations involving the acrocentrics localize to Yq12. Of these 1.1 percent are onto chromosome 15 and 0.4 percent are with chromosome 22.[64] The origin of translocation chromosomes was paternal in most cases. There are a few reports of infertile individuals with breakpoints in Yq12 heterochromatin.[33,65] Apart from a few exceptions associated with fertile or subfertile individuals,[33,66] Y-autosome translocations usually cause impaired meiosis leading to male infertility. The individuals who retain the SRY gene on the short arm during the translocations are males. However, presence of regions outside the SRY locus on the Y-chromosome results in a female phenotype.

Complex chromosome rearrangements (CCRs) are structural aberrations involving at least 3 chromosomes and three or more breakpoints.[67] The case of an azoospermic male, studied by analysis of synaptonemal complex involving chromosomes 12, 15 and Y showed spermatogenic arrest at pachytene leading to cell death of vast majority of spermatocytes. Pentavalents and univalents were observed at pachytene and primary infertility appeared to be due to arrest of spermatogenesis at the spermatocyte level, mainly at late pachytene. Fluorescence *in situ* hybridization (FISH) on synaptonemal complex detect the presence of CCRs in subfertile men more efficiently.[68] The worst prognosis for spermatogenesis completion occurs when the aberrations include the sex chromosomes.

Twelve percent of the azoospermic/severe oligospermic males have a karyotypic abnormality[69] that comprises of numerical, Robertsonian or reciprocal translocations. A review on meiotic studies by De Braekeleer and Dao[69] showed that 8 percent of infertile males had some kind of cytogenetic error. Therefore, mitotic and meiotic studies are indicated in males with severe gamete impairment when the other possible causes have been eliminated. Robertsonian translocations show different level of spermatogenic impairment and are more in

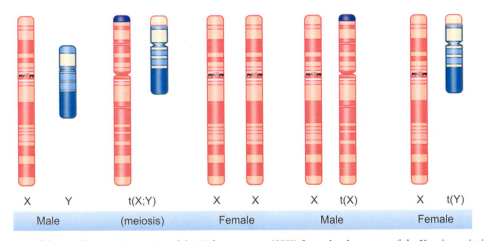

Figure 34.4: Translocation of the sex determining region of the Y chromosome (SRY) from the short arm of the Y to its meiotic pairing partner, the X, leads to male development in the Xt(X) individual owing to the presence of SRY. Deletion of the SRY from the Y chromosome on the other hand results in the development of a XY female (*Source*: Hiller B, Bradtke J, Balz H and Rieder H (2004): "CyDAS Online Analysis Site", http://www.cydas.org/OnlineAnalysis)

severe oligozoospermy than azoospermy. Usually male relatives carrying the same rearrangement and are fertile are found within the family. The utilization of FISH for characterization of rearrangements, allowed a detailed definition and resolution of breakpoints. Failure of pairing between the X and Y-chromosome was reported in a few cases of Y-chromosome structural rearrangements, including a dicentric Y-chromosome, ring Y, and pericentric inversion Y.

Involvement of chromosomal aberrations in male infertility has been reported from 1957 onwards with the observation of a Barr body in 47,XXY (Klinefelter's) males. Kjessler[70] showed a correlation between mean sperm concentration of the ejaculate and chromosome abnormalities. With the advent of the banding techniques large-scale cytogenetic analysis of infertile couples were done. These studies elucidated numerical anomalies and autosomal structural abnormalities. Many of these studies establish a correlation between sperm concentration in ejaculate and the frequency of chromosome abnormality.[69] Spermatogenic activity in XYY men shows great diversity, ranging from severe impairment to apparent normality. The short and long Y-chromosomes (Yq− and Yq+) were seen in azoospermics and severe oligozoospermics and hence the postulation of factor AZF on Yq euchromatin.

Cytogenetic errors during male meiosis can be responsible for the birth of a child with an abnormal karyotype, and male infertility. An arrest at any stage of spermatogenesis is found in many infertile men.[71] Gametogenic or early zygotic origins of dicentrics result in a nondetectable 46,XY cell line, even if the patient is a mosaic. But a late postzygotic event will present a normal cell line. At least 97 percent of patients with dicentric isochromosomes of Y are mosaics without a normal cell line.[33] 45,X cell line is usually found in these patients.[33,72,73] Relatively stable isodicentric Y-chromosomes have been reported from few patients.[73,74] Patients carrying a dicentric Y-chromosome have a wide range of somatic, genital, and gonadal phenotypic manifestations, depending on the structure of the dicentric Y-chromosome, the Yq and Yp breakpoints and the types of mosaicism. As previously reviewed 40.9 percent of the affected subjects are phenotypic females, 31.8 percent phenotypic males and 27.3 percent show different degrees of intersexuality.[73]

The human Y-chromosome includes a male specific Y region (MSY) that is 95 percent of the entire Y, flanked by 2 pseudoautosomal regions (PARs) on the two ends of it that is ~5 percent. The functions of most PAR genes are unknown although PAR1 deletions and translocations have been associated with infertility.[75-78] Rearrangements in PAR are also seen in infertile men with Y-chromosomal microdeletions, detected using Real Time PCR assays. All AZFbc microdeletions with abnormal karyotypes had more CNVs in PARs.[79] It is surprising that gains and losses were observed in PAR1 genes, whereas PAR2 genes demonstrated only losses. A few patients with microdeletions and normal karyotype also showed CNV of PAR but the frequency of loss was more in individuals with Y aberrations. The genetic aberrations in these regions could have a profound effect on the health of these individuals and their potential offspring.

For some men with Y-chromosome microdeletions, IVF/ICSI offers the opportunity to father children. Y-chromosome microdeletions must be checked and genetic counseling offered prior to this, for fear of transmitting aberrations to the male offspring. As microdeletions can affect the copy number of genes present in PARs, risk of transmitting congenital abnormalities exist. Function of several PAR genes is not known, but several are associated with psychiatric disorders like bipolar affective disorder (PAR1 and polymorphisms in two PAR2 genes), autism and other medical conditions.

Y-chromosomal Rearrangements in Infertile Males

Structural aberrations of the human Y-chromosome include deletions, rings, Y-autosomal translocations, Y-X translocations, isochromosomes, and dicentrics. Dicentric chromosomes are of the most frequent structural aberrations of the human Y-chromosome. Structurally, some dicentric Y-chromosomes have the breakpoint in the long arm with duplication of the proximal long arm and the entire short arm, including SRY. Other dicentric Y's result from breakpoints in the short arm and thus have the entire long arm and proximal short arm duplicated. These may or may not carry SRY. The presence of SRY in the dicentric would initiate testis development. A number of cases of Yq isochromosomes have been reported from 1965. These patients display at least two cell lines 46,X,i(Yq)/45,XO. These patients may vary from Turner like females to normal males most of whom are azoospermic, depending on the ratio of Y-bearing cells.[80] Isodicentrics with two centromeres are found in 25 percent of isodicentric Y [i(Y)] and pseudoisodicentric i(Y) in 75 percent cells. Pseudoisodicentrics have a single primary constriction, giving the chromosome a submetacentric appearance. Although these have two centric bands, one of the centromeres is inactivated and thus these are functional monocentrics. Very few i(Y) chromosomes are structural monocentrics with only a single centric band. The iso-Y gives rise to both 45,X cells and cells with different Y rearrangements, which are presumably postzygotic events. Prezygotic events harbor paternal X in XXY cases.[74] Dicentric chromosomes are generally unstable and cause bridge formation during anaphase. The azoospermic status could be due to aberrant meiotic pairing and improper segregation.[81,82] Mitotic nondisjunction, chromosome breakage, somatic recombination and centromere deletion may jointly account for the different cell populations. Bias in assessment is a major problem in the interpretation of data from these patients because of the wide phenotypic variation in karyotype found among patients with dicentric Y-chromosomes. Genetic counseling of patients with prenatal or postnatal detection of dicentrics regarding risk of gonadoblastoma and sexual development poses a problem because of the mosaicism.[72] Non-mosaic isodicentric Y-chromosome (47,XX,+idic(Y)(pter->q12::q12->pter) which exhibited phenotype as described for individuals with 48,XXYY karyotype has been described by Heinritz et al.[74] Unstable i(Y) can lead to a spectrum of events like mitotic nondisjunctions, tricentric Y, marker Ys and supernumerary Y-chromosomes as was reported by Haaf and Schmid.[81]

Hsu who described 350 cases with abnormal Y-chromosomes characterized using conventional cytogenetic techniques has reviewed Y-chromosome aneuploidy.[33] As these were analyzed by karyotyping no detailed molecular information on the Y sequences present are available. Fluorescence *in situ* hybridization (FISH) technique is more useful for revealing the detailed structure and content of abnormal chromosomes. FISH in combination with PCR analysis determines the molecular events more accurately. Among the Y-chromosomal rearrangements, i(Yp) appears to be the most uncommon.[83]

Reciprocal Translocations Involving the Y-chromosome

Structural chromosomal anomalies are more common in infertile men compared to the general population.[84,85] Of the chromosomal anomalies, Robertsonian translocations and numerical sex chromosome aberrations are the most common. Robertsonian translocations are formed by centric fusions of two acrocentric chromosomes, resulting in a 45, chromosome karyotype. Earlier on it was believed that testicular dysfunctions are associated with sex chromosome anomalies like classic and variant types of Klinefelter's. Defective spermatogenesis was found to occur in individuals with different translocations. Carriers of reciprocal translocations have reduced fertility and/or are at increased risk of having a spontaneous abortion or chromosomally unbalanced offspring (reviews by[69,86]). Many male carriers with reduced fertility have a decreased number of gametes, of which a variable fraction has unbalanced chromosomal constitution.

A correlation exists between sperm morphological abnormalities and genetic aberrations.[87-90] Giltay et al.,[66] showed that morphologically normal and total sperms from a t(Y;16) patient scheduled for ICSI had 49 and 92 percent chromosomal translocations respectively. In general sex chromosome/autosome translocations have a stronger fertility-reducing effect when compared to autosome/autosome translocations. All males with X/autosome translocations[86] and 80 percent of the males with Y/autosome translocations[33] have azoospermia or they produce sperm with a high percentage of spermatozoa bearing the translocations.[66] Meiotic studies with t(Y;6) and azoospermia[65] showed asynapsis within the quadrivalent at the pachytene stage in some cells and dragging of chromosome 6 into sex vesicle in others.

There exists a correlation between increased frequencies of disomic and diploid spermatozoa and recurrent abortion.[91,92] Most of the numerical chromosome anomalies and *de novo* structural rearrangements originate at meiosis by spermatogenic impairment.[93-95] Translocations between different chromosomes could disrupt meiotic pairing, leading to late spermatocyte arrest and azoospermia.[96]

Chromosomal rearrangements that occur during meiosis could result in mutations of any of the genes involved in the complex gametogenesis pathway[95, 97-99] or alternately the regulatory regions of these genes. Majority of the rearrangements reported in male infertility are from studies of peripheral blood leukocytes. Chromosome abnormalities limited to spermatogenic cells will not be detectable through the study of the somatic cells.[100]

There is discernible relationship between chromosome aberrations and the morphology of spermatozoa.[56,90,101,102] Deletions of the long arm of the mouse Y-chromosome produces sperm head morphological abnormalities and motility related problems, the severity of which depends on the extent of Yq deletion.[101] When all aspects are considered it seems likely that all males with Y/autosome translocations produce few or no sperms or they produce sperms with a high percentage of unbalanced spermatozoa.[65]

Spermatogenesis and X-chromosome

Though Y is directly involved in male sex determination, paradoxically there is enrichment of testis-specific genes on X chromosome and accretion of certain male beneficial genes.[103-106] There is an over-representation of testis-expressed genes on the X chromosome in mouse and human.[104,107-109] It has been hypothesized that male beneficial genes tend to accumulate on the X chromosome during evolution because of its hemizygosity in male.[110,111] Rice[111] proposed that recessive mutations on the X chromosome that result in enhanced male reproductive fitness should rapidly accumulate in the population because the hemizygous nature of such mutations in males causes them to be immediately expressed thus conferring an immediate male benefit.

X-autosome Translocations and Male Infertility

Robertsonian translocations involving different chromosomes can lead to improper chromosome pairing and segregation at meiosis leading to azoospermy or severe oligozoospermy resulting in infertility. The effects of such translocations appear to be more severe when the X or the Y-chromosomes (gonosomes) are involved in such translocations.[112] Incompatibilities between X and Y-chromosomes have been found to bring about sterility due to very high frequency of X-Y dissociation in first meiotic metaphase in spermatocytes of mouse hybrids.[113,114] According to Miklos,[115] ineffective meiotic pairing may lead to disruption of X-inactivation and inappropriate expression of genes in the unpaired chromosomes, leading to disruption of spermatogenesis.

Spermatogenesis and Autosomal Genes

Thus genes involved in spermatogenesis are present not solely on the Y-chromosome, which has been set aside for the male sex determination, spermatogenesis and fertility. Vast majority of genes required for spermatogenesis and spermiogenesis are non-Y linked. Studies have shown that 2300 genes (4% of the mouse genome) are dedicated to male germ cell specific expression. Approximately 99 percent of these are first expressed during or after meiosis.[116] Different germ cell type-specific libraries identified 11–20 percent testis specific genes. These genes are involved in transcriptional regulation during spermatogenesis and fertilization, sperm morphology, nuclear activity in spermatogenic cells, meiotic division and metabolism in sperm.[117,118] The transcription profiling of mouse testis at six different time points revealed the expression of 2058 spermatogenesis related genes.[119] These had functions in physiological processes, cellular processes, development, regulation, behavior, signal transduction, transporter activity, transcription regulator activity, chaperone activity, enzyme regulator activity, antioxidant activity and translation regulator activity.

Fertility Factors on the Y-chromosome and Hybrid Male Sterility

The Y-chromosomes from different species harbor repeats that are specific to the species. These species-specific repeats evolve rapidly and vary to different degrees between geographically isolated populations. These geographically isolated populations gradually attain greater variation in the repeats on the Y-chromosomes, leading to reproductive isolation finally ending up as new species altogether. The molecular drive inherent in repetitive DNAs contributes to hybrid incompatibilities and speciation.[120,121] When males and females from different strains or species interbreed, it results in a phenomenon called hybrid dysgenesis or cytoplasmic male sterility. This is the result of incompatibility between the Y-chromosome and cytoplasm of the female egg invoking the presence of factors on the Y-chromosome, which interact with the cytoplasmic milieu of the egg. It is generally the males that are infertile in such interspecific or inter-strain crosses suggesting a Y-chromosome that has drifted away owing to the variation in the species-specific repeats. Thus the repeats on the Y-chromosome apparently harbor factors responsible for fertility.

Y is the only functionally specialized chromosome within a genetic complement of an organism, set aside for sex determination and spermatogenesis. All the other chromosomes carry an assorted package of genes for different functions. The Y-chromosome is an interesting paradigm, as it is not essential for the survival of the individual, as the females do very well, without the Y. On the other hand Y-chromosome is indispensible for the propagation of the species. The organism in its quest for self-propagation is often at loggerheads with nature, which prefers to eliminate the weak and unfit in order to preserve the best for posterity. If only the fascination of mankind would stop meddling with Nature, even if it were in his quest for artificial assistance to the desperate desire for an offspring, would posterity be less morbid.

■ REFERENCES

1. Vergnaud G, Page DC, Simmler MC, Brown L, Rouyer F, Noel B, et al. A deletion map of the human Y-chromosome based on DNA hybridization. Am J Hum Genet 1986;89:491-6.

2. Morton NE. Parameters of the human genome. Proc Natl Acad Sci USA 1991;88:7474-6.

3. Skaletsky H, Kuroda-Kawaguchi T, Minx PJ, Cordum HS, Hillier L, Brown LG, et al. The male-specific region of the human Y-chromosome is a mosaic of discrete sequence classes. Nature 2003;423:825-37.

4. Neil DL, Villasante A, Fisher RB, Vetric D, Cox B, Tyler-Smith C. Structural instability of human tandemly repeated DNA

sequences cloned in yeast artificial chromosome vectors. Nucl Acids Res 1990;18:1421-8.

5. Slim R, Le Paslier D, Compain S, Levilliers J, Ougen P, Billault A, et al. Construction of a yeast artificial chromosome contig spanning the pseudoautosomal region and isolation of 25 new sequence-tagged sites. Genomics 1993;16:691-7.

6. Bardoni B, Zuffardi O, Guioli S, Ballabio A, Simi P, Cavalli P, et al. A deletion map of the human Yq11 region: implications for the evolution of the Y-chromosome and tentative mapping of a locus involved in spermatogenesis. Genomics 1991;11:443-51.

7. Vogt PH, Edelmann A, Kirsch S, Henegariu O, Hirscmann P, Kiesewetter F, et al. Human Y-chromosome azoospermia factors (AZF) mapped to different sub-regions in Yq11. Hum Mol Genet 1996;5:933-43.

8. Elliott DJ, Millar MR, Oghene K, Ross A, Kiesewetter F, Pryor J, et al. Expression of RBM in the nuclei of human germ cells is dependent on a critical region of the Y-chromosome long arm. Proc Natl Acad Sci USA 1997;94:3848-53.

9. Duell T, Mathews S, Wunderlich B, Mittermuller J, Schmetzer H. Interstitial and terminal deletion of chromosome Y in a male individual with cryptozoospermia. Mol Hum Repro 1998;4:325-31.

10. Bühler EM. A synopsis of the human Y-chromosome. Hum Genet 1980;55:145-75.

11. Foote S, Vollrath D, Hilton A, Page DC. The human Y-chromosome: overlapping DNA clones spanning the euchromatic region. Science 1992;258:60-6.

12. Stevens NM. Studies in spermatogenesis with special reference to the accessor Y-chromosome. Publication of the Carnegies Institution of Washington 1905;36:1-74.

13. Wilson EB. The chromosomes in relation to the determination of sex in insects. Science 1905;22:500-2.

14. Morgan TH. The scientific work of Miss. N. M. Stevens. Science 1912;36:468-70.

15. Page DC, Mosher R, Simpson EM, Fisher EM, Mardon G, Pollack J, et al. The sex-determining region of the human Y-chromosome encodes a finger protein. Cell 1987;51:1091-104.

16. Sinclair AH, Berta P, Palmer MS, Hawkins JR, Griffiths BL, Smith MJ, et al. A gene from the human sex-determining region encodes a protein with homology to a conserved DNA-binding motif. Nature 1990;346:240-4.

17. Page DC, Fisher EM, McGillivray B, Brown LG. Additional deletion in sex-determining region of human Y-chromosome resolves paradox of X,t(Y;22) female. Nature 1990;346:279-81.

18. Vollrath D, Foote S, Hilton A, Brown LG, Beer-Romero P, Bogan JS, Page DC. The human Y-chromosome: a 43-interval map based on naturally occurring detions. Science 1992;258:52-8.

19. Kirsch S, Weiss B, de Rosa M, Ogata T, Lombardi G, Rappold GA. FISH deletion mapping defines a single location for the Y-chromosome stature gene, GCY. J Med Genet 2000;37:593-9.

20. Duzcan F, Atmaca M, Cetin GO, Bagci H. Cytogenetic studies in patients with reproductive failure. Acta Obstet Gynecol Scand 2003;82:53-6.

21. Aho M, Harkonen K, Suikkari AM, Juvonen V, Anttila L, Lahdetie J. Y-chromosomal microdeletions among infertile men. Acta Obstet Gynecol Scand 2001;80:652-6.

22. Kamp C, Hirschmann P, Voss H, Huellen K, Vogt PH. Two long homologous retroviral sequence blocks in proximal Yq11 cause

AZFa microdeletions as a result of intrachromosomal recombination events. Hum Mol Genet 2000;12:2563-72.

23. Repping S, Skaletsky H, Lange J, Silber S, Van DerVeen F, Oates RD, et al. Recombination between palindromes P5 and P1 on the human Y-chromosome causes massive deletions and spermatogenic failure. Am J Hum Genet 2002;71:906-22.

24. Kuroda-Kawaguchi T, Skaletsky H, Brown LG, Minx PJ, Cordum HS, Waterston RH, et al. The AZFc region of the Y-chromosome features massive palindromes and uniform recurrent deletions in infertile men. Nat Genet 2001;29:279-86.

25. Vogt PH. Genomic heterogeneity and instability of the AZF locus on the human Y-chromosome. Mol Cell Endocrinol 2004;224:1-9.

26. The Y-chromosome Consortium. A nomenclature system for the tree of human Y-chromosomal binary haplogroups. Genome Res 2002;12:339-48.

27. Repping S, Skaletsky H, Brown L, van Daalen SK, Korver CM, Pyntikova T, et al. Polymorphism for a 1.6-Mb deletion of the human Y-chromosome persists through balance between recurrent mutation and haploid selection. Nat Genet 2003;35:247-51.

28. Lahn BT, Page DC. Functional coherence of the human Y-chromosome. Science 1997;278:675-80.

29. Vogt PH, Affara N, Davey P, Hammer M, Jobling MA, Lau YF, et al. Report of the Third International Workshop on Y-chromosome Mapping 1997. Cytogenet Cell Genet 1997;79:1-20.

30. Vogt PH. Human chromosome deletions in Yq11, AZF candidate genes and male infertility: history and update. Mol Hum Reprod 1998;4:739-44.

31. Jaruzelska J, Korcz A, Wojda A, Jedrzejczak P, Bierla J, Surmacz T, et al. Osaicism for 45,X cell line may accentuate the severity of spermatogenic defects in men with AZFc deletion. J Med Genet 2001;38:798-802.

32. Siffori JP, Le Bourhis C, Krausz C, Barbaux S, Quintana-Murci L, Kanafani S, et al. Sex chromosome mosaicism in males carrying Y-chromosome long arm deletions. Hum Reprod 2000;15:2559-62.

33. Hsu. LYF Phenotype/genotype correlations of Y-chromosome aneuploidy with emphasis on structural aberrations in postnatally diagnosed cases. Am J Med Genet 1994;53:108-40.

34. Krausz C, McElreavey K. Y-chromosome and male infertility. Front Biosci 1999;4:E1-8.

35. Krausz C, Forti G, McElreavey K. The Y-chromosome and male fertility and infertility. Int J Androl 2003;26:70-5.

36. Najmabadi H, Huang V, Yen P, Subbarao MN, Bhasin D, Banaag L, et al. Substantial prevalence of microdeletions of the Y-chromosome in infertile men with idiopathic azoospermia and oligozoospermia detected using a sequence-tagged site-based mapping strategy. J Clin Endocrinol Metab 1996;81:1347-52.

37. Foresta C, Ferlin A, Garolla A, Rossato M, Barbaux S, De Bortoli A. Y-chromosome deletions in idiopathic severe testiculopathies. J Clin Endocrinol Metab 1997;82:1075-80.

38. Sandberg AA. The Y-chromosome. Part B. Clinical aspects of Y-chromosome abnormalities. Alan R Liss Inc., New York, 1985.

39. Vogt PH, Fernandes S. Polymorphic DAZ gene family in polymorphic structure of AZFc locus: Artwork or functional for human spermatogenesis? APMIS 2003;111:115-27.

40. Kent-First MG, Kol S, Muallem A, Ofir R, Manor D, Blazer S, et al. The incidence and possible relevance of Y-linked microdeletions in babies born after intracytoplasmic sperm injection and their infertile fathers. Mol Hum Reprod 1996;2:943-50.

41. Page DC, Silber S, Brown LG. Men with infertility caused by AZFc deletion can produce sons by intracytoplasmic sperm injection, but are likely to transmit the deletion and infertility. Hum Reprod 1999;14:1722-6.

42. Oates RD, Silber S, Brown LG, Page DC. Clinical characterization of 42 oligospermic or azoospermic men with microdeletion of the AZFc region of the Y-chromosome, and of 18 children conceived via ICSI. Hum Reprod 2002;17:2813-24.

43. In't Veld P, Brandenburg H, Verhoeff A, Dhont M, Los F. Sex chromosomal abnormalities and intracytoplasmic sperm injection. Lancet 1995;346:773.

44. Van Opstal D, Los FJ, Ramlakhan S, Van Hemel JO, Van Den Ouweland AM, Brandenburg H, et al. Determination of the parent of origin in nine cases of prenatally detected chromosome aberrations found after intracytoplasmic sperm injection. Hum Reprod 1997;12:682-6.

45. Martínez-Pasarell O, Templado C, Vicens-Calvet E, Egozcue J, Nogués C. Paternal sex chromosome aneuploidy as a possible origin of Turner syndrome in monozygotic twins: case report. Hum Reprod 1999;14:2735-8.

46. Lazebnik N, Filkins KA, Jackson CL, Linn KB, Doshi NN, Hogge WA. 45,X/46,XY mosaicism: the role of ultrasound in prenatal diagnosis and counselling. Ultrasound Obstet Gynecol 1996;8:325-8.

47. Bostock CJ, Gosden JR, Mitchell AR. Localization of a male-specific DNA fragment to a sub-region of the human Y-chromosome. Nature 1978;272:324-8.

48. Jehan Z, Vallinayagam S, Tiwari S, Pradhan S, Singh L, Suresh A, et al. Novel noncoding RNA from human Y distal heterochromatic block (Yq12) generates testis-specific chimeric CDC2L2. Genome Res 2007;17:433-40.

49. Van den Berghe H, Petit P, Fryns JP. Y to X translocation in man. Hum Genet 1977;36:129-41.

50. Khudr G, Benirschke K, Judd HL, Strauss J. Y to X translocation in a woman with reproductive failure. JAMA 1973;226:544-9.

51. Borgaonkar DS, Sroka BM, Flores M. Y-to-X translocation in a girl. Lancet 1974;1:68-9.

52. Bernstein R, Wagner J, Isdale J, Nurse GT, Lane AB, Jenkins T. X-Y translocation in a retarded phenotypic male. J Med Genet 1978;15:466-74.

53. Bernstein R, Pinto MR, Almeida M, Solarsh SM, Meck J, Jenkins T. X;Y translocation in an adolescent mentally normal phenotypic male with features of hypogonadism. J Med Genet 1980;17:437-43.

54. Evans HJ, Buckton KE, Spowart G, Carothers AD. Heteromorphic X chromosomes in 46,XX males: evidence for the involvement of X-Y interchange. Hum Genet 1979;49:11-31.

55. Hecht T, Cooke HJ, Cerrillo M, Meer B, Reck G, Hameister H. A new case of Y to X translocation in a female. Hum Genet 1980;54:303-7.

56. Morel F, Fellmann F, Roux C, Bresson JL. Meiotic segregation analysis by FISH investigation of spermatozoa of a 46,Y,der(X),t(X;Y)(qter-p22::q11-qter) carrier. Cytogenet Cell Genet 2001;92:63-8.

57. Tiepolo L, Zuffardi O, Rodewald A. Nullisomy for the distal portion of Xp in a male child with a X/Y translocation. Hum Genet 1977;39:277-81.

58. Akesson HO, Hagberg B, Wahlstrom J. Y-to-X chromosome translocation observed in two generations. Hum Genet 1980;55:39-42.

59. Pfeiffer RA. Observations in a case of an X/Y translocation, t(X;Y)(p22;q11), in a mother and son. Cytogenet Cell Genet 1980;26:150-7.

60. Yamada K, Nanko S, Hattori S, Isurugi K. Cytogenetic studies in Y-to-X translocation observed in three members of one family, with evidence of infertility in male carriers. Hum Genet 1982;60:85-90.

61. Gardner RJ, Suhterland GR. Sex Chromosome Translocations. In: Gardner RJ, Suhterland GR (Eds). Chromosome Abnormalities and Genetic Counselling. New York: Oxford University Press; 1996.pp.95-114.

62. Powell C. Sex chromosomes and sex abnormalities. In: Gersen SL, Keagle MB (Eds). The Principles of Clinical Cytogenetics. Totowa, NJ: Humana Press, 1999.pp.229-58.

63. Smith A, Fraser IS, Elliott G. An infertile male with balanced Y;19 translocation. Review of Y; autosome translocations. Ann Genet 1979;22:189-94.

64. Kalz L, Schwanita G. Investigations in probands with rearrangements in the acrocentric chromosomes. Int J Hum Genet 2007;7:252-62.

65. Delobel B, Djlelati R, Gabriel-Robez O, Croquette M-F, Rousseaux-Prevost R, Rousseaux J, et al. Y-autosome translocation and infertility: usefulness of molecular, cytogenetic and meiotic studies. Hum Genet 1998;102:98-102.

66. Giltay JC, Kastrop PM, Tiemessen CH, van Inzen WG, Scheres JM, Pearson PL. Sperm analysis in a subfertile male with a Y;16 translocation, using four-color FISH. Cytogenet Cell Genet 1999;84:67-72.

67. Pai GS, Thomas GH, Mahoney W, Migeon BR. Complex chromosome rearrangements. Report of a new case and literature. Clin Genet 1980;18:436-44.

68. Coco R, Rahn MI, Estanga PG, Antonioli G, Solari AJ. A constitutional complex chromosome rearrangement involving meiotic arrest in an azoospermic male: case report. Hum Repro 2004;19:2784-90.

69. De Braekeleer M, Dao TN. Cytogenetic studies in male infertility: a review. Hum Repro 1991;6:245-50.

70. Kjessler B. In: Karger SL (Ed). Karyotype, meiosis and spermatogenesis in a sample of men attending an infertility clinic. Basel, Switzerland: Monographs in Human Genetics 1966.pp.1-93.

71. Yoshida A, Nakahori Y, Kuroki Y, Motoyama M, Araki Y, Miura K, et al. Dicentric Y-chromosome in an azoospermic male. Mol Hum Repro 1997;3:709-12.

72. Tuck-Muller CM, Chen H, Martinez JE, Shen C-C, Li S, Kusyk C, et al. Isodicentric Y-chromosome: cytogenetic, molecular and clinical studies and review of the literature. Hum Genet 1995;96:119-29.

73. Codina-Pascual M, Oliver-Bonet M, Navarro J, Starke H, Liehr T, Gutierrez-ateo C, et al. FISH characterization of a dicentric Yq (p11.32) isochromosome in an azoospermic male. Am J Med Genet 2004;127A:302-6.

74. Heinritz W, Kotzot D, Heinze S, Kujar A, Kleemann WJ, Forster UG. Molecular and cytogenetic characterization of a non-mosaic isodicentric Y-chromosome in a patient with Klinefelter Syndrome. Am J Med Genet 2005;132A:198-201.

75. Quack B, Speed RM, Luciani JM, Noel B, Guichaoua M, Chandley AC. Meiotic analysis of two human reciprocal X-autosome translocations. Cytogenet Cell Genet 1988;48:43-7.

76. Gabriel-Robez O, Rumpler Y, Ratomponirina C, Petit C, Levilliers J, Croquette MF, et al. Deletion of the pseudoautosomal region and lack of sex-chromosome pairing at pachytene in two infertile men carrying an X;Y translocation. Cytogenet Cell Genet 1990;54:38-42.

77. Mohandas TK, Speed RM, Passage MB, Yen PH, Chandley AC, Shapiro LJ. Role of the pseudoautosomal region in sex chromosome pairing during male meiosis: meiotic studies in a man with a deletion of distal Xp. Am J Hum Genet 1992;51:526-33.

78. Lee S, Lee SH, Chung TG, Kim HJ, Yoon TK, Kwak IP, et al. Molecular and cytogenetic characterization of two azoospermic patients with X-autosome translocation. J Asst Reprod Genet 2003;20:385-9.

79. Jorgez CJ, Weedin JW, Sahin A, Tannour-Louet M, Han S, Bournat JC, et al. Aberrations in pseudoautosomal regions (PARs) found in infertile men with Y-chromosome microdeletions. J Clin Endocrinol Metab 2011;96:E674-9.

80. Therman E, Susman M. Human sex determination and the Y-chromosome. In: Therman E, Susman M (Eds). Human Chromosomes: structure, Behaviour and Effects. 3rd edn. New York: Springer-Verlag; 1993.pp.203-9.

81. Haaf T, Schmid M. Y isochromosome associated with a mosaic karyotype and inactivation of the centromere. Hum Genet 1990;85:486-90.

82. Guttenbach M, Muller U, Schmid M. Cytogenetic and molecular analysis of Yq isochromosome. Hum Genet 1990;86:147-59.

83. Lin YH, Chuang L, Lin YM, Lin YH, Teng YN, Kuo PL. Isochromosome of Yp in a man with Sertoli-cell-only syndrome. Fertil Steril 2005;83:764-6.

84. Van Assche E, Bonduelle M, Tournaye H, Joris H, Verheyen G, Devroey P, et al. Cytogenetics of infertile men. Hum Reprod 1996;11:Suppl 4:1-24; discussion 25-26.

85. Kalantari P, Sepehri H, Behjati F, Ashtiani ZO, Akbari MT. Chromosomal studies in infertile men. Tsitol Genet 2001;35:50-4.

86. Chandley AC. Infertility. In: Emery AE, Riomoin DL, (Eds). Principles and practices of Medical Genetics. 3rd edn. Edinburgh: Churchill Livingstone 1996.pp.1-9.

87. Chandley AC, Maclean N, Edmond P, Fletcher J, Watson GS. Cytogenetics and fertility in man. II. Testicular histology and meiosis. Ann Hum Genet 1976;40:165-76.

88. In't Veld PA, Broekmans FJ, de Fracne HF, Pearson PI, Pieters MH, van Kooij RJ. Intracytoplasmic sperm injection (ICSI) and chromosomally abnormal spermatozoa. Hum Reprod 1997;12:752-4.

89. Ogawa S, Araki S, Ohno M, Sato I. Chromosome analysis of human spermatozoa from an oligoasthenozoospermic carrier for a 13:14 Robertsonian translocation by their injection into mouse oocytes. Hum Reprod 2000;15:1136-9.

90. Baccetti B, Collodel G, Marzella R, Moretti E, Poimboni P, Scapigliati G, et al. Ultrastructural studies of spermatozoa from

infertile males with Robertsonian translocations and 18, X, Y aneuploidies. Hum Repro 2005;20:2295-300.

91. Giorlandino C, Calugi G, Iaconianni L, Santoro ML, Lippa A. Spermatozoa with chromosomal abnormalities may result in a higher rate of recurrent abortion. Fertil Steril 1998;70:576-7.

92. Rubio C, Simón C, Blanco J, Vidal F, Mínguez Y, Egozcue J, et al. Implications of sperm chromosome abnormalities in recurrent miscarriage. J Assist Reprod Genet 1999;16:253-8.

93. Jacobs PA, Hassold TJ. The origin of numerical chromosome abnormalities. Adv Genet 1995;33:101-33.

94. Olson SB, Magenis RE. Preferential paternal origin of de novo structural chromosome rearrangements. In: Daniel A (Ed). The cytogenetics of mammalian autosomal rearrangements. New York: Alan R Liss 1988;583-99.

95. Egozcue S, Blanco J, Vendrell JM, Garcia F, Veiga A, Aran B, et al. Human male infertility: chromosome anomalies, meiotic disorders, abnormal spermatozoa and recurrent abortion. Hum Reprod. Update 2000;6:93-105.

96. Gazvani MR, Wilson EDA, Richmond DH, Howard PJ, Kingland CR, Lewis Jones DI. Evaluation of the role of mitotic instability in karyotypically normal men with oligozoospermia. Fertil Steril 2000;73:51-5.

97. Barlow AL, Hultén MA. Combined immunocytogenetic and molecular cytogenetic analysis of meiosis I human spermatocytes. Chromosome Res 1996;4:562-73.

98. Edelmann W, Cohen PE, Kane M, Lau K, Morrow B, Bennett S, et al. Meiotic pachytene arrest in MLH1-deficient mice. Cell 1996;85:1125-34.

99. Hassold TJ. Mismatch repair goes meiotic. Nat Genet 1996;13: 261-2.

100. Robinson DO, Dalton P, Jacobs PA, Moses K, Power MM, Skuse DH, et al. A molecular and FISH analysis of structurally abnormal Y-chromosomes in patients with Turner syndrome. J Med Genet 1999;36:279-84.

101. Burgoyne PS, Mahadevaiah SK, Sutcliffe MJ, Palmer SJ. Fertility in mice requires X-Y pairing and a Y-chromosomal 'spermiogenesis' gene mapping to the long arm. Cell 1992;71:391-8.

102. Styrna J, Imai HT, Moriwaki K. An increased level of sperm abnormalities in mice with a partial deletion of the Y-chromosome. Genet Res 1991;57:195-9.

103. Zechner U, Wilda M, Kehrer-Sawatzki H, Vogel W, Fundele R, Hameister H. A high density of X linked genes for general cognitive ability: A run-away process shaping human evolution? Trends Genet 2001;17:697-701.

104. Wang PJ, McCarrey JR, Yang F, Page DC. An abundance of X-linked genes expressed in spermatogonia. Nat Genet 2001;27: 422-6.

105. Lercher MJ, Urrutia AO, Hurst LD. Evidence that the human X chromosome is enriched for male-specific but not for female-specific genes. Mol Biol Evol 2003;20:1113-6.

106. Torgerson DG, Singh RS. Enhanced adaptive evolution of sperm-expressed genes on the mammalian X chromosome. Heredity 2006;96:39-44.

107. Khil PP, Smirnova NA, Romanienko PJ, Camerini-Otero RD. The mouse X chromosome is enriched for sex-biased genes not subject to selection by meiotic sex chromosome inactivation. Nat Genet 2004;36:642-6.

108. Vallender EJ, Pearson NM, Lahn BT. The X chromosome: not just her brother's keeper. Nat Genet 2005;37:343-5.

109. Muller JL, Mahadevaiah SK, Park PJ, Warburton PE, Page DC, Turner JM. The mouse X chromosome is enriched for multi-copy testis genes showing postmeiotic expression. Nat Genet 2008;40:794-9.

110. Rice WR. Sex chromosomes and evolution of sexual dimorphism. Evolution 1984;38:735-42.

111. Rice WR. Sexually antagonistic genes: experimental evidence. Science 1992;256:1436-9.

112. Perrin A, Douet-Guilbert N, Le Bris MJ, Keromnes G, Langlois ML, Barriere P, et al. Segregation of chromosomes in sperm of a t(X;18)(q11;p11.1) carrier inherited from his mother: case report. Hum Repro 2008;23:227-30.

113. Matsuda Y, Hirobe T, Chapman VM. Genetic basis of X-Y-chromosome dissociation and male sterility in interspecific hybrids. Proc Natl Acad Sci USA 1991;88:4850-4.

114. Hale DW, Washburn LL, Eicher EM. Meiotic abnormalities in hybrid mice of the C57BL/6J x Mus spretus cross suggest a cytogenetic basis for Haldane's rule of hybrid sterility. Cytogenet Cell Genet 1993;63:221-34.

115. Miklos GLG. Sex-chromosome pairing and male fertility. Cytogenet Cell Genet 1974;13:558-77.

116. Schultz N, Hamra FK, Garbers DL. A multitude of genes expressed solely in meiotic or postmeiotic spermatogenic cells offers a myriad of contraceptive targets. Proc Natl Acad Sci USA 2003;100:12201-6.

117. Choi E, Lee J, Park I, Han C, Yi C, Kim do H, et al. Integrative characterization of germ cell-specific genes from mouse spermatocyte UniGene library. BMC Genomics 2007;8:256.

118. Hong S, Choi I, Woo JM, Oh J, Kim T, Choi E, et al. Identification and integrative analysis of 28 novel genes specifically expressed and developmentally regulated in murine spermatogenic cells. J Biol Chem 2005;280:7685-93.

119. Xiao P, Tang A, You Z, Cai A. Gene expression profile of 2058 spermatogenesis-related genes in mice. Biol Pharm Bull 2008;31:201-6.

120. Dover G. Molecular drive: a cohesive mode of species evolution. Nature 1982;299:111-7.

121. Henikoff S, Ahmad K, Malik HS. The centromere paradox: stable inheritance with rapidly evolving DNA. Science 2001;293: 1098-1102.

35

The Biological Clock of Male Fertility

Fábio Firmbach Pasqualotto, Eleonora Bedin Pasqualotto

ABSTRACT

Couples are waiting longer to have children, and advances in reproductive technology are allowing older men and women to consider having children. The lack of appreciation among both medical professionals and the lay public for the reality of a male biological clock makes these trends worrisome. The age-related changes associated with the male biological clock affect sperm quality, fertility, hormone levels, libido, erectile function, and a host of non-reproductive physiological issues. The effects of paternal age on a couple's fertility are real and may be greater than has previously been thought. Age is a further factor to be taken into account when deciding the prognosis for infertile couples.

Cellular aging can manifest itself at several levels. Changes to mitochondria are among the most remarkable features observed in aging cells and several theories place mitochondria at the hub of cellular events related to aging, namely in terms of the accumulation of oxidative damage to cells and tissues, a process in which these organelles may play a prominent role, although alternative theories have also emerged. Furthermore, mitochondrial energy metabolism is also crucial for male reproductive function and mitochondria may therefore constitute a common link between aging and fertility loss.

Recent reports have raised concern about decreasing male fertility caused by genomic abnormalities. There are reports of increased congenital anomalies and testicular cancer in children. Sperm DNA is known to contribute one half of the genomic material to offspring. Thus, normal sperm genetic material is required for fertilization, embryo and fetal development and postnatal child well being. The abnormality or defect in the genomic material may take the form of condensation or nuclear maturity defects, DNA breaks or DNA integrity defects and sperm chromosomal aneuploidy. Fathering at older ages may have significant effects on the viability and genetic health of human pregnancies and offspring, primarily as a result of structural chromosomal aberrations in sperm.

INTRODUCTION

Approximately 15 percent of couples of reproductive age experience infertility, and approximately one-third to half of infertility cases may be attributed to male factors.[1] It is well-known that maternal age is a significant contributor to human infertility,[2] due primarily to the precipitous loss of functional oocytes in women by their late thirties.[3] Human spermatogenesis, on the other hand, continues well into advanced ages, allowing men to reproduce during senescence. Although very little is known about the topic, paternal age may also contribute to human infertility.

In contrast to the female, male reproductive functions do not cease abruptly, but androgen production and spermatogenesis continue lifelong. However, to evaluate a possible decline in the semen quality is a little bit difficult. Some men are reluctant to provide semen samples unless actively concerned about their fertility. For instance, population based studies typically recruit at least 20 percent of young men willing to provide semen samples[4,5] constituting an inevitable participation bias in such studies.[6,7] In addition, the majority of the published studies about sperm output in older men are largely restricted to patients attending infertility clinics, where few are older than 50 years.[8] An uncertain, but probably high proportion of such men have unrecognized defects in sperm production and/or function. Furthermore, access to such specialized medical services may be strongly influenced by non-biological factors, and the results from infertility clinics may not be reliably extrapolated to the general male population.

Anyway, the effects of paternal age on a couple's fertility are real and may be greater than has previously been thought. Ford et al. stated that, after adjustments for other factors, the probability that a fertile couple will take >12 months to conceive nearly doubles from 8 percent when the man is <25 years to 15 percent when he is >35 years; thus paternal age is a further factor to be taken into account when deciding the prognosis for infertile couples.[9]

To explain the age-dependent changes observed in semen quality two issues should be considered.[8-11] First, cellular or physiological changes due to aging have been described in testicles, seminal vesicles, prostate and epididymis. Age-related narrowing and sclerosis of the testicular tubular lumen, decreases in spermatogenic activity, increased degeneration of germ cells, and decreased numbers and function of Leydig cells have been found in autopsies of men who died from accidental causes.[12] Smooth muscle atrophy and a decrease in protein and water content, which occur in the prostate with aging, may contribute to decreased semen volume and sperm motility. Also, the epididymis, a hormonally sensitive tissue, may undergo age-related changes. The hormonal or epididymal senescence may lead to decreased motility in older men. Secondly, increasing age implies more frequent exposure to exogenous damage or disease.[8] In addition to age per se, factors such as urogenital infections, vascular diseases or an accumulation of toxic substances (cigarettes) may be responsible for worsening semen parameters. Indeed, a retrospective cross-sectional study in 3698 infertile men showed an infection rate of the accessory glands in 6.1 percent in patients aged <25 years but in 13.6 percent of patients >40 years, and total sperm counts were significantly lower in patients with an infection of the accessory glands.[13] In addition, an age-dependent increase of polychlorinated biphenyls (PCB) in men has been described and in men with normal semen parameters the PBC concentration is inversely correlated with sperm count and progressive motility.[14] The concentration of cadmium also increases with age in the human testis, epididymis and prostate, although lead and selenium remain constant over the whole age range in reproductive organs.[15,16]

Handelsman and Staraj demonstrated that, after exclusion of men with different diseases associated with diminishing testicular size, the specific effects of age on testicular volume appears only in the 8th decade of life.[17] In healthy men of this age group, the testis volume is 31 percent lower than in 18–40 year old men.[18] However, recently a study showed a decline in testicular volume over time, specially after the age of 45 years old.[19]

Morphological characteristics of aging testes vary from Sertoli cells accumulating cytoplasmic lipid droplets and are reduced in number,[20] to Leydig cells[21] undergoing the same changes and possibly being multinucleated.[22] Tubule involution is associated with an enlargement of the tunica propria, leading to progressive sclerosis parallel to a reduction of the seminiferous epithelium with complete tubular sclerosis as an endpoint.[23] Testicular sclerosis is associated with defective vascularization of the testicular parenchyma and with systemic arteriosclerosis of affected men.[24] Arteriographic patterns of the epididymis and the testes support these findings and are correlated with the degree of systemic arteriosclerosis.[24] In addition, age-dependent alterations of the prostate are well-known[25] and are detectable histologically in 50 percent of 50-year-old men, but in 90 percent of men aged >90 years.[26]

SEMEN ANALYSIS

Considering the age-dependent changes in reproductive organs of men, variations in semen parameters over time are not surprising; however, only few studies are controlled for abstinence time and other possible factors that may influence semen quality such as hypertension or smoking habits. Most studies are retrospective and rarely include males more than 60 or 70-years-old. Pasqualotto et al. recently described a decrease in semen volume across the groups evaluated in the study.[19] In fact, reports in the literature have shown a decrease in semen volume with aging.[8,27,28] The higher number of days' abstinence in men over 50 years old could explain these results. In the studies where the analyses were adjusted for days' abstinence, a decrease in semen volume of 3–22 percent was observed.[9]

Regarding sperm motility, many studies adjusted for time of abstinence found a significant decrease in sperm motility associated with age and a yearly decrease ranging between 0.17[29] and 0.7 percent.[30] However, these studies were performed in sperm donors[29-32] as well as in infertile patients.[33,34] Pasqualotto et al. are on the same page as others showing that sperm motility tends to decrease as time goes by. Those studies that have been adjusted for duration of abstinence have reported statistically significant effects, such as negative linear relationships and decreases in motility ranging from 0.17–0.6 percent for each year of age.[8,29,35,36]

A computer-assisted semen analysis (CASA) has been developed as a specific tool to make the assessment of semen quality more objective and detailed.[37] Several specific motility parameters describing the movements of spermatozoa in a more detailed manner can be obtained with CASA. In addition, the classification into motile and immotile spermatozoa can be based on well-defined velocity thresholds. However, no correlations are detected between specific motion parameters as evaluated with CASA and the aging effect in the study by Pasqualotto et al.[19]

When focusing on sperm concentration, abstinence-adjusted studies do not provide a uniform picture. Even though some studies have reported a decrease in sperm concentration with increased age, several other studies have reported an increase in sperm concentration with age or found little or no association between age and sperm concentration.[9,11,35,38] In fact, there are two different populations that we have to consider before evaluating the results: fertile versus infertile men. A significant age-dependent decrease[30,32] as well as constant values over the age range[31] or even a non-significant age-dependent increase with age[29] has been detected in healthy men. Regarding the infertile population, sperm concentration increases[33,34] or remains unaltered,[13] as indicated in abstinence-adjusted studies.

One of the good indicators of the germinal epithelium status is the sperm morphology. Degenerative changes in the germinal epithelium because of aging may affect spermatogenesis and thus sperm morphology. Pasqualotto et al., based on a linear regression analysis, stated that normal sperm morphology tends to decrease by 0.039 percent each year.[19] Auger et al. in a linear regression model, have shown that the normal sperm morphology decreases 0.9 percent yearly.[32] Thus, as compared to the average 30-year-old man, an average 50-year-old had a 18 percent decrease in normally shaped sperm.[33] Ng et al. showed that older men had more abnormal sperm morphology with decreasing numbers of normal forms and reduced vitality, as well as increased numbers of cytoplasmic droplets and sperm tail abnormalities (30 versus 17%) compared to younger men.[28] The aberrant sperm morphology in older men was most evident in defects of tail morphology, possibly reflecting the complex cellular structural assembly process of the axoneme. Such increasing proportion of defects may reflect degenerative changes with aging in the germinal epithelium and/or in the intrinsic program directing spermiogenesis. In fact, the decrease per year varies from 0.2[36] to 0.9 percent.[32]

All reported changes of histological and seminal parameters develop gradually without a sudden age threshold. The alterations in semen parameters fall within normal ranges. Nevertheless, the age-dependent alterations of testicular histology and semen parameters are accompanied by a significant increase in follicle-stimulating hormone (FSH)[19,39] and a slight but significant decrease in inhibin B,[18,40] which are also found in men with apparently normal semen parameters.

SPERM DNA DAMAGE

Understanding the effects of male age on sperm DNA damage is especially relevant for men attending reproductive clinics because of the increasing reliance on modern technologies, especially among marginally fertile older men. Intracytoplasmic sperm injection (ICSI) and *in vitro* fertilization (IVF) enhance the probability of achieving fatherhood, yet they also circumvent the natural barriers against fertilization by damaged sperm.

Schmid et al. demonstrated an association between male age and sperm DNA strand damage in a non-clinical sample of active healthy non-smoking workers and retirees.[41] Sperm of older men had significantly higher frequencies of sperm with DNA damage measured under alkaline conditions, which is thought to represent alkalilabile DNA sites and single-strand DNA breaks. However, age was not associated with sperm DNA damage under neutral conditions, which is thought to represent double-strand DNA breaks. The observations of differential effects of age on genomic damage is consistent with the recent finding of Wyrobek et al. who reported age-related effects on DNA fragmentation and achondroplasia mutations but not aneuploidy, Apert syndrome mutations or sex ratio.[42]

The finding of age-related increases in DNA strand damage under alkaline conditions is consistent with the findings of Morris and colleagues who studied 60 men participating in an IVF program.[43] They reported that sperm DNA damage was positively correlated with donor age and with impairment of post-fertilization embryo cleavage following ICSI, indicating an overall decline in the integrity of sperm DNA in older men. The findings by Schmid et al. of no association between age and sperm DNA damage under neutral conditions is in contrast with the study of Singh and colleagues, who studied 66 men, aged 20–57 years, from an infertility clinic and a non-clinical group.[41] However, Singh et al.[44] did not investigate sperm DNA damage under alkaline conditions in sperm, and Morris et al. did not investigate sperm damage under neutral conditions.[43] Using a different assay for measuring DNA strand damage in sperm, the sperm chromatin structure assay (SCSA), Spano et al.[45] found a strong association of DNA fragmentation index (DFI) with age among men aged 18–55 years old, a finding confirmed by Wyrobek et al.[42] using a larger group of men that spanned 20–80 years of age.

Older men may produce more sperm with DNA damage as a consequence of age-associated increased oxidative stress in their reproductive tracts.[46,47] Oxidative stress can damage sperm DNA as well as mitochondrial and nuclear membranes.[48,49] Kodama et al. reported an association between oxidative DNA damage in sperm and male infertility.[49] Alternatively, apoptotic functions of spermatogenesis may be less effective in older males resulting in the release of more sperm with DNA damage.[50,51] While apoptosis has been identified in the testes of elderly men, there have been no comparisons on rates of apoptosis among men of different ages.[50] Increased sperm DNA damage has been associated with chromosomal abnormalities, developmental loss and birth defects in mouse model systems[51,52] and with increases in the percentage of human embryos that failed to develop after ICSI.[49]

Increasing oxidative stress levels associated with aging might be responsible for this increase in DNA damage with age.[53] Oxidative stress-mediated DNA damage may be an etiology for repeated assisted reproductive technology failures in older men. Increasing male age may have an influence on DNA fragmentation in the form of single-strand breaks. This may not have any effect on fertilization because the oocyte can repair single-strand breaks. However, if the oocyte repair mechanisms are dysfunctional, this may result in poor, if not failed, blastocyst formation. Thus, oxidative stress-induced DNA damage can lead to various genomic defects.[54,55] Therefore, reactive oxygen species (ROS) might play a central role in decreased male fertility with aging.[56-58] This hypothesis provides guidance for future study and experiments, focusing on specific biomarkers of aging in men (telomere function, lipofuscin, amyloid) and their comparison with semen parameters and male fertility.

Also, there are some conditions that may affect the elderly, such as chronic use of alcohol and cigarette smoking, as well as some medications.

ALCOHOL

Long-term effects of chronic alcohol use include erectile dysfunction, reduced libido, and gynecomastia.[59] One mechanism of these effects is a reduction in serum testosterone caused by decreased testicular production and increased metabolic clearance in the liver. It is thought that alcoholism and hepatic cirrhosis cause alterations in the hypothalamic pituitary gonadal (HPG) axis, resulting in testicular dysfunction. In addition, the oxidation of alcohol competes with testicular production of testosterone. These mechanisms lead to subsequent decrease in semen volume and sperm density. Another factor appears to be an elevation in serum estrogen caused by peripheral conversion of testosterone to estrogen through increased activity of the enzyme aromatase, which is present both in the liver and in peripheral fat cells.[60]

"Social" or light alcohol ingestion does not appear to interfere with semen quality.[61] However, excessive acute alcohol intake does have adverse effects on male fertility by causing decreased serum testosterone concentrations. Impairment of spinal reflexes, also caused by excessive alcohol abuse, leads to reduced sensation and innervation of the penis, and thus may also contribute to erectile dysfunction.[59]

CIGARETTE SMOKING

Many studies have examined the effects of cigarette smoking on fertility, and cumulative evidence suggests that it has a significant negative impact on sperm production, motility, and morphology.[61,62] Several reports demonstrated that the mutagenic and carcinogenic components of cigarette smoke have adverse effects on rapidly dividing cells, including germ cells in the testis.[63] However, recently we observed that no differences were seen in testicular volume, FSH and testosterone levels, sperm concentration, motility and morphology in a population of fertile patients who smoke or drink coffee compared to patients that do not have these habits.[64]

Animal studies have show that nicotine, cigarette smoke, and/or polycyclic aromatic hydrocarbons can cause testicular atrophy, poor sperm morphology, and overall impaired spermatogenesis, leading to the presence of oligospermia and teratospermia (<4% normal sperm forms). Serum levels of prolactin and estradiol (E2) are also elevated in smokers. This was most pronounced in smokers who had low sperm counts compared to smokers who had normal sperm counts. E2 impairs spermatogenesis via several different mechanisms, including alteration of the HPG axis. Studies have also shown that elevated E2 levels can cause increased catecholamine levels, which in turn can produce ischemia of the seminiferous tubules. While the exact mechanism for the apparent elevation in E2 in smokers is unknown, it appears to be due to increased production of this hormone rather than to decreased metabolic clearance.

It has been reported that cigarette smoking causes increased serum levels of norepinephrine, which in turn can increase aromatization of testosterone to E2 in Sertoli cells *in vitro*.[65] While it is unclear exactly how smoking directly affects spermatogenesis, overwhelming evidence suggests that it has an unfavorable impact on fertility. Thus, every effort should be made to counsel both partners to stop the use of tobacco as part of their infertility treatment.

■ ILLICIT DRUGS

Several illicit drugs are detrimental to male fertility and should be avoided, especially in men trying to establish a pregnancy.[66] Marijuana interferes with spermatogenesis by decreasing sperm density and motility and would not increasing the number with morphologic abnormalities[67] be a good thing rather than an interference. High doses of opiates lead to a decline in libido and erectile function. Opiates suppress the luteinizing hormone (LH) and luteinizing hormone releasing factor (LH-RH), leading to a decline in testosterone production. The pituitary gland itself may also be directly suppressed by opiates. High doses of cocaine impair erectile function, and high doses of amphetamines have been shown to cause diminished libido.[61]

■ ANTIHYPERTENSIVES

While medical treatment of hypertension is important, urologists treating male infertility must be knowledgeable about the agents that cause the most significant impairments in testicular function.[61,66] While fertility remains desirable, men using these medications can often be switched to another class of antihypertensive medications while attempting pregnancy.

Most antihypertensive agents exert a deleterious effect on fertility by impairing sexual function. However, it is important to keep in mind that hypertension occurs more commonly in the older population, a group known to have a higher incidence of erectile dysfunction in general. The use of antihypertensives in conjunction with vascular insufficiency may exacerbate inadequate blood flow to the male genitals.[67]

Diuretics such as the thiazides decrease blood flow to the penis by reducing vascular resistance.[61,66] Propranolol has been noted to cause a decrease in both libido and erectile function.[61,66,67] Cardioselective agents such as atenolol and metoprolol appear to have less deleterious effects on male sexual function. Vasodilators themselves do not inhibit sexual function because they do not interfere with sympathetic reflexes. However, they are often used in conjunction with blockers and diuretics that do affect potency and libido. Efforts should be made to refer patients back to their clinicians to change B-blockers to other agents such as angiotensin converting enzyme (ACE) inhibitors.

Due to its effect on the HPG axis, spironolactone may cause profound fertility problems. This agent also prevents the binding of dihydrotestosterone (DHT) to its receptor and inhibits the production of testosterone, which may result in reduced libido, erectile dysfunction, and significantly decreased sperm production.[61,67]

■ CALCIUM CHANNEL BLOCKERS

Calcium influx is critical for the normal acrosome reaction to occur.[68] Thus, calcium channel blocking (CaCB) medications have recently received particular attention as potential inhibitors of the normal fertilization process. The calcium influx required during the acrosome reaction may be impaired directly by the effects of CaCBs or by insertion of the CaCBs into the plasma membrane of the sperm head. This insertion causes an alteration in the surface molecules expressed on the sperm head that are also required for normal fertilization to occur.[68,69]

Clinical studies have shown that cessation of the CaCB may reverse this process and restore the fertility in some otherwise infertile men. Other reports, however, have failed to show any adverse effect of CaCBs on male fertility.[70] While the effects of CaCBs on male fertility remain unclear, it may be prudent to discuss a switch to another antihypertensive agent with patients who are taking these medications and who desire fertility.

■ α-ADRENERGIC BLOCKERS

Agents such as alfuzosin, tamsulosin, terazosin, and doxazosin are commonly prescribed for the treatment of benign prostatic hyperplasia, and are also used in younger men with voiding complaints. They function by blocking the motor sympathetic adrenergic nerve supply to the prostate, resulting in a reduction in urethral pressure.[70] Differences in affinity for the α-receptor subtypes determine the side-effect profile for the individual agents.

The more selective α-blocking agents, by reducing smooth muscle tone at the bladder neck, can cause retrograde ejaculation.[61] While patients tend to better tolerate and are more compliant with alfuzosin and tamsulosin than doxazosin, terazosin, and prazosin, retrograde ejaculation is more commonly associated with tamsulosin, occurring in about 8.5 percent of men. While ganglion blockers (methyldopa, guanethidine, and reserpine) can have similar side effects on male sexual function, they are rarely used clinically.[71]

ANGIOTENSIN CONVERTING ENZYME INHIBITORS

Agents such as captopril and enalapril have not been associated with male sexual dysfunction or infertility, nor have direct vaso-dilators effects such as hydralazime and minoxidil.[61]

PSYCHOTHERAPEUTIC AGENTS

These agents exert much of their effect on male fertility by inhibiting sexual function and libido.

ANTIPSYCHOTICS

Most antipsychotics block dopamine in the central nervous system (CNS), leading to suppression of the HPG axis and decreased libido. Some antipsychotics agents also have α-adrenergic blocking agents that block innervation of the internal genital organs. In addition, some are vasodilators that can redirect blood away from the penis and cause erectile dysfunction. It is important to realize, however, that antipsycothics can bring about important changes in overall well-being that may far outweigh any of the deleterious effects above.[59,67]

TRICYCLIC ANTIDEPRESSANTS

The use of tricyclic antidepressants or selective serotonin reuptake inhibitors (SSRIs) can lead to erectile dysfunction and reduced libido through their anticholinergic and sedative side effects.[61,59,67] They have also been shown to impair ejaculation. Because these agents cause a delay in ejaculation, they have been used to treat men with premature ejaculation.

Perhaps the most significant side effect of antidepressants, however, is the potential for substantial elevation in serum prolactin concentrations. Hyperprolactinemia suppresses secretion of gonadotropin releasing hormone (GnRH) from the hypothalamus and the high prolactin levels inhibit LH from binding to Leydig cells in the testes. These actions lead to significant but reversible suppression of spermatogenesis. If fertility is desired, the initial treatment of hyperprolactinemia caused by antidepressant use is a change to another class of medication. However, if this is not possible, cabergoline or bromocriptine can be administered.

OTHER PSYCHOTHERAPEUTIC AGENTS

Phenothiazines can cause hyperprolactinemia and negatively affect male fertility in the same way as tricyclic antidepressants, thus, treatment is similar.[66,67] Monoamine oxidase inhibitors, another prominent class of antidepressants, can cause erectile dysfunction or ejaculatory problems. Finally, lithium carbonate has been shown to decrease the action of dopamine in the CNS, causing decreased libido and potency.

Testosterone Production

With the increasing availability of safe, well-tolerated treatment methods, testosterone replacement therapy has become more common in clinical medicine. However, the use of exogenous androgens impairs spermatogenesis by inhibiting the HPG axis.[59,61,67] Testosterone is also converted to estrogen in peripheral fat cells by the enzyme aromatase, increasing the negative feedback on the HPG axis. In men with decreased serum testosterone concentrations who wish to remain fertile, testosterone replacement in its various forms should not be used. An alternative in younger men with decreased serum testosterone concentrations is treatment with gonadotropins (such as hCG) or with the centrally-acting antiestrogen, clomiphene citrate. This agent has the advantage of being available in an oral form, while human chorionic gonadotropin (hCG) requires repeated subcutaneous feedback inhibition. However, both of these treatments will improve serum and intratesticular testosterone concentrations without decreasing gonadotropin levels through feedback inhibition.

OTHER HORMONAL THERAPIES

Estrogens have been used in the past to treat advanced prostate cancer in men. Effects on sexual function include decreased libido, feminization, erectile dysfunction and testicular atrophy. Finasteride is frequently used by men of reproductive age for its preventative effects on male-pattern baldness.[72] While the use of this medication could conceivably alter intratesticular testosterone concentrations, there appears to be no evidence for any alteration in semen quality.

Saw palmetto is a commonly used herbal agent for symptoms of bladder outlet obstruction. While its mechanisms of action are largely unknown, it appears that it may exert some of its beneficial effect through slight estrogenic activity or by blocking the conversion of testosterone to DHT.[73,74] While these effects could theoretically impair sperm production or function, no studies have yet been performed to evaluate this.

FERTILITY OF AGING MEN

Without any type of doubt, male fertility is basically maintained until very late in life, and it has been documented scientifically up to more than 90 years old.[74] Besides female age, further confounders, such as reduced coital frequency, an increasing incidence of erectile dysfunction and smoking habits have to be considered in studies analyzing male fertility. All studies focused on a non-clinical population found a significant negative relationship between male age and couples' fertility.

A retrospective study of a large sample of European couples analyzed the risk of difficulties (due to adverse pregnancy outcome, such as ectopic pregnancy, miscarriage or stillbirth or due to delayed conception) and the risk of delay in pregnancy onset.[75] Age-related changes were also found in a prospective study that estimated day-specific probabilities for pregnancy relative to ovulation.[76] Frequency of sexual intercourse was monitored by sexual diaries and ovulation was based on basal body temperature measurements. According to this study, fertility for men aged >35 years is significantly reduced and the age effect of men aged 35–40 years is about the same as when intercourse frequency drops from twice per week to once per week.[77] In studies dealing with subfertile couples, a significant decrease in pregnancy rates[33] or increase in time to get pregnant (TTP)[78] were observed with female but not with male age, possibly indicating that male age-dependent alterations are masked by the infertility as such.

With methods of assisted reproduction, prerequisites for natural conception such as motility or fertilizing capacity are circumvented. In fact, the more invasive the treatment, the less important male age appears. Therefore, the success rates of ICSI[79] or IVF[80-82] are not associated with male age. On the other hand, the success rate of intrauterine insemination (IUI), a method requiring much higher quality and capability of sperm, is without question related to male age.[83,84]

Genetic Risks of the Aging Male

A maternal age effect has been found for all trisomy conditions but varies among chromosomes, with an exponential increase of chromosome 21 and a linear increase, for instance, for chromosome 16.[85] Early observations also associate paternal age with certain syndromes.[86] Meanwhile it has become evident that some mutations, consisting of single base substitutions in three different genes: FGFR2 (fibroblast growth factor receptor 2) and FGFR3 (fibroblast growth factor receptor 3), are exclusively of paternal origin and may increase with male age.[87]

A possible explanation for this male-specific age effect is the much higher number of germ cell divisions in males than in females: in the fetal ovary, germ cells undergo 22 mitotic divisions before they enter the meiotic prophase.[88] They remain in meiotic arrest and continue meiosis in adulthood when ovulation has taken place. Thus, while it was formerly believed that in women germ cell divisions are completed before birth, a recent publication suggests that adult mouse ovaries still possess mitotically active germ cells.[89]

On the other hand, male germ cells divide continuously. It has been estimated that 30 spermatogonial stem cell divisions take place before puberty, when they begin to undergo meiotic divisions. From then on, 23 mitotic divisions per year occur, resulting in 150 replications by the age of 20 years and 840 replications by the age of 50 years.[87] Therefore, due to these numerous divisions of stem cells, older men may have an increased risk of errors in DNA transcription. Consequently, the association between elevated paternal age and serious birth defects is the reason why the age of semen donors is limited to 40 years in certain countries.[90,91] On the other hand, male age is not an indicator for prenatal diagnosis.

■ NUMERICAL CHROMOSOME DISORDERS

Aneuploidy, the presence of an extra or missing chromosome, is the leading genetic cause of pregnancy loss. Aneuploidies are detected in 35 percent of spontaneous abortions, in 4 percent of stillbirths and in 0.3 percent of live births.[92] Among spontaneous abortions, Turner's syndrome (45,X) and trisomy 16, 21 and 22 are the most prevalent aneuploidies. In general, aneuploidies arise by the process of non-disjunction, for instance, the failure of paired chromosomes to separate in the first meiotic division of maternal meiosis.[93,94] Sperm reveal an aneuploidy incidence of 2 percent with a high variability of disomy frequency of individual sperm from different fluorescence *in situ* hybridization (FISH) studies.[93] The disomy frequency was calculated to be 0.26 percent for the sex-chromosomes and 0.15 percent for the autosomes with an exception for chromosomes 14, 21 and 22 which display higher disomy frequencies.[95]

Studies analyzing the age-dependent alteration of aneuploidy frequency in chromosomes are highly limited due to low case numbers. Interestingly, the age-dependent increase of XY disomy was also detected in sperm from fathers of boys with Klinefelter's syndrome,[96-98] irrespective of paternal or maternal inheritance of the extra X-chromosome.[30] Fifty percent of Klinefelter's syndrome cases are of paternal origin and other gonosomal aneuploidies are even more often paternally inherited in live births, as are 80 percent of Turner's syndrome cases (45,X) and 100 percent of XYY karyotypes.[99] However, none of these syndromes is related to paternal age.[99] Similarly, the incidence of autosomal aneuploidies, such as trisomy 13, 16 and 18, is independent of paternal age.[98,100] Therefore, the paternal age effect for trisomy 21 remains to be elucidated.

Early studies with small sample sizes reflect different results in the same study population depending on the method of statistical analysis.[100,101] In spontaneous abortions a non-significant paternal age effect was detected[102] and in live births, no age effect[102,103] or a significant paternal age effect[104,105] were evident. It should be kept in mind that only 10 percent of Down's syndrome patients receive the excess chromosome from their father,[106] so that an age effect could be confined to this small category of cases and subtle age effects might go undetected unless those derived paternally are considered separately. However, with respect to paternally inherited Down's syndrome cases, no paternal age effect became evident.[107] Paternal age effect was seen in association with a maternal age lower than 35 years, so that a paternal age effect in aged couples can no longer be neglected concerning trisomy 21, whereas other autosomal or sex chromosomal aneuploidies are not associated with increased paternal age.[104]

Structural Chromosomal Anomalies

Structural chromosomal anomalies result from chromosomal breakage and the following abnormal rearrangement within the same or within different chromosomes. In 84 percent of cases, *de novo* structural aberrations are of paternal origin[108] and they are found in 2 percent of spontaneous abortions and in 0.6 percent of live births.[109] Cytogenetic studies on structural chromosomal anomalies in sperm are rare but consistently describe an increase of mutations with age.[110]

FISH was used for the structural analysis of individual chromosomes: duplications and deletions for the centromeric and subtelomeric regions of chromosome 9 increase significantly with age.[111] In spite of these age-dependent structural alterations in sperm, no increase of *de novo* structural chromosomal anomalies has been detected in newborns from older fathers.[107]

Autosomal Dominant Diseases

Achondroplasia, the most common form of dwarfism, is the first genetic disorder that was hypothesized to have a paternal age component.[86] Apert's syndrome and achondroplasia have been amenable to direct sperm DNA mutation analysis[112,113] and both are characterized by an age-dependent increase of mutations in sperm, but there are some peculiarities. For sporadic cases of Crouzon's or Pfeiffer's syndrome, 11 different mutations of the FGFR 2 gene are responsible, indicating that, unlike Apert's syndrome or achondroplasia, these are genetically heterogeneous conditions.[114] These mutations also arise in the male germ line and advanced paternal age was noted for fathers of those patients.

The relationship between mutation frequency and paternal age is heterogeneous among autosomal dominantly inherited diseases.[115] In contrast to the above-mentioned diseases, osteogenesis imperfecta, neurofibromatosis or bilateral retinoblastoma show a weak paternal age effect.[116] This may be due to the fact that a significant fraction of new mutations are not base substitutions.[87] Many of the mutations of the neurofibromatosis gene are intragenic deletions. These deletions are not age-dependent because they occur by mechanisms other than the base substitutions and are maternally derived in 16 of 21 cases.[117]

Due to this heterogeneity of the paternal age effect in autosomal dominant diseases, the risk estimates proposed by Friedman for paternal age and autosomal dominant mutations may be overestimated.[118] Friedman calculated a risk for autosomal dominant diseases of 0.3–0.5 percent among offspring of fathers aged >40 years. This risk is comparable with the risk of Down's syndrome for 35–40 year old women. However, the calculation was based on the assumption that the paternal age effect found in achondroplasia is typical of all autosomal dominant diseases.

There are conflicting data for Alzheimer's disease. Few studies conclude that paternal age is a risk factor.[119] However, the inconsistent results may be due to small sample sizes of the studies or due to the genetic heterogeneity of the disease.

Regarding schizophrenia, there are more conclusive data. In fact, the studies identified an increased risk of schizophrenia with paternal age.[120] Patients without a family history of schizophrenia had significantly older fathers than familial patients, so that de novo mutations were considered responsible.[121] Pre-eclampsia, which is considered to be a risk factor for schizophrenia, is also associated with paternal age.[122]

One very important point we should never forget is that advanced paternal age increases the risk of other cancers in offspring. According to the Swedish Family-Cancer Database,

there is an effect of paternal age on the incidence of sporadic breast and sporadic nervous system cancer in offspring.[123] Interestingly, an association between paternal age and the son's risk of prostate cancer was found.[124] The association of paternal age with early onset prostate cancer (<65 years) was greater than that with late onset.

CONCLUSION

Although based on a small number of cases, the data presented for testicular morphology, semen parameters and fertility in aging males are conclusive and reflect a gradual deterioration with age within a broad individual spectrum. Most studies suggest that reduced fertility begins to become evident in the late thirties in men. Increased male age is associated with an increased risk of miscarriages and both the risk of infertility and the risk of miscarriage strongly depend on female age. Advancing paternal age is associated with an increased risk for trisomy 21 and with diseases of complex etiology such as schizophrenia.

Couples should be aware of these age-dependent alterations in fertility and predisposition to genetic risks. Although at the moment increased paternal age is not an indication for prenatal diagnosis, there may be further developments in the future.

REFERENCES

1. Templeton A. Infertility-epidemiology, etiology and effective management. Health Bull (Edinb) 1995;53(5):294-8.
2. Joffe M, Li Z. Male and female factors in fertility. Am J Epidemiol 1995;141(11):1107-8.
3. Lansac J. Delayed parenting. Is delayed childbearing a good thing? Hum Reprod 1995;10(5):1033-5.
4. Lubna P, Santoro N. Age-related decline in fertility. Endocrinol Metab Clin N Am 2003;32:669-88.
5. Jensen TK, Jorgensen N, Punab M, Haugen TB, Suominen J, Zilaitiene B, Horte A, Andersen AG, Carlsen E, Magnus O, et al. Association of *in utero* exposure to maternal smoking with reduced semen quality and testis size in adulthood: a cross-sectional study of 1770 young men from the general population in five European countries. Am J Epidemiol 2004;159:49-58.
6. Handelsman DJ. Sperm output of healthy men in Australia: magnitude of bias due to self-selected volunteers. Hum Reprod 1997;12:2701-5.
7. Cohn BA, Overstreet JW, Fogel RJ, Brazil CK, Baird DD, Cirillo PM. Epidemiologic studies of human semen quality: considerations for study design. Am J Epidemiol 2002;155:664-71.
8. Kidd SA, Eskenazi B, Wyrobek AJ. Effects of male age on semen quality and fertility: a review of the literature. Fertil Steril 2001;75:237-48.
9. Ford WCL, North K, Taylor H, Farrow A, Hull MGR, Golding J and the ALSPAC Study Team. Increasing paternal age is associated with delayed conception in a large population of fertile couples: evidence for declining fecundity in older men. Hum Reprod 2000;15:1703-8.
10. Eskenazi B, Wyrobek AJ, Sloter E, Kidd SA, Moore L, Young S, Moore D. The association of age and semen quality in healthy men. Hum Reprod 2003;18:447-54.

11. Hassan MAM, Killick SR. Effect of male age on fertility: evidence for the decline in male fertility with increasing age. Fertil Steril 2003;79:1520-7.

12. Neaves WB, Johnson L, Porter JC, Parker CR, Petty S. Leydig cell numbers, daily sperm production and serum gonadotropin levels in aging men. J Cl Endocrinol Metab 1984;59:756-63.

13. Rolf C, Kenkel S, Nieschlag E. Age-related disease pattern in infertile men: increasing incidence of infections in older patients. Andrologia 2002;34:209-17.

14. Dallinga JW, Moonen EJ, Dumoulin JC, Evers JL, Geraedts JP, Kleinjans JC. Decreased human semen quality and organochlorine compounds in blood. Hum Reprod 2002;17:1973-99.

15. Oldereid NB, Thomassen Y, Attramadal A, Olaisen B, Purvis K. Concentrations of lead, cadmium and zinc in the tissues of reproductive organs of men. J Reprod Fertil 1993;99:421-55.

16. Oldereid NB, Thomassen Y, Purvis K. Selenium in human male reproductive organs. Hum Reprod 1998;13:2172-6.

17. Handelsman DJ, Staraj S. Testicular size: the effects of aging, malnutrition, and illness. J Androl 1985;6:144-51.

18. Mahmoud AM, Goemaere S, El-Garem Y, Van Pottelbergh I, Comhaire FH, Kaufman JM. Testicular volume in relation to hormonal indices of gonadal function in community-dwelling elderly men. J Clin Endocrinol Metab 2003;88:179-84.

19. Pasqualotto FF, Sobreiro BP, Hallak J, Pasqualotto EB, Lucon AM. Sperm concentration and normal sperm morphology decrease and follicle-stimulating hormone level increases with age. BJU International 2005;96:1087-91.

20. Harbitz TB. Morphometric studies of the Sertoli cells in elderly men with special reference to the histology of the prostate. Acta Pathol Microbiol Scand Sect A Pathol 1973;81:703-17.

21. Johnson L. Spermatogenesis and aging in the human. J Androl 1986;7:331-54.

22. Paniagua R, Amat P, Nistal M, Martin A. Ultrastructure of Leydig cells in human aging testes. J Anat 1986;146:173-83.

23. Paniagua R, Nistal M, Amat P, Rodriguez MC, Martin A. Seminiferous tubule involution in elderly men. Biol Reprod 1987;36:939-47.

24. Regadera J, Nistal M, Paniagua R. Testis, epididymis, and spermatic cord in elderly men. Correlation of angiographic and histologic studies with systemic arteriosclerosis. Arch Pathol Lab Med 1985;109:663-7.

25. Hermann M, Untergasser G, Rumpold H, Berger P. Aging of the male reproductive system. Exp Gerontol 2000;35:1267-79.

26. Coffey DS, Berry SJ, Ewing LL. An overview of current concepts in the study of benign prostate hyperplasia. In: Rodgers CH, Coffey DS, Cunha G, Grayhack JT, Hinman F, Horton R (Eds) Benign Prostatic Hyperplasia, Vol II. NIH publication No. 1987;2881.pp.1-13.

27. Kühnert B, Nieschlag E. Reproductive functions of the aging male. Hum Reprod Update 2004;10:327-39.

28. Ng KK, Donat R, Chan L, Lalak A, Di Pierro I, Handelsman DJ. Sperm output of older men. Hum Reprod 2004;8:1811-5.

29. Fisch H, Goluboff ET, Olson JH, Feldshuh J, Broder SJ, Barad DH. Semen analysis in 1,283 men from the United States over a 25-year period: no decline in quality. Fertil Steril 1996;65:1009-14.

30. Eskenazi B, Wyrobek AJ, Kidd SA, Lowe X, Moore D 2nd, Weisiger K, Aylstock M. Sperm aneuploidy in fathers of children

with paternally and maternally inherited Klinefelter syndrome. Hum Reprod 2002;17:576-83.

31. Schwartz D, Mayaux MJ, Spira A, Moscato ML, Jouannet P, Czyglik F, David G. Semen characteristics as a function of age in 833 fertile men. Fertil Steril 1983;39:530-5.

32. Auger J, Kunstmann JM, Czyglik F, Jouannet P. Decline in semen quality among fertile men in Paris during the past 20 years. N Engl J Med 1995;332:281-5.

33. Rolf C, Behre HM, Nieschlag E. Reproductive parameters of older couples compared to younger men of infertile couples. Int J Androl 1996;19:135-42.

34. Andolz P, Bielsa MA, Vila J. Evolution of semen quality in Northeastern Spain: a study in 22759 infertile men over a 36 year period. Hum Reprod 1999;14:731-5.

35. Berling S, Wolner-Hanssen P. No evidence of deteriorating semen quality among men in infertile relationships during the last decade: a study of males from southern Sweden. Hum Reprod 1997;12:1002-5.

36. Carlsen E, Giwercman A, Keiding N, Skakkebaek NE. Evidence for decreasing quality of semen during past 50 years. BMJ 1992;305:609-13.

37. Agarwal A, Ozturk E, Loughlin KR. Comparison of semen analysis between the two Hamilton-Thorn semen analysers. Andrologia 1992;24:327-9.

38. Hommonai ZT, Fainman N, David MP, Paz GF. Semen quality and sex hormone pattern of 29 middle aged men. Andrologia 1982;14:164-70.

39. Nieschlag E, Lammers U, Freischem CW, Langer K, Wickings EJ. Reproductive functions in young fathers and grandfathers. J Clin Endocrinol Metab 1982;55:676-81.

40. Baccarelli A, Morpurgo PS, Corsi A, Vaghi I, Fanelli M, Cremonesi G, Vaninetti S, Beck-Peccoz P, Spada A. Activin A serum levels and aging of the pituitary–gonadal axis: a cross-sectional study in middle-aged and elderly healthy subjects. Exp Gerontol 2001;36:1403-12.

41. Schmid TE, Eskenazi B, Baumgartner A, Marchetti F, Young S, Weldon R, Anderson D, Wyrobek AJ. The effects of male age on sperm DNA damage in healthy non-smokers. Hum Reprod 2007;22(1):180-7.

42. Wyrobek AJ, Evenson D, Arnheim N, Jabs EW, Young S, Pearson F, Glasser RLF, Thiegmann I, Eskenazi B. Advancing male age increase the frequencies of sperm with DNA fragmentation and certain gene mutations, but not aneuploidies or diploidies. Proc Natl Acad Sci USA 2006;103(25):9601-6.

43. Morris ID. Sperm DNA damage and cancer treatment. Int J Androl 2002;25(5):255-61.

44. Singh NP, Muller CH, Berger RE. Effects of age on DNA doublestrand breaks and apoptosis in human sperm. Fertil Steril 2003;80(6):1420-30.

45. Spano M, Kolstad AH, Larsen SB, Cordelli E, Leter G, Giwercman A, Bonde JP. The applicability of the flow cytometric sperm chromatin structure assay in epidemiological studies. Hum Reprod 1998;13(9):2495-2505.

46. Barnes CJ, Hardman WE, Maze GL, Lee M, Cameron IL. Age-dependent sensitization to oxidative stress by dietary fatty acids. Aging (Milano) 1998;10(6):455-62.

47. Barroso G, Morshedi M, Oehninger S. Analysis of DNA fragmentation, plasma membrane translocation of phosphatidylserine

and oxidative stress in human spermatozoa. Hum Reprod 2000;15(6):1338-44.

48. Aitken RJ, Baker MA, Sawyer D. Oxidative stress in the male germ line and its role in the etiology of male infertility and genetic disease. Reprod Biomed Online 2003;7(1):65-70.

49. Kodama H, Yamaguchi R, Fukuda J, Kasai H, Tanaka T. Increased oxidative deoxyribonucleic acid damage in the spermatozoa of infertile male patients. Fertil Steril 1997;68(3):519-24.

50. Brinkworth MH, Weinbauer GF, Bergmann M, Nieschlag E. Apoptosis as a mechanism of germ cell loss in elderly men. Int J Androl 1997;20(4):222-8.

51. Print CG, Loveland KL. Germ cell suicide: new insights into apoptosis during spermatogenesis. Bioessays 2000;22(5):423-30.

52. Marchetti F, Lowe X, Bishop J, Wyrobek J. Induction of chromosomal aberrations in mouse zygotes by acrylamide treatment of male germ cells and their correlation with dominant lethality and heritable translocations. Environ Mol Mutagen 1997;30:410-7.

53. Marchetti F, Bishop JB, Cosentino L, Moore D II, Wyrobek AJ. Paternally transmitted chromosomal aberrations in mouse zygotes determine their embryonic fate. Biol Reprod 2004;70:616-24.

54. Barratt CLR, Aitken J, Bjorndahl L, Carrell DT, de Boer P, Kvist U, Lewis SEM, Perreault SD, Perry MJ, Ramos L, Robaire B, Ward S, Zini A. Sperm DNA: organization, protection and vulnerability: from basic science to clinical applications—a position report. Human Reproduction 2010;25(4):824-38.

55. Desai N, Sabanegh E Jr, Kim T, Agarwal A. Free Radical Theory of Aging: Implications in Male Infertility. Urology 2010;75(1):14-9.

56. Pasqualotto FF, Sharma RK, Nelson DR, Thomas AJ Jr, Agarwal A. Relationship between oxidative stress, semen characteristics and clinical diagnosis in men undergoing infertility investigation. Fertil Steril 2000;73:459-64.

57. Pasqualotto FF, Sharma RK, Kobayashi H, Nelson DR, Thomas AJ Jr, Agarwal A. Oxidative stress in normospermic men undergoing fertility evaluation. J Androl 2001;22:316-22.

58. Sharma RK, Pasqualotto FF, Nelson DR, Thomas AJ Jr, Agarwal A. ROS-TAC is a novel marker of oxidative stress. Hum Reprod 1999;14:2801-7.

59. Buffum J. Pharmacosexology: the effects of drugs on sexual function a review. J Psychoactive Drugs 1983;14:5-44.

60. Purohit V. Can alcohol promote aromatization of androgens to estrogens? A review. Alcohol 2000;22(3):123-7.

61. Monoski M, Nudell DM, Lipshultz LI. Effects of medical therapy, alcohol, and smoking on male fertility. Contemporary Urology June 2002.pp.57-63.

62. Pasqualotto FF, Sobreiro BP, Hallak J, Pasqualotto EB, Lucon AM. Cigarette smoking is related to a decrease in semen volume in a population of fertile men. British Journal of Urology 2006;97:324-6.

63. Stillman RJ, Rosemberg MJ, Sachs BP. Smoking and reproduction. Fertil Steril 1986;46(4):545-66.

64. Lucon AM, Pasqualotto FF, Peng BC, Hallak J, Arap S. Do tobacco and caffeine impair semen characteristics in men with fertility proved? [Abstract 1394]. J Urol 2002;167(4):351.

65. Klaiber EL, Broverman DM. Dynamics of estradiol and testosterone and seminal fluid indexes in smokers and nonsmokers. Fertil Steril 1988;4:630-4.

66. Thompson ST. Prevention of male infertility: an update. Urol Clin North Am 1994;21(3):365-76.

67. Buffum J. Pharmacosexology update: prescription drugs and sexual function. J Psychoactive Drugs 1986;18(2):97-106.

68. Hershlag A, Cooper GW, Benoff S. Pregnancy following discontinuation of a calcium channel blocker in the male partner. Hum Reprod 1995;10(3):599-606.

69. Benoff S, Jacob A, Hurley I. Male infertility and environmental exposure to lead and cadmium. Hum Reprod Update 2000;6:107-21.

70. Katsoff D, Check JH. A challenge to the concept that the use of calcium channel blockers causes reversible male infertility. Hum Reprod 1997;12(7):1480-2.

71. Debruyne FM. Alpha blockers: are all created equal? Urology 2000;56:20-2.

72. Overstreet JW, Fuh VL, Gould J, Howards SS, Lieber MM, Hellstrom W, et al. Chronic treatment with finasteride daily does not affect spermatogenesis or semen production in young men. J Urol 1999;162(4):1295-1300.

73. Marks LS, Partin AW, Epstein JI, Tyler VE, Simon I, Macairan ML, et al. Effects of a saw palmetto herbal blend in men with symptomatic benign prostatic hyperplasia. J Urol 2000;163(5):1451-6.

74. Seymour FI, Duffy C, Koerner A. A case of authenticated fertility in a man, aged 94. J Am Med Assoc 1935;105:1423-4.

75. De la Rochebrochard E, Thonneau P. Paternal age and maternal age are risk factors for miscarriage; results of a multicentre European study. Hum Reprod 2002;17:1649-56.

76. Dunson DB, Colombo B, Baird D. Changes with age in the level and duration of fertility in the menstrual cycle. Hum Reprod 2002;17:1399-1403.

77. Dunson DB, Baird DD, Colombo B. Increased infertility with age in men and women. Obstet Gynecol 2004;103:51-6.

78. Olson J. Subfecundity according to the age of the mother and the father. Dan Med Bull 1990;37:281-2.

79. Spandorfer SD, Avrech OM, Colombero LT, Palermo GD, Rosenwaks Z. Effect of parental age on fertilization and pregnancy characteristics in couples treated by intracytoplasmic sperm injection. Hum Reprod 1998;13:334-8.

80. Piette C, de Mouzon J, Bachelot A, Spira A. In-vitro fertilization: influence of women's age on pregnancy rates. Hum Reprod 1990;5:56-9.

81. Gallardo E, Simón C, Levy M. Effect of age on sperm fertility potential: oocyte donation as a model. Fertil Steril 1996;66:260-4.

82. Paulson RJ, Milligan RC, Sokol RZ. The lack of influence of age on male fertility. Am J Obstet Gynecol 2001;184:818-22.

83. Mathieu C, Ecochard R, Bied V, Lornage J, Czyba JC. Cumulative conception rate following intrauterine artificial insemination with husband's spermatozoa: influence of husband's age. Hum Reprod 1995;10:1090-7.

84. Brzechffa PR, Buyalos RP. Female and male partner age and menotrophin requirements influence pregnancy rates with human menopausal gonadotrophin therapy in combination with intrauterine insemination. Hum Reprod 1997;12:29-33.

85. Wyrobek AJ, Aardema M, Eichenlaub-Ritter U, Ferguson L, Marchetti F. Mechanisms and targets involved in maternal and paternal age effects on numerical aneuploidy. Environ Mol Mutagen 1996;28:254-64.

86. Penrose LS. Parental age and mutation. Lancet 1955;269:312-3.

87. Crow JF. The origins, patterns and implications of human spontaneous mutation. Nat Rev Genet 2000;1:40-7.

88. Drost JB, Lee WR. Biological basis of germline mutation: comparisons of spontaneous germline mutation rates among drosophila, mouse, and human. Environ Mol Mutagen 1995;25(Suppl 26):48-64.

89. Johnson J, Canning J, Kaneko T, Pru JK, Tilly JL. Germline stem cells and follicular renewal in the postnatal mammalian ovary. Nature 2004;428:145-50.

90. American Society for Reproductive Medicine. Guidelines for therapeutic donor insemination: sperm. Fertil Steril 1998;70(Suppl 3):1S-3S.

91. British Andrology Society. British Andrology Society guidelines for the screening of semen donors for donor insemination. Hum Reprod 1999;14:1823-6.

92. Hassold T, Hunt P. To err (meiotically) is human: the genesis of human aneuploidy. Nat Rev Genet 2001;2:280-91.

93. Griffin DK. The incidence, origin, and etiology of aneuploidy. Int Rev Cytol 1996;167:263-96.

94. Eichenlaub-Ritter U. Parental age-related aneuploidy in human germ cells and offspring: a story of past and present. Environ Mol Mutagen 1996;28:211-36.

95. Shi Q, Martin RH. Aneuploidy in human sperm: a review of the frequency and distribution of aneuploidy, effects of donor age and lifestyle factors. Cytogenet Cell Genet 2000;90:219-26.

96. Lowe X, Eskenazi B, Nelson DO, Kidd S, Alme A, Wyrobek AJ. Frequency of XY sperm increases with age in fathers of boys with Klinefelter syndrome. Am J Hum Genet 2001;69:1046-54.

97. Lorda-Sanchez I, Binkert F, Maechler M, Robinson WP, Schinzel AA. Reduced recombination and paternal age effect in Klinefelter syndrome. Hum Genet 1992;89:524-30.

98. Hatch M, Kline J, Levine B, Hutzler M, Wartburton D. Paternal age and trisomy among spontaneous abortions. Hum Genet 1990;85:355-61.

99. Bordson BL, Leonardo VS. The appropriate upper age limit for semen donors: a review of the genetic effects of paternal age. Fertil Steril 1991;56:397-401.

100. Stene E, Stene J, Stengel-Rutkowski S. A reanalysis of the New York State prenatal diagnosis data on Down's syndrome and paternal age effects. Hum Genet 1987;77:299-302.

101. Hook EB, Cross PK. Paternal age and Down's syndrome genotypes diagnosed prenatally: no association in New York state data. Hum Genet 1982;62:167-74.

102. De Michelena MI, Burstein E, Lama JR, Vasquez JC. Paternal age as a risk factor for Down syndrome. Am J Med Genet 1993;45:679-82.

103. Stoll C, Alembik Y, Dott B, Roth MP. Study of Down syndrome in 238942 consecutive births. Ann Genet 1998;41:44-51.

104. Fisch H, Hyun G, Golden R, Hensle TW, Olsson CA, Liberson GL. The influence of paternal age on Down syndrome. J Urol 2003;169:2275-8.

105. McIntosh GC, Olshan AF, Baird PA. Paternal age and the risk of birth defects in offspring. Epidemiology 1995;6:282-8.

106. Hassold T, Sherman S. Down syndrome: genetic recombination and the origin of the extra chromosome 21. Clin Genet 2000;57:95-100.

107. Hook EB, Regal RR. A search for a paternal-age effect upon cases of 47, þ 21 in which the extra chromosome is of paternal origin. Am J Hum Genet 1984;36:413-21.

108. Olsen SD, Magenis RE. Preferential paternal origin of de novo structural chromosome rearrangements. In: Daniel A (Ed). The Cytogenetics of Mammalian Autosomal Rearrangements. Alan R. Liss, New York 1988.pp.583-99.

109. Jacobs PA. The chromosome complement of human gametes. Oxf Rev Reprod Biol 1992;14:47-72.

110. Sartorelli EM, Mazzucatto LF, de Pina-Neto JM. Effect of paternal age on human sperm chromosomes. Fertil Steril 2001;76:1119-23.

111. Bosch M, Rajmil O, Martinez-Pasarell O, Egozcue J, Templado C. Linear increase of diploidy in human sperm with age: a four-color FISH study. Eur J Hum Genet 2001;9:533-8.

112. Glaser RL, Broman KW, Schulman RL, Eskenazi B, Wyrobek AJ, Jabs EW. The paternal-age effect in Apert syndrome is due, in part, to the increased frequency of mutations in sperm. Am J Hum Genet 2003;73:939-47.

113. Goriely A, McVean GA, Rojmyr M, Ingemarsson B, Wilkie AO. Evidence for selective advantage of pathogenic FGFR2 mutations in the male germ line. Science 2003;301:643-6.

114. Glaser RL, Jiang W, Boyadjiev SA, Tran AK, Zachary AA, Van Maldergem L, Johnson D, Walsh S, Oldridge M, Wall SA, et al. Paternal origin of FGFR2 mutations in sporadic cases of Crouzon syndrome and Pfeiffer syndrome. Am J Hum Genet 2000;66:768-77.

115. Risch N, Reich EW, Wishnick MM, McCarthy JG. Spontaneous mutation and parental age in humans. Am J Hum Genet 1987;41:218-48.

116. Sivakumaran TA, Ghose S, Kumar HAS, Kucheria K. Parental age in Indian patients with sporadic hereditary retinoblastoma. Ophthal Epidemiol 2000;7:285-91.

117. Lazaro C, Gaona A, Ainsworth P, Tenconi R, Vidaud D, Kruyer H, Ars E, Volpini V, Estivill X. Sex differences in the mutation rate and mutational mechanism in the NF gene in neurofibromatosis type 1 patients. Hum Genet 1996;98:696-9.

118. Friedman JM. Genetic disease in the offspring of older fathers. Obstet Gynecol 1981;57:745-9.

119. Bertram L, Busch R, Spiegl M, Lautenschlager NT, Müller U, Kurz A. Paternal age is a risk factor for Alzheimer disease in the absence of a major gene. Neurogenetics 1998;1:277-80.

120. Dalman C, Allebeck P. Paternal age and schizophrenia: further support for an association. Am J Psychiatry 2002;159:1591-2.

121. Malaspina D, Corcoran C, Fahim C, Berman A, Harkavy-Friedman J, Yale S, Goetz D, Goetz R, Harlap S, Gorman J. Paternal age and sporadic schizophrenia: evidence for de novo mutations. Am J Med Genet 2002;114:299-303.

122. Harlap S, Paltiel O, Deutsch L, Knaanie A, Masalha S, Tiram E, Caplan LS, Malaspina D, Friedlander Y. Paternal age and pre-eclampsia. Epidemiology 2002;13:660-7.

123. Hemminki K, Kyyronen P. Parental age and risk of sporadic and familial cancer in offspring: implications for germ cell mutagenesis. Epidemiology 1999;10:747-51.

124. Zhang Y, Kreger BE, Dorgan JF, Cupples LA, Myers RH, Splansky GL, Schatzkin A, Ellison RC. Parental age at child's birth and son's risk of prostate cancer. The Framingham Study. Am J Epidemiol 1999;150:1208-12.

36

Ethical Dilemma in Infertility

Pasquale Patrizio, Marcia C Inhorn

INTRODUCTION

Infertility is defined as the inability to conceive after a year of regular unprotected intercourse and in about 50 percent of the cases, the male is identified as responsible for the reproductive failure,[1] either exclusively (about 30%) or coresponsible (about 20%).[2]

Physicians who care for infertile couples must thus know how to perform a basic evaluation of the male reproductive function and, furthermore, need to recognize men who require more extensive evaluation by fertility specialists. The initial screening relies on at least two semen analyses performed at six week intervals. Of note, although far from being ideal, the results of the semen analyses are still universally used as indicators of male fertility. Currently, the reference values for normal males include a minimum volume of 2.0 mL, a pH between 7.2–7.8, a concentration of 20×10^6 spermatozoa/mL or greater, and a total sperm number of at least 40×10^6 spermatozoa per ejaculate.[2] Additional parameters are motility of 50 percent or more, vitality of at least 50 percent, and white blood cell counts of fewer than 1×10^6/mL. Sperm morphology is also considered part of the standard semen analysis and can be assessed according to the WHO manual or to strict criteria. In absence of an absolute specific value, it is accepted that as normal-sperm morphology falls below 30 percent, the rate of *in vitro* fertilization (IVF) decreases.

Although it is widely recognized that a number of causes are responsible for male infertility, a considerable percentage of cases are still of unknown etiology. Summary of the most commonly known causes of male infertility, reported according to the results of the semen analysis and categorized into four groups:

1. Azoospermia, which means no sperm in the ejaculate, affecting 25 percent of infertile males.
2. Oligoasthenozoospermia, which means low sperm count and low motility, affecting 60 percent of infertile males.
3. Teratozoospermia, which means all sperm are non-viable or with severe abnormal morphology, affecting 5 percent of infertile males.
4. Coital factors, including men with paraplegia, men with retroperitoneal lymph node dissection because of prostatic cancer, and men with retrograde ejaculation, together affecting 10 percent of infertile males.

The field of male infertility, as with the corresponding female counterpart, is constantly developing policies and guidelines to preserve the desire for paternity and the methods available to maintain reproductive options. These strategies are subject to ethical debates. Some of these ethical debates have been inspired by the increasing survival rates of patients stricken by cancers during their reproductive years. Fertility preservation by sperm banking is a reasonable and effective option for men requiring chemotherapy or radiation treatment and can serve as a 'backup' in the event that spermatogenesis does not rebound after treatment. However, it is important to discuss, at the time of sperm banking, the directives for disposal of the specimens, should a patient die. Equally important to recognize are experimental approaches versus established practices, particularly when children are the subjects of research studies aimed at protecting their future reproductive options.

The ethical dilemmas discussed in this chapter are:

- The use of donor sperm and its associated paternal ambivalence, especially for men from particular religious traditions
- Transmission through intracytoplasmic sperm injectiojn (ICSI) of male infertility and other genetic anomalies to offspring of genetically infertile men;
- Disclosing donor sperm identities to the future offspring
- The number of offspring that each sperm donor should be allowed to sire
- Issues surrounding fertility preservation, including in children with cancer
- Issues surrounding posthumous procreation (i.e. children from dead fathers).

USE OF DONOR SPERM TO PROCREATE

Thanks to the 1991 advent of ICSI for the treatment of infertile males with very low sperm counts and motility, the requests for donor sperm insemination (DI) have been drastically reduced. For example, in 1987 there were about 170,000 recorded donor inseminations per year, but in 2004 there were only 80,000 inseminations with donor sperm, or less than half.[3] Nonetheless, these 2004 figures translate into about 30,000 births per year due to DI.

The practice of DI raises a number of ethical issues:

- How do religious restrictions on DI affect infertile male patients' decisions?

- What should be offered to infertile men whose religion prohibits DI?
- Should disclosure to children conceived with donor sperm be optional or mandatory?
- Should there be a maximum number of pregnancies achieved by the same donor?

How do Religious Restrictions on DI Affect Infertile Male Patients' Decisions?

Two of the major monotheistic religious traditions, namely Catholicism and Sunni Islam, have formally opposed DI. Within the Catholic Church, the opposition to DI is part of the Church's doctrine opposing *all* forms of reproductive technology (including contraception and abortion). With regard to DI and other forms of assisted reproductive technology (ART), the Catholic Church's disapproval is based on the disassociation of procreation from sex, both of which are intended to occur only within the holy covenant of matrimony. According to the Catholic doctrine of "natural law," no artificial barriers or aids to conception are to be used during the procreative act. Replacing loving intercourse with the masturbation and surgical procedures required in IVF will necessarily erode marital unity.[4] A life that is created by medical practitioners—rather than through an act of conjugal love between two married people—"establishes the domination of technology over the origin and destiny of the human person".[5] The technology of DI, therefore, threatens the unity of marriage; IVF physicians themselves become "third parties" to a marriage, intruding into the marital functions of sex and procreation.

Similarly, all forms of third-party donation—of eggs, sperm, embryos, or uteri, as in surrogacy—are seen as "offenses" to the conjugal unity of the couple, introducing an "emotional and spiritual wedge between husband and wife both symbolized by and enacted in sexual infidelity".[6] In this regard, the Catholic Church's opposition to ARTs and the practice of third-party donation has resulted in legal bans in some Catholic countries. For example, ARTs are outlawed altogether in Costa Rica, and the 2004 Vatican-inspired "Medically Assisted Reproduction Law" in Italy prohibits the use of third-party gamete donation (eggs, sperm, embryos) and surrogacy.[7] Thus, Catholic men who follow Church doctrine closely may reject DI as a solution to male infertility.

Similarly, more than half of the world's population of nearly 80 million infertile people is estimated to live in Muslim countries, where, for the most part, third-party donation, including DI, is strictly prohibited.[8] In the Muslim world, attitudes toward family formation are closely tied to religious teachings that stress the importance of "purity of lineage".[9] Islam is a religion that privileges—even mandates—biological descent and inheritance. Preserving the "origins" of each child, meaning his or her relationships to a known biological mother and father, is considered not only an ideal in Islam, but a moral imperative.[10] In Islamic *fiqh* (jurisprudence), the tie by *nasab* (that is, filiation, lineage, relations by blood) is considered to be one of God's great gifts to his worshippers. The preservation of *nasab* is emphasized

through Qur'anic rules designed to ensure the sanctity of the family and the society; by preserving *nasab*, personal and social immorality are prevented, thus leading to the maintenance of society as a whole.[11]

In the face of such religious edicts, the concept of "social parenthood"—of either an adopted or donor child—is considered untenable in most of the Muslim world.[12] The vast majority of infertile Muslim men do not accept the idea of DI as a solution to their childlessness. Sperm donation is seen as particularly abhorrent. Men's moral concerns revolve around four sets of related issues.[13]

With regard to the first issue, Islam is a religion that can be said to privilege—even mandate—heterosexual marital relations. Reproduction outside of marriage is considered *zina*, or adultery, which is strictly forbidden in Islam. Although DI does not involve the sexual body contact ("touch or gaze") of adulterous relations, nor presumably the desire to engage in an extramarital affair, it is nonetheless considered by most Islamic religious scholars to be a form of adultery, by virtue of introducing a third party into the sacred dyad of husband and wife. It is the very fact that another man's sperm enter a place where they do not belong that makes DI inherently wrong and threatening to the marital bond.

The second aspect of third-party donation that troubles marriage is the potential for incest among the offspring of anonymous donors. If an anonymous sperm donor "fathers" hundreds of children, the children could grow up, unwittingly meet each other, fall in love and marry. Thus, moral concerns have been raised about the potential for incest to occur among sperm donor children who are biological half-siblings.

A third moral concern has to do with issues of family incest, or how parents and donor children should comport themselves in daily family life. To wit, a donor child is *halal*, or religiously permitted to marry a person who is not related by blood ties. Thus, feelings of attraction might develop between donor parents and their non-biologically-related offspring, especially in the intimate conditions of household life, where individuals are revealed to each other. An infertile father who is not biologically related to a donor daughter could, theoretically, marry her when she reaches the age of maturity. Thus, in Muslim family life, proper comportment would have to revolve around the diminution of erotic feelings toward a donor child. This would complicate matters such as bathing, praying, veiling, and all matters pertaining to "touch and gaze."

The final moral concern voiced by Muslim men is that third-party donation confuses issues of kinship, descent, and inheritance. As with marriage, Islam is a religion that can be said to privilege—even mandate—biological inheritance. Preserving the *nasab* of each child—meaning its genealogical relationship to a known biological father and mother—is considered not only an ideal in Islam, but a moral imperative. The problem with third-party donation, therefore, is that it destroys a child's *nasab* and violates the child's legal rights to known parentage, which is considered immoral, cruel, and unjust.

Muslim men use the term "mixture of relations" (*ikhtilat il-ansab*) to describe this untoward outcome. Such a mixture of relations, or the literal confusion of lines of descent introduced by third-party donation, is described as being very "dangerous," "forbidden," "against nature," "against God"—in a word, *haram,* or morally unacceptable. It is argued that donation, by allowing a "stranger to enter the family," confuses lines of descent in Islamic societies. For men in particular, ensuring paternity and the "purity" of lineage through "known fathers" is of paramount concern. This is because most Muslim societies are organized patrilineally—that is, descent and inheritance are traced through fathers and the "fathers of fathers" through many generations. Thus, knowing paternity is of critical concern.[14]

Mothers, too, share kinship relations with their children through gestation and especially the sharing of milk through breastfeeding (often thought of as "milk kinship"). However, descent itself is traced through the patriline, flowing through males to successive generations. Thus, sperm donation in particular threatens not only a child's *nasab*, but a man's patrilineage. Not surprisingly, then, Muslim men feel strongly about the importance of patriliny and paternity, claiming that a sperm donor child "won't be my son."[15] Coupled with men's feelings that such children are created through *zina*, or adultery—"It's as if my wife slept with another man!"—the child conceived through sperm donation is considered to be of questionable moral character. Together, questions of *nasab* and *zina* lead to strong rejection of sperm donation.

Bringing such donor children into the world is considered unfair to the children themselves, who would never be treated with the love and concern parents feel for their "real" children. Such a child could only be viewed as a bastard—a *walad il-zina,* "a child of illicit sex," or an *ibn haram,* literally "son of the forbidden." Thus, a child of third-party donation starts its life off as an "illegal" child. It is deemed illegitimate and stigmatized even in the eyes of its own parents, who will therefore lack the appropriate parental sentiments.

As a result, the vast majority of Muslims, of both the Sunni (90%) and Shia (10%) branches of Islam, reject DI out of hand. Although the Supreme Leader of the Islamic Republic of Iran, Ayatollah Ali Husayn Al-Khamene'i, allowed sperm donation for his followers as of 1999, sperm donation is not a popular option, even in the ayatollah's own country of Iran.[16] This is partly because Ayatollah Khamene'i deemed naming, inheritance, and biological descent to rest with the sperm donor, not the infertile man. The problems of naming and inheritance are critical in understanding Iranian men's aversions to DI. As shown by anthropologist Soraya Tremayne, Iranian men who have chosen to use donor sperm may later regret their decisions, taking out their angst and anger on hapless wives and donor children.[17] Furthermore, the Royan Institute, one of the major ART research centers in Tehran, has conducted survey research on attitudes toward sperm donation among infertile men.[18] Despite Ayatollah Khamene'i's approval of sperm donation, Iranian men continue to be morally ambivalent about the practice, finding it much less acceptable than either egg or embryo donation. At the time of this writing, Iran has outlawed sperm donation and encourages embryo donation, but both practices—as well as egg donation and gestational surrogacy—continue to be practiced in the country.[19] In the rest of the Muslim world (which stretches

from Morocco to Malaysia), sperm donation is practiced only in Lebanon, but there, too, it meets with ardent resistance on the part of most men.[20]

What Should be Offered to Infertile Men Whose Religion Prohibits DI?

Given the resistance to DI in most Muslim countries, and in some Catholic countries as well, clinicians must respect men's moral concerns, instead of attempting to convince religiously pious patients to "accept" DI when they register their religious opposition. Instead, ICSI can be offered to infertile men as a treatment, as long as viable spermatozoa are found in the ejaculate or through testicular aspiration or biopsy. Unfortunately, ICSI is not always successful, especially in cases of severe male-factor infertility and among men with non-obstructive azoospermia (i.e., no spermatozoa found in the testis). High rates of non-obstructive azoospermia are found among Arab including Arab-American men. These non-obstructive azoospermia cases may be due to three major causes:

1. Undescended testicles which are not surgically corrected early in a male infant's life
2. Genetic causes, which may be linked to high rates of consanguineous marriage in the region[21]
3. Cancer treatment in which male fertility preservation through semen collection prior to chemotherapy or radiation therapy is not offered.

Due to advances in the field of genetics, it is now realized that a significant percentage of male infertility cases, particularly those that are severe, are due to genetic abnormalities. Indeed, "a virtual explosion in the identification of genes affecting spermatogenesis has occurred" in recent years.[22] A variety of abnormalities in both the Y and X chromosomes, as well as genetic abnormalities of the hypothalamic-pituitary-gonadal axis involved in the production of reproductive hormones, are now well-established causes of male infertility.[23] Probably the most frequent genetic cause of infertility in men involves microdeletions of the long arm of the Y chromosome, which are associated with spermatogenic failure.[24] In men with such Y microdeletions, the spermatozoa will always be infertile, because these genetic alterations are incurable and will be present throughout a man's lifetime.[25] Such deletions are manifest in a variety of sperm defects, including defects of the sperm head (e.g., round heads, heads with craters) and sperm tail (e.g., stunted, immotile, or detached tails).

If most male infertility is, indeed, genetically based, then the use of ICSI as the major technological solution to overcome male infertility problems is also ethically questionable.[26] Through the use of ICSI, genetic defects of sperm will be transferred to male offspring, who will also be infertile. Conceiving infertile male offspring will thus require the intervention of ICSI generation after generation.[27] To prevent this from happening, some IVF practitioners and ethicists are recommending the "culling" of all male embryos in severe male infertility cases, before they are ever implanted. This way, only female offspring, who do not carry the Y-chromosome, are born to such infertile men.[28] This may be ethically sensitive in Muslim and other societies (e.g., South and East Asia) where male heirs are highly desired.

Ideally, in all cases of severe male-factor infertility, genetic counseling prior to initiation of ICSI is highly desirable. Unfortunately, across the Middle East, genetic screening and counseling are still in their infancy. However, the need for genetic medicine in association with fertility medicine across the Middle East is clear. In one Turkish study—which showed relatively high frequencies of both chromosomal abnormalities and Y-chromosome microdeletions in a genetic survey of 1,935 Turkish men—the authors advised "the need for genetic screening and proper genetic karyotyping before initiation of assisted reproduction treatment".[29]

Should Disclosure to Children Conceived with Donor Sperm be Optional or Mandatory?

The resistance to DI described above—and men's desire to use ICSI even in the face of genetic male infertility—are not unique to Muslim societies. Even though DI is the "oldest" ART—having been practiced in the United States and Europe for nearly a century[30]—anthropologists have revealed the stigma and secrecy incumbent in this practice.[31] In the West, men seem to have less trouble donating sperm—usually for a nominal fee—than "accepting" it from another man. In order to accept DI, infertile men must find ways to reframe their sense of fatherhood, convincing themselves that they are able to feel deep love for individuals who are not biologically related to them.

Moreover, infertile men and their spouses must make difficult decisions regarding donor disclosure. For example, should friends and family be notified that a child is the product of sperm donation? Should parents disclose this information to a donor child, and at what point in the child's life? Do a child's rights to medical knowledge trump parental desires for secrecy? As shown in anthropologist Gay Becker's work on DI in the United States, "to tell or not to tell" becomes a major ethical dilemma in the local moral worlds of infertile American men and their wives.[32] Some couples choose absolute secrecy, while others deem disclosure necessary to prevent dishonesty and deception. In some cases, couples choose the path of least resistance by "delaying" the decision indefinitely.

In the United States, most, if not all, sperm bank and DI programs offer to recipients the option of using "open identity" donors (i.e., donors who consent to have their identities revealed to a future child resulting from the use of their sperm). In other countries such as Sweden and the UK,[33] recipients are required to use open identity donors. An immediate consequence of open identity donation has been a sharp decrease in the availability of donors. In addition, there has been a shift in the characteristics of men donating sperm: they are older with families of their own, and have become more aware of the consequences of their "donation" and are accepting this increased responsibility.

An important factor in deciding whether donor anonymity should be removed is the well-being of the child. For parents who plan to tell their child about his or her conception, having as much information as possible may help answer a child's

questions as they arise. For example, about half the children in a sample of lesbian-headed families wanted more information about their donor.[34]

Testimonials from DI youth and adults who learned of their origins before adulthood also indicate that individuals feel less resentment toward their family, but the desire and need to know more about the donor remains.[35] However, some have argued that, for the well-being of the children, disclosure should be mandatory and that children resulting from gamete donation should be compared to children from adoption (who are almost universally told of their origins). At the moment, however, there is no conclusive evidence to support forced disclosure and, furthermore, it is incorrect to compare the practice of gamete donation as being identical to adoption. With sperm donation, one of the parents—the mother—is the biological parent, while the father is the social parent. With adoption, both parents are social parents.

Furthermore, if a policy requiring disclosure is to be truly effective, various conditions must be satisfied. These include:

- A couple willing to reveal the origin of the gametes to their offspring
- A donor who is willing to donate his spermatozoa knowing that he may be later identified
- A system of enforcement to ensure that the couple will reveal the source of the gametes (perhaps through the use of a special notation on the birth certificate)
- Health providers who will restrict reproductive services only to couples who agree to sign a consent for disclosure
- Assurance that the provider of obstetric care, usually a different physician, is informed by the couple of the means by which reproduction was achieved and is made aware of the existence of consent to disclose in order to complete the birth certificate. This list, by no means complete, makes the issue of disclosure quite complicated. Furthermore, forcing potential parents to tell their child of his/her genetic origin as a requirement for admission into an infertility program is discriminatory.[36]

Actually, forcing disclosure instead of protecting the child's best interests has the risk of not creating a child at all, since potential parents and clinics may find the burden of controlling disclosure too heavy to overcome and forgo the process altogether. In countries where the identification of the donor is required by law, namely, Netherlands and Sweden, the pool of sperm donors has substantially decreased. Many clinics have ceased operations or have such long waiting lists that couples are giving up.

Despite this concern, the UK passed legislation in April 2005 that imposes mandatory disclosure for donor sperm. As a result of donors' unwillingness to be identified, there has been a marked reduction in the frequency of sperm donations and inseminations. For example, a BBC survey in September 2006 found that 90 percent of UK sperm donors were recruited in just 10 of 87 licensed clinics for DI and that after the removal of donor anonymity, the cost of purchasing sperm rose very substantially—about an eight-fold increase. Between 2004 and 2006, there was a 30 percent reduction in patients requiring DI, but a much larger reduction, about 45 percent, in the number of treatment cycles. A recent survey of DI services by the British Fertility Society found that:

- 37 percent of clinics are finding it harder to recruit donors
- 94 percent of clinics are finding it harder to purchase donor sperm
- 89 percent charge more for treatment because of the increased cost of the sperm they are able to purchase
- 74 percent of clinics have increased their waiting lists for DI treatment
- 86 percent of clinics are able to offer less donor choice and are only able to match for racial group alone
- 60 percent of clinics have introduced rationing of treatment cycles
- 9 percent have closed their DI services.

The impact of the legislation to remove donor anonymity has confirmed those concerns expressed by the opponents of a mandatory disclosure law. A possible solution to this problem would be to review and amend the current legislation to give donors the choice of:

- Retaining complete anonymity
- Disclosing non-identifying information only
- Becoming identifiable in the way the law currently requires. Couples needing DI treatment would then, at the very least, have the choice of deciding whether they really want sperm from a donor who is prepared to be identified in the future.

Should There be a Maximum Number of Pregnancies Achieved by the Same Donor?

It is very important to maintain detailed medical records of the number of pregnancies for which a given donor is responsible and to try to establish a limit. It is difficult, however, to provide a precise number of times that a given donor can be used, because one must take into consideration the population base from which the donor is selected and the geographic area that may be served by a given donor. According to American Society for Reproductive Medicine (ASRM) guidelines, it has been suggested that in a population of 800,000, limiting a single donor to no more than 25 births would avoid any significant increased risk of inadvertent consanguineous conception.[37] This suggestion may require modification if the population using DI represents an isolated subgroup or if the specimens are distributed over a wide geographic area. In the future, keeping in mind the issues of patient confidentiality, providers of reproductive care and sperm banks should devise a data base tracking system to avoid the recruitment of the same sperm donor in excess of the limit set for pregnancies within a particular geographic area. This, however, is a very difficult task.

■ FERTILITY PRESERVATION

The contemporary use of powerful chemotherapeutic and radiotherapy protocols are procuring the cure, or significantly extending the survival, of many patients with cancer. As a result of this progress, quality-of-life issues after cancer are emerging. Included in this quality-of-life paradigm is protection of fertility from the toxicity of cancer treatments. Five-year survival rates with testicular cancer, hematological malignancies, breast cancer, and other cancers that strike young people may be in the 90 percent to 95 percent range. However, treatment of these cancers is often highly detrimental to male reproductive function, and as a consequence 20 to 25 percent of these patients become irreversibly sterile.[38] The testis is highly susceptible to the toxic effects of radiation and chemotherapy at all stages of life. Cytotoxic chemotherapy and radiotherapy may produce long-lasting or persistent damage to spermatogonial (primordial) cells, leading to oligo- or azoospermia.

One of the most effective and established methods for preserving fertility in males affected by cancer is sperm banking by cryopreservation. However, in some other circumstances, such as prepubertal boys or adolescents unable to produce a sample by ejaculation, gonadal tissue biopsy may also help to preserve fertility. Surveys of cancer patients reveal a very strong desire to be informed of available options for fertility preservation and future reproduction.[39]

Role of Cancer Specialists in Preserving Fertility

Physicians treating younger patients for cancer should be aware of the adverse effects of treatment on fertility and of ways to minimize those effects. If gonadal toxicity is unavoidable, they should also be knowledgeable about options for fertility preservation and offer referrals to patients.[40]

Oncologists traditionally have focused on providing the most effective treatments available to prolong life, but sometimes they need to consider the fertility preservation in cases of younger persons with treatable cancers. This involves informing patients and/or their families of options, benefits, and risks, and referring them to fertility specialists, if appropriate. Unless patients are informed or properly referred before treatment, options for later reproduction may be lost. Thus, fertility specialists and patient organizations should be working with cancer specialists.

Role of Fertility Specialists in Preserving Fertility

Fertility specialists are constantly involved in developing and using procedures to preserve gametes, embryos, and gonadal tissue before cancer treatment. Their role is to assist cancer survivors in understanding the limits of each technology and to counsel patients while providing hope and assistance to protect future fertility. As suggested above, consultation with the patient's oncologist is often essential. The fertility specialist must ask the cancer specialist about the patient's health and prognosis, and decide with the patient when and how to undergo a fertility preservation procedure.[41]

From an ethical standpoint, the key reason for pursuing fertility protection is to restore personal autonomy to those who are unable to conceive. However, since many of the technologies are innovative but experimental, it is difficult to design clinical trials: how to provide a proper informed consent and respect for autonomy? Who to include or exclude in the trials? How to assess the risks? Can the moral principle of beneficence be upheld if testicular tissue cryopreservation poses future risks to any children who might result from this technique? Ideally, the decision about who is a candidate for fertility preservation should be rendered by a team including a medical oncologist, reproductive endocrinologist, a pathologist and a psychologist, all guided by written protocols which can be shared with patients. Patients should not be provided with false hopes, and alternative plans, such as no intervention, should also be part of the discussion. It is reasonable in the absence of special grant funds, to seek reimbursement from patients to cover the expenses of the research, but there should be no charge for clinical fees. Finally, for the time being, fertility preservation involving testicular harvesting for freezing should be performed only in a few specialized centers working with proper IRB-approved consent protocols.

Preserving Fertility in Children with Cancer

Unfortunately, the modalities that are available to children to preserve their fertility are limited by their sexual immaturity and are essentially experimental. For boys who cannot produce mature sperm, harvesting and cryopreservation of testicular stem cells with the hope of future autologous transplantation or *in vitro* maturation represents a promising method of fertility preservation. However, it is difficult for children to conceptualize impaired future fertility as another potential consequence of exposure to cancer therapies, which will potentially be traumatic to them as adults. In addition, given the uncertainty of predicting fertility outcomes and the experimental nature of the options available, it is also difficult to counsel parents.

Care and tact should be taken in discussing all the options with families, both with and without the presence of the child. If children cannot ejaculate or are too young, then testicular biopsy for sperm extraction or biopsy to use as a germ cell repository can be done under IRB experimental conditions. Child assent and parental consent should always be sought. If children are too young to give assent, no procedure involving more than minimal risk or for their proven benefit should be permitted. The consent should cover the possible use of the reproductive tissue, the duration of storage, and the disposal of the tissue in the event of mental incapacitation or death. According to some rulings of the Human Fertilization and Embryo Authority (HFEA) in the UK, parental control over the stored gametic material is restricted to storage only, thus allowing the patient greater control over his genetic material. Transition of absolute control was discussed by the HFEA, and it was anticipated that this would normally occur at the point of that child's maturity.[42]

Additional risks associated with fertility preservation are more difficult to assess due to the lack of data to quantify them. For instance, the potential risk of reintroduction of malignant cells to the patient when gonadal tissue is re-transplanted cannot be estimated since only limited animal data exist. Moreover, the risk to offspring conceived through such technologies, such as inheritance of genetic predisposition to cancer or other unforeseen genetic risks, are currently unknown.

POSTHUMOUS USE OF STORED REPRODUCTIVE TISSUE AND GAMETES

A relevant question is whether the deceased has consented to posthumous use of his stored tissue or gametes in a consent form, advance directive, or other reliable indicator of consent before death. The American legal system has recognized that the person's prior wishes about disposition of reproductive material is controlling after death. Instructions that all such material shall be destroyed or not used after death should be honored. Similarly, United States law permits gametes and embryos to be used after death if the person has given such directives or if the partner or next of kin has dispositional control of them. Courts have also accepted that children born after posthumous conception or implantation are the legal offspring of the deceased if he gave instructions that gametes or embryos may be used after his death for reproduction.

The programs that are storing gametes, embryos, or gonadal tissue for cancer patients inform patients of the options for disposition of those materials at a future time; this assumes that the depositor may be unable to consent to disposition in the future due to death, incompetency, or unavailability. Whether offspring conceived posthumously will be recognized under the deceased's will or state inheritance laws will depend on the law of the state where the event occurs.[43] Of recent interest is that the service of sperm cryopreservation has been utilized by soldiers going to war (Iraq and Afghanistan), and specific directives about sperm disposal issues have been left in the hands of their spouses.

Who Gives Consent, According to What Guidelines, in Postmortem Sperm Retrieval?

There are more significant questions to consider prior to performing postmortem sperm retrieval (PMSR). Consideration of postmortem conception is rarely anticipated and thus prospective authorization is not likely to occur. The decision to perform a postmortem usually has to occur within a short time frame (within 24 hours of death), because recovery of viable sperm appears relatively uncommon at a later time unless the body has been cooled. A reasonable expectation that the recently deceased would consent to having his sperm used for procreation would best be determined by his actions and discussions prior to death with respect to intended pregnancy. Therefore, only men undergoing fertility treatment, actively attempting conception, or who had specifically expressed their plans to attempt conception in the immediate future would be suitable candidates for retrieval. This is why it is best to determine the intentions of the deceased man for conception, and to give procedural consent only to his wife.[44] The wife must understand that assisted reproduction would be required to use these specimens and generally a period of six months quarantine prior to its use is recommended. If the wife should decide not to proceed with an attempt at conception, as is expected to occur in most cases, this decision would invalidate any intended paternity provided by the couple together.

CONCLUSION

As shown in this chapter, knowledge of male infertility—its causes, treatment, and prevention—continues to evolve. With these emerging understandings come many new ethical debates. Some of these debates are based in religious traditions, which condemn human intervention into procreation and/or forbid the use of donor gametes to assist conception. Furthermore, the ART which has been designed to overcome male infertility—namely, ICSI—may lead to the transmission of genetic infertility to future male offspring. Whether male children should be protected from such known reproductive impairments is a serious ethical question. The rights and protection of children also come to the fore in cancer treatment. Namely, male fertility preservation techniques in childhood cancer may involve experimental protocols as well as parental consent. When male fertility cannot be preserved, or male infertility cannot be overcome through the use of ICSI, donor insemination remains an option. However, as shown in this chapter, DI is accompanied by a number of ethical dilemmas surrounding forced disclosure and the recent movement, at least in some Western nations, toward open identity donation. The rights of children to knowledge of biological paternity must be weighed against the rights of adults (both donors and parents) to privacy. Finally, death of a husband or male partner raises the possibility of posthumous procreation. However, as shown in this chapter, this decision is difficult in the absence of what might be called "advanced fertility directives." Whenever possible, clinicians treating men with life-threatening illnesses should seek such advanced directives—in writing—to prevent difficult posthumous fertility decisions on the part of grieving loved ones.

REFERENCES

1. Galan JJ, De M, et al. Association of genetic markers within the *KIT* and *KITLG* genes with human male infertility. Human Reproduction 2006;21:3185-92.
2. Oehninger Sergio, Kruger Thinus. Male Infertility Diagnosis and Treatment. United Kingdom: Informa Healthcare.
3. Payne, Michael AMS, Emmet J Lamb. Use of frozen semen to avoid human immunodeficiency virus type 1 transmission by donor insemination: a cost-effectiveness analysis. Fertility and Sterility 2004;81:81-92.
4. Traina C, et al. Compatible contradictions: religion and the naturalization of assisted reproduction. In: Altering Nature (Eds.) Lustig BA, Brody BA, McKenny GP. New York: Springer 2008.
5. Richards J. A Roman Catholic perspective on fertility issues: objective truths, moral absolutes and the natural law. In: Faith and Fertility: Attitudes towards Reproductive Practices in Different Religions from Ancient to Modern Times (Eds.) Blyth E, Landau R. London: Jessica Kingsley 2009.
6. Traina C, et al. Compatible contradictions: religion and the naturalization of assisted reproduction. In: Altering Nature (Eds.) Lustig BA, Brody BA, McKenny GP. New York: Springer 2008.
7. Inhorn MC, Patrizio P, Serour GI. Third-party assisted conception around the Mediterranean: comparing Sunni Egypt, Catholic Italy, and multi-sectarian Lebanon. Reproductive BioMedicine Online 2010;21:848-53.
8. Inhorn MC. Local Babies, Global Science: Gender, Religion, and *in vitro* Fertilization in Egypt. New York: Routledge, 2003.
9. Serour GI. Bioethics in reproductive health: a Muslim's perspective. Middle East Fertility Society Journal 1996;1:30-5.
10. Sonbol AA Adoption in Islamic society: a historical survey. In: Children in the Muslim Middle East (Ed.) Fernea EW. Austin: University of Texas Press 1995.
11. Sonbol AA Adoption in Islamic society: a historical survey. In: Children in the Muslim Middle East (Ed.) Fernea EW. Austin: University of Texas Press 1995.
12. Sonbol AA Adoption in Islamic society: a historical survey. In: Children in the Muslim Middle East (Ed.) Fernea EW. Austin: University of Texas Press 1995.
13. Inhorn MC. The New Arab Man: Emergent Masculinities, Technologies, and Islam in the Middle East. Princeton, NJ: Princeton University Press 2012.
14. Clarke M. Islam and New Kinship: Reproductive Technology and the Shariah in Lebanon. New York: Berghahn, 2009.
15. Inhorn MC. "He won't be my son": Middle Eastern men's discourses of adoption and gamete donation. Medical Anthropology Quarterly 2006;20(1):94-120.
16. Tremayne S. Law, ethics and donor technologies in Shia Iran. In: Birenbaum-Carmeli D, Inhorn MC (Eds). Assisting Reproduction, Testing Genes: Global Encounters with New Biotechnologies. New York: Berghahn, 2009.
17. Tremayne S. The "down side" of gamete donation: challenging "happy family" rhetoric in Iran. In: Islam and Assisted Reproductive Technologies: Sunni and Shia Perspectives (Eds.) Inhorn MC, Tremayne S. New York: Berghahn 2012.
18. Reza Samani, Royan Institute, personal communication.
19. Inhorn MC, Tremayne S (Eds). Islam and Assisted Reproductive Technologies: Sunni and Shia Perspectives. New York: Berghahn, in press, 2012.
20. Inhorn MC. The New Arab Man: Emergent Masculinities, Technologies, and Islam in the Middle East. Princeton, NJ: Princeton University Press 2012.
21. Inhorn MC, Kobeissi L, Nassar Z, Lakkis D, Fakih MH. Consanguinity and family clustering of male infertility in Lebanon. Fertility and Sterility 2009;91:1104-8.
22. Maduro MR, Lamb DJ. Understanding the new genetics of male infertility. Journal of Urology 2002;168:2197-2205.
23. Maduro MR, Lo KC, Chuang WW, Lamb DJ. Genes and male infertility: what can go wrong? Journal of Andrology 2003;24:485-93.
24. Krauz C, Forti G, McElreavey K. The Y-chromosome and male fertility and infertility. International Journal of Andrology 2003;26:570-5.
25. Baccetti B, et al. Genetic sperm defects and consanguinity. Human Reproduction 2001;16:1365-71.
26. Chan P. "Practical genetic issues in male infertility management." Paper presented at American Society for Reproductive Medicine 2007.p.13.
27. Baccetti B, et al. Genetic sperm defects and consanguinity. Human Reproduction 2001;16:1365-71.
28. Birenbaum-Carmeli D. Increased prevalence of Mediterranean and Muslim populations in mutation-related research literature. Community Genetics 2004;279:1-5.
29. Kumtepe Y, et al. A genetic survey of 1935 Turkish men with severe male factor infertility. Reproductive BioMedicine Online 2009;18:465-574.

30. Becker G. Deciding whether to tell children about donor insemination: an unresolved question in the United States. In: Infertility around the Globe: New Thinking on Childlessness, Gender, and Reproductive Technologies (Eds.) Inhorn MC, van Balen F. Berkeley: University of California Press 2002.

31. Becker B. The Elusive Embryo: How Women and Men Approach New Reproductive Technologies. Berkeley: University of California Press, 2000.

32. Becker G. Deciding whether to tell children about donor insemination: an unresolved question in the United States. In: Infertility around the Globe: New Thinking on Childlessness, Gender, and Reproductive Technologies (Eds.) Inhorn MC, van Balen F. Berkeley: University of California Press 2002.

33. Scheib JE, et al. Adolescents with open-identity sperm donors: reports from 12–17 year olds. Human Reproduction 2005;20:239-52.

34. American Society for Reproductive Medicine. Open-identity donor insemination in the United States: is it on the rise? Fertility and Sterility 2007;88:231-2.

35. (Franz and Allen, 2001; Blyth, 2002; Hewitt, 2002; Shanner and Harris, 2002; Lorbach 2003).

36. Patrizio P, et al. Disclosure to children conceived with donor gametes should be optional. Human Reproduction 2001;16: 2036-8.

37. American Society for Reproductive Medicine. Guidelines for gamete and embryo donation. Fertility and Sterility 2006;86:38-50.

38. The Ethics Committee of the American Society for Reproductive Medicine. Fertility preservation and reproduction in cancer patients. Fertility and Sterility 2005;83:1622-8.

39. Oehninger Sergio. Strategies for Fertility Preservation in Female and Male Cancer Survivors. Journal of the Society for Gynecologic Investigation 2005;12:222-31.

40. Lee SJ, Schover LR, Partridge AH, Patrizio P, et al. American Society of Clinical Oncology Recommendations on Fertility Preservation in Cancer Patients. J Clin Oncol 2006;24(18):2917-31.

41. Robertson, John A. Cancer and Fertility: Ethical and Legal Challenges. Journal of the National Cancer Institute Monographs 2005;34:104-6.

42. Bahadur G, Chatterjee R, Ralph D. Testicular tissue cryopreservation in boys. Ethical and legal issues. Human reproduction 2000;15:1416-20.

43. Pennings G, et al. ESHRE Task Force on Ethics and Law 11: Posthumous assisted reproduction. Human Reproduction 2006;21:3050-3.

44. Tash J, et al. Postmortem sperm retrieval: the effect of instituting guidelines. The Journal of Urology 2003;170:1922-5.

37

Ethics and Human-assisted Reproductive Technology

Martin Olsen

Any discussion of procreation has the potential to stimulate strong emotions in individuals and society at large. Scientific advances in assisted reproductive technology therefore may be controversial. This chapter will attempt to assist the practitioner in ethical decision making. A brief overview of medical ethics will be followed by a discussion of some specific ethical issues currently receiving attention in human assisted reproductive technology.

INTRODUCTION

The 2009 birth of octuplets in California prompted discussion on the responsibilities of reproductive endocrinologists to society. While reproductive endocrinologists focused their attention on the number of embryos transferred, the public's focus was on the economic considerations and the well-being of the children.[1] Dialogue was thus directed toward the concept of restricting access to assisted reproductive technology.

Physicians are not always able to agree upon restrictions. A survey of United States Obstetricians and Gynecologists outlines some of these disagreements.[2] In this study, eighty percent of the physicians surveyed would discourage a pregnancy if the patient were 56 years old. Seventy-three percent would discourage a pregnancy if the patient had human immunodeficiency virus. Twenty-four percent of the physicians surveyed would discourage a patient from the use of assisted reproductive technology if she already had five healthy biological children. Seventeen percent would discourage a woman who planned to be a single parent from accessing assisted reproductive technology options. Fourteen percent of physicians would discourage patients from assisted reproductive technology if her sexual partner was a female. Male physicians and physicians who were seen as religious physicians would more likely discourage the use of assisted reproductive technology for lesbian, single, or unmarried patients. Almost three percent of these Obstetrics and Gynecology (OB/GYN) physicians would decline to help any patient obtain treatment with artificial insemination using donor sperm or *in vitro* fertilization with donor sperm.[2]

These observations highlight the fact that a patient may receive very different levels of assistance depending on which OB/GYN practice she accesses.

Physicians do struggle with some ethical decision-making in their patients with infertility.

ETHICAL DECISION-MAKING

The most common stratagem used in medical ethics decision making has been the concept of principle based ethics. Principle based ethics have three components which include:
- Patient autonomy
- Beneficence/Nonmaleficence
- Justice.

Before delving into principle based ethics, however, it is appropriate to briefly discuss alternative ethical stratagems. The careful ethical decision maker may want to use components of multiple stratagems in order to come to the decision which is best for the patient, the patient's family and potentially the community. These alternative ethical systems include the following concepts:
- Virtue ethics attempt to provide guidance by asking what a good morally virtuous physician would do in specific circumstances.[3]
- Care based ethics emphasize moral attention, sympathetic understanding, relationship awareness, accommodation and response.[4]
- Feminist ethics can expose androcentric reasoning in clinical care and public policy. An example of this androcentric reasoning would be the previous exclusion of women from participation in many clinical research trials. Feminist ethics are concerned with oppression as a pervasive and insidious moral wrong.[5] Feminist ethics can help to challenge dominance and oppression not only of women but also of other groups who have received discrimination based on race, class or other characteristics.[3]
- Communitarian ethics emphasize a community's shared values, ideals, and goals. This ethical framework suggests that the needs of the larger community may take precedence in some cases over the rights and desires of individuals.[3]
- Case-based reasoning ethical decision making builds on precedents set in prior specific ethical cases.[6]
- Finally, Principle based ethics describe major principles that are commonly used as guides for ethical decision making including autonomy, beneficence, nonmaleficence, and justice. Other principles such as fidelity, honesty, privacy, and confidentiality may also have roles.

Autonomy is the principle of respect for the personal rule of the self. The patient should be free from the controlling influences of others and from personal limitations that prevent meaningful choice, such as inadequate understanding.[7] The principle of autonomy is strongly emphasized in an informed consent. Like all ethical principles, autonomy is not absolute and at times may conflict with other principles or ethical systems.[3]

Beneficence and nonmaleficence are similar with subtle distinctions and describes beneficence but does not refer to nonmaleficence. Beneficence is the obligation to promote the patient's well-being. Beneficence can conflict with the principle of autonomy when the physician feels that the patient is making a choice that is not in her best interest.[3]

The principle of justice demands that people receive what is due to them. Justice demands that individuals receive equal treatment unless a solid reason establishes that they are different from other patients in ways that are relevant to the treatment in question.[3]

Informed consent is the willing acceptance of a medical intervention by a patient after adequate disclosure by the physician of the nature of the intervention with its risks and benefits and of the alternatives with their risks and benefits.[8] Informed consent involves three steps:

1. Disclosure by the physicians to the patient of an adequate amount of information.
2. Understanding of that information by the patient.
3. A voluntary choice by the patient regarding the management of her condition.[9]

A consent form documents the process; the primary purpose of the process is to maintain patient autonomy. A patient's ability to understand depends upon her maturity, state of consciousness, mental status, education, cultural background, native language, and the opportunity and ability to ask questions. Diminished capacity to understand is not the same as legal incompetence.[3]

Conflict of Interest

Society's trust in physicians can be diminished even by perceived conflicts of interest. It is therefore important for health care providers to avoid even the appearance of a conflict of interest. A conflict of interest occurs when a physician has two or more obligations that may "conflict". An example would be obligation to patients and an obligation to a managed care organization. A conflict exists when one interest, such as a patient's well being, conflicts with another interest, such as a physician's financial well-being.[3]

A conflict of interest is not in itself unethical but it creates the occasion and temptation for the physician to behave in an unethical fashion.

When difficult ethical decision making events arise, more than one course of action may be morally justifiable. It can therefore be very difficult for the physician to choose the best option.

A framework for ethical decision-making is described in ACOG committee opinion #390 Ethical Decision Making In Obstetrics and Gynecology.[3]

SPECIFIC ETHICAL ISSUES

The remainder of the chapter will discuss specific ethical issues of interest to the infertility team. One area left undiscussed is the issue of providing infertility care to patients with significant medical morbidity. The author believes this is an area in need of future ethical work.

The positive right to reproduce is not recognized in international law.[10]

Documents such as United Nations Universal Declaration of Human Rights and the European Convention for the Protection of Human and Fundamental Freedoms protect the rights of human beings to be left alone. Persons have a right to found a family.[11] This is not the same as a right to claim entitlement to a service. There is no definite right of each person to reproduce.[10]

Issues Involved in the Care of Post-menopausal Women Who Desire Conception

Today's reproductive technology options could be visualized as a mechanism to level the reproductive options of the genders. Older men have been having children with younger women for millennia. But one significant difference is that men are not placed at medical risk during pregnancy. Another difference is that the death of an older man during the progeny's childhood could be compensated to some extent by the likely continued survival of the younger mother. In many cases postmenopausal women either have older partners themselves or no life partner.

Recent advances such as oocyte donation, improved medications, and *in vitro* fertilization provide opportunities for postmenopausal women to give birth. The ethical issues involved in these recent advances include:

- The safety of pregnancy for older women.
- Risks posed to the fetus if carried by an older mother.
- Safety issues for a child relative to the age of the parents.
- The importance of a guarantee that someone will serve in the parental role should an older parent or parents become disabled or die.[10]

In the United States, for the year 2002, there were 263 births reported from women between the ages of 50 and 54.[12]

Increased maternal age is associated with increased obstetrical and perinatal complications. Maternal complications include increased risk of gestational diabetes, hypertension, pregnancy-induced hypertension, and spontaneous early abortion. Fetal complications for offspring of older mothers include stillbirth, low-birth weight, and increased perinatal morbidity and mortality[13] and chromosome abnormalities.

The Royal College of Obstetrics and Gynecology of the United Kingdom does advocate that women should be supported in their life choices, but points out that women and society need to be aware of the possible problems that older women may encounter. Women should therefore be encouraged to have families during the period of optimum fertility.[14]

Concern about the care of older mothers includes not only the unease that the child might be orphaned at an early age but also the apprehension that older mothers may not have the energy and the stamina to care for young children.[14]

The American Society of Reproductive Medicine (ASRM) has stated that oocyte donation to postmenopausal women should be discouraged. There seems to be no medical or ethical reason compelling enough, however, to judge the practice unethical in every case.[15] The ethics committee of ASRM has commented that oocyte donation to menopausal women should be discouraged but should not be considered unethical in every case.[16]

Patient with Mental Illness

A patient with mental illness may have complications that would exacerbate her condition during and following her pregnancy. Both prematurity and postpartum psychoses have been associated with pregnancy in patients with schizophrenia.[17] A case can be made however that a failure to offer assisted reproductive technology to a patient with mental illness would constitute discrimination.[18]

In New Zealand, The Human Rights Act and the New Zealand Bill of Rights indicate that in no case will it be acceptable to refuse infertility treatment solely on the basis of mental illness. The court argued that one may have general concerns about the welfare of a future child or the health of a mother but unless such reasons are weighted in good evidence they are unlikely to meet the high standards that will be required to be able to discriminate by exception.[18]

Providers of ART must be cognizant of the rights of these patients while also remaining aware of the risks to these patients and their potential children.

Ethical Issues in Single/Gay/Lesbian/Transgender Patients

Single women requesting artificial insemination by donor sperm may not be single mothers by choice. Many mothers may prefer to have a child within a partner relationship but their circumstance has forced them to decide between single motherhood or unwanted childlessness.[19]

One program has described its exclusionary criteria for denying assisted reproductive technology to single women. This program has treated single women but set up a mental health assessment process to assist the program in deciding which women would be best served by the program's services. Criteria for denial of a single woman's request to receive artificial insemination by donor sperm included:

- Problems involving the family in origin. These include traumatic childhood experiences, other conflicts within the family and a symbiotic relationship with a parent.
- Problems with partner relationships. These include a failure to build intimate relationships, failure to overcome a broken relationship, or a confused ongoing relationship.
- Instability of the applicant's life including lack of financial resources, unclear living conditions, and ongoing psychiatric

problems. (It should be noted that arguments have been made that denying fertility services to most mentally ill patients is inappropriate, see above).

- Lack of a constructive social network on which the patients could rely.

Those single women accepted enjoyed a stable socioeconomic situation in which they could call on a large social network in case they needed emotional or practical support. The accepted individuals functioned independently.[19]

An argument could be made that fairness would mandate that similar criteria be used to assess all patients, not just single patients, before declining treatment.

The ethics committee of the American Society of Reproductive Medicine (ASRM) has stated that fertility treatment should be offered to single individuals, unmarried heterosexual couples, and gay and lesbian couples with interests in having and rearing children. Programs should treat all requests for assisted reproduction equally without regard to marital status or sexual orientation.[20] The ethics committee has stated "we believe that the ethical duty to treat persons with equal respect requires that fertility programs treat single persons and gay and lesbian couples equally to heterosexual married couples in determining which services to provide".[20]

The majority of offspring in the US are born to heterosexual married couples but variations from this status do not generally harm offspring or society.[20] Therefore concerns about welfare of the children or promotion of marriage do not justify the denial of reproductive services to unmarried individuals or couples including those who are gay or lesbians.[20]

The California Supreme Court has ruled that physicians who provide assisted reproductive technology must be willing to provide that treatment to lesbian women (or find a colleague who is willing to do so) even if this provision is in contradiction with the physician's religious commitment.[21]

One study indicated that lesbian and bisexual women who were trying to conceive report levels of depression and anxiety comparable to lesbian and bisexual women in the postpartum period. These women did report largely positive experiences with their healthcare professionals.[22]

The American Psychological Association has reviewed the data on offspring of gay and lesbian couples. They have concluded that research suggests that the development and well being of children with lesbian and gay parents do not differ from that of children of heterosexual parents.[23]

The sharing of motherhood with biological lesbian co-mothers has been advocated as an *in vitro* fertilization indication. It is important to point out that when traditional insemination is used, the partner of the inseminated woman lacks legal recognition or participation in some jurisdictions. Taking the eggs from one lesbian partner and implanting a resulting embryo in the uterus of the other partner allows both partners to participate biologically in the creation of the family. The ethics of carrying out such a technique with two fertile women in a lesbian couple have been questioned and challenged but the techniques have been stated as legal in Spain and in the United States.[24]

A transgender man legally married to a woman has given birth with the assistance of ART.[25] The potential psychologic risk to a child in families raised by a transgender man who has given birth to a newborn is a poorly studied area. There is a lack of data on the potential for a transgender identity to weaken family bonds. There is a lack of information on potential gender confusion for the children. There is a lack of data on how society might perceive this child.[25] A recommendation has been made that fertility clinicians may offer their help to people wanting children as long as they are healthy enough and prepared for the work of child-rearing. This standard does not exclude men and women with unconventional identities.[25]

Surrogate Motherhood

The use of a surrogate mother in procreation efforts continues to be controversial. Arguments can be made that surrogacy is a contractual relationship for all parties; the loss of this ability would limit the options of infertile couples and would limit the capabilities of women who wish to provide assistance to infertile couples. Other arguments indicate that when surrogates are contracted this gives wealthy individuals the opportunity to take advantage of women in other socioeconomic classes by shifting the risk of pregnancy from wealthy individuals to less wealthy women. In some United States jurisdictions, legal descriptions surrounding surrogate motherhood are not clearly defined and may vary between different states.[26,27]

Multiple types of surrogacy exist. In one type, the surrogate mother is artificially inseminated with sperm provided by the male partner of a couple seeking her surrogacy services. In this format, the genetic component of the child may consist of genetic contributions from the father who plans to raise the child; no genetic contribution from the woman who will raise the child is present. Variations of this model include others who contract with surrogate mothers such as homosexual couples or single individuals of either gender with donor sperm.

In another type of surrogacy arrangement, *in vitro* fertilization and ovum transfer are combined in a fashion such that the surrogate mother becomes a "gestational carrier" and does not have any genetic contribution to the fetus; the parents who will raise the child could comprise all genetic contributions.

Ethical arguments against surrogate motherhood concern potential harms that may occur. These harms could include: harm to the child that was born, harm to the surrogate mother, or harm to the existing children and family of the surrogate mother.[26]

From a larger social perspective, an argument could be made that surrogacy arrangements can depersonalize pregnant women. According to this argument, using one woman as a vehicle for the genetic perpetuation of others may harm not only the surrogate mother but also the status of women in society as a whole.[26]

A lack of evidence exists concerning the mechanisms of the surrogacy process and its impact upon the people involved.[28] Therefore, no solid foundations for ethical conclusions can be accessed from the data.[26] It is appropriate to take precautions to prevent medical, psychologic and legal harm to the intended parents, the surrogate mother and the prospective child.

Surrogacy arrangements often take place between parties who have unequal power, education, and/or economic status.[29]

For these reasons, surrogate mothers may be vulnerable to exploitation. Some jurisdictions specifically prohibit surrogacy contracts that involve payment.[26]

Opponents of surrogate motherhood have argued that financial payments create a financial barrier to surrogacy services such that only the affluent will be able to access this technology. This barrier of course exists for many infertility services.[26]

Physician involvement in surrogacy arrangements fall into four different categories:

1. The counseling of potential surrogate mothers.
2. The advisement of infertile couples who consider surrogacy.
3. Providing an obstetric service for a pregnant surrogate mother.
4. Offering ART related to a planned surrogate pregnancy.

Given the four different potentially divergent interests, one physician should not represent the interest of both major parties in a surrogacy arrangement.[26]

Recommendations for infertility programs working with surrogate mothers or couples considering surrogacy include the following:

- Surrogacy should not be done for convenience only.
- A physician may decline to participate in surrogacy arrangements.
- A physician should be sure that appropriate procedures have been followed to screen the prospective parents and the surrogate mother.
- Mental health counseling should be provided to both the surrogate mother and the intended parents.
- The surrogacy arrangement should be overseen by private nonprofit agencies. These nonprofit agencies should have thorough processes similar to an adoption agency.
- The physician should receive compensation only for medical services.
- The physician should refuse to refer patients to any surrogacy program in which the financial arrangements are likely to exploit either the surrogate mother or prospective parents.
- Possible contingencies should be addressed in advance. These contingencies include: health behaviors of the surrogate mother, potential prenatal diagnosis of a fetal abnormality, death of one of the intended parents, dissolution of the couple's marriage during the pregnancy, the birth of an infant with a disability, a decision by a surrogate mother to abrogate the contract and attempt to obtain custody of the infant conceived with sperm of the intended father.
- Both the surrogate mother and the couple facing infertility issues should be encouraged to have independent legal representation.
- Compensation to the surrogate mother for providing this service should be based solely on her time and effort; it must not be conditional on the success of the delivery or on the health of the child.[26]

Known Donor *vs* Anonymous Donor Gamete Donation

In Canada, the Assisted Human Reproduction Act prohibits the use of financial compensation for gamete donation. All gamete donations in Canada since 2005 are therefore only the result of altruistic donation. The resulting lack of compensation has drastically reduced the number of donor gametes. Canadians are now traveling aboard to seek donor oocytes in other countries such as the United States where such treatments are available.

A Canadian study followed women who donated oocytes for altruistic reasons in Canada. The oocyte donors were relatives or friends of the infertile couple.[30] Subjects of this study overwhelmingly indicated that mandatory psychologic counseling was an important part of the oocyte donation experience. Negative emotional experiences did occur for some donors. Donors experienced devastated feelings when the cycle failed. When cycles were successful, some donors found difficulty in setting appropriate boundaries between themselves and the resulting child. One subject described a negative change in the relationship with her life time partner. One donor found it very upsetting to be around the resulting child. This study was small but it is noteworthy that less than 25 percent of the recipients would ever donate again and these would only donate to the same couple.[30]

The use of known oocyte donation does not allow recipient couples privacy to deal with their own infertility. This may increase the pressure on infertile couples. An anonymous donation, therefore improves the privacy of the experience for the infertile couple. On the other hand, the potential child has increased ability to know the donor and the donor's genetic heritage with a known donor. This potential advantage is useful only if the child is told about the use of oocyte donation.

In a program that offers both directed donor and anonymous donor oocyte programs, a difference was noted in the rate of disclosure of the oocyte donation. Ninety-seven percent of the recipients who used a directed donor choose to tell others about their participation in an oocyte donation program while only fifty-eight percent of those who used anonymous donors desired to tell others about their participation.[31]

In the United Kingdom (UK), gamete donor anonymity is no longer legally permitted. This removes the ability of anonymous egg sharing donation programs. Under such a program, a donor shares her eggs in exchange for a significant reduction in her treatment cost. Under the recent UK law, an egg-sharing donor would either agree to being identified or be unable to undergo treatment.[32] (Some *in vitro* fertilization programs do not participate in egg sharing donor programs due to the concerns about potential for conflict and decision making between caring for the two individual patients. For example, if only a few eggs are high quality, will the program proceed to attempt embryo creation for the couple paying for the process or the egg-sharing donor?).

It has been argued that the gamete donation plan that offers the greatest justice is a dual-track system where the prospective parents chose whether they want to know the identity of the gamete donor or not know the gamete donor. The parents can then make this choice based on their own belief system on what is best for their child.[32] Education is of course important to maximize the ability of the parents to make this decision. Placing a value judgment on known vs anonymous gamete donation implies that one form is good and one form is bad. Recommendations have been made, however, that in cases of both known donor and anonymous donor gamete donation, it seems desirable that resulting children are aware of the donor conception prior to adolescence.[33]

Cross-border Reproductive Care

In some countries, single women, postmenopausal women, homosexual couples and unmarried couples are not eligible for infertility treatment. Other reasons for seeking cross border infertility care include long waiting lists or inability to access specific procedures in the home country.[34] The United States of America offers ready access to infertility treatment and provides more fertility services to non-residents than any other country. The Indian government promotes medical tourism; this brings valuable dollars into the country.[35]

Ethical concerns have been raised about the globalization of human ART when individuals and couples from wealthy countries begin accessing the facilities in less wealthy countries. It has been felt that such actions may utilize the reproductive capacities of poor women in order to compliment the reproductive deficiencies of people in affluent societies.[35] Such actions may embody stereotypical conceptions in poor women. A social obligation may exist such that those who have power and influence or derive the greatest benefit from a medical system bear the greater share of responsibility for any unjust outcomes which may occur.[35] Cross border reproductive care may therefore exploit the vulnerabilities of participating women in less wealthy societies.[35] A comparison between surrogacy and prostitution has been discussed.[29]

Impoverished women in poor economies may prefer to sell their bodily resources rather than sink further into poverty. The surrogacy trade, however, can intersect structures of inequality and social subordination that exploit the vulnerabilities of participating women. (It should also be noted that the infertile women travelers also have vulnerabilities). Surrogate mothers do not necessarily feel exploited.

In one Indian clinic, each surrogate was paid between $5,000 and $7,000, which is the equivalent of up to ten years' salary for a rural Indian citizen.[36]

Legal protections available to prospective mothers in their home country may not apply abroad. Equality of the medical treatment may not be the same standard as the home country. Genetic tests may be unreliable and reliable data on complication rates during the pregnancy may not be available.[35]

Another ethical concern is that the less wealthy country's health care resources may be directed towards the treatment of patients from wealthy countries as opposed to improving the medical care of citizens of the less wealthy country.

The couple or individual and infertility providers who participate in cross border reproductive care must be aware of local laws. In Romania, 30 people were arrested on suspicion of removing and purchasing human eggs from indigent Romanian women. The women apparently were paid a few hundred Euros while their oocytes were sold for thousands of Euros.[37]

At the current time there is no international certification or accreditation for fertility clinics.

Advertising

Patients with infertility may be desperate to have a child. They are often willing to pursue expensive treatments or unproven treatments. They are, therefore, a vulnerable group. Accurate reporting of data assists in the formation of realistic expectations.[38] Medical advising is unethical when it contains material that is unsubstantiated, misleading, deceptive, or false.[39] A paid advertisement promoting a medical practice must be clearly identified as an advertisement. It is not ethical to compensate the communication media in any way for publicity in a news item. If a television infomercial is used it should be very clear that this is paid advertising.[39]

It is appropriate to make sure that the information is dispensed in an appropriate form of communication. Short television and radio advertisements may require the omission of so much information that the advertisement could become misleading. Advertisers must be careful to avoid any implications of subspecialty training when none exists. Actively approaching specific individuals in person or by phone with an intention to attract patients is usually unethical. The physician or clinic must be able to substantiate all claims in advertisement.[39]

Any efforts to mislead or attract vulnerable patients must be avoided. If rankings are used the advertiser must describe how these rankings were established. Any advertisements that relate to a ranking which involved payment by a physician must state so in the advertisement. No advertisement which denigrates the competence of another group of professionals is considered ethical. If a physician has carefully verified that he or she is the only practitioner to offer a certain treatment in a particular geographic area this information may be dispensed; any claims that a physician has a unique skill or a unique treatment would otherwise be considered deceptive. Advertisements which involve success rates or other outcomes must be supported by valid, reproducible data.

Fee structures and costs may be advertized as long as the information is complete and does not encourage inaccurate assumptions. For example, a money-back guarantee may be misleading because only a portion of the patient's money is refunded if the patient does not experience the desired outcome. "Do one get one free" treatments usually result in additional expenses for the initial treatment and may not truly save the patient any money.[39,40]

Ethical Issues Between Cultures

Patients from non–Western cultures who present for infertility treatment may have different expectations than patients from Western cultures. For example, the use of ART is widely accepted in Islamic countries[41] but infertility practices are generally acceptable only for married heterosexual couples and surrogacy

arrangements are not acceptable.[42] No gamete donations are allowed under Islamic law; procreation is limited to husband and wife.[43] Preimplantation genetic diagnosis (PGD) is permitted but there is some ambiguity among professionals with respect to sex selection.[42] Sex selection can be performed in a case of medical necessity but the use of PGD for family balancing is controversial.[42]

Role of Ethics Committees

In the United States, all hospitals which are accredited by the Joint Commission are required to have a mechanism in place for addressing ethical issues.[44] The formation of these committees was initially driven in the past by well-publicized cases involving end-of-life decision-making.[44]

Ethics committees' roles include educational efforts which should include self education, education of health professionals, education of staff, and community outreach.

The purpose of an ethics consultation is to address value conflict or uncertainty and to build consensus among decision makers about how to move forward in an ethically acceptable way. A historic linkage exists between the original development of ethical committees and palliative care.[44] It is therefore imperative that clinicians familiarize themselves with the strengths and weaknesses of the respective services at their own institutions. An ethics committee which does an excellent job with end-of-life decision making may be unprepared to delve into issues that are unfamiliar to that particular ethics committee. Conflicts with ethical decision making for patients desiring reproduction may not be well managed by a committee that is not familiar with the issues involved.

■ CONCLUSION

Human ART can be controversial. The desire for procreation is a very powerful human drive which can make infertility patients and their families extremely vulnerable. It is therefore important for programs which provide infertility care to ensure that their actions and policies are consistent with existing ethical principles and guidelines.

■ REFERENCES

1. Minkoff H, Ecker J. The California octuplets and the duties of reproductive endocrinologists. Am J Obstet Gynecol 2009;201(1):3-4.
2. Lawrence RE, Rasinski KA, Yoon JD, Curlin FA. Obstetrician-gynecologists' beliefs about assisted reproductive technologies. Obstet Gynecol 2010;116(1):127-35.
3. ACOG Committee Opinion No. 390. Ethical decision making in obstetrics and gynecology. American College of Obstetricians and Gynecologists. Obstet Gynecol 2007;110:1479-87.
4. Manning RC. A care approach. In: Kuhse H, Singer P (Eds). A companion to bioethics. Malden (MA): Blackwell 1998.pp.98-105.
5. Tong R. Feminist approaches to bioethics. In: Wolf SM (Ed). Feminism and bioethics: beyond reproduction. New York (NY): Oxford University Press 1996.pp.67-94.

6. Jonsen AR. Casuistry: an alternative or complement to principles? Kennedy Inst Ethics J 1995;5:237-51.

7. Beauchamp TL, Childress JF. Principles of biomedical ethics. 5th edn. New York (NY): Oxford University Press 2001.pp.57-112.

8. Jonsen AR, Siegler M, Winslade WJ. Clinical ethics: a practical approach to ethical decisions in clinical medicine. 6th edn. New York (NY): McGraw-Hill; 2006.

9. McCullough LB, Chervenak FA. Ethics in obstetrics and gynecology. New York (NY): Oxford University Press 1994.p.138.

10. Caplan AL, Patrizio P. Are you ever too old to have a baby? The ethical challenges of older women using infertility services. Semin Reprod Med 2010;28(4):281-6. Epub 2010 Aug 3.

11. United Nations Universal Declaration of Human Rights (1948). Available at: http://www.un.org/en/documents/udhr/.

12. Heffner LJ. Advanced Maternal Age—How Old Is Too Old? N Engl J Med 2004;351(19):1927-9.

13. Franz M, Husslein P. Obstetrical management of the older gravida. Womens Health (Lond Engl) 2010;6(3):463-8.

14. Royal College Obstetrics Gynecology Statement on later maternal age (2009). Available at: http://www.rocg.org.uk/what-we-do/campaigning-and-opinions/statement/rcog-statement-later-maternal-age.

15. American Society of Reproductive Medicine. Guidelines for gamete and embryo donation: a practice committee report. Fertil Steril 2007;90(Suppl 3):530-44.

16. Ethics Committee of the American Society for Reproductive Medicine. Oocyte donation to postmenopausal women. Fertil Steril 2004;82(Suppl 1):S254-5.

17. Matevosyan NR. Pregnancy and postpartum specifics in women with schizophrenia: a meta-study. Arch Gynecol Obstet 2011;283(2):141-7.

18. Fancourt N. Assisted reproduction and metal illness: a human rights perspective from New Zealand. J Law Med 2010;18(1):124-9.

19. Baetens P, Ponjaert-Kristoffersen I, Devroey P, Van Steirteghem AC. Artificial insemination by donor: an alternative for single women. Hum Reprod 1995;10(6):1537-42.

20. Ethics Committee of the American Society for Reproductive Medicine. Access to fertility treatment by gays, lesbians, and unmarried persons. Fertil Steril 2009;92(4):1190-3.

21. First amendment-California Supreme Court holds that free exercise of religion does not give fertility doctors right to deny treatment to lesbians. North Coast Women's Care Medical Group, Inc. v. San Diego County Superior Court, 189 P. 3d 959 (Cal. 2008). Harv Law Rev 2008;122:787-94.

22. Yager C, Brennan D, Steele LS, Epstein R, Ross LE. Challenges and mental health experiences of lesbian and bisexual women who are trying to conceive. Health Soc Work 2010;35(3):191-200.

23. American Psychological Association 2004. Available at: http://www.apa.org/pi/lgbc/policy/parents.html. Accessed Sept 27, 2006.

24. Marina S, Marina D, Marina F, Fosas N, Galiana N, Jové I. Sharing motherhood: biological lesbian co-mothers, a new IVF indication. Hum Reprod 2010;25(4):938-41.

25. Murphy TF. The ethics of helping transgender men and women have children. Perspect Biol Med 2010;53(1):46-60.

26. American College Obstetrics and Gynecology Committee Opinion No. 397. Surrogate Motherhood. American College of Obstetricians and Gynecologists. Obstet Gynecol 2008;111:465-70.

27. National Conference of Commissioners on Uniform State Laws. Gestational agreement. Article 8. In: Uniform parentage act. Chicago (IL): NCCUSL 2002.pp.68-78.

28. Surrogate mothers. American Fertility Society. Fertil Steril 1994;62(suppl 1):71S-77S.

29. Harrison M. Financial incentives for surrogacy. Womens Health Issues 1991;1:145-7.

30. Yee S, Hitkari JA, Greenblatt EM. A follow-up study of women who donated oocytes to known recipient couples for altruistic reasons. Human Reprod 2007;22(7):2040-50.

31. Greenfeld DA, Greenfeld DG, Mazure CM, Keefe DL, Olive DL. Do attitudes toward disclosure in donor oocyte recipients predict the use of anonymous versus directed donation? Fertil Steril 1998;70(6):1009-14.

32. De Jonge C, Barratt CL. Gamete donation: a question of anonymity. Fertil Steril 2006;85(2):500-1.

33. Kirkman M. Parents' contributions to the narrative identity of offspring of donor-assisted conception. Soc Sci Med 2003;57:2229-42.

34. Ferraretti AP, Pennings G, Gianaroli L, Natali F, Magli MC. Cross-border reproductive care: a phenomenon expressing the controversial aspects of reproductive technologies. Reprod BioMed Online 2010;20:261-6.

35. Donchin A. Reproductive tourism and the quest for global gender justice. Bioethics 2010;24(7):323-32.

36. Haworth A. Marie Claire Article-Surrogate Mothers: Womb for Rent http://www.marieclaire.com/print-this/world-report/news/international/surrogate-mothers-india.

37. Siegel-Itzkovich J. Romanian police raid clinic run by Israelis, accusing them of buying women's eggs and selling them for profit. BMJ 2009;339:b3003.

38. The Practice Committee, Society for Assisted Reproductive Technology; American Society for Reproductive Medicine. Guidelines for advertising by ART programs. Fertil Steril 2004;82(2):527-8.

39. American College Obstetrics and Gynecology Committee Opinion No. 341. Ethical ways for physicians to market a practice. American College of Obstetricians and Gynecologists. Obstet Gynecol 2006;108:239-42.

40. The Jacobs Institute of Women's Health—Naber Conference. Accountability in the advertising and marketing of assisted reproduction. Womens Health Issues 1997.pp.167-71.

41. Eskandarani HA. A code of practice is overdue for assisted reproductive technology in the GCC Countries: some comments and suggestions. Qatar Med J 2007;16(1):16-9.

42. Eskandarani HA. Preimplantation genetic diagnosis in the Gulf Cooperative Council countries: utilization and ethical attitudes. Hum Reprod Genet Ethics 2009;15(2):68-74.

43. Albar MA. Ethical considerations in the prevention and management of genetic disorders with special emphasis on religious considerations Saud Med J 2002;23(6):627-32.

44. Aulisio MP, Arnold RM. Role of the ethics committee: helping to address value conflicts or uncertainties. Chest 2008;134(2):417-24.

38

Repopulating the Testes: Are Stem Cells a Reality?

Trustin Domes, Kirk C Lo

INTRODUCTION

Over the last decade, there has been considerable hype in the main stream media regarding stem cell research and its clinical applications. Being able to unlock the restorative potential of stem cells to potentially cure previously incurable diseases and conditions such as Parkinson's disease, diabetes mellitus, spinal cord injuries and even male infertility has increased the profile and funding for this research, as evidenced by US President's Barack Obama's executive order in 2009 to overturn previous National Institute of Health (NIH) funding restrictions on embryonic stem cells.[1] Although, the use of stem cells has tremendous promise, we have to respect the current limitations of this technology and be cognizant of the ethical dilemmas that may arise by conducting and applying the research in this area.

With the advent of stem cell research, there have been tremendous advances in knowledge regarding the mechanisms responsible for spermatogenesis and the testicular microenvironment. Despite this, trying to recreate spermatogenesis outside of the testicular environment continues to elude andrologists. Having the ability to "grow" human sperm would be a tremendous advance in reproductive biology with multiple possible clinical applications, such as a treatment option for men with testicular failure and azoospermia of multiple etiologies. Currently, there are both *in vitro* and *in vivo* spermatogenesis model systems that have been pivotal in our understanding of male reproductive biology. This chapter will first provide a brief primer on stem cells and the spermatogenesis cycle and then will discuss the basic methodologies, possible clinical applications, and benefits and limitations of the *in vitro* and *in vivo* spermatogenesis model systems. Although our understanding of human spermatogenesis has been greatly enhanced through stem cell research and spermatogenesis model systems, practical clinical applications of this research has not yet reached prime time.

STEM CELL PRIMER

Stem cells are unique compared to other cells because of their ability to self-renew, proliferate indefinitely and differentiate into specialized tissues depending on the source of the stem cells.[2] Stem cells can be categorized as totipotent, pluripotent/embryonic and somatic.

A fertilized oocyte and a blastomere (up to the 8 cell stage embryo) are considered totipotent because they can differentiate and generate a complete organism. Pluripotent stem cells, such as embryonic stem cells (ESC), are derived from the inner cell mass of a blastocyst and retain the property of self-renewal and the ability to differentiate into cells and tissues from all 3 germ layers (ectoderm, endoderm and mesoderm).[3] The only tissue that ESC cannot form is the placenta. Somatic stem cells persist into adulthood and are responsible for the regenerative properties of several organ systems.[4] Tissues with regenerative potential include the gastrointestinal, integumentary, hematopoietic and spermatogenic systems. The spermatogonial stem cell (SSC) is responsible for the replenishment of sperm throughout postpubertal life and is the source of cells responsible for the recovery of spermatogenesis after a toxic insult to the testes.

HUMAN SPERMATOGENESIS PRIMER

In humans, primordial germ cells (PGCs) are formed from extraembryonic mesoderm and travel from the yolk sac through the dorsal mesentery of the developing embryo to reach the genital ridges approximately four to five weeks after conception.[5] The PGCs become gonocytes once they are incorporated into the genital cords by being surrounded by Sertoli cells (future seminiferous tubules). The diploid (2n) gonocytes migrate to the basement membrane of the seminiferous tubule and become spermatogonia, which remain relatively quiescent in the G0/G1 stage, with only low levels of mitotic activity until puberty.[6]

At puberty, the hypothalamic-pituitary-gonadal hormonal axis is activated to stimulate spermatogenesis (**Fig. 38.1**). The Ad (dark) spermatogonia are the true SSC of the testicle, which have a low mitotic index except during testicular development.[7] The Ad spermatogonia are resistant to cellular damage and the low rate of mitosis preserves the genomic integrity of the germ line. The Ad spermatogonium is the precursor to the Ap (pale) spermatogonium, which acts as a self-renewing progenitor and as the functional reserve in the adult testis. The Ap spermatogonium commits to final differentiation when it becomes a type B spermatogonium, which later differentiates into the primary spermatocyte. The first stage of meiosis, and the production of haploid gametes, occurs between the primary (diploid, 2n) and secondary spermatocyte (haploid, 1n) stage. The second stage of

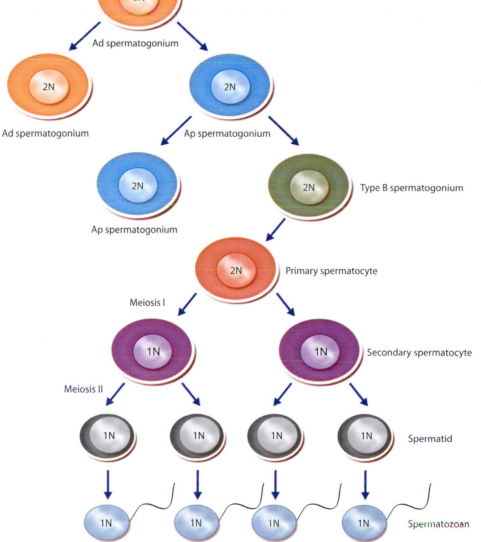

Figure 38.1: Process of human spermatogenesis

meiosis occurs between the secondary spermatocyte and spermatid (round and elongated) stage. Spermatids differentiate into spermatozoa through the process of spermiogenesis. The entire spermatogenic cycle in humans takes approximately 64 days.[8]

IN VITRO SPERMATOGENESIS MODELS

Having the ability to foster the developmental maturation of ESC and/or SSC extragonadally is not only a matter of scientific curiosity but also is a quest for the treatment of male infertility. A well characterized model for human spermatogenesis is critical to our understanding of the physiological and genetic pathways of male reproduction and the clinical applications extend to the study of

human reproductive toxicology and preservation of fertility in treated cancer patients.

Simple testicular tissue culture has been attempted and maintained in a variety of species in the early twentieth century,[9-11] however, gonocyte development and progression in these models arrested at meiosis. It was soon determined that the supporting cells or the "microenvironment of the testicle" was critical to spermatogenesis. The challenge of creating an *in vitro* testicular model has been trying to replicate the microenvironment to successfully recreate spermatogenesis. Novel conventional and 3-dimensional (3D) culture systems have since been developed to foster the maturation of sperm. Using a 3-D culture system to spatially arrange germ cells, Stukenborg and colleagues showed that by co-culturing premeiotic germ cells with somatic testicular tissue from mice in the presence of gonadotropin, complete maturation of germ cells into morphologically normal spermatozoa can be accomplished.[12]

Currently, there is a paucity of literature addressing *in vitro* germ cell maturation in humans. Cremades and colleagues co-cultured testicular biopsy samples from azoospermic men with Vero cells and reported *in vitro* maturation of round spermatids to elongated spermatids and mature sperm.[13] This was the first time spermatogenetic development occurred *in vitro* under conventional culture conditions in humans. An argument to the validity of this experiment is the fact that sperm can be found in approximately 50 percent of men with non-obstructive azoospermia at time of microsurgical testicular sperm extraction[14] and the sperm recovered may represent the heterogeneous population of germ cells instead of true maturation of spermatids. Despite this, Tanaka and colleagues have shown that a single human spermatocyte can undergo meiosis and differentiate into round spermatids when co-cultured with Vero cells, but the maturation does not continue past this stage.[15] Further research efforts are required to reveal the applicability of *in vitro* culture technique for human germ cells and the functionality of the cultured spermatozoa for generating offspring.

Embryonic Stem Cells

To further understand the genetic and epigenetic programming responsible for germ cell development, embryonic stem cell (ESC) cultures from both murine and human sources have been studied. In a landmark paper, Geijsen et al. reported the derivation of mouse PGCs by adding retinoic acid to an ESC culture media.[16] The primordial germ cells retain their self renewal properties and further differentiate into haploid male gametes. The function of these germ cells was eloquently confirmed when intracytoplasmically injected into oocytes, which restored a somatic diploid chromosomal complement with a 20 percent blastocyst formation rate. To investigate this process further, Nayernia and his group in 2006 reported the generation of offspring mice from male gametes derived from *in vitro* differentiated ESC.[17] Human ESC also have the capacity to differentiate into PGCs *in vitro*, even spontaneously, as determined by surface markers and gene expression profiles.[18,19] Growth factors such as bone morphogenetic protein (BMP) and others play a critical role in inducing germ cell differentiation from human ESC.[20,21] To date, the limits of *in vitro* models using human ESC has been halted at the production of postmeiotic spermatids.[22] *In vitro* development of human stem cells into mature sperm has yet to be reported.

The future of human ESC research has become contentious and controversial due to the ethics and availability of these pluripotent cells. The availability of human ESC and embryonic germ cells is dependent on tissue from an excess human embryo and an aborted fetus, respectively.[23] Ethically, opponents of human stem cell research and use believe that since the embryo and unborn fetus are unable to grant consent for use, their rights are violated.[24] On the other hand, proponents of this technology

argue that it is reasonable to use the excess embryos generated during *in vitro* fertilization (IVF) instead of destroying or storing them indefinitely.[25] Amidst these debates, current guidelines on human ES research in the United States have to meet strict criteria, which were established in August 2001 by President Bush:

- Stem cells must be derived from an embryo that was created for reproductive purposes
- The embryo is no longer needed for this purpose
- Informed consent must be obtained for the donation of the embryo
- No financial inducements are provided for donation of the embryo.

Induced Pluripotent Stem Cells

In order to avoid the ethical dilemmas surrounding human ESC, induced pluripotent stem cells (iPSCs) have been developed. The derivation of iPSCs involves the use of easily acquired cultured adult somatic cells instead of embryonic tissues. The somatic cells are induced into pluripotency with viral transfection or the non-viral delivery of reprogramming factor transgenes, such as Yamanaka factors (Oct3/4, Sox2, Klf4, c-Myc).[26,27] These approaches have been performed in human cells using the same approaches,[28,29] and the reprogrammed human iPSC display similar potential as human ESC in their developmental capacity to generate PGCs.[30]

These investigations are still preliminary, and the impact of this new discovery in human reproductive studies remains to be seen. However, the genetic and epigenetic defects resulted in the derivation of iPSCs have raised the question of safety and their eventual use in the clinical setting. A series of recent articles suggest that iPSCs display more abnormalities than do ESCs and fibroblasts. Chromosomal abnormalities appear earlier in iPSCs cultures,[31] and higher frequency of mutations and greater number of novel copy number variants (CNVs) are also present in iPSCs.[31,32] Aberrant DNA methylation and retention of epigenetic markers from the cell of origin also suggest significant reprogramming variability in human iPSCs.[33] In summary, safety of iPSCs application in humans should certainly raise concerns, and be the focus of future studies.

■ *IN VIVO* SPERMATOGENESIS MODELS

In vivo models have several advantages over *in vitro* models, in particular they provide the testicular microenvironment, or niche, that facilitates the development of germ cells. There are two established *in vivo* experimental models:

- SSC transplantation
- Testis xenograft transplantation.

Spermatogonial Stem Cell Transplantation

Breakthroughs in SSC transplantation in the early 1990's inspired a new wave of testicular stem cell research. Ground-breaking research by Brinster evaluated the transplantation of normal SSC into the testes of chemotherapy-treated mice with the goal of restoring spermatogenesis.[34] His technique first isolated SSC from wild type (normal) mouse testes which were retrogradely injected into a chemotherapy-treated recipient testis (devoid of germ cells) via the efferent duct into the seminiferous tubules. The benefit of this design is that Sertoli and other supporting cells are resilient to most chemotherapies, hence, retain their structure and function. This cellular scaffold provides a home for the injected normal SSC, which have the ability to migrate pass the testis-blood barrier formed by the gap junctions between Sertoli cell cytoplasm. Finally, the transplanted SSC can then proliferate and differentiate to form mature sperm and restore spermatogenesis in the recipient testis.[34] This theoretical model has successfully restored spermatogenesis with both fresh and cryopreserved mouse SSC and has been successfully expanded into other animal models.

While SSC transplantation has been successfully applied to fertility preservation in rodent and farm animals, this technique has not been tested in humans due to both technical and health concerns. First, the quantity of SSC that can be harvested from a pre-pubertal testis is very limited, and may not be sufficient to re-colonize the donor testis to re-establish fertility. Recent cell culture work by Sadri-Ardekani and colleagues may ameliorate this situation, as they reported a >18,000 fold increase in SSC numbers over 64 days in their post-pubertal human germline stem cell culture system.[35] Although it seems feasible to expand the SSC population prior to transplantation, it remains unknown if pre-pubertal human SSC will react in a similar fashion to the post-pubertal SSC used in the Sadri-Ardekani assay and if clonally expanded SSC will repopulate the testis in the same fashion as *de novo* SSC directly from the testis. Second, autologous SSC transplanted back to a treated cancer patient harbors the theoretical risk of also re-introducing malignant cells. In a rat model, transplantation of testicular cells from leukemic rats led to transmission of leukemia in the recipient rat.[35] Several strategies are currently being studied to overcome this limitation, including flow cytometry cell sorting and immunomagnetic separation techniques, which have yielded variable results.[36,37]

Although the amplification and purification techniques applied to SSC are promising, none are yet validated and safe enough for human clinical use. In the future, clinical application of the SSC transplantation may become a reality for the fertility preservation of treated prepubertal male cancer patients. In prepubertal patients, their spermatogenic potential is contained within the SSC. A clinical strategy proposed would be to harvest SSC from testicular tissue, which could be cryopreserved prior to gonadotoxic cancer therapy. At a later date, these SSC could then be injected back into the testicle if the cancer survivor wishes to have his own genetic children in the future.

■ TESTIS XENOGRAFT TRANSPLANTATION MODEL

Xenotransplantation is the transplantation of living cells, tissues or organs from one species to another. Grafting immature (neonatal) donor testicular tissue onto an immunodeficient recipient mouse has lead to testicular maturation and demonstration of complete spermatogenesis with the production of offspring by using the mature sperm obtained from the graft. Successful xenografts of fresh and cryopreserved testicular tissue have been reported in a variety of species, including: mouse,[38] hamster,[39] rabbit,[40] pig,[41] sheep,[38] cattle,[42] cat,[43] horse,[44] and non-human primates.[45]

Testicular tissue suitable for xenografting must be from an immature testicular source, as for still unknown reasons mature testis tissue grafts do not support germ cell differentiation.[46] In animal models, xenografts made from immature testis tissue has better survival and accelerated maturation once transplanted compared to mature testicular tissues.[45] In humans, xenografting adult testicular tissue from biopsies obtained from infertile patients unfortunately demonstrated poor survival and failure to support spermatogenesis.[47]

The study of xenograft transplantation models in humans has been limited primarily due to the lack of donor tissues. Nevertheless, preliminary work that has been conducted with human testicular xenograft models has been promising. Yu and colleagues transplanted fetal (20–26 weeks) human testicular tissue onto an immunodeficient nude mouse and demonstrated that the xenograft could survive for more than 135 days.[48] These fetal grafts did extremely well, with increased graft weight, Sertoli cells differentiation and germ cell migration was demonstrated over time. Similarly, Sato et al. transplanted human testicular tissue from a 3-month-old patient to an immunodeficient nude mouse and reported progression of germ cell differentiation from the spermatogonia stage to pachytene spermatocyte formation.[49] As well, Wyns and colleagues transplanted testicular tissue harvested from five prepubertal cancer patients prior to chemotherapy into the scrotums of nude mice and showed that the xenograft survived greater than 6 months.[50] These xenografts produced numerous pre-meiotic spermatocytes, a few spermatocytes at the pachytene stage and spermatid-like cells, but complete regeneration of normal spermatogenesis with mature sperm cells was not observed.

Despite the encouraging results from human testicular xenograft models, there are significant limitations. To date, there have been no reports of complete spermatogenesis with mature sperm demonstrated in a human testis xenograft model. Additionally, the risk of contamination of germ line cells with that of foreign species will likely prohibit the use of gametes derived from this model for human clinical use. However, the major advantage of this *in vivo* model is the potential for human reproductive toxicology studies. Currently, the reproductive effect and toxicity of novel pharmaceuticals and chemicals are tested on healthy volunteers, with significant expense and inherent risk to the subjects. A safer and more efficient preclinical platform to study reproductive toxicology in humans would involve the utilization of a xenografted testis model.

■ CONCLUSION

Successes of both *in vitro* and *in vivo* germ cell maturation animal studies have given us hope, but due to ethical, safety and experimental limitations, direct human applications have yet to reach

Table 38.1: Overview of the benefits and limitation on current models available for the study of spermatogenesis and male fertility preservation

Model	Benefits	Limitations
In vitro germ cell maturation	• Minimal tissue retrieval/banking required • No cross contamination from using animal surrogates • Potential to derive germ cell from somatic cells	• Requires co-culturing with Vero cells and/or growth factors • Potential epigenetic changes in the cultured germ cells • Ethical implications regarding stem cells • Limited supply and availability of pluripotent stem cells
Spermatogonial stem cell (SSC transplantation)	• Potential autologous germ cell stem cell • Minimize risk of rejection • If successful, could lead to repopulation of germ cells in recipient and allow natural conception	• Limited quantity of SSCs can be harvested • Invasive nature of testicular tissue retrieval • Potential for relapse of malignancy from autologous transplantation
Testis xenography transplantation	• Intact testicular tissue provides optimal microenvironment for germ cell development • Consistent graft recovery in animal and human models • Platform to perform human toxicology studies	• Invasive nature of testicular tissue retrieval • Contamination of gametes with xenogenic proteins and/or retroviruses • Applicable to immature testicular tissue only

prime time. There are potential benefits and limitations of the currently available *in vitro* and *in vivo* spermatogenesis model systems (**Table 38.1**). The challenge for the future andrologists and reproductive biologists is to develop strategies to overcome these limitations within an ethical framework. Clearly more basic, translational, and clinical research is required before this technology can be applied to the many men with infertility that will one day benefit from it.

■ REFERENCES

1. Removing barriers to responsible scientific research involving human stem cells. Federal Register 2009;74(46):10667.
2. Robey PG. Stem cells near the century mark. J Clin Invest 2000;105(11):1489-91.
3. Thomson JA, Itskovitz-Eldor J, Shapiro SS, Waknitz MA, Swiergiel JJ, Marshall VS, et al. Embryonic stem cell lines derived from human blastocysts. Science 1998;282(5391):1145-7.
4. Katsumoto K, Shiraki N, Miki R, et al. Embryonic and adult stem cell systems in mammals: ontology and regulation. Dev Growth Differ 2010;52(1):115-29.
5. Ostrer H, Huang HY, Masch RJ, et al. A cellular study of human testis development. Sex Dev 2007;1(5):286-92.
6. Orth J. Cell biology of testicular development in the fetus and neonate. In: Desjardins C, Ewing L (Eds). Cell and molecular biology of the testis. New York: Oxford University Press 1993. pp.3-43.
7. Meistrich M, van Beek M. Spermatogonial Stem Cells. In: Desjardins C, Ewing L (Eds). Cell and molecular biology of the testis. New York: Oxford University Press 1993.pp.266-95.
8. Heller CG, Clermont Y. Spermatogenesis in man: an estimate of its duration. Science 1963;12(140):184-6.
9. Goldschmidt R. Some experiments on spermatogenesis in vitro. Proc Natl Acad Sci USA 1915;1:220-2.
10. Champy C. Quelques résultats de la méthode de culture des tissus. ARch Zool Exp Gen 1920;60:461-500.
11. Michailow M. Experimentell-histologische untersuchungen über die elemente der hodenkanälchen. Z Zellforsch 1937;26:174-201.
12. Stukenborg JB, Schlatt S, Simoni M, Yeung CH, Elhija MA, Luetjens CM, et al. New horizons for in vitro spermatogenesis? An update on novel three-dimensional culture systems as tools for meiotic and post-meiotic differentiation of testicular germ cells. Mol Hum Reprod 2009;15(9):521-9.
13. Cremades N, Bernabeu R, Barros A, et al. *In vitro* maturation of round spermatids using co-culture on Vero cells. Hum Reprod 1999;14(5):1287-93.
14. Schlegel PN. Testicular sperm extraction: microdissection improves sperm yield with minimal tissue excision. Hum Reprod 1999;14(1):131-5.
15. Tanaka A, Nagayoshi M, Awata S, Mawatari Y, Tanaka I, Kusunoki H. Completion of meiosis in human primary spermatocytes through in vitro coculture with Vero cells. Fertil Steril 2003;79(1):795-801.
16. Geijsen N, Horoschak M, Kim K, Gribnau J, Eggan K, Daley GQ. Derivation of embryonic germ cells and male gametes from embryonic stem cells. Nature 2004;427(6970):148-54.
17. Nayernia K, Nolte J, Michelmann HW, Lee JH, Rathsack K, Drusenheimer N, et al. *In vitro* differentiated embryonic stem cells give rise to male gametes that can generate offspring mice. Dev Cell 2006;11(1):125-32.
18. Clark AT, Bodnar MS, Fox M, Rodriquez RT, Abeyta MJ, Firpo MT, et al. Spontaneous differentiation of germ cells from human embryonic stem cells in vitro. Hum Mol Genet 2004;13(7):727-39.
19. Aflatoonian B, Moore H. Human primordial germ cells and embryonic germ cells, and their use in cell therapy. Curr Opin Biotechnol 2005;16(5):530-5.
20. Kee K, Gonsalves JM, Clark AT, et al. Bone morphogenetic proteins induce germ cell differentiation from human embryonic stem cells. Stem Cells Dev 2006;15(6):831-7.
21. Park TS, Galic Z, Conway AE, Lindgren A, van Handel BJ, Magnusson M, et al. Derivation of primordial germ cells from human embryonic and induced pluripotent stem cells is

significantly improved by coculture with human fetal gonadal cells. Stem Cells 2009;27(4):783-95.

22. Moore H, Aflatoonian B. From stem cells to spermatozoa and back. Soc Reprod Fertil Suppl 2007;65:19-32.

23. Lo KC, Chuang WW, Lamb DJ. Stem cell research: the facts, the myths and the promises. J Urol 2003;170(6 Pt 1):2453-8.

24. Ruiz-Canela M. Embryonic stem cell research: the relevance of ethics in the progress of science. Med Sci Monit 2002;8(5):SR21-6.

25. McLaren A. Ethical and social considerations of stem cell research. Nature 2001;414(6859):129-31.

26. Okita K, Ichisaka T, Yamanaka S. Generation of germline-competent induced pluripotent stem cells. Nature 2007; 19;448(7151):313-7.

27. Woltjen K, Michael IP, Mohseni P, Desai R, Mileikovsky M, Hamalainen R, et al. piggyBac transposition reprograms fibroblasts to induced pluripotent stem cells. Nature 2009;9:458(7239);766-70.

28. Takahashi K, Tanabe K, Ohnuki M, Narita M, Ichisaka T, Tomoda K, et al. Induction of pluripotent stem cells from adult human fibroblasts by defined factors. Cell 2007;30:131(5):861-72.

29. Park IH, Zhao R, West JA, Yabuuchi A, Huo H, Ince TA, et al. Reprogramming of human somatic cells to pluripotency with defined factors. Nature 2008;10:451(7175):141-6.

30. Clark AT. Egg-citing advances in generating primordial germ cells in the laboratory. Biol Reprod Feb;82(2):233-4.

31. Laurent LC, Ulitsky I, Slavin I, Tran H, Schork A, Morey R, et al. Dynamic changes in the copy number of pluripotency and cell proliferation genes in human ESCs and iPSCs during reprogramming and time in culture. Cell Stem Cell 2011;7:8(1):106-18.

32. Hussein S, Batada N, Vuoristo S, Ching R, Autio R, Narva E, et al. Copy number variation and selection during reprogramming to pluripotency. Nature 2011;471:58-62.

33. Lister R, Pelizzola M, Kida YS, Hawkins RD, Nery JR, Hon G, et al. Hotspots of aberrant epigenomic reprogramming in human induced pluripotent stem cells. Nature 2011;471:68-73.

34. Brinster RL, Zimmermann JW. Spermatogenesis following male germ-cell transplantation. Proc Natl Acad Sci USA 1994;22:91(24):11298-302.

35. Sadri-Ardekani H, Mizrak SC, van Daalen SK, Korver CM, Roepers-Gajadien HL, Koruji M, et al. Propagation of human spermatogonial stem cells in vitro. JAMA 2009;18:302(19):2127-34.

36. Fujita K, Ohta H, Tsujimura A, Takao T, Miyagawa Y, Takada S, et al. Transplantation of spermatogonial stem cells isolated from leukemic mice restores fertility without inducing leukemia. J Clin Invest 2005;115(7):1855-61.

37. Hou M, Andersson M, Zheng C, Sundblad A, Soder O, Jahnukainen K. Immunomagnetic separation of normal rat testicular cells from Roser's T-cell leukaemia cells is ineffective. Int J Androl 2009;32(1):66-73.

38. Honaramooz A, Snedaker A, Boiani M, Scholer H, Dobrinski I, Schlatt S. Sperm from neonatal mammalian testes grafted in mice. Nature 2002;15:418(6899):778-81.

39. Schlatt S, Kim SS, Gosden R. Spermatogenesis and steroidogenesis in mouse, hamster and monkey testicular tissue after cryopreservation and heterotopic grafting to castrated hosts. Reproduction 2002;124(3):339-46.

40. Shinohara T, Inoue K, Ogonuki N, Kanatsu-Shinohara M, Miki H, Nakata K, et al. Birth of offspring following transplantation of cryopreserved immature testicular pieces and *in vitro* microinsemination. Hum Reprod 2002;17(12):3039-45.

41. Honaramooz A, Megee SO, Dobrinski I. Germ cell transplantation in pigs. Biol Reprod 2002;66(1):21-8.

42. Rathi R, Honaramooz A, Zeng W, et al. Germ cell fate and seminiferous tubule development in bovine testis xenografts. Reproduction 2005;130(6):923-9.

43. Snedaker AK, Honaramooz A, Dobrinski I. A game of cat and mouse: xenografting of testis tissue from domestic kittens results in complete cat spermatogenesis in a mouse host. J Androl 2004;25(6):926-30.

44. Rathi R, Honaramooz A, Zeng W, et al. Germ cell development in equine testis tissue xenografted into mice. Reproduction 2006;131(6):1091-8.

45. Honaramooz A, Li MW, Penedo MC, et al. Accelerated maturation of primate testis by xenografting into mice. Biol Reprod 2004;70(5):1500-3.

46. Arregui L, Rathi R, Zeng W, Honaramooz A, Gomendio M, Roldan ER, et al. Xenografting of adult mammalian testis tissue. Anim Reprod Sci 2008;106(1-2):65-76.

47. Schlatt S, Honaramooz A, Ehmcke J, Goebell PJ, Rubben H, Dhir R, et al. Limited survival of adult human testicular tissue as ectopic xenograft. Hum Reprod 2006;21(2):384-9.

48. Yu J, Cai ZM, Wan HJ, Zhang FT, Ye J, Fang JZ, et al. Development of neonatal mouse and fetal human testicular tissue as ectopic grafts in immunodeficient mice. Asian J Androl 2006;8(4):393-403.

49. Sato Y, Nozawa S, Yoshiike M, Arai M, Sasaki C, Iwamoto T. Xenografting of testicular tissue from an infant human donor results in accelerated testicular maturation. Hum Reprod May;25(5):1113-22.

50. Wyns C, Van Langendonckt A, Wese FX, et al. Long-term spermatogonial survival in cryopreserved and xenografted immature human testicular tissue. Hum Reprod 2008;23(11):2402-14.

Index

Page numbers followed by *f* refer to figure and *t* refer to table